Royal Liverpool University Hos

Retinal Degenerative Diseases

Laboratory and Therapeutic Investigations

Advances in Experimental Medicine and Biology

A Continuation Order Plan is available for this series. A continuation order will bring delivery of each new volume immediately upon publication. Volumes are billed only upon actual shipment. For further information please contact the publisher.

Robert E. Anderson · Matthew M. LaVail
Joe G. Hollyfield
Editors

Md Nawajes A. Mandal
Associate Editor

Retinal Degenerative Diseases

Laboratory and Therapeutic Investigations

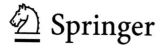 Springer

Editors
Robert E. Anderson
University of Oklahoma
Health Science Center
Dean A. McGee Eye Inst.
608 Stanton L. Young Blvd.
Oklahoma City OK 73104
USA
robert-anderson@ouhsc.edu

Matthew M. LaVail
University of California, San
  Francisco
School of Medicine
Beckman Vision Center
10 Kirkham St.
San Francisco CA 94143
USA
matthew.lavail@ucsf.edu

Joe G. Hollyfield
Cleveland Clinic Foundation
Division of Ophthalmology
9500 Euclid Ave.
Cleveland OH 44195
USA
hollyfj@ccf.org

ISSN 0065-2598
ISBN 978-1-4419-1398-2   e-ISBN 978-1-4419-1399-9
DOI 10.1007/978-1-4419-1399-9
Springer New York Dordrecht Heidelberg London

Library of Congress Control Number: 2009943262

Printed on acid-free paper

Springer is part of Springer Science+Business Media (www.springer.com)

Dedication

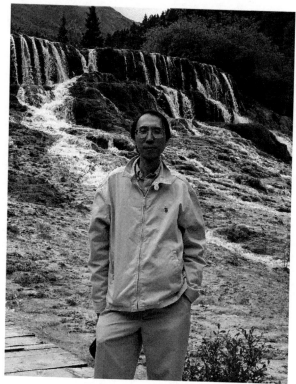

Wei Cao, M.D., Ph.D.
(May 3, 1957 – October 10, 2007)

The editors acknowledge the strong support of our friend, colleague, and collaborator Wei Cao, MD, PhD in this and past RD meetings. Wei was an excellent scientist, a gifted musician, and a talented artist. He was also the person solely responsible for finding the site and making the arrangements for us to hold this meeting at Emeishan. We dedicate this volume to Wei in recognition of his outstanding career in retinal degeneration research.

Dedication

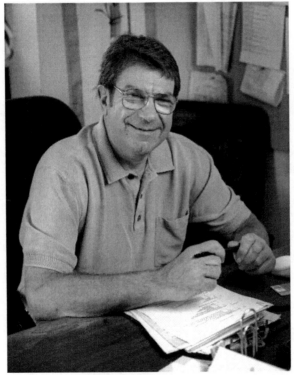

Ruben Adler, M.D.
(November 10, 1940 – December 31, 2007)

The editors acknowledge the strong support of our friend and colleague Ruben Adler, MD who participated in many of our previous Retinal Degeneration Symposia. He was a plenary lecturer at the 2006 meeting in San Carlos de Bariloche, Argentina. This volume is dedicated to Ruben in recognition of his outstanding career in developmental biology and retinal degeneration research.

Preface

The International Symposium on Retinal Degeneration has been held in conjunction with the biennial International Congress of Eye Research (ICER) since 1984. These RD Symposia have allowed basic and clinician scientists from around the world to convene and present their new research findings. They have been organized to allow sufficient time for discussions and one-on-one interactions in a relaxed atmosphere, where international friendships and collaborations can be fostered.

The XIII International Symposium on Retinal Degeneration (also known as RD2008) was held from September 18–23, 2008 at the Hong Zhu Shan Hotel at the foot of Emei Mountain in the Sichuan Province of China, near Chengdu. The meeting brought together 152 basic and clinician scientists, retinal specialists in ophthalmology, and trainees in the field from all parts of the world. In the course of the meeting, 42 platform and 88 poster presentations were given, and a majority of these are presented in this proceedings volume. New discoveries and state of the art findings from most research areas in the field of retinal degenerations were presented. The RD2008 meeting was highlighted by three special lectures. The first was given by **Glen Prusky**, PhD, Weill Cornell Medical College of Cornell University, New York City, NY. Dr. Prusky discussed the measures of vision in rodents as a tool for evaluating the treatment of retinal degenerative diseases. The second was given by **Kang Zhang**, MD, PhD, on the molecular genetics of Stargardt's Disease. Dr. Zhang's undergraduate degree in biochemistry is from West China University in Chengdu, and he currently is at the Shiley Eye Center, University of California at San Diego, San Diego, CA. The third plenary lecture was given by **Peter Campochiaro**, MD, of the Wilmer Eye Institute, Johns Hopkins University, Baltimore, MD. Dr. Campochiaro discussed the role of oxidant stress in macular degeneration.

This Symposium would not have been possible without the support of our colleagues at the Sichuan People's Provincial Hospital and the Department of Ophthalmology of West China Hospital, Sichuan University. **Fan Ying Chuan**, MD, Vice Chairman, Sichuan Ophthalmology Society, Director of Ophthalmology Department, Sichuan Academy of Medical Science & Sichuan Provincial People's Hospital and **Chen Xiao Ming**, MD, Chairman, Sichuan Ophthalmology Society, Director of West China Eye Center, West China Hospital, Sichuan University, gave tirelessly to our effort from the beginning. We are especially grateful to the administration of the Sichuan People's Provincial Hospital, which provided the financial guarantees necessary to secure the meeting venue. The assistance of **Chen Hui (Robert)**, MD, of the SPPH throughout the planning and the meeting itself were of enormous help to us. We appreciate all of the officers of various medical associations who gave support or participated in the Welcoming Ceremony. These include: **Li Yuan Feng**, MD, President, Sichuan Academy of Medical Science & Sichuan Provincial People's Hospital; **Cai Li**, MD, Vice President, Sichuan Academy of Medical Science & Sichuan Provincial People's Hospital; **Xiong Jun Hao**, MD, Assistant President, Sichuan Academy of Medical Science & Sichuan Provincial People's Hospital; **Fang Yong**, MD, General Secretary, Sichuan Medical Association; **Wang Wei**, MD, Vice General Secretary, Sichuan Medical Association; and **Shi Ying Kang**, MD, President, West China Hospital, Sichuan University.

We were pleasantly surprised that our old friend and colleague Dominic Lam, PhD attended and spoke at our Opening Ceremonies. Dominic is well known in ophthalmology circles in China. As President and CEO of the World Eye Organization, he has been responsible for establishing a number of eye clinics throughout China to provide care for those who cannot afford it. Most recently he established the Thorsten Wiesel Research Institute at West China University in Chengdu, in honor of his mentor Nobel Laureate Thorsten Wiesel.

We also thank the management and staff of the beautiful Hong Zhu Shan Hotel for all of their assistance in making this a truly memorable experience for all of the attendees. We are especially grateful to **Walton Wang**, the hotel representative who worked with us from the outset to make sure that everything went smoothly.

The Symposium received international financial support from a number of organizations. We are particularly pleased to thank The Foundation Fighting Blindness, Owings Mills, Maryland, for its continuing support of this and the previous biennial Symposia, without which we could not have held these important meetings. In addition, for the fourth time, the National Eye Institute of the National Institutes of Health contributed to the meeting. Funds from these two organizations allowed us to provide 35 Travel Awards to young investigators and trainees working in the field of retinal degenerations. The response to the Travel Awards program was extraordinary, with 74 applicants.

We also acknowledge the diligent and outstanding efforts of Ms. **Holly Whiteside**, who carried out most of the administrative aspects of the RD2008 Symposium, designed and maintained the meeting website, and organized and edited the production of this volume. Holly is the Administrative Manager of Dr. Anderson's laboratory at the University of Oklahoma Health Sciences Center, and she has become the permanent Coordinator for the Retinal Degeneration Symposia. Her dedicated efforts with the Symposia since RD2000 have provided continuity not available previously, and we are deeply indebted to her. We are also indebted to Dr. **Md. Nawajes A. Mandal**, who served as the Associate Editor of this volume. Dr. Mandal read every manuscript and organized them into thematic blocks.

Finally, we honor the memory of two colleagues who died in 2007. **Ruben Adler** was a great friend to most who attend our RD meetings. He was our keynote speaker in Argentina, where he gave an extraordinary lecture on the hope, reality, and challenges of using stem cells to treat blinding diseases. **Wei Cao** was a colleague at the Dean McGee Eye Institute and also a great friend to many of our attendees. Wei was solely responsible for arranging for this meeting to be held in Sichuan Provence and in securing the support of the local organizers. We dedicate this volume to Ruben and Wei.

Robert E. Anderson
Matthew M. LaVail
Joe G. Hollyfield

Contents

Contributors

Toshiaki Abe Division of Clinical Cell Therapy, Center for Translational and Advanced Animal Research, 1-1 Seiryomachi, Aobaku, Miyagi, Sendai 980-8574, Japan, toshi@oph.med.tohoku.ac.jp

Martin-Paul Agbaga Department of Cell Biology and Ophthalmology, Dean McGee Eye Institute, University of Oklahoma Health Sciences Center, 608 Stanton L.Young Blvd, DMEI 409, Oklahoma, OK 73104, USA, martin-paul-agbaga@ouhsc.edu

Jae H. Ahn Jules Stein Eye Institute, UCLA, Los Angeles, CA 90095, USA

N.B. Akhmedov Jules Stein Eye Institute, UCLA School of Medicine, 100 Stein Plaza, Los Angeles, CA 90095-7000, USA

John Alexander Department of Pathology, College of Medicine, University of Florida, Gainesville, FL, USA

Muayyad R. Al-Ubaidi Department of Cell Biology, BMSB 781, 940 Stanton L. Young Blvd., Oklahoma City, OK 73104, USA, muayyad-al-ubaidi@ouhsc.edu

Robert E. Anderson Department of Cell Biology and Ophthalmology, University of Oklahoma Health Sciences Center, Oklahoma City, OK, USA; Dean A. McGee Eye Institute, Oklahoma City, OK, USA; Department of Cell Biology, University of Oklahoma Health Sciences Center, Oklahoma City, OK, USA

Rajendra S. Apte Ophthalmology and Visual Sciences, Developmental Biology, Barnes Retina Institute, Washington University School of Medicine, 660 South Euclid Avenue Box 8096, St. Louis, MO 63110 USA, apte@vision.wustl.edu

Claudia Aruta Department of Biomedical Sciences, University of Modena and Reggio Emilia, Modena, Italy

John D. Ash Oklahoma Center for Neuroscience, University of Oklahoma Health Sciences Center, Oklahoma City, OK, USA; Department of Ophthalmology, University of Oklahoma Health Sciences Center, Oklahoma City, OK, USA; Department of Cell Biology, University of Oklahoma Health Sciences Center, Oklahoma, OK 73104, USA; Dean A. McGee Eye Institute, Oklahoma, OK 73104, USA, john-ash@ouhsc.edu

Jaya Badhwar Department of Ophthalmology and Visual Sciences, University of Michigan/Kellogg Eye Center, Ann Arbor, MI, USA

Wolfgang Baehr Department of Biology, University of Utah, Salt Lake City, UT 84132, USA; Department of Ophthalmology, University of Utah Health Science Center, Salt Lake City, UT 84132, USA; Department of Neurobiology and Anatomy, University of Utah Health Science Center, Salt Lake City, UT 84132, USA; John A. Moran Eye Center, University of Utah Health Science Center, Salt Lake City, UT 84132, USA, wbaehr@hsc.utah.edu

Peter Barabas Department of Ophthalmology and Visual Sciences, Moran Eye Center, University of Utah School of Medicine, Salt Lake City, UT 84132, USA

Colin J. Barnstable Department of Neural and Behavioral Sciences, Penn State College of Medicine, 500 University Drive, Hershey, PA 17033, USA, cbarnstable@psu.edu

Frank Bart Department of Cell Biology, BMSB 781, 940 Stanton L. Young Blvd., Oklahoma City, OK 73104, USA

Nicolas G. Bazan Neuroscience Center of Excellence and Department of Ophthalmology, Louisiana State University Health Sciences Center, 2020 Gravier Street, Suite D, New Orleans, LA 70112, USA, nbazan@lsuhsc.edu

Srilaxmi Bearelly The Duke Center for Macular Diseases and Albert Eye Research Institute, Duke University Eye Center, Durham, NC, USA, beare002@mc.duke.edu

S. Patricia Becerra NEI-NIH, Building 6, Room 134, 6 Center Dr., MSC 0608, Bethesda, MD 20892-0608, USA

N.T. Bech-Hansen Department Medical Genetics, Faculty of Medicine, University of Calgary, Calgary, Alberta T2N4N1, Canada; Division of Ophthalmology, Department of Surgery, University of Calgary, Calgary, Alberta T2N4N1, Canada; Lions Centre for Retinal Degeneration Research, University of Calgary, Calgary, Alberta T2N4N1, Canada; Institute of Maternal and Child Health, University of Calgary, Calgary, Alberta T2N4N1, Canada

Susanne C. Beck Division of Ocular Neurodegeneration, Institute for Ophthalmic Research, Centre for Ophthalmology, University of Tuebingen, Tuebingen, Germany

James Bena Lerner Research Institute, Cleveland, OH, USA; Department of Quantitative Health Sciences, Cleveland Clinic Foundation, Cleveland, OH, USA

Martin Biel Munich Center for Integrated Protein Science, CIPSM and Department Pharmazie, Zentrum für Pharmaforschung, Ludwig-Maximilians-University, Munich, Germany

David G. Birch Retina Foundation of the Southwest, Dallas, TX, USA

S. Bonfield Lions Centre for Retinal Degeneration Research, University of Calgary, Calgary, Alberta T2N4N1, Canada

Michael Bonin Microarray Facility Tuebingen, Institute of Human Genetics, University of Tuebingen, Tuebingen, Germany

C. Bonnin-Arias Optic II, University Complutense de Madrid, Madrid, Spain

Sara J. Bowne The University of Texas Health Science Center Houston, Human Genetics Center, 1200 Herman Pressler, Houston TX, 77030, USA

Richard S. Brush Department of Ophthalmology, University of Oklahoma Health Sciences Center, Oklahoma City, OK, USA; Dean A. McGee Eye Institute, Oklahoma City, OK, USA; Department of Cell Biology, University of Oklahoma Health Sciences Center, Oklahoma, OK, USA

Marie Burstedt Department of Ophthalmology, Clinical Sciences, Umeå University, 901 85, Umeå, Sweden

M.T. Cahill

Xue Cai Department of Cell Biology, University of Oklahoma Health Sciences Center, Oklahoma City, OK 73104, USA

Jorgelina M. Calandria Neuroscience Center of Excellence and Department of Ophthalmology, Louisiana State University Health Sciences Center, 2020 Gravier Street, Suite D, New Orleans, LA 70112, USA

Matthew Campbell The Ocular Genetics Unit, Department of Genetics, Trinity College Dublin, Dublin 2, Ireland, matthew.campbell@tcd.ie

Wei Cao Dean A McGee Eye Institute, 608 Stanton L. Young Blvd., Oklahoma City, OK 73104, USA

Guiqun Cao Torsten Wiesel Research Institute and Department of Ophthalmology, West China Hospital, Sichuan University, Chengdu, China

Joseph Caprioli Jules Stein Eye Institute, UCLA, Los Angeles, CA 90095, USA

Joseph Carroll Department of Ophthalmology, Medical College of Wisconsin, The Eye Institute, Milwaukee, WI, USA; Department of Cell Biology, Neurobiology, and Anatomy, Medical College of Wisconsin, The Eye Institute, Milwaukee, WI, USA; Department of Biophysics, Medical College of Wisconsin, The Eye Institute, Milwaukee, WI, USA, jcarroll@mcw.edu

L. Cassidy

J.M. Benitez-del Castillo San Carlos University Hospital, University Complutense de Madrid, Madrid, Spain

Michael Centola Department of Cell Biology, BMSB 781, 940 Stanton L. Young Blvd., Oklahoma City, OK 73104, USA

Naomi Chadderton The Ocular Genetics Unit, Department of Genetics, Trinity College Dublin, Dublin 2, Ireland

Dibyendu Chakraborty Department of Cell Biology, University of Oklahoma Health Sciences Center, Oklahoma, OK 73126-0901, USA

Bo Chang The Jackson Laboratory, Bar Harbor, ME, USA

Michael E. Cheetham UCL Institute of Ophthalmology, London, EC1V 9EL, UK, michael.cheetham@ucl.ac.uk

Enid Chelva Department of Medical Technology and Physics, Sir Charles Gairdner Hospital, Hospital Avenue, Nedlands, WA, 6009, Australia

Haoyu Chen Joint Shantou International Eye Center, Shantou University and the Chinese University of Hong Kong, North Dongxia Road, Shantou, 515041 China; Moran Eye Center, University of Utah, Salt Lake City, Utah 84112, USA, drchenhaoyu@gmail.com

Xigui Chen Preclinical Medical College, Gannan Medical University, Ganzhou, Jiangxi Province 341000, China

Y. Chen Faculty of Medicine, University of Toronto, Toronto, ON, Canada

Wei Chen Torsten Wiesel Research Institute and Department of Ophthalmology, West China Hospital, Sichuan University, Chengdu, China

Srinivas Chollangi Department of Bioengineering, University of Oklahoma, Norman, OK, USA

Vicki Chrysostomou Research School of Biological Sciences, The Australian National University, Canberra, Australia; ARC Centre of Excellence in Vision Science, The Australian National University, Canberra, Australia, vicki.chrysostomou@anu.edu.au

Lei Chuntao Department of Ophthalmology, Sichuan Provincial People's Hospital, Chengdu, Sichuan, 610072, China, hblct@163.com

Garrett Cobb Brandeis University, Waltham, MA, USA

Ross F. Collery UCD School of Biomolecular and Biomedical Science, UCD Conway Institute of Biomolecular and Biomedical Research, University College Dublin, Dublin, Ireland, rcollery@mcw.edu

Shannon M. Conley Department of Cell Biology, University of Oklahoma Health Sciences Center, Oklahoma City, OK 73104, USA

Scott W. Cousins The Duke Center for Macular Diseases and Albert Eye Research Institute, Duke University Eye Center, Durham, NC, USA; Department of Ophthalmology, Duke University, Durham, NC, USA

John W. Crabb Cole Eye Institute, Cleveland, OH, USA; Lerner Research Institute, Cleveland, OH, USA; Department of Chemistry, Case Western Reserve

University, Cleveland, OH, USA; Department of Ophthalmology, Cleveland Clinic Lerner College of Medicine of Case Western Reserve University, Cleveland, OH, USA, crabbj@ccf.org

Rosalie K. Crouch Department of Ophthalmology, Medical University of South Carolina, Charleston, SC, USA, crouchrk@musc.edu

Stephen P. Daiger The University of Texas Health Science Center Houston, Human Genetics Center, 1200 Herman Pressler, Houston TX, 77030, USA stephen.p.daiger@uth.tmc.edu

Dong Dandan Department of Ophthalmology, Sichuan Academy of Medical Sciences and Sichuan Provincial People's Hospital, Sichuan 610072, China

Anna De Marzo Department of Biomedical Sciences, University of Modena and Reggio Emilia, Modena, Italy, anna.demarzo@unimore.it

Monte A. Del Monte Department of Ophthalmology and Visual Sciences, University of Michigan/Kellogg Eye Center, Ann Arbor, MI, USA, madm@umich.edu

M.E. del Valle Morphology and Cell Biology, Universidad de Oviedo, Oviedo, Spain

Wentao Deng Department of Ophthalmology, College of Medicine, University of Florida, Gainesville, FL, USA

Sorcha Ni Dhubhghaill Ocular Genetics Unit, Department of Genetics, Trinity College Dublin, Dublin 2, Ireland, nidhubs@tcd.ie

Xi-Qin Ding Department of Cell Biology, University of Oklahoma Health Sciences Center, 940 Stanton L. Young Blvd., BMSB 781, Oklahoma City, OK 73126-0901, USA, xi-qin-ding@ouhsc.edu

C.J. Doering Hotchkiss Brain Institute, University of Calgary, Calgary, Alberta T2N4N1, Canada; Department of Physiology and Biophysics, University of Calgary, Calgary, Alberta T2N4N1, Canada

Dongsheng Duan Department of Molecular Microbiology and Immunology, University of Missouri, Columbia, MO, USA

Adam M. Dubis Department of Cell Biology, Neurobiology, and Anatomy, Medical College of Wisconsin, The Eye Institute, Milwaukee, WI, USA

Eric M. Dufour Centre de Recherche Institut de la Vision, UMR_S968, Inserm, UPMC University of Paris 06, 17 rue Moreau, 75012 Paris, France

J.L. Duncan Department of Ophthalmology, University of California, San Francisco, CA, USA, duncanj@vision.ucsf.edu

Mary Dwyer Department of Pharmacology, Duke University, Durham, NC, USA

Michael H. Elliott Department of Ophthalmology, University of Oklahoma Health Sciences Center, Oklahoma City, OK, USA; Department of Cell Biology, Dean A. McGee Eye Institute, Oklahoma City, OK, USA

Yingchuan Fan Department of Ophthalmology, Sichuan Academy of Medical Sciences & Sichuan Provincial People's Hospital, Sichuan 610072, China, lucyjeffersonqu@hotmail.com

Cheng Fang Preclinical Medical College, Gannan Medical University, Ganzhou, Jiangxi Province 341000, China

Debora B. Farber Jules Stein Eye Institute, UCLA School of Medicine, 100 Stein Plaza, Los Angeles, CA 90095-7000, USA, farber@jsei.ucla.edu

G. Jane Farrar The Ocular Genetics Unit, Department of Genetics, Trinity College Dublin, Dublin 2, Ireland

A. Fernandez-Balbuena Optic School, University Complutense de Madrid, Madrid, Spain

Silvia C. Finnemann Department of Biological Sciences, Fordham University, Bronx, NY 10458, USA, finnemann@fordham.edu

M. Dominik Fischer Division of Ocular Neurodegeneration, Institute for Ophthalmic Research, Centre for Ophthalmology, University of Tuebingen Schleichstr. 12–16, 72070 Tuebingen, Germany, dominik.fischer@med.uni-tuebingen.de

J. Browning Fitzgerald Department of Cell Biology, University of Oklahoma Health Sciences Center, 940 Stanton L. Young Blvd., Oklahoma, OK 73104, USA

Erica L. Fletcher Department of Anatomy and Cell Biology, University of Melbourne, Parkville, Australia

Steven J. Fliesler Veterans Administration Western New York Healthcare System, and the Department of Ophthalmology and Biochemistry, University at Buffalo (State University of New York), Buffalo, NY 14215, USA, fliesler@buffalo.edu

Arkasubhra Ghosh Department of Molecular Microbiology and Immunology, University of Missouri, Columbia, MO, USA

Pooja Godara Department of Ophthalmology, Medical College of Wisconsin, The Eye Institute, Milwaukee, WI, USA

Irina Golovleva Department of Medical and Clinical Genetics, Medical Biosciences, Umeå University, 901 85, Umeå, Sweden, irina.golovleva@medbio.umu.se

Douglas B. Gould Departments of Ophthalmology and Anatomy and Institute for Human Genetics, University of California at San Francisco, San Francisco, CA 94143, USA, gouldd@vision.ucsf.edu

C. Grimm Lab for Retinal Cell Biology, Department Ophthalmology, University of Zurich, Zurich, Switzerland; Zurich Center for Integrative Human Physiology (ZIHP), Zurich, Switzerland

Alecia K. Gross University of Alabama at Birmingham, WORB 618, 924 18th Street South, Birmingham, AL 35295, USA, agross@uab.edu

Gregory H. Grossman Department of Ophthalmic Research, Cole Eye Institute, Cleveland Clinic, 9500 Euclid Avenue, Cleveland, OH 44195, USA

Jiayin Gu Cole Eye Institute, Cleveland, OH, USA; Lerner Research Institute, Cleveland, OH, USA; Department of Chemistry, Case Western Reserve University, Cleveland, OH, USA

Xiaorong Gu Cole Eye Institute, Cleveland, OH, USA; Lerner Research Institute, Cleveland, OH, USA

Stephanie A. Hagstrom Department of Ophthalmic Research, Cole Eye Institute, Cleveland, OH, USA; Lerner Research Institute, Cleveland, OH, USA; Department of Ophthalmology, Cleveland Clinic Lerner College of Medicine of Case Western Reserve University, Cleveland, OH, USA, hagstrs@ccf.org

Cynthia S. Harry Department of Cell Biology, University of Oklahoma Health Sciences Center, 940 Stanton L. Young Blvd., Oklahoma, OK 73104, USA

William W. Hauswirth Department of Ophthalmology, College of Medicine, University of Florida, Gainesville, FL, USA

Yuan He Department of Neural and Behavioral Sciences, Pennsylvania State University College of Medicine, Hershey, PA, USA, openji7127@hotmail.com

John R. Heckenlively Kellogg Eye Center, University of Michigan, Ann Arbor, MI, USA

Lizbeth Hedstrom Brandeis University, Waltham, MA, USA

Kimberly R. Henry Department of Ophthalmology, University of Oklahoma Health Sciences Center, Oklahoma City, OK, USA; Dean A. McGee Eye Institute, Oklahoma City, OK, USA

V. Michael Holers Department of Medicine, University of Colorado Denver School of Medicine, Denver, CO 80045, USA

Peng Hu Department of Ophthalmology, Duke University, Durham, NC, USA

Zhihua Huang Preclinical Medical College, Gannan Medical University, Ganzhou, Jiangxi Province 341000, China

Gesine Huber Division of Ocular Neurodegeneration, Institute for Ophthalmic Research, Centre for Ophthalmology, University of Tuebingen, Tuebingen, Germany

Chen Hui Department Ophthalmology of Physical Center, The 1st Affiliated Hospital of Chongqing Medical University, Chongqing, 400016, China; Department of Ophthalmology, Sichuan Provincial People's Hospital, Chengdu, Sichuan Province, 610072, China, chenhuicq@yahoo.com.cn

Marian M. Humphries The Ocular Genetics Unit, Department of Genetics, Trinity College Dublin, Dublin 2, Ireland

Pete Humphries The Ocular Genetics Unit, Department of Genetics, Trinity College Dublin, Dublin 2, Ireland

Jianbin Hu Department of Ophthalmology, Sichuan Academy of Medical Sciences and Sichuan Provincial People's Hospital, Sichuan 610072, China, jbinhy@hotmail.com

Hu Jianbin Department of Ophthalmology, Sichuan Provincial People's Hospital, Chengdu, Sichuan, 610072, China

Li Jiang Department of Biology, University of Utah, Salt Lake City, UT 84132, USA

Zeng Jing Pharmaceutic College, Gannan Medical University, Ganzhou, Jiangxi Province 341000, China, zengjing61@hotmail.com

Yogita Kanan Department of Cell Biology, BMSB 781, 940 Stanton L. Young Blvd., Oklahoma City, OK 73104, USA

Manabu Kaneda Department of Molecular Neurobiology, University of Kanazawa, Kanazawa 920-8640, Japan

Satoru Kato Department of Molecular Neurobiology, University of Kanazawa, Kanazawa 920-8640, Japan, satoru@med.kanazawa-u.ac.jp

Paul F. Kenna The Ocular Genetics Unit, Department of Genetics, Trinity College Dublin, Dublin 2, Ireland

Breandán N. Kennedy UCD School of Biomolecular and Biomedical Science, UCD Conway Institute of Biomolecular and Biomedical Research, University College Dublin, Dublin, Ireland

Hemant Khanna Department of Ophthalmology and Visual Sciences, Kellogg Eye Center, Ann Arbor, MI 48105, USA, hkhanna@med.umich.edu

Anna-Sophia Kiang The Ocular Genetics Unit, Department of Genetics, Trinity College Dublin, Dublin 2, Ireland

Seok H. Kim Jules Stein Eye Institute, UCLA, Los Angeles, CA 90095, USA

Linda Köhn Department of Medical and Clinical Genetics, Medical Biosciences, Umeå University, 901 85, Umeå, Sweden

Yoshiki Koriyama Department of Molecular Neurobiology, University of Kanazawa, Kanazawa 920-8640, Japan

Piyush C. Kothary Department of Ophthalmology and Visual Sciences, University of Michigan/Kellogg Eye Center, Ann Arbor, MI, USA

Timothy W. Kraft University of Alabama at Birmingham, WORB 618, 924 18th Street South, Birmingham, AL 35295, USA

David Krizaj Department of Ophthalmology and Visual Sciences, Moran Eye Center, University of Utah School of Medicine, Salt Lake City, UT 84132, USA, david.krizaj@hsc.utah.edu

James A. Kuchenbecker Department of Ophthalmology, University of Washington, Seattle, WA, USA

Kannan Kunchithapautham Department of Ophthalmology and Neurosciences, Division of Research, Medical University of South Carolina, Charleston, SC 29425, USA

Jacky M.K. Kwong Jules Stein Eye Institute, UCLA, Los Angeles, CA 90095, USA

Dominic Man-Kit Lam World Eye Organization, 1209 6 Harbor Road, Hong kong, China

Tina Lamey Department of Medical Technology and Physics, Sir Charles Gairdner Hospital, Hospital Avenue, Nedlands, WA, 6009, Australia

C. Lange Lab for Retinal Cell Biology, Department Ophthalmology, University of Zurich, Zurich, Switzerland; Zurich Center for Integrative Human Physiology (ZIHP), Zurich, Switzerland, christina.lange@usz.ch

Sarina Laurin Department of Medical Technology and Physics, Sir Charles Gairdner Hospital, Hospital Avenue, Nedlands, WA, 6009, Australia

Matthew M. LaVail Department of Anatomy and Ophthalmology, University of California, San Francisco, CA 94143, USA

Yun-Zheng Le Departments of Medicine, University of Oklahoma Health Sciences Center, Oklahoma, OK 73104, USA; Cell Biology and Ophthalmology, University of Oklahoma Health Sciences Center, Oklahoma, OK 73104, USA; Harold Hamm Oklahoma Diabetes Center, University of Oklahoma Health Sciences Center, Oklahoma, OK 73104, USA; Dean A. McGee Eye Institute, Oklahoma, OK 73104, USA, yun-le@ouhsc.edu

Bo Lei Department of Ophthalmology, The First Affiliated Hospital of Chongqing Medical University, Chongqing Key Laboratory of Ophthalmology, Chongqing, China; Department of Veterinary Medicine & Surgery and Department of Ophthalmology, Mason Eye Institute, University of Missouri, Columbia, MO, USA, bolei99@126.com

Dean Y. Li Department of Oncological Sciences and Medicine and Program in Human Molecular Biology and Genetics, University of Utah, Salt Lake City, Utah 54112, USA

Liangdong Li Preclinical Medical College, Gannan Medical University, Ganzhou, Jiangxi Province 341000, China

Qiuhong Li Department of Ophthalmology, College of Medicine, University of Florida, Gainesville, FL, USA

Xiong Liang Department of Preventive Medicine, Gannan Medical College, Ganzhou, China

Li Liangdong Preclinical Medical College, Gannan Medical University, Ganzhou, Jiangxi Province 341000, China

Richard T. Libby Department of Ophthalmology and Biomedical Genetics, University of Rochester Eye Institute, University of Rochester Medical School, Rochester, NY 14642, USA

Ying Lin Sichuan Provincial Key Laboratory for Human Disease Gene Study, Sichuan Academy of Medical Sciences & Sichuan Provincial People's Hospital, Sichuan 610072, China

Jonathan H. Lin Department of Pathology, University of California, San Diego, La Jolla, CA 92093-0612, USA, matthew.lavail@ucsf.edu

Hu Liqun Department of Ophthalmology, People Hospital of Ganzhou City, Ganzhou, China

Xuyang Liu Torsten Wiesel Research Institute and Department of Ophthalmology, West China Hospital, Sichuan University, Chengdu, China, xliu1213@yahoo.com.cn

Qin Liu F.M. Kirby Center for Molecular Ophthalmology, University of Pennsylvania School of Medicine, Philadelphia, PA, USA, qinliu3@mail.med.upenn.edu

N. Lodha Department Medical Genetics, Faculty of Medicine, University of Calgary, Calgary, Alberta T2N4N1, Canada; Division of Ophthalmology, Department of Surgery, University of Calgary, Calgary, Alberta T2N4N1, Canada; Lions Centre for Retinal Degeneration Research, University of Calgary, Calgary, Alberta T2N4N1, Canada, nlodha@ucalgary.ca

Nyall R. London Department of Oncological Sciences and Medicine and Program in Human Molecular Biology and Genetics, University of Utah, Salt Lake City, Utah 54112, USA

Ke Ma Torsten Wiesel Research Institute and Department of Ophthalmology, West China Hospital, Sichuan University, Chengdu, China

Jia Ma Torsten Wiesel Research Institute and Department of Ophthalmology, West China Hospital, Sichuan University, Chengdu, China

Goldis Malek Department of Ophthalmology, Duke University, Durham, NC, USA, gmalek@duke.edu

Mallika Mallavarapu Program in Physiology, Biophysics and Systems Biology, Graduate School of Medical Sciences, Weill Cornell Medical College, New York, USA

Anna P. Malykhina Department of Physiology, University of Oklahoma Health Sciences Center, 940 Stanton L. Young Blvd., Oklahoma, OK 73104; Division of Urology, Department of Surgery, University of Pennsylvania, 500 S. Ridgeway Ave, Glenolden, PA, 19036, USA

Katherine Mancuso Department of Ophthalmology, University of Washington, Seattle, WA, USA, kmancuso@u.washington.edu

Md Nawajes A. Mandal Department of Ophthalmology, Dean McGee Eye Institute, University of Oklahoma Health Sciences Center, 608 Stanton L.Young Blvd, DMEI 409, Oklahoma, OK 73104, USA

Valeria Marigo Department of Biomedical Sciences, University of Modena and Reggio Emilia, Modena, Italy, valeria.marigo@unimore.it

Toru Matsukawa Department of Molecular Neurobiology, University of Kanazawa, Kanazawa 920-8640, Japan

Matthew C. Mauck Department of Ophthalmology, Medical College of Wisconsin, Milwaukee, WI, USA

Kazuhiro Mawatari Division of Health Sciences, Graduate School of Medicine, University of Kanazawa, Kanazawa 920-8640, Japan

Suzanne D. McAlear University of Alabama at Birmingham, WORB 618, 924 18th Street South, Birmingham, AL 35295, USA

J.E. McRory Hotchkiss Brain Institute, University of Calgary, Calgary, Alberta T2N4N1, Canada; Department of Physiology and Biophysics, University of Calgary, Calgary, Alberta T2N4N1, Canada

S.C. Mema Department of Ophthalmology and Physiology, Hotchkiss Brain Institute, University of Alberta, Calgary, Alberta T2N4N1, Canada

Hugo F. Mendes UCL Institute of Ophthalmology, London, EC1V 9EL, UK

Stylianos Michalakis Munich Center for Integrated Protein Science, CIPSM and Department Pharmazie, Zentrum für Pharmaforschung, Ludwig-Maximilians-University, Munich, Germany

Dong Minghua Department of Preventive Medicine, Gannan Medical College, Ganzhou, China

Yusuke Mori Department of Molecular Neurobiology, University of Kanazawa, Kanazawa 920-8640, Japan; Information Engineering, Graduate School of Natural Science, University of Kanazawa, Kanazawa 920-8640, Japan

Orson L. Moritz Department of Ophthalmology and Visual Sciences, University of British Columbia, Vancouver, BC, Canada, olmoritz@interchange.ubc.ca

Yasunari Munemasa Jules Stein Eye Institute, UCLA, Los Angeles, CA 90095, USA

Kenichiro Muramoto Information Engineering, Graduate School of Natural Science, University of Kanazawa, Kanazawa 920-8640, Japan

Carlos Murga-Zamalloa Department of Ophthalmology and Visual Sciences, Kellogg Eye Center, Ann Arbor, MI 48105, USA

Muna I. Naash Department of Cell Biology, University of Oklahoma Health Sciences Center, 940 Stanton L. Young Blvd., BMSB 781, Oklahoma, OK 73126-0901, USA, muna-naash@ouhsc.edu

Taka Nagasaki Department of Ophthalmology, Columbia University, New York, NY 10032, USA

Mikiko Nagashima Department of Molecular Neurobiology, University of Kanazawa, Kanazawa 920-8640, Japan; Division of Health Sciences, Graduate School of Medicine, University of Kanazawa, Kanazawa 920-8640, Japan

Emeline F. Nandrot Centre de Recherche Institut de la Vision, UMR_S968, Inserm, UPMC University of Paris 06, 17 rue Moreau, 75012 Paris, France, emeline.nandrot@inserm.fr

Umadevi Narendra Department of Ophthalmic Research, Cole Eye Institute, Cleveland Clinic, 9500 Euclid Avenue, Cleveland, OH 44195, USA; Lerner Research Institute, Cleveland, OH, USA

Riccardo Natoli School of Biology and ARC Centre of Excellence in Vision Science, The Australian National University, RSBS, Bldg 46, Biology Place, Canberra, ACT2601, Australia

Maureen Neitz Department of Ophthalmology, University of Washington, Seattle, WA, USA

Jay Neitz Department of Ophthalmology, University of Washington, Seattle, WA, USA

Anh Thi Hong Nguyen Ocular Genetics Unit, Department of Genetics, Trinity College Dublin, Dublin 2, Ireland

Patricia M. Notario Georgetown University Medical School, 3700 Reservoir Rd. NW, Washington, D.C., 20007, USA

Tomoya Nunome Department of Molecular Neurobiology, University of Kanazawa, Kanazawa 920-8640, Japan; Information Engineering, Graduate School of Natural Science, University of Kanazawa, Kanazawa 920-8640, Japan

N.C. Orton Department Medical Genetics, Faculty of Medicine, University of Calgary, Calgary, Alberta T2N4N1, Canada; Lions Centre for Retinal Degeneration Research, University of Calgary, Calgary, Alberta T2N4N1, Canada; Hotchkiss Brain Institute, University of Calgary, Calgary, Alberta T2N4N1, Canada

Ji-Jing Pang Department of Ophthalmology, College of Medicine, University of Florida, Gainesville, FL, USA, jpang@ufl.edu

Ryan O. Parker Department of Neurosciences, Medical University of South Carolina, Charleston, SC, USA, parkerry@musc.edu

Gayle J.T. Pauer Department of Ophthalmic Research, Cole Eye Institute, Cleveland Clinic, 9500 Euclid Avenue, Cleveland, OH 44195, USA; Lerner Research Institute, Cleveland, OH, USA

Neal S. Peachey Cole Eye Institute, Cleveland, OH, USA; Lerner Research Institute, Cleveland, OH, USA; Louis Stokes VA Medical Center, Cleveland, OH, USA; Department of Ophthalmology, Cleveland Clinic Lerner College of Medicine of Case Western Reserve University, Cleveland, OH, USA

Carolee Cutler Peck Department of Ophthalmology and Visual Sciences, Moran Eye Center, University of Utah School of Medicine, Salt Lake City, UT 84132, USA

Eric A. Pierce F.M. Kirby Center for Molecular Ophthalmology, University of Pennsylvania School of Medicine, Philadelphia, PA, USA

Ma Ping ChengDu University of Traditional Chinese Medicine, Sichuan 610072, China

Carolina Pinzon-Guzman Department of Neural and Behavioral Sciences, Penn State College of Medicine, 500 University Drive, Hershey, PA 17033, USA

Natik Piri Jules Stein Eye Institute, UCLA, Los Angeles, CA 90095, USA, piri@jsei.ucla.edu

Scott M. Plafker University of Oklahoma Health Sciences Center, Oklahoma City, OK, 73104, USA, scott-plafker@ouhsc.edu

Theresa Puthussery Department of Ophthalmology, Casey Eye Institute, Oregon Health & Science University, Portland, OR, USA, puthusse@ohsu.edu

Chao Qu Department of Ophthalmology, Sichuan Academy of Medical Sciences and Sichuan Provincial People's Hospital, Sichuan 610072, China

Alexander B. Quiambao Department of Cell Biology, University of Oklahoma Health Sciences Center, 940 Stanton L. Young Blvd., Oklahoma, OK 73104, USA

R. Rehak Hotchkiss Brain Institute, University of Calgary, Calgary, Alberta T2N4N1, Canada; Department of Physiology and Biophysics, University of Calgary, Calgary, Alberta T2N4N1, Canada

Brandon Renner Department of Medicine, University of Colorado Denver School of Medicine, Denver, CO 80045, USA

Jungtae Rha Department of Ophthalmology, Medical College of Wisconsin, The Eye Institute, Milwaukee, WI, USA

Kun Do Rhee Jules Stein Eye Institute, Molecular Biology Institute, University of California, Los Angeles, CA, USA, kdrhee@ucla.edu

Olaf Riess Department of Medical Genetics, University of Tuebingen, Tuebingen, Germany

John De Roach Department of Medical Technology and Physics, Sir Charles Gairdner Hospital, Hospital Avenue, Nedlands, WA, 6009, Australia

Bärbel Rohrer Department of Ophthalmology and Neurosciences, Division of Research, Medical University of South Carolina, Charleston, SC 29425, USA, rohrer@musc.edu

A. Roorda School of Optometry, University of California, Berkeley, CA, USA

M. Saghizadeh Jules Stein Eye Institute, UCLA School of Medicine, 100 Stein Plaza, Los Angeles, CA 90095-7000, USA

Junichi Saito Department of Molecular Neurobiology, University of Kanazawa, Kanazawa 920-8640, Japan; Division of Health Sciences, Graduate School of Medicine, University of Kanazawa, Kanazawa 920-8640, Japan

Robert G. Salomon Department of Chemistry, Case Western Reserve University, Cleveland, OH, USA

M. Samardzija Lab for Retinal Cell Biology, Department Ophthalmology, University of Zurich, Zurich, Switzerland

C. Sanchez-Ramos Optic II, Neurocomputing and Neurorobotic Group, University Complutense de Madrid, Madrid, Spain, celiasr@opt.ucm.es

Ola Sandgren Department of Ophthalmology, Clinical Sciences, Umeå University, 901 85, Umeå, Sweden

Y. Sauvé Departments of Ophthalmology and Physiology, University of Alberta, T5H 3V9, Calgary, Edmonton, Canada

Karin Schaeferhoff Microarray Facility Tuebingen, Institute of Human Genetics, University of Tuebingen, Tuebingen, Germany

Brett Schroeder Department of Ophthalmology, Medical College of Wisconsin, The Eye Institute, Milwaukee, WI, USA

Mathias W. Seeliger Division of Ocular Neurodegeneration, Institute for Ophthalmic Research, Centre for Ophthalmology, University of Tuebingen, Tuebingen, Germany

Li Shumei Department of Preventive Medicine, Gannan Medical College, Ganzhou, China, gnyxylsm@163.com

Li Sisi Department of Preventive Medicine, Gannan Medical College, Ganzhou, China

Janet R. Sparrow Department of Ophthalmology, Columbia University, New York, NY 10032, USA; Department of Pathology and Cell Biology, Columbia University, New York, NY 10032, USA, jrs88@columbia.edu

Catherine J. Spellicy The University of Texas Health Science Center Houston, Human Genetics Center, 1200 Herman Pressler, Houston TX, 77030, USA, catherine.j.spellicy@uth.tmc.edu

W.K. Stell Division of Ophthalmology, Department of Surgery, University of Calgary, Calgary, Alberta T2N4N1, Canada; Lions Centre for Retinal Degeneration Research, University of Calgary, Calgary, Alberta T2N4N1, Canada; Hotchkiss Brain Institute, University of Calgary, Calgary, Alberta T2N4N1, Canada; Department of Cell Biology and Anatomy, University of Calgary, Calgary, Alberta T2N4N1, Canada

Kimberly Stepien Department of Ophthalmology, Medical College of Wisconsin, The Eye Institute, Milwaukee, WI, USA

Jonathan Stone Research School of Biological Sciences, The Australian National University, Canberra, Australia; ARC Centre of Excellence in Vision Science, The Australian National University, Canberra, Australia; Save Sight Institute and Discipline of Physiology, University of Sydney, Sydney, Australia

Gwen M. Sturgill Louis Stokes VA Medical Center, Cleveland, OH, USA

Liu Su Department Ophthalmology of Physical Center, The 2nd Affiliated Hospital of Chongqing Medical University, Chongqing, 400016, China

Preeti Subramanian NEI-NIH, Building 6, Room 134, 6 Center Dr., MSC 0607, Bethesda, MD 20892-0608, USA

Kayo Sugitani Department of Molecular Neurobiology, University of Kanazawa, Kanazawa 920-8640, Japan; Division of Health Sciences, Graduate School of Medicine, University of Kanazawa, Kanazawa 920-8640, Japan

Lori S. Sullivan The University of Texas Health Science Center Houston, Human Genetics Center, 1200 Herman Pressler, Houston TX, 77030, USA

Anand Swaroop Neurobiology-Neurodegeneration and Repair laboratory (N-NRL), National Eye Institute, National Institutes of Health, Bethesda, MD 20892, USA

Diane M. Tait Department of Ophthalmology, Medical College of Wisconsin, The Eye Institute, Milwaukee, WI, USA

Beatrice M. Tam Department of Ophthalmology and Visual Sciences, University of British Columbia, Vancouver, BC, Canada

Lawrence C.S. Tam The Ocular Genetics Unit, Department of Genetics, Trinity College Dublin, Dublin 2, Ireland, lawrenct@tcd.ie

Shibo Tang State Key Laboratory of Ophthalmology, Zhongshan Ophthalmic Center, Sun Yat-sen University, 54S, Xianlie Road, Guangzhou, China

Naoyuki Tanimoto Division of Ocular Neurodegeneration, Institute for Ophthalmic Research, Centre for Ophthalmology, University of Tuebingen, Tuebingen, Germany

Masaki Tanito Department of Ophthalmology, University of Oklahoma Health Sciences Center, Oklahoma City, OK, USA; Dean A. McGee Eye Institute, Oklahoma City, OK, USA, tanito-oph@umin.ac.jp

W. Rowland Taylor Department of Ophthalmology, Casey Eye Institute, Oregon Health & Science University, Portland, OR, USA

The Clinical Genomic and Proteomic AMD Study Group Cole Eye Institute, Cleveland, OH, USA; Louis Stokes VA Medical Center, Cleveland, OH, USA; Department of Quantitative Health Sciences, Cleveland Clinic Foundation, Cleveland, OH, USA; Department of Ophthalmology, Cleveland Clinic Lerner College of Medicine of Case Western Reserve University, Cleveland, OH, USA; Department of Ophthalmology, School of Medicine, Case Western Reserve University, Cleveland, OH, USA

V.P. Theendakara Jules Stein Eye Institute, UCLA School of Medicine, 100 Stein Plaza, Los Angeles, CA 90095-7000, USA

M. Thiersch Lab for Retinal Cell Biology, Department Ophthalmology, University of Zurich, Zurich, Switzerland

Joshua M. Thurman Department of Medicine, University of Colorado Denver School of Medicine, Denver, CO 80045, USA

Chun Yu Tian Southwest Hospital, Southwest Eye Hospital, Third Military Medical University, Chongqing 400038, China

R. Tobias Department Medical Genetics, Faculty of Medicine, University of Calgary, Calgary, Alberta T2N4N1, Canada; Lions Centre for Retinal Degeneration Research, University of Calgary, Calgary, Alberta T2N4N1, Canada

Yumi Tokita-Ishikawa Division of Clinical Cell Therapy, Center for Translational and Advanced Animal Research, 1-1 Seiryomachi, Aobaku, Miyagi, Sendai 980-8574, Japan

Joyce Tombran-Tink Department of Neural and Behavioral Sciences, Pennsylvania State University College of Medicine, Hershey, PA, USA, jttink@aol.com

Deepti Trivedi Jules Stein Eye Institute, University of California, 200 Stein Plaza, Los Angeles, CA 90095, USA, dtrivedi@ucla.edu

Yumi Ueki Oklahoma Center for Neuroscience, University of Oklahoma Health Sciences Center, Oklahoma, OK 73104, USA; Dean A. McGee Eye Institute, Oklahoma, OK 73104, USA

Krisztina Valter Research School of Biological Sciences, The Australian National University, Canberra, Australia; ARC Centre of Excellence in Vision Science, The Australian National University, Canberra, Australia

J.A. Vega Morphology and Cell Biology, Universidad de Oviedo, Oviedo, Spain

Kirstan A. Vessey Department of Anatomy and Cell Biology, University of Melbourne, Parkville, Australia

Melissa Wagner-Schuman Department of Biophysics, Medical College of Wisconsin, The Eye Institute, Milwaukee, WI, USA

Ryosuke Wakusawa Department of Ophthalmology and Visual Science, Graduate School of Medicine, Tohoku University, 1-1 Seiryomachi, Aobaku, Miyagi, Sendai 980-8574, Japan

Yun Wang Torsten Wiesel Research Institute and Department of Ophthalmology, West China Hospital, Sichuan University, Chengdu, China

Michelle M. Ward Department of Anatomy and Cell Biology, University of Melbourne, Parkville, Australia, m.ward@unimelb.edu.au

Dong Wei Department of Ophthalmology, Sichuan Academy of Medical Sciences and Sichuan Provincial People's Hospital, Sichuan 610072, China

George M. Weinstock Genome Sequencing Center, Washington University, St. Louis, MO, USA

Chuan Chuang Weng Southwest Hospital, Southwest Eye Hospital, Third Military Medical University, Chongqing 400038, People's Republic of China

Christina Weng Department of Ophthalmology and Visual Sciences, University of Michigan/Kellogg Eye Center, Ann Arbor, MI, USA

Lea D. Wicker Department of Ophthalmology, University of Oklahoma Health Sciences Center, Oklahoma City, OK, USA; Dean A. McGee Eye Institute, Oklahoma City, OK, USA

Albert Wielgus Department of Ophthalmology, Duke University, Durham, NC, USA

David S. Williams Jules Stein Eye Institute, University of California, 200 Stein Plaza, Los Angeles, CA 90095, USA

Bernd Wissinger Molecular Genetics Laboratory, Institute for Ophthalmic Research, Centre for Ophthalmology, University of Tuebingen, Tuebingen, Germany

Li Wu Department of Ophthalmology, Columbia University, New York, NY 10032, USA

Huang Xi Department of Physical Center, The 1st Affiliated Hospital of Chongqing Medical University, Chongqing, Sichuan Province, 400016, China, doctorhyh@hotmail.com

Zeng Xiangyun Department of Ophthalmology of the 1st Affiliated Hospital, Gannan Medical College, Ganzhou, China

Hai Xiao Preclinical Medical College, Gannan Medical University, Ganzhou, Jiangxi Province 341000, China

Li Xiao Preclinical Medical College, Gannan Medical University, Ganzhou, Jiangxi Province 341000, China

Luo Xiaoting Department of Biochemistry and Molecular Biology, Gannan Medical College, Ganzhou, China

Wu Xiaoyun Medical Records and Statistics Department, Shenzhen People's Hospital, Shenzhen, Guangdong, 518020, China

Dong Xu Brandeis University, Waltham, MA, USA

Naihong Yan Torsten Wiesel Research Institute and Department of Ophthalmology, West China Hospital, Sichuan University, Chengdu, China

Xian-Jie Yang Jules Stein Eye Institute, Molecular Biology Institute, University of California, Los Angeles, CA, USA

Zheng Qin Yin Southwest Hospital, Southwest Eye Hospital, Third Military Medical University, Chongqing 400038, People's Republic of China, qinzyin@yahoo.com.cn

Fan Yingchuan Department Ophthalmology of Physical Center, The 1st Affiliated Hospital of Chongqing Medical University, Chongqing, 400016, China

Fan Yingchuan Department of Ophthalmology, Sichuan Provincial People's Hospital, Chengdu, Sichuan, 610072, China

Yufeng Yu ChengDu University of Traditional Chinese Medicine, Sichuan 610072, China

Xiuzhen Yue Cole Eye Institute, Cleveland, OH, USA; Lerner Research Institute, Cleveland, OH, USA

Yongping Yue Department of Molecular Microbiology and Immunology, University of Missouri, Columbia, MO, USA

Raffaella Zaccarini UCL Institute of Ophthalmology, London, EC1V 9EL, UK

Jing Zeng Pharmaceutic College, Gannan Medical University, Ganzhou, Jiangxi Province 341000, China, zengjing61@hotmail.com

Mingzhi Zhang Joint Shantou International Eye Center, Shantou University and the Chinese University of Hong Kong, North Dongxia Road, Shantou, 515041 China

Ji Zhang Department of Ophthalmology, The Second Affiliated Hospital of Soochow University, Suzhou, Jiangsu Province, 215004, China

Kang Zhang Moran Eye Center, University of Utah, Salt Lake City, Utah 84112 USA; Institute for Genomic Medicine and Shiley Eye Center, University of California at San Diego, La Jolla, CA 92093-0838

Keqing Zhang Departments of Veterinary Medicine, Surgery and Ophthalmology, University of Missouri-Columbia, Columbia, MO, USA

Samuel Shaomin Zhang Department of Neural and Behavioral Sciences, Penn State College of Medicine, 500 University Drive, Hershey, PA 17033, USA

Qi Zhang F.M. Kirby Center for Molecular Ophthalmology, University of Pennsylvania School of Medicine, Philadelphia, PA, USA

Tong Tao Zhao Southwest Hospital, Southwest Eye Hospital, Third Military Medical University, Chongqing 400038, China

Lixin Zheng Department of Ophthalmology, University of Oklahoma Health Sciences Center, Oklahoma, OK 73104, USA; Dean A. McGee Eye Institute, Oklahoma, OK 73104, USA

Huang Zhihua Preclinical Medical College, Gannan Medical University, Ganzhou, Jiangxi Province 341000, China

Meili Zhu Department of Medicine, University of Oklahoma Health Sciences Center, Oklahoma, OK 73104, USA; Harold Hamm Oklahoma Diabetes Center, University of Oklahoma Health Sciences Center, Oklahoma, OK 73104, USA

Yuan Zhu School of Biology and ARC Centre of Excellence in Vision Science, The Australian National University, RSBS, Bldg 46, Biology Place, Canberra, ACT2601, Australia, yuan.zhu@anu.edu.au

Travel Awards

We gratefully acknowledge Foundation Fighting Blindness and National Eye Institute for their generous support of 35 travel fellowships to attend this meeting. The travel awardees are listed below. Each awardee submitted a chapter to this proceedings volume and is identified by an asterisk in the Table of Contents.

Martin-Paul Agbaga
Rajendra Apte
Srilaxmi Bearelly
Joseph Carroll
Haoyu Chen
Ross Collery
Shannon M. Conley
Anna de Marzo
M. Dominik Fischer
Doug Gould
Alecia Gross
Gregory H. Grossman
Xiaorong Gu
Li Jiang
Hemant Khanna
Christina Lange
Bo Lei
Jonathan H. Lin

Qin Liu
Mallika Mallavarapu
Katherine Mancuso
Orson Moritz
Mikiko Nagashima
Ji-jing Pang
Ryan Parker
Scott M. Plafker
Theresa Puthussery
Kun Do Rhee
Catherine J. Spellicy
Lawrence Tam
Masaki Tanito
Deepti Trivedi
Yumi Ueki
Michelle Ward
Yuan Zhu

About the Editors

Robert E. Anderson, MD, PhD, is George Lynn Cross Research Professor, Dean A. McGee Professor of Ophthalmology, and Adjunct Professor of Biochemistry & Molecular Biology and Geriatric Medicine at The University of Oklahoma Health Sciences Center in Oklahoma City, Oklahoma. He is also Director of Research at the Dean A. McGee Eye Institute. He received his Ph.D. in Biochemistry (1968) from Texas A&M University and his M.D. from Baylor College of Medicine in 1975. In 1968, he was a postdoctoral fellow at Oak Ridge Associated Universities. At Baylor, he was appointed Assistant Professor in 1969, Associate Professor in 1976, and Professor in 1981. He joined the faculty of the University of Oklahoma Health Sciences Center in January of 1995. He has received several honorary appointments including Visiting Professor, West China School of Medicine, Sichuan University, Chengdu, China; Honorary Professorship, Xi'an Jiaotong University, Xi'an, China; and Honorary Professor of Sichuan Medical Science Academy, Sichuan Provincial People's Hospital, Sichuan, China. Dr. Anderson has received the Sam and Bertha Brochstein Award for Outstanding Achievement in Retina Research from the Retina Research Foundation (1980), and the Dolly Green Award (1982) and two Senior Scientific Investigator Awards (1990 and 1997) from Research to Prevent Blindness, Inc. He received an Award for Outstanding Contributions to Vision Research from the Alcon Research Institute (1985), and the Marjorie Margolin Prize (1994). He has served on the editorial boards of *Investigative Ophthalmology and Visual Science*, *Journal of Neuroscience Research*, *Neurochemistry International*, *Current Eye Research*, and *Experimental Eye Research*. Dr. Anderson has published extensively in the areas of lipid metabolism in the retina and biochemistry of retinal degenerations. He has edited 14 books, 13 on retinal degenerations and 1 on the biochemistry of the eye. Dr. Anderson has received grants from the National Institutes of Health, The Retina Research Foundation, the Foundation Fighting Blindness, and Research to Prevent Blindness, Inc. He has been an active participant in the program committees of the Association for Research in Vision and Ophthalmology (ARVO) and was a trustee representing the Biochemistry and Molecular Biology section. He was named a Gold Fellow by ARVO in 2009. He has served on the Vision Research Program Committee and Board of Scientific Counselors of the National Eye Institute and the Board of the Basic and Clinical Science Series of The

American Academy of Ophthalmology. Dr. Anderson is a past Councilor, Treasurer, and President of the International Society for Eye Research.

Matthew M. LaVail, PhD, is Professor of Anatomy and Ophthalmology at the University of California, San Francisco School of Medicine. He received his Ph.D. degree in Anatomy (1969) from the University of Texas Medical Branch in Galveston and was subsequently a postdoctoral fellow at Harvard Medical School. Dr. LaVail was appointed Assistant Professor of Neurology-Neuropathology at Harvard Medical School in 1973. In 1976, he moved to UCSF, where he was appointed Associate Professor of Anatomy. He was appointed to his current position in 1982, and in 1988, he also became director of the Retinitis Pigmentosa Research Center at UCSF, later named the Kearn Family Center for the Study of Retinal Degeneration. Dr. LaVail has published extensively in the research areas of photoreceptor-retinal pigment epithelial cell interactions, retinal development, circadian events in the retina, genetics of pigmentation and ocular abnormalities, inherited retinal degenerations, light-induced retinal degeneration, and pharmaceutical and gene therapy for retinal degenerative diseases. He has identified several naturally occurring murine models of human retinal degenerations and has developed transgenic mouse and rat models of others. He is the author of more than 150 research publications and has edited 13 books on inherited and environmentally induced retinal degenerations. Dr. LaVail has received the Fight for Sight Citation (1976); the Sundial Award from the Retina Foundation (1976); the Friedenwald Award from the Association for Research in Vision and Ophthalmology (ARVO, 1981); two Senior Scientific Investigators Awards from Research to Prevent Blindness (1988 and 1998); a MERIT Award from the National Eye Institute (1989); an Award for Outstanding Contributions to Vision Research from the Alcon Research Institute (1990); the Award of Merit from the Retina Research Foundation (1990); the first John A. Moran Prize for Vision Research from the University of Utah (1997); the first Trustee Award from The Foundation Fighting Blindness (1998); and the Llura Liggett Gund Award from the Foundation Fighting Blindness (2007). He has served on the editorial board of *Investigative Ophthalmology and Visual Science* and as an Executive Editor of *Experimental Eye Research*. Dr. LaVail has been an active participant in the program committee of ARVO and has served as a Trustee (Retinal Cell Biology Section) of ARVO. He was named a Gold Fellow of ARVO in 2009. He has been a member of the program committee and a Vice President of the International Society for Eye research. He has also served on the Scientific Advisory Board of the Foundation Fighting Blindness since 1973.

Joe G. Hollyfield, PhD, is the Llura and Gordon Gund Professor of Ophthalmology Research in the Cole Eye Institute at The Cleveland Clinic Foundation, Cleveland, Ohio. He received a Ph.D. from the University of Texas at Austin and did postdoctoral work at the Hubrecht Laboratory in Utrecht, The Netherlands. He has held faculty positions at Columbia University College of Physicians and Surgeons in New York City and at Baylor College of Medicine in Houston, Texas. He was Director of the Retinitis Pigmentosa Research Center in The Cullen Eye Institute at Baylor from 1978 until his move to The Cleveland Clinic Foundation in 1995. He is currently Director of the Foundation Fighting Blindness Research Center at The Cleveland Clinic Foundation. Dr. Hollyfield has published over 200 papers in the area of cell and developmental biology of the retina and retinal pigment epithelium in both normal and retinal degenerative tissue. He has edited 14 books, 13 on retinal degenerations and 1 on the structure of the eye. Dr. Hollyfield received the Marjorie W. Margolin Prize (1981, 1994), the Sam and Bertha Brochstein Award (1985) and the Award of Merit in Retina Research (1998) from the Retina Research Foundation; the Olga Keith Weiss Distinguished Scholars' Award (1981) and two Senior Scientific Investigator Awards (1988, 1994) from Research to Prevent Blindness, Inc.; an award for Outstanding Contributions to Vision Research from the Alcon Research Institute (1987); the Distinguished Alumnus Award (1991) from Hendrix College, Conway, Arkansas; the Endre A. Balazs Prize (1994) from the International Society for Eye Research (ISER); and the Proctor Medal (2009) from the Association for Research in Vision and Ophthalmology (ARVO). He was named a Gold Fellow by ARVO in 2009. He is currently Editor-in-Chief of the journal, *Experimental Eye Research* published by Elsevier. Dr. Hollyfield has been active in the Association for Research in Vision and Ophthalmology (ARVO) serving on the Program Committee (1976), as Trustee (Retinal Cell Biology, 1989–1994), as President (1993–1994) and as Immediate Past President (1994–1995). He was also President (1988–1991) and Secretary (1984–1987) of the International Society of Eye Research. He is Chairman of the scientific review panel for the Macular Degeneration program of the American Health Assistance Foundation (Clarksburg, MD), serves on the scientific advisory boards of the Foundation Fighting Blindness (Owings Mills, MD), the Knights Templar Eye Research Foundation (Chicago, IL), the Helen Keller Eye Research Foundation (Birmingham, AL), the South Africa Retinitis Pigmentosa Foundation (Johannesburg, South Africa), and is Co-Chairman of the Medical and Scientific Advisory Board of Retina International (Zurich, Switzerland).

Part I
Basic Science Underlying Retinal Degeneration

Chapter 1
Analysis of Genes Differentially Expressed During Retinal Degeneration in Three Mouse Models

Yogita Kanan, Michael Centola, Frank Bart, and Muayyad R. Al-Ubaidi

Abstract An estimated 100,000 people in the US alone have retinitis pigmentosa. This disease, caused by the loss of rods and cones, results in blindness. With the intention of identifying common cell death pathways that result in RP, the pattern of global gene expression in three different mouse models of retinal degeneration was analyzed using DNA arrays. The models used were $opsin^{\Delta 255-256}$, a transgenic mouse line that expresses a mutant form of opsin with a deletion of an isoleucine at either position 255 or 256; the Bouse C mouse, whereby normal opsin is over-expressed by over 2 folds; *MOT1*, a model that expresses SV-40 T antigen downstream of opsin promoter and leads to retinal degeneration. We found that, at least in the 2 models of retinal degeneration that are characterized by rhodopsin abnormalities, death is due to the TNF pathway. In addition, there are a number of unknown genes not yet annotated in each of the models that could be promising in revealing novel functions in photoreceptors.

1.1 Introduction

Millions worldwide suffer from the blinding disorder retinitis pigmentosa (RP) (Hartong et al. 2006). This condition is characterized by a gradual loss, through cell death, of rods and cones. To understand the cell death process in RP and in the hope of identifying genes that can be targets for therapy, we analyzed differential gene expression during photoreceptor death by performing microarray analysis between age matched C57Bl/6 mice and three mouse models of retinal degeneration. These models are Bouse C, a model where the opsin protein is over-expressed

M.R. Al-Ubaidi (✉)
Department of Cell Biology, BMSB 781, 940 Stanton L. Young Blvd., Oklahoma City, OK 73104, USA
e-mail: muayyad-al-ubaidi@ouhsc.edu

R.E. Anderson et al. (eds.), *Retinal Degenerative Diseases*, Advances in Experimental Medicine and Biology 664, DOI 10.1007/978-1-4419-1399-9_1,
© Springer Science+Business Media, LLC 2010

by 2.2 folds of the levels measured in non-transgenic animals (Tan et al. 2001), *opsin* $^{\Delta 255-256}$, a model with a deletion in an isoleucine in opsin either at position 255 or 256 (Gryczan et al. 1995) and *MOT1*$^{-/-}$ a model that expresses SV-40 T antigen downstream of opsin promoter and leads to retinal degeneration (Al-Ubaidi et al. 1992).

1.2 Methods

1.2.1 RNA Preparation and cDNA Labeling

Retinas were removed at postnatal days (P) 10, 12 and 14 and the retinal pigment epithelium was dissected away under a microscope. Total RNA was prepared using Trizol (Invitrogen, Carlsbad, CA). Genomic DNA contamination was removed by treatment of the samples with RQ1 RNase free DNase (Promega, Madison, WI). cDNA was synthesized using CyScribe First-Strand cDNA Labeling Kit (GE Healthcare, Piscataway, NJ). Microarrays were made using a 70-mer oligonucleotide library from Qiagen/Opern (Mouse genome set, version 2.0). The library contains 70-mer, gene specific oligonucleotides representing about 16,463 mouse genes.

1.2.2 Hybridization of Slides, Image Acquisition and Bioinformatics

Cy-3-labeled transgenic mouse cDNA, and the Cy-5-labeled age matched C57Bl/6 mouse were dissolved in Hybridization Buffer (Clontech, San Jose, CA) and hybridized at 42°C for 8 h in a microarray hybridization station (Ventana Medical Systems, Tucson, AZ). Fluorescent intensity was analyzed by a dual-channel scanner (Affymetrix, Santa Clara, CA). An associative analysis approach was used to identify genes that are differentially expressed between the transgenic mouse models and wild type mice (Dozmorov and Centola 2003). Only genes up-regulated or down-regulated by about 2-folds were analyzed further.

1.2.3 Real-Time PCR

Real-time quantitative PCR was performed as described before (Kanan et al. 2008). Real time PCR confirmed all gene modulations observed on the arrays and presented herein.

1.3 Results

1.3.1 Microarray Analysis of Opsin $^{\Delta 255-256}$ $^{-/-}$ Model

One of the first opsin mutations observed in humans was the rhodopsin I255/256 mutations (Inglehearn et al. 1991). This mutation eliminates one of 2 sequential isoleucines at rhodopsin position 255, 256, which are present in the transmembrane helix 6. Transgenic mice expressing the *opsin* $^{\Delta 255-256}$ were previously generated (Gryczan et al. 1995). Histological comparisons of the homozygous I255/256 strain of mice with the age matched wild type mice C57/Bl6 show a fast rate of photoreceptor loss (Penn et al. 2000). At P10, *opsin* $^{\Delta 255-256}$ retinas exhibit early degenerative changes, and by P15, the outer nuclear layer is reduced to half that of the wild type mice. We analyzed RNA samples from homozygous *opsin* $^{\Delta 255-256}$ strain of mice at P10, P12 and P14 retina and compared it to age matched retinas from C57/BL mice by microarray. At P10, all the genes on the array were comparable in expression levels to wild type mice. Array analysis at P12 and P14 showed 56 genes differentially modulated, with 37 genes down-regulated and 19 up-regulated (Table 1.1). The down-regulated genes belonged mainly to the categories of structural proteins (8%), proteins involved in metabolism (8%), protein transport (8%), phototransduction (33%) and transcription factors (19%). About 24% of the proteins down-regulated were unknown proteins. Up-regulated genes belonged to the categories of apoptosis (10%), protein degradation (16%), signal transduction (16%), lipid metabolism (21%), transcription factors (10%) while 27% of the proteins were unknown.

Table 1.1 List of genes differentially regulated in the *Opsin* $^{\Delta 255-256}$ model

Genes down-regulated in the *opsin* $^{\Delta 255-256}$ model

Gene modulated	P12	P14
Phototransduction genes		
Guanine nucleotide binding protein, alpha transducing 1	0.08	0.0
Guanylyl cyclase	0.12	0.08
ROM1	0.41	0.07
Retinitis pigmentosa 1	0.50	0.06
Cyclic nucleotide-gated channel beta subunit 1	0.37	0.02
Guanine nucleotide binding protein, beta 1	0.38	0.09
Recoverin	0.26	0.08
Retinitis pigmentosa GTPase regulator interacting protein 1	0.37	0.13
Unc119 homolog	0.42	0.36
Similar to retinol-binding protein 3	0.40	0.14
Prominin	0.69	0.26
Cyclic nucleotide gated channel, cGMP gated	0.30	0.0
Structural genes		
Adiponectin receptor 1	0.42	0.22
Elovl4	0.53	0.23
Photoreceptor cadherin	0.77	0.25

Table 1.1 (continued)

Genes down-regulated in the *opsin*$^{\Delta 255-256}$ model

Gene modulated	P12	P14
Metabolism genes		
Lactate dehydrogenase 1	0.74	0.41
Hexokinase 1	0.59	0.47
Ornithine decarboxylase antizyme	0.79	0.50
Protein binding or transport genes		
Karyopherin (importin) alpha 2	0.52	0.27
Rab5ef-pending|Rab5 exchange factor	0.45	0.45
PH domain containing protein in retina 1	0.80	0.48
Transcription factor genes		
N-myc downstream regulated 1	0.87	0.39
High mobility group nucleosomal binding domain 2	0.79	0.23
Neurogenic differentiation 1	0.82	0.38
Hematopoietic zinc finger	0.61	0.40
Signal recognition particle 54 kDa	1.35	0.43
Cold shock domain protein A	0.52	0.07
Cone-rod homeobox containing gene	0.60	0.15
Unknown genes		
RIKEN cDNA 2900052E22 gene	0.38	0.20
Mus musculus, Similar to hypothetical protein FLJ13993	0.30	0.12
Retbindin	0.35	0.22
Coiled-coil domain containing 96	0.47	0.11
Aryl-hydrocarbon interacting protein-like 1	0.38	0.10
RIKEN full-length enriched library, clone:2310065B16	0.60	0.28
Glutamate receptor, ionotropic, N-methyl D-asparate-associated protein 1	0.71	0.48
RIKEN full-length enriched library, clone:9030405D14 product	0.45	0.48
Emopamil binding protein-like	0.63	0.34
Genes up-regulated in the *opsin*$^{\Delta 255-256}$ model		
Apoptosis genes		
Shugoshin-like 2 tumor necrosis factor-alpha-induced protein B12 – human	1.45	5.25
Similar to Death-associated protein 1 (DAP-1)The ubiquitin-homology protein	1.96	2.30
Protein degradation genes		
Ring finger 38, lippopolysaccharide induced ubiquitin ligase	1.53	2.09
Histone deacetylase 6	1.09	2.60
Transcription factor genes		
Zinc finger protein 95	1.03	3.34
RIKEN cDNA 2310028D20 gene, positive regulation of transcription from Pol II promote	0.93	2.28

Table 1.1 (continued)

Genes down-regulated in the $opsin^{\Delta255-256}$ model

Gene modulated	P12	P14
Signal transduction genes		
Par-6 partitioning defective 6 homolog gamma	1.02	5.40
Ppab2b|Phosphatidic acid phosphatase type 2B	1.02	2.38
Calmodulin 1	1.28	2.29
Lipid metabolism genes		
RIKEN cDNA 2300002D11 gene, lipid binding activity	1.15	2.28
Sterol O-acyltransferase 1	1.45	2.38
Peroxiredoxin 5	1.48	2.26
Apolipoprotein E	1.67	2.88
Unknown genes		
HAI-2 related small protein	1.2	10.72
RIKEN clone:6330411I15	1.4	2.46
F-box protein 16	0.89	2.93
RIKEN clone:5730419O14	2.28	3.55
RIKEN clone:6230410I01	0.74	2.92

1.3.2 Microarray Analysis of Bouse C Model

To determine whether cell death in other models of retinal degeneration follows the same pattern, modulated genes in the Bouse C that over-expresses opsin were studied. We analyzed RNA samples from homozygous Bouse C strain of mice at P10, P12 and P14 retina and compared it to that of age matched C57/BL. At P10 all the genes on the array were comparable in expression levels to wild type mice except opsin, which is up-regulated 4-fold. However, at P12 and P14, there was significant modulation of expression compared to wild type controls (Table 1.2). There were a total of 78 genes that were differentially regulated, with 15 genes down-regulated and 63 genes up-regulated. Down-regulated genes fell into the groups of phototransduction (53%), transcription factors (13%), metabolic (20%) and ion transport (13%). Up-regulated genes belonged to the classes of apoptosis (3%), protein biosynthesis (6%), transferase activity (5%), lipid metabolism (3%), carbohydrate metabolism (3%), transcription factor (19%), electron transport (3%), protein transport (5%), neurotransmitter secretion (3%), and unknown genes (50%).

Table 1.2 List of genes differentially regulated in the Bouse C model

Genes down-regulated in the Bouse C model

Gene modulated	P12	P14
Phototransduction genes		
Guanine nucleotide binding protein, alpha transducing 1	0.26	0.14
Cyclic nucleotide-gated channel beta subunit 1	0.78	0.38

Table 1.2 (continued)

Genes down-regulated in the Bouse C model

Gene modulated	P12	P14
Cyclic nucleotide gated channel, cGMP gated	0.61	0.25
Guanylate cyclase activator 1B	0.16	0.16
Guanine nucleotide binding protein, beta 1	0.60	0.39
Retinitis pigmentosa 1 homolog (human)	0.86	0.36
Cone-rod homeobox containing gene	0.87	0.37
Prominin	0.89	0.48
Ion transport genes		
ATPase, Na$^+$K$^+$ transporting, alpha 3 subunit	0.71	0.36
ATPase, H$^+$ transporting, lysosomal (vacuolar proton pump), beta 56/58 kDa, isoform 2	0.88	0.37
Transcription factor genes		
Aryl hydrocarbon receptor nuclear translocator	1.00	0.34
B lymphoma Mo-MLV insertion region 1	1.19	0.37
Metabolism genes		
Glucose phospha-te isomerase 1 complex	0.67	0.33
Phosphofructokinase, liver, B-type	0.45	0.33
Pyruvate kinase 3	0.77	0.38
Genes up-regulated in the Bouse C model		
Transcription factor genes		
Zinc finger with KRAB and SCAN domains 6	0.87	5.61
Zinc finger and BTB domain containing 7C	0.95	2.34
Chromobox homolog 2 (Drosophila Pc class)	1.01	2.33
Zinc finger protein of the cerebellum 1	0.95	4.46
Fetal liver zinc finger 1	2.22	77.22
Mlx interactor MIR	1.2	4.2
Hypothetical transcription factor nuclear regulation homolog polymerase RNA alternative containing protein	0.47	2.39
Early development regulator 1 (homolog of polyhomeotic 1)	0.86	2.82
Upstream transcription factor 2	0.87	3.16
Homeo box A10	0.73	77.09
High mobility group box 2-like 1	1.18	3.56
Kruppel-like factor 16	0.81	3.99
Protein biosynthesis genes		
Ribosomal protein S27a	1.24	3.74
Ribosomal protein S19	1.28	31.72
Mitochondrial ribosomal protein S16	1.24	2.25
Ribosomal protein S27-like (Rps27l)	1.27	2.42
Apoptosis genes		
Tumor necrosis factor receptor superfamily, member 1b	0.73	1086127
Tumor necrosis factor receptor superfamily, member 23	1.08	3.04
Neurotransmittor release genes		
Histamine N-methyltransferase	0.77	2.16
Synapsin I	1.27	3.24

Table 1.2 (continued)

Genes down-regulated in the Bouse C model

Gene modulated	P12	P14
Lipid metabolism genes		
Patatin-like phospholipase domain containing 3	1.00	5.23
Protein kinase, AMP-activated, gamma 1 non-catalytic subunit	1.68	2.06
Carbohydrate metabolism genes		
N-acetylneuraminate pyruvate lyase	0.90	2.74
Mannosidase 1, beta	0.61	40.23
Transferase activity genes		
Williams Beuren syndrome chromosome region 22	0.97	2.15
Dihydrolipoamide S-succinyltransferase	0.86	2.48
Dolichol-phosphate (beta-D) mannosyltransferase 1	1.26	4.64
Electron transport genes		
Cytochrome c oxidase, subunit VIIa 3	1.34	3.15
ATPase inhibitor	1.25	2.21
Protein transport genes		
ADP-ribosylation factor 5	0.83	6.67
ADP-ribosylation factor-like 8B	0.90	2.03
RAB1, member RAS oncogene family	0.97	2.3
Unknown genes		
Glycoprotein 38	2.01	0.99
Transmembrane protein 16A	0.71	13.77
cDNA, RIKEN clone:4921511C04	5,540	2,363
cDNA, RIKEN clone:6230414M07	0.73	2336671
cDNA, RIKEN clone:4632407G05	0.64	10.26
cDNA, RIKEN clone:4930423O20	0.78	12.85
cDNA, RIKEN clone:B230110O18	0.94	8.62
cDNA, RIKEN clone:1200014H14	0.79	9.68
cDNA, RIKEN clone:4921518G09	1.02	19.09
cDNA, RIKEN clone:1700097M23	1.02	4.03
cDNA, RIKEN clone:4930512M02	1.03	5.08
	0.81	1712243
cDNA, RIKEN clone:3000002G13	1.01	168
cDNA, RIKEN clone:4930569F06	0.73	24.13
cDNA, RIKEN clone:4933405L10	6.02	20.20
cDNA, RIKEN clone:5530401N18	1.15	2.30
cDNA, RIKEN clone:2600001G24	0.91	4.12
cDNA, RIKEN clone:4933400F21	1.39	3.57
cDNA, RIKEN clone:4933417C20	5.14	1204875
cDNA, RIKEN clone:9530097N15	0.84	8.74
cDNA RIKEN 9630055N22 gene	0.73	1514470
cDNA, RIKEN clone:1700016M24	0.77	4.62
cDNA, RIKEN clone:2210021I22	0.93	2.00
cDNA, RIKEN clone:3110006I21	1.16	2.08
Golgi autoantigen, golgin subfamily a, 7	0.89	3.65

Table 1.2 (continued)

Genes down-regulated in the Bouse C model

Gene modulated	P12	P14
Mus musculus mg53d08.r1 mRNA	19.08	17.38
cDNA, RIKEN clone:1700027D21	3.88	79.15
cDNA, RIKEN clone:2310015L07	1.24	3.01
cDNA, RIKEN clone:4632426C10	1.06	2.27
Mus musculus plakophilin 4	1.29	2.67
cDNA, RIKEN clone:1110001H19	1.05	2.25
cDNA, RIKEN clone:6230409E21	2.26	223
cDNA, RIKEN clone:4933431J24	1.13	9.89

1.3.3 Microarray Analysis of MOT1 Mouse

MOT1 is a model that expresses SV-40 T antigen under the opsin promoter (Al-Ubaidi et al. 1992). The expression of the viral oncogene forces the postmitotic photoreceptors to re-enter the cell cycle and then undergo apoptosis. At P10 there is no photoreceptor loss. However at P15, there is a loss of 50% rod photoreceptors and only cone photoreceptors survive by P25 (Al-Ubaidi et al. 1992). In this model, we observed gene modulations as early as P10 whereby, 36 genes were differentially expressed (Table 1.3). Out of these, 20 genes were down-regulated and 16 genes were up-regulated. Down regulated genes belonged to the categories of phototransduction (65%), transport protein (16%) and unknown genes (20%) while Up-regulated genes fell into the categories of DNA binding proteins (25%), transcription factors (13%), protein binding (25%), cell cycle (13%), ubiquitin cycle (13%) and unknown genes (13%).

Table 1.3 List of genes differentially regulated in the *MOT1* model

Genes down-regulated in the *MOT1* model

Gene modulated	P10	P12	P14
Phototransduction genes			
Rod opsin	0.16	0.13	0.09
Guanine nucleotide binding protein, alpha transducing 1	0.14	0.07	0.05
Retinitis pigmentosa 1 homolog (human)	0.60	0.39	0.26
Rod photoreceptor 1	0.63	0.33	0.23
Retinol dehydrogenase 12	0.59	0.36	0.25
Guanine nucleotide binding protein, beta 1	0.61	0.41	0.41
Retinol-binding protein 3, interstitial	0.51	0.35	0.28
Guanine nucleotide binding protein, beta 5	0.37	0.32	0.25

Table 1.3 (continued)

Genes down-regulated in the *MOT1* model			
Gene modulated	P10	P12	P14
Unc119 homolog	0.54	0.39	0.49
Retinitis pigmentosa GTPase regulator interacting protein 1	0.40	0.32	0.18
Similar to cyclic nucleotide-gated channel beta subunit 1	0.47	0.38	0.26
Rod outer segment membrane protein 1	0.64	0.44	0.34
Recoverin	0.23	0.19	0.22
Transport genes			
Potassium inwardly-rectifying channel, subfamily J, member 14	0.37	0.0	0.03
Cyclic nucleotide gated channel, cGMP gated	0.48	0.33	0.12
Vesicular glutamate transporter 1	0.50	0.34	0.21
Unknown genes			
RIKEN cDNA 9630013K17 gene	0.01	0.0	0.25
Oxysterol binding protein 2	0.55	0.44	0.29
RIKEN cDNA 4921513E08 gene	0.51	0.43	0.26
RIKEN cDNA 9030405D14 gene	0.66	0.44	0.74
Genes up-regulated in the *MOT1* model			
DNA binding genes			
Topoisomerase (DNA) II alpha	644038	761293	798278
Breakpoint cluster region protein 1	2.46	1.89	1.95
H2A histone family, member Z	2.91	2.96	4.77
Nucleosome assembly protein 1-like 1	1.21	2.10	0.96
Transcription factor genes			
Homeo box B1	2.46	3.59	6.89
Zinc finger protein 467	2.17	1.04	1.52
Protein binding genes			
Non-SMC condensin II complex, subunit G2	2.98	1.85	1.97
PDZ binding kinase	14.65	30.72	14.20
EMI domain containing 2	2.25	1.46	1.48
Solute carrier family 3 (activators of dibasic and neutral amino acid transport), member 2	2.65	1.42	1.54
Cell cycle genes			
Antigen identified by monoclonal antibody Ki 67	4.69	6.54	7.04
Similar to acidic protein rich in leucines	96.42	708217	3.41
Ubiquitin genes			
Ubiquitin-conjugating enzyme E2C	82623	460584	61924
ubiquitin-conjugating enzyme E2S	2.14	5.32	2.07
Unknown genes			
RIKEN cDNA 2510015F01 gene	2.49	3.33	2.50
RIKEN cDNA 2610008F03 gene	16.58	419236	8.09

1.4 Discussion

To uncover common genes that will be modulated in different retinal degenerative mouse models, we performed microarray analysis on 3 mouse models of retinal degeneration. Two of these models are related to rhodopsin, of which one of the models has a deletion of isoleucine at position 255 or 256 ($opsin^{\Delta 255-256}$). The second rhodopsin model, over expresses opsin by over two folds (Bouse C). The third model expresses the oncogene SV-40 T antigen (*MOT1*) downstream of opsin promoter. The first phototransduction gene to be severely affected in all the models is guanine nucleotide binding protein, alpha transducing 1.

In the $opsin^{\Delta 255-256\,-/-}$ model, we observed up-regulation of 2 proteins involved with cell death, Shugoshin-like 2 tumor necrosis factor-alpha-induced protein B12 and death-associated protein 1 (DAP-1), which causes TNF mediated cell death by the recruitment of FADD death effector (Liou and Liou 1999). The Bouse model of retinal degeneration up-regulates 2 death genes, the tumor necrosis factor receptor superfamily, member 1b and tumor necrosis factor receptor superfamily, member 23 suggesting that in these 2 models of retinal degeneration that are characterized by rhodopsin abnormalities, death is due to the extrinsic TNF pathway.

In the *MOT1* model of retinal degeneration, we observed up-regulation of genes involved in DNA binding, DNA replication and ubiquitin mediated degradation. Since *MOT1* is a model for cell-cycle dependant cell death, an intracellular event, it is very likely that the intrinsic mitochondrial pathway is activated. In addition, there are several unknown genes not yet annotated in each of the models that could be promising in revealing novel functions in photoreceptors.

In summary, the three models of retinal degeneration show very few similarities regarding modulation of retinal gene expression during degeneration. In conclusion, although the degenerative process appears very similar by histologic examination, the initially activated cell death pathway may be totally different.

References

Al-Ubaidi MR, Hollyfield JG, Overbeek PA et al (1992) Photoreceptor degeneration induced by the expression of SV40 T antigen in the retina of transgenic mice. Proc Natl Acad Sci 89: 1194–1198

Dozmorov I, Centola M (2003) An associative analysis of gene expression array data. Bioinformatics 19:204–211

Gryczan CW, Kuszak JR, Novak L et al (1995) A transgenic mouse model for autosomal dominant retinitis pigmentosa caused by a three base pair deletion in codon 225/256 of the opsin gene. Invest Ophthalmol Vis Sci 36:S423.

Hartong DT, Berson EL, Dryja TP (2006) Retinitis pigmentosa. Lancet 368:1795–1809

Inglehearn CF, Bashir R, Lester DH et al (1991) A 3-bp deletion in the rhodopsin gene in a family with autosomal dominant retinitis pigmentosa. Am J Hum Genet 48:26–30

Kanan Y, Kasus-Jacobi A, Moiseyev G et al (2008) Retinoid processing in cone and Müller cell lines. Exp Eye Res 86:344–354

Liou ML, Liou HC (1999) The ubiquitin-homology protein, DAP-1, associates with tumor necrosis factor receptor (p60) death domain and induces apoptosis. J Biol Chem 274:10145–10153

Penn JS, Li S, Naash MI (2000) Ambient hypoxia reverses retinal vascular attenuation in a transgenic mouse model of autosomal dominant retinitis pigmentosa. Invest Ophthalmol Vis Sci 41:4007–4013

Tan E, Wang Q, Quiambao AB et al (2001) The relationship between opsin overexpression and photoreceptor degeneration. Invest Ophthalmol Vis Sci 42:589–600

Chapter 2
Regulation of Angiogenesis by Macrophages

Rajendra S. Apte

Abstract Abnormal angiogenesis is a cardinal feature in the pathophysiology of several diseases of the retina including retinopathy of prematurity, diabetic retinopathy and choroidal neovascularization associated with age-related macular degeneration. Recent evidence has implicated macrophages as components of the innate immune system that play a key role in regulating angiogenesis in the retina and choroid. This review will focus on the role of macrophages in regulating ocular angiogenesis.

Immune vascular interactions are important role in regulating angiogenesis during development and in disorders of aging such as cancers, atheromatous heart disease and blinding eye disease such as age-related macular degeneration (AMD) (Apte et al. 2006; Espinosa-Heidmann et al. 2002; Hansson 2005; Kelly et al. 2007; Nakao et al. 2005; Taylor et al. 2005). AMD is the leading cause of blindness in North America in people over 50 years of age and blindness in AMD occurs largely from the exudative (wet) form of the disease that is characterized by the development of abnormal blood vessels underneath the retina i.e. CNV (Klein et al. 2004; van Leeuwen et al. 2003). Strong evidence has implicated macrophages in this process. Macrophages have been demonstrated to be necessary and sufficient in order to induce regression of lens vasculature during development and in inhibiting the growth of abnormal blood vessels in the eye in AMD (Ambati et al. 2003; Apte et al. 2006; Dace et al. 2008; Lobov et al. 2005). On the other hand, alternative lines of evidence have also implicated macrophages in promoting abnormal blood vessel growth in AMD (Espinosa-Heidmann et al. 2003; Sakurai et al. 2003).

Recent studies have demonstrated that cytokines can influence macrophage polarization and their regulation of angiogenesis. Mice that lack interleukin-10 (IL-10–/–) are significantly impaired in their ability to generate CNV after laser-induced tissue injury (Apte et al. 2006; Kelly et al. 2007). In the eye, IL-10 promotes

R.S. Apte (✉)
Ophthalmology and Visual Sciences, Developmental Biology, Barnes Retina Institute, Washington University School of Medicine, 660 South Euclid Avenue Box 8096, St. Louis, MO 63110, USA
e-mail: apte@vision.wustl.edu

R.E. Anderson et al. (eds.), *Retinal Degenerative Diseases*, Advances in Experimental Medicine and Biology 664, DOI 10.1007/978-1-4419-1399-9_2,
© Springer Science+Business Media, LLC 2010

angiogenesis by altering macrophage function. Polarization of macrophages can play a pivotal role in determining the ultimate effector function of these cells (Mosser 2003). Macrophages stimulated in presence of IFN-γ, LPS or GM-CSF produce high levels of cytokines such as IL-12, IL-23, IL-6, TNF-α and iNOS2 with low levels of IL-10, TGF-β and arginase 1(Arg-1). This signature defines a classically activated, anti-angiogenic macrophage (M1) that is also important in anti-bacterial and inflammatory functions. Our laboratory has previously demonstrated that GM-CSF cultured macrophages polarize to an M1 phenotype and can inhibit laser-induced CNV upon injection in to the eyes of host mice (Apte et al. 2006; Kelly et al. 2007). In presence of IL-10, IL-4, or IL-13, macrophages become alternatively activated and polarized to a pro-angiogenic phenotype (M2) characterized by high levels of IL-10, TGF-β and Arg-1 and low levels of pro-inflammatory cytokines such IL-6 and TNF-α. This is especially relevant as aging in mice leads to a drift in the macrophage population to a pro-angiogenic phenotype (Kelly et al. 2007). Although classification of macrophages in to two distinct compartments such as M1 and M2 might be too simplistic, there is clearly a spectrum of macrophage phenotype as it pertains to angiogenic function.

It is important to elucidate factors that regulate macrophage-mediated regulation of developmental and post-developmental angiogenesis especially since abnormal angiogenesis in the aged eye in AMD and in the young eye in ROP leads to blindness. VEGF-A is an important factor in inducing CNV in patients with AMD. Currently, a number of treatments directed at exudative AMD and neovascularization from diabetic retinopathy are focused on neutralization of VEGF-A activity in the eye (Brown et al. 2006). These treatments have offered physicians an ability to intervene in this difficult disease and significantly reduced the risk of severe vision loss from complications of unbridled angiogenesis. They have also enhanced the likelihood of improving vision in patients affected by the disease. Unfortunately, VEGF inhibitors have to be delivered directly in to the eye with multiple, frequent intraocular injections, a process that is highly unpalatable to the patient and one that may be associated with serious ocular adverse events such as infections, hemorrhage and retinal detachments (Brown et al. 2006; Rosenfeld et al. 2006). It has been shown that anti-VEGF agents delivered in to the eye can reach the systemic circulation and that chronic systemic inhibition of VEGF may be associated with significant cardiovascular and cerebrovascular risk. In addition, anti-VEGF therapy, although relatively effective in treating neovascular processes in the eye has not been proven efficacious as a) prophylactic therapy to reduce disease progression and the possibility of developing CNV in AMD or b) curative in successfully inhibiting CNV without sustained therapy. Although complement factor H polymorphisms are also associated with AMD, there is no data that suggests a role for complement in macrophage function and its regulation of angiogenesis (Edwards et al. 2005).

We are now in an era where identifying signaling pathways within macrophages that stimulate abnormal angiogenesis is critical in advancing the gains achieved with anti-VEGF therapy and in order to develop preventive therapies. Also, it is crucial to identify safe and effective modalities of targeted delivery of potential therapeutic agents to the site of disease processes in order to maximize sustained treatment benefit and minimize local or systemic adverse events.

2.1 Macrophage Polarization and Its Role in Angiogenesis

Polarization of macrophages can play a pivotal role in determining the ultimate effector functions of these cells (Mosser 2003). Macrophages stimulated in presence of IFN-γ, LPS or GM-CSF undergo classical activation and produce high levels of IL-12, IL-23, IL-6, TNF-α, iNOS2 and low levels of IL-10, TGF-β and Arg-1. This signature highlights an M1 macrophage that has important anti-bacterial and inflammatory functions and has also been shown to be anti-angiogenic. Our laboratory has previously demonstrated that GM-CSF cultured macrophages can inhibit CNV upon injection in to the eyes of host mice at the time of tissue injury (Apte et al. 2006). In presence of IL-10 or IL-4, macrophages undergo alternative activation and become polarized to a pro-angiogenic phenotype characterized by high levels of IL-10, TGF- β and Arg-1 and low levels of M1 cytokines. This alternatively activated macrophage has also been called an M2 macrophage. We have also demonstrated that senescence and IL-10 can influence the macrophage phenotype. Aging and high levels of IL-10 in the micromilieu (as seen with senescence) can independently influence macrophages to become pro-angiogenic.

In non-ocular tumors, it has been shown that the tumor micromilieu can influence the polarization and activation of the tumor associated macrophages (TAM) to a pro-angiogenic M2 phenotype. The M2 TAM has been shown to promote the growth and proliferation of several non-ocular tumors while the M1 TAM has pro-inflammatory and anti-angiogenic properties. It is clear that the combined effect of the cytokine profile is what drives the angiogenic phenotype of the macrophage e.g. although TNF-α has been shown to be pro-angiogenic in cancers, it is also secreted at functionally significant levels by the anti-angiogenic M1 macrophages (Sethi et al. 2008). Although we have shown that the level of FasL on the surface of the macrophage can be regulated by aging (and IL-10) and may represent a membrane-bound marker for defining macrophage polarization, it is unclear what other factors, especially signaling intermediates, play a role in the drifting macrophage phenotype and its downstream effects on immune surveillance function. This is especially important in the light of published data that FasL on the macrophage and the RPE are critical in regulating angiogenesis (Apte et al. 2006; Kaplan et al. 1999).

Immune privilege can be characterized as a subversion of the effector immune response that is unique to the eye, the central nervous system and the fetal-maternal interface in the uterus (Niederkorn 2006). Evolutionarily, it may have evolved to protect delicate tissues in the eye from innocent bystander damage and necrotic cell death that are part of a vigorous cell-mediated immune response to antigen. Immune privilege in the eye is orchestrated by membrane-bound molecules such as FasL and TRAIL as well as soluble factors such as TGF-β, VIP, α-MSH and MIF among others (Apte et al. 1997; Apte and Niederkorn 1996; Niederkorn 2006). The deviant immune response in privileged settings such as the eye is highly complex and is ultimately characterized by the suppression of delayed type hypersensitivity (DTH). The F4/80+ macrophage is essential for induction of immune privilege (Lin et al. 2005). Although there is apparent loss of privilege in retinal degenerate [rd] mice as they age, the effect of normal aging on immune privilege and immune deviation is not reported (Welge-Lussen et al. 1999). Formation of blood vessels in the eye after birth i.e. post-developmental angiogenesis is always pathologic and is associated with diseases of the eye such as ROP, DR and AMD. Teleologically, the anti-angiogenic function of young, healthy ocular macrophages can potentially be perceived as an extension of immune privilege in order to inhibit the destructive effects of abnormal blood vessel growth on visual function. We have demonstrated that aging, IL-10 and hypoxia unmasks the pro-angiogenic phenotype in a macrophage.

References

Ambati J, Anand A, Fernandez S et al (2003) An animal model of age-related macular degeneration in senescent Ccl-2- or Ccr-2-deficient mice. Nat Med 9:1390–1397

Apte RS, Mayhew E, Niederkorn JY (1997) Local inhibition of natural killer cell activity promotes the progressive growth of intraocular tumors. Invest Ophthalmol Vis Sci 38:1277–1282

Apte RS, Niederkorn JY (1996) Isolation and characterization of a unique natural killer cell inhibitory factor present in the anterior chamber of the eye. J Immunol 156:2667–2673

Apte RS, Richter J, Herndon J et al (2006) Macrophages inhibit neovascularization in a murine model of age-related macular degeneration. PLoS Med 3:310–320

Brown DM, Kaiser PK, Michels M et al (2006) Ranibizumab versus verteporfin for neovascular age-related macular degeneration. N Engl J Med 355:1432–1444

Dace DS, Khan AA, Kelly J et al (2008) Interleukin-10 promotes pathological angiogenesis by regulating macrophage response to hypoxia during development. PLoS ONE 3:e3381

Edwards AO, Ritter R 3rd, Abel KJ et al (2005) Complement factor H polymorphism and age-related macular degeneration. Science 308:421–424

Espinosa-Heidmann DG, Suner I, Hernandez EP et al (2002) Age as an independent risk factor for severity of experimental choroidal neovascularization. Invest Ophthalmol Vis Sci 43:1567–1573

Espinosa-Heidmann DG, Suner IJ, Hernandez EP et al (2003) Macrophage depletion diminishes lesion size and severity in experimental choroidal neovascularization. Invest Ophthalmol Vis Sci 44:3586–3592

Hansson GK (2005) Inflammation, atherosclerosis, and coronary artery disease. N Engl J Med 352:1685–1695

Kaplan HJ, Leibole MA, Tezel T et al (1999) Fas ligand (CD95 ligand) controls angiogenesis beneath the retina. Nat Med 5:292–297

Kelly J, Khan AA, Yin J et al (2007) Senescence regulates macrophage activation and angiogenic fate at sites of tissue injury in mice. J Clin Invest 117:3421–3426

Klein R, Peto T, Bird A et al (2004) The epidemiology of age-related macular degeneration. Am J Ophthalmol 137:486–495

Lin HH, Faunce DE, Stacey M et al (2005) The macrophage F4/80 receptor is required for the induction of antigen-specific efferent regulatory T cells in peripheral tolerance. J Exp Med 201:1615–1625

Lobov IB, Rao S, Carroll TJ et al (2005) WNT7b mediates macrophage-induced programmed cell death in patterning of the vasculature. Nature 437:417–421

Mosser DM (2003) The many faces of macrophage activation. J Leukoc Biol 73:209–212

Nakao S, Kuwano T, Tsutsumi-Miyahara C et al (2005) Infiltration of COX-2-expressing macrophages is a prerequisite for IL-1beta-induced neovascularization and tumor growth. J Clin Invest 115:2979–2991

Niederkorn JY (2006) See no evil, hear no evil, do no evil: the lessons of immune privilege. Nat Immunol 7:354–359

Rosenfeld PJ, Brown DM, Heier JS et al (2006) Ranibizumab for neovascular age-related macular degeneration. N Engl J Med 355:1419–1431

Sakurai E, Anand A, Ambati BK et al (2003) Macrophage depletion inhibits experimental choroidal neovascularization. Invest Ophthalmol Vis Sci 44:3578–3585

Sethi G, Sung B, Aggarwal BB (2008) TNF: a master switch for inflammation to cancer. Front Biosci 13:5094–5107

Taylor PR, Martinez-Pomares L, Stacey M et al (2005) Macrophage receptors and immune recognition. Annu Rev Immunol 23:901–944

Welge-Lussen U, Wilsch C, Neuhardt T et al (1999) Loss of anterior chamber-associated immune deviation (ACAID) in aged retinal degeneration (rd) mice. Invest Ophthalmol Vis Sci 40: 3209–3214

van Leeuwen R, Klaver CC, Vingerling JR et al (2003) Epidemiology of age-related maculopathy: a review. Eur J Epidemiol 18:845–854

Chapter 3
Protein Kinase C Regulates Rod Photoreceptor Differentiation Through Modulation of STAT3 Signaling

Carolina Pinzon-Guzman, Samuel Shaomin Zhang, and Colin J. Barnstable

Abstract The molecular signals governing retinal development remain poorly understood, but some key molecules that play important roles have been identified. Activation of STAT3 by cytokines such as LIF and CNTF specifically blocks differentiation of rod photoreceptors. Here we test the hypothesis that PKC activation promotes development of rod photoreceptors by inhibiting STAT3. Explant cultures of mouse retina were used to study the effects of PKC activation on rod development. The expression of opsin, a rod specific marker, is induced at an early stage in retina explants cultured in the presence of PMA and this effect is prevented by the PKC inhibitor Go7874. Histological experiments show that there is expression of PKC beta1, but not PKC-alpha in the outer nuclear layer between E17.5 and PN5. In vitro data derived from cell lines shows that activation of PKC results in reduction of STAT3 phosphorylation. In addition, inhibition of PKC results in increase STAT3 phosphorylation. We suggest that cross talk of signals between STAT3 and PKC may determine the differentiation of rods from retinal progeitors.

3.1 Introduction

Rod photoreceptors are among the last cell types to differentiate from multipotential retinal progenitors. Much of the information necessary to generate rod photoreceptors is intrinsic to the retinal epithelium since explants of embryonic retinas are capable of forming all the major classes of cells (Sparrow et al. 1990). Within the retinal epithelium, however, photoreceptor differentiation can clearly be influenced by a number of cell interactions mediated by either direct cell-cell contacts or through soluble factors released from cells (Watanabe and Raff 1990; 1992; Reh 1992; Altshuler and Cepko 1992). Several of these factors have been

C.J. Barnstable (✉)
Department of Neural and Behavioral Sciences, Penn State College of Medicine, 500 University Drive, Hershey, PA 17033, USA
e-mail: cbarnstable@psu.edu

R.E. Anderson et al. (eds.), *Retinal Degenerative Diseases*, Advances in Experimental Medicine and Biology 664, DOI 10.1007/978-1-4419-1399-9_3,
© Springer Science+Business Media, LLC 2010

identified that can promote the formation of rods but the mechanisms by which these signals regulate the transition from progenitor to postmitotic neuron are only partially understood (Altshuler et al. 1993; Levine et al. 2000; Yang 2004).

One of the most robust findings by many groups has been that signal transducer and activator of transcription 3 (STAT3) is a key signaling protein that regulates rod formation. STAT3 is tyrosine phosphorylated in response to a range of factors including epidermal growth factor (EGF), granulocyte colony-stimulating factor (G-CSF), leptin and IL-6 family cytokines such as ciliary neurotrophic factor (CNTF), oncostatin M and leukemia inhibitory factor (LIF). In addition to activating STAT3, the IL-6 family of ligands causes activation of the ERK1/2 members of the MAPK family. We, and others, have shown that IL-6 family ligands are potent inhibitors of rod differentiation (Neophytou et al. 1997; Ezzedine et al. 1997; Zhang et al. 2004). By using adenovirus constructs controlling expressing of dominant negative or constitutively active forms of STAT3, and inhibitors of ERK activation, we showed that the inhibitory action of CNTF was mediated entirely by STAT3 (Zhang et al. 2004). Similar results have been obtained in a number of other studies (Rhee et al. 2004). Because STAT3 is found in proliferating progenitors and then rapidly lost from the postmitotic rods, we suggested that a major action of CNTF and related ligands might be to inhibit exit of daughter cells from the progenitor pool into a differentiation path (Zhang et al. 2005).

There is much less information about the mechanism by which rod formation is induced.

Although a number of factors, as diverse as taurine and IL-4, can increase the number of rods formed in vitro, little is know about the ways in which these effects are achieved (Altshuler et al. 1993; da Silva et al. 2008). We have recently found that protein kinase C (PKC) is a key signal molecule in this process. PKC is a cyclic nucleotide-independent enzyme that phosphorylates serine and threonine residues in many target proteins. There are a number of isozymes of PKC and one group of these shares the property of activation by phorbol esters. Since PKC was first identified, its involvement in many biological processes has been demonstrated, including development, memory, and carcinogenesis. It also triggers several pathways signaling cell proliferation and differentiation.

In this study we show that activation of PKC by phorbol esters leads to an increase in the number of rod photoreceptors in retinal explants. We examined the expression of the phorbol-ester activated isoforms of PKC in the developing retina and found that PKC-beta1, but not PKC alpha or PKC beta2, is present at the right time in the right place to regulate rod formation. One of the ways in which PKC may exert its action is blocking the activation of STAT3.

3.2 Materials and Methods

3.2.1 Reagents

Recombinant mouse LIF was purchased from Chemicon (Temecula, CA), STAT3 (C20) polyclonal antibodies were from Santa Cruz Biotechnology (Santa Cruz,

CA). Phosphorylated STAT3 (P-Tyr705) polyclonal antibodies were purchased from Cell Signaling Technology (Boston, MA). Antibodies recognizing isoforms of PKC were obtained from various suppliers. Ret-P1 monoclonal antibody recognizes an epitope on the N-terminus of opsin of rod photoreceptor (Hicks and Barnstable 1987).

3.2.2 Animals and Retina Explant Culture

Timed-pregnant C57Bl/6 J mice were purchased from Jackson Laboratories (Bar Harbor, ME). All mouse protocols were in accordance with ARVO guidelines and were approved by the IACUC of PSU. Most of the litters were born on E19.5, which was considered equivalent to postnatal day 0 (PN0). E17.5 embryos were dissected in cooled phosphate-buffered saline (PBS). Retinas were isolated and cultured in serum free medium supplied with L-glutamine and antibiotics. The phorbol ester PMA (12-O-tetradecanoylphorbol 13-acetate), dissolved in 100% DMSO, and/or LIF were added in the culture medium 5 h after isolation and kept for 1 or 5 days. Every 2 or 3 days half of the total medium was replaced by fresh medium. Treated and control (Blank control and DMSO control) retina samples were collected after 1 or 7 days. Immunocytochemistry and western blots were performed to detect the changes of rod photoreceptor marker expression and the protein levels of PKC, phospho-PKC, STAT3, and phospho-STAT3.

3.2.3 Cell Culture

3T3 cells were maintained in DMEM supplemented with 10% fetal bovine serum, 10 μg/ml gentamycin and 2 mM glutamine.

3.2.4 Western Blot Assay

Retinas from embryonic and postnatal mice or explanted retina were suspended in a whole cell extract buffer. The tissues were frozen and thawed three times to lyse the cells. The supernatant was collected by micro-centrifugation, and protein concentrations were measured. Twenty to 40 μg of the whole cell extract were separated by SDS-polyacrylamide gel electrophoresis and transferred to Immun-BlotTM polyvinylidene difluoride membrane (Bio-Rad). After blocking with 1–5% non-fat milk in washing buffer, membranes were incubated with primary antibodies. Following washes, they were incubated in anti-rabbit or anti-mouse IgG coupled to horseradish peroxidase. The immunoreactive bands were visualized using SuperSignalR Chemiluminescent Substrate (Pierce).

3.3 Results

3.3.1 Phorbol Esters Increase Rod Generation

Retinal explants from neonatal mice were maintained in culture with no additions, with PMA or with LIF. After 96 h of culture explants were fixed, sectioned and labeled with an antibody against opsin to identify rod photoreceptors (Fig. 3.1). In the control explants we observed a few opsin-labeled rods. LIF treatment blocked even this low level of rod formation and no opsin-expressing cells were found. Treatment with PMA, however, substantially increased the number of opsin-expressing rods in the explants. To confirm that the rod-promoting effect of PMA was due to its action on PKCs we carried out the same type of experiment in the presence of the broad-spectrum PKC inhibitor Go7874. Go7874 blocked the effect of PMA and reduced the number of detectable rod photoreceptors to control levels (Fig. 3.2). Together these experiments indicate that activation of PKC promote the production of rod photoreceptors from progenitor cells in the developing retinal epithelium.

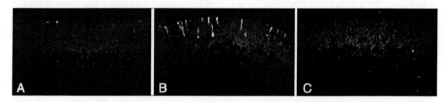

Fig. 3.1 Rod photoreceptor expression in P1 retinal explant cultures. Retinas were placed in culture in the presence of 100 nM PMA, or 20 ng/mL LIF. Retinas were fixed after 96 h in culture, paraffin embedded and IHC was used to identify rod photoreceptors with Ret-P1 antibody specific for opsin. Retinas cultured in PMA develop more rod photoreceptors than control retinas. LIF treatment inhibited rod photoreceptor development

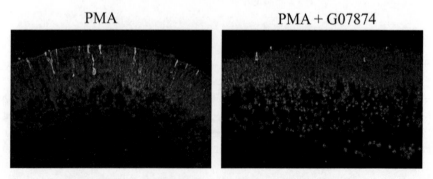

Fig. 3.2 Rod photoreceptor expression in P1 retinal explant cultures. Retinas were placed in culture in the presence of 100 nM PMA, or PMA plus 100 nM Go7874 (pan inhibitor of PKC). Retinas were fixed after 96 h in culture, paraffin embedded and IHC was used to identify rod photoreceptors. PMA induction of rod photoreceptor development was blocked with 100 nM of Go7874

3.3.2 Expression of PKC Isoforms in Developing Retina

We examined expression of PKC alpha, Beta1, and Beta2 isoforms of PKC by immunocytochemistry in sections of retina from E17.5, PN1, and PN5 animals. These ages span the period of major rod photoreceptor formation in the mouse. No expression of PKC Beta2 was found at any age. PKC alpha was also absent at these ages and only became detectable in a population of bipolar cells as these developed (not shown). PKC Beta 1 was expressed both in the inner retina and in a strong band at the Outer Limiting Membrane. From the timing and location of expression we suggest that PKC Beta1 may be responsible for the action of phorbol esters in stimulating rod photoreceptor differentiation.

3.3.3 Activation of PKC Decreases Phosphorylation of STAT3

We tested the interaction of PKC and STAT3 using mouse 3T3 cells and western blots probed with antibodies selective for the activated forms of the proteins. When cells were treated with PMA for 15 min we detected an increase in PKC activation but no change in STAT3 activation. This increase was blocked by the addition of the PKC inhibitor Go7874. When cells were treated for 15 min with LIF we detected an increase in STAT3 activation but no change in PKC activation. When cells were treated with both PMA and LIF the increase in STAT3 activation was reduced and, when PKC was inhibited by Go7874, LIF elicited a larger increase in activated STAT3. Together these results suggest an interaction between PKC and STAT3 such that activation of PKC is able to inhibit STAT3 activation (Figs. 3.3 and 3.4).

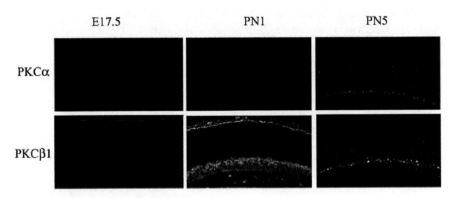

Fig. 3.3 Immunocytochemical detection of PKC isoforms in the developing retina. Retinas were isolated at the ages indicated and fixed, embedded in paraffin and 5 μm sections prepared. No expression of PKC alpha was detected at the ages shown. PKC Beta 1 was detectable at the outer edge of the retina at E17.5 and was strongly expressed in both the inner and outer retina at PN1. The labeling declined dramatically by PN5

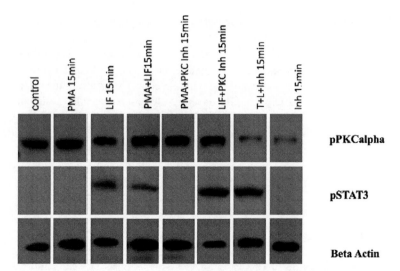

Fig. 3.4 Activation of PKC reduces the LIF-induced activation of STAT3 in 3T3 cells. Incubation of 3T3 cells with 100 nM PMA for 15 min activated PKC but not STAT3. Incubation with 20 ng/ml LIF for 15 min activated STAT3 but not PKC. Pre-treatment with PMA reduced the activation of STAT3 induced by LIF and this effect was removed by the PKC inhibitor Go7874

3.4 Discussion

There is clear evidence that the progression of progenitor cells into differentiated rod photoreceptors can blocked by the activation of STAT3. There remains some doubt as to the actual stage of development at which this block takes place (Neophytou et al. 1997; Zhang et al. 2004). Nevertheless, it seems likely that a critical step in commitment to rod formation is the relief of this block by decreased activation of STAT3. The data presented above clearly show that activation of at least one isoform of PKC results in decreased STAT3 activation and increased formation of rod photoreceptors.

Previous studies have also demonstrated that PKC activation rapidly decreases the levels of CNTF-induced STAT3 tyrosine phosphorylation, but not serine phosphorylation, and causes a slower decrease in STAT3 protein levels (Malek and Halvorsen 1999; Yokogami et al. 2000). This effect shows specificity because while the PKC activator PMA reduced STAT3 protein levels it did not affect the levels of several other STAT proteins (Malek and Halvorsen 1999). The mechanism by which PKC achieves this effect is unclear.

We suggest that movement of retinal progenitors into a rod photoreceptor differentiation pathway is normally blocked by the action of STAT3 and only occurs when STAT3 activity is decreased. Whether PKC is the only signal molecule that can regulate STAT3 activity is not clear. Also, the natural regulators of PKC activity in the developing retina have yet to be identified. Finally, it is intriguing to consider whether these interactions are of more general applicability in the developing retina. STAT3 is expressed in the inner retina during embryonic development and then appears in the outer retina at the time when rod photoreceptors are being generated (Zhang et al. 2003). Perhaps other retinal cell types can only differentiate when their STAT3 block is overcome by the actions of other factors, possibly also acting through isoforms of PKC.

Acknowledgments This work was supported by grants from the NIH and the Macular Vision Research Foundation.

References

Altshuler D, Cepko C (1992) A temporally regulated, diffusible activity is required for rod photoreceptor development in vitro. Development 114:947–957

Altshuler D, Lo Turco JJ, Rush J, Cepko C (1993) Taurine promotes the differentiation of a vertebrate retinal cell type in vitro. Development 119:1317–1328

da Silva AG, Campello-Costa P, Linden R, Sholl-Franco A (2008) Interleukin-4 blocks proliferation of retinal progenitor cells and increases rod photoreceptor differentiation through distinct signaling pathways. J Neuroimmunol 196:82–93

Ezzeddine ZD, Yang X, DeChiara T, Yancopoulos G, Cepko CL (1997) Postmitotic cells fated to become rod photoreceptors can be respecified by CNTF treatment of the retina. Development 124:1055–1067

Hicks D, Barnstable CJ (1987) Different rhodopsin monoclonal antibodies reveal different binding patterns on developing and adult retina. J Histochem Cytochem 35:1317–1328

Levine EM, Fuhrmann S, Reh TA (2000) Soluble factors and the development of rod photoreceptors. Cell Mol Life Sci 57:224–234

Malek RL, Halvorsen SW (1999) Ciliary neurotrophic factor and phorbol ester each decrease selected STAT3 pools in neuroblastoma cells by proteasome-dependent mechanisms. Cytokine 11:192–199

Neophytou C, Vernallis AB, Smith A, Raff MC (1997) Müller-cell-derived leukaemia inhibitory factor arrests rod photoreceptor differentiation at a postmitotic pre-rod stage of development. Development 124:2345–2354

Reh TA (1992) Cellular interactions determine neuronal phenotypes in rodent retinal cultures. J Neurobiol 23:1067–1083

Rhee KD, Goureau O, Chen S, Yang XJ (2004) Cytokine-induced activation of signal transducer and activator of transcription in photoreceptor precursors regulates rod differentiation in the developing mouse retina. J Neurosci 24:9779–9788

Sparrow JR, Hicks D, Barnstable CJ (1990) Cell commitment and differentiation in explants of embryonic rat retina. Comparison to the developmental potential of dissociated retina. Dev Brain Res 51:69–84

Watanabe T, Raff MC (1990) Rod photoreceptor development in vitro: intrinsic properties of proliferating neuroepithelial cells change as development proceeds in the rat retina. Neuron 4:461–467

Watanabe T, Raff MC (1992) Diffusible rod-promoting signals in the developing rat retina. Development 114:899–906

Yang XJ (2004) Roles of cell-extrinsic growth factors in vertebrate eye pattern formation and retinogenesis. Semin Cell Dev Biol 15:91–103

Yokogami K, Wakisaka S, Avruch J, Reeves SA (2000) Serine phosphorylation and maximal activation of STAT3 during CNTF signaling is mediated by the rapamycin target mTOR. Curr Biol 10:47–50

Zhang SS, Liu M-G, Kano A, Zhan C, Fu X-Y, Barnstable CJ (2005) STAT3 activation in response
    to growth factors or cytokines participates in retina precursor proliferation. Exp Eye Res 81:
    103–115
Zhang SS, Wei JY, Kano R, Qin H, Zhang L, Xie B, Hui P, Deisseroth AB, Barnstable CJ, Fu XY
    (2004) STAT3-mediated signaling in the determination of rod photoreceptor cell fate in mouse
    retina. IOVS 45:2407–2412
Zhang SS, Wei J-Y, Lia C, Barnstable CJ, Fu X-Y (2003) Expression and activation of STAT
    proteins during mouse retina development. Exp Eye Res 76:421–431

Chapter 4
Pigment Epithelium-derived Factor Receptor (PEDF-R): A Plasma Membrane-linked Phospholipase with PEDF Binding Affinity

Preeti Subramanian, Patricia M. Notario, and S. Patricia Becerra

Abstract Pigment epithelium-derived factor (PEDF), a multifunctional protein, acts in retinal differentiation, survival and maintenance by interacting with high affinity receptors on the surface of target cells. We have recently identified PEDF-R, a new member of the patatin-like phospholipase domain-containing 2 (PNPLA2) family with characteristics of a PEDF receptor. The PEDF-R sequence reveals a patatin-like phospholipase domain toward its amino-end, and four transmembrane domains interrupted by two extracellular loops and three intracellular regions along its polypeptide sequence. This newly identified protein is present on the surface of retina and RPE cells, and has the expected transmembrane topology. It has specific and high binding affinity for PEDF, and exhibits a potent phospholipase A_2 activity that liberates fatty acids. Most importantly, PEDF binding stimulates the enzymatic phospholipase A_2 activity of PEDF-R. In summary, PEDF-R is a novel component of the retina that is a phospholipase-linked membrane protein with high affinity for PEDF. The results suggest a molecular pathway by which PEDF ligand/receptor interactions on the cell surface could generate a cellular signal. These conclusions enhance our understanding of the role of PEDF as a neurotrophic survival factor.

4.1 Introduction

Pigment epithelium-derived factor (PEDF), a non-inhibitory member of the serine protease inhibitor superfamily (SERPIN), is a multifunctional protein involved in neuronal survival and differentiation (Barnstable and Tombran-Tink 2004; Becerra 2006; Bouck 2002). It was discovered as a 50-kDa protein released by cultured pigment epithelial cells from fetal human retina (Tombran-Tink et al. 1991). PEDF is ubiquitously expressed and distributed in the human body (Singh et al. 1998).

S.P. Becerra (✉)
NEI-NIH, Building 6, Room 134, 6 Center Dr., MSC 0608, Bethesda, MD 20892-0608, USA
e-mail: becerrap@nei.nih.gov

R.E. Anderson et al. (eds.), *Retinal Degenerative Diseases*, Advances in Experimental Medicine and Biology 664, DOI 10.1007/978-1-4419-1399-9_4,
© Springer Science+Business Media, LLC 2010

The retinal pigment epithelium (RPE) expresses the highest levels of *PEDF* transcripts among ocular tissues (Becerra et al. 2004; Perez-Mediavilla et al. 1998) and secretes the protein product into the interphotoreceptor matrix (Tombran-Tink et al. 1995; Wu et al. 1995). PEDF acts to promote photoreceptor and retinal neuron cell survival (Cayouette et al. 1999; Takita et al. 2003), and prevents the pathological invasion of neovessels (Dawson et al. 1999). Decreased levels of PEDF have been linked to several retinal diseases, such as age-related macular degeneration (AMD), diabetic retinopathy, and neuroretinal dystrophies (Duh et al. 2004; Holekamp et al. 2002; Ogata et al. 2004). The importance of PEDF in the development, maintenance, and function of the retina and CNS is evident in animal models for inherited and light-induced retinal degeneration, elevated intraocular pressure, retinopathy of prematurity, as well as for degeneration of spinal cord motor neurons (Bilak et al. 1999; Cao et al. 2001; Cayouette et al. 1999; Dawson et al. 1999; Duh et al. 2002). The above observations have prompted development of clinical trials on the efficacy of PEDF in the context of AMD (Chader 2005). Although the mechanisms of neuroprotection and angiogenesis inhibition remain unknown, it has been implied that they are associated with receptor interactions at cell-surface interfaces.

4.2 Identification of a PEDF Receptor

The surface of normal and tumor retina cells exhibit high affinity binding for PEDF ligands ($K_D = 2$–8 nM) (Alberdi et al. 1999; Aymerich et al. 2001). Plasma membranes of retina cells from different species contain specific PEDF-binding components that migrate as 80–85-kDa proteins by SDS-PAGE (Alberdi et al. 1999; Aymerich et al. 2001). Yeast 2-hybrid experiments performed using a commercial fetal human liver cDNA library as target and human PEDF plasmids as bait, reveal about 50 clones with potential PEDF interacting genes, but only a few of the sequences are of interest (Notari et al. 2006). One of them, clone 12c, contains a cDNA with 100% identity to a fragment of a new mRNA transcript isolated from the RPE of a human eye, which we have termed *PEDF-R*.

4.3 *In Silico* Information

The newly identified *PEDF-R* transcript has a coding capacity of 504 amino acids and four *N*-glycosylation consensus sites. The sequence shares strong homology with members of the Ca^{2+}-independent PLA_2 ($iPLA_2$)/desnutrin/patatin-like phospholipase domain-containing protein 2 (PNPLA2) family (Jenkins et al. 2004; Notari et al. 2006). Members of the PNPLA2 family have demonstrable triglyceride lipase, triacylglycerol transacylase and phospholipase activities. The *PEDF-R* nucleotide and its derived amino acid sequences match those of human TTS-2.2 and iPLA2ζ, and share high identity to mouse desnutrin and ATGL, all of which are synonyms of PEDF-R. The *PEDF-R* gene contains 10 exons with the initiating methionine codon in the second exon (Fig. 4.1, top panel). The structure of the exon/intron junctions reflects to a certain degree the proposed domain structure of

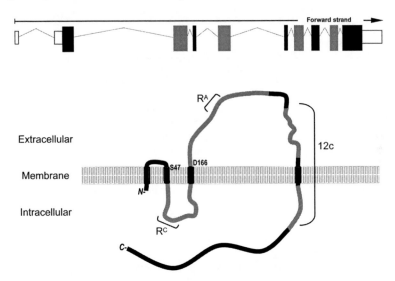

Fig. 4.1 *In silico* information of gene, transcript and protein structure of PEDF-R. (**Top**) Transcript summary information for human PEDF-R obtained from http://www.ensembl.org for ENST00000336615 (Hubbard et al. 2005). PEDF-R gene has 10 exons (*top line*), the transcript length is 2,071 bps (exons are illustrated by *boxes*; coding regions are *black* and *grey*; introns are *lines flanking boxes*); and the translation length is 504 amino acid residues. (**Bottom**) Computer programs predict a transmembrane topology for PEDF-R. Exons are mapped on the illustration and are coded as in **Top Panel**. Features illustrated are: the coding region corresponding to the yeast-2 hybrid clone p12c; the locations of peptide antigens for antibodies Ab-R[A] and Ab-R[C], and the Ser[47]-Asp[166] catalytic dyad

the protein (Fig. 4.1, bottom panel). Hydrophobicity plots predict a transmembrane nature for the PEDF-R polypeptide product with 4 transmembrane (TM) domains interrupted by 2 extracellular loops and 3 intracellular regions. The region of the first two TM domains plus the smallest extracellular loop located between them is flanked by introns. Each of the other TM domains and the smallest intracellular loop are also flanked by introns; while the longest extracellular loop and the last intracellular region are composed entirely of exons.

4.4 Expression and Distribution in the Retina

Most tissues of several species express *PEDF-R* transcripts (Notari et al. 2006). Although adipose tissues express the highest levels among tissues, *PEDF-R* mRNA is clearly expressed in ocular tissues, especially in the neural retina and the RPE (Table 4.1). The RPE cell lines ARPE-19 and H-Tert, and the retina precursor cell lines R28 and RGC-5 also express significant levels of *PEDF-R* transcripts. In the native retina PEDF-R protein is distributed in the RPE and in the inner segments of the photoreceptors, and at lower levels, in the inner nuclear and retinal ganglion cell layers (Notari et al. 2006). It partitions with plasma membrane proteins by

Table 4.1 PEDF-R expression survey includes sources of interest. Selected cDNA sources from the UniGene reported expression survey fall into three main categories, as related to the key functions of PEDF

Ocular sources	Neuronal sources	Tumorigenic sources
Retinal pigment epithelium (RPE)	White matter	Retinoblastoma, adenocarcinoma, chondrosarcoma, germ cell tumors, pooled,
Choroid	Hypothalamus	squamous cell carcinoma, pituitary
Optic nerve	Brain	adenomas, serous papillary carcinoma,
Fetal eye	Hippocampus	choriocarcinoma, epithelioid carcinoma,
Lens	Medulla	leiomyosarcoma cell line, anaplastic
Retina		oligodendroglioma, epithelioid carcinoma
Eye anterior segment		cell line, renal carcinoma, myeloma,
Lacrimal gland		astrocytoma grade IV, hepatocellular
		carcinoma, ductal carcinoma, duodenal
		adenocarcinoma, chronic lymphotic
		leukemia, meningioma, melanoma, adrenal
		adenoma

biochemical cell fractionation. Western blots with a specific antiserum to PEDF-R clearly demonstrate the presence of a single immunoreacting band that migrates as an 83-kDa protein in RPE, retina, ARPE-19, RGC-5 and R28 cell membrane fractions (Fig. 4.2).

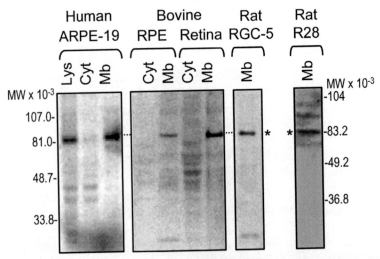

Fig. 4.2 Subcellular localization of PEDF-R in retinal cells. Cell lysates (Lys) were fractionated by high speed centrifugation ($80,000 \times g$) into cytosolic (cyt) and membrane fractions (Mb). Western blots of fractions were immunostained with anti-PEDF-R[A] antibody. Total protein loaded in lanes were as follows: (ARPE-19, Lys) 19.8 μg; (ARPE-19, Cyt) 12 μg; (ARPE-19, Mb) 6.5 μg; (RPE, Cyt) 67 μg; (RPE, Mb) 10 μg; (Retina, Cyt) 71 μg; (Retina, Mb) 10 μg; (RGC-5, Mb) 9.5 μg; and (R29, Mb) 5.7 μg respectively. The *asterisks* point to the migration position of PEDF-R

4.5 Transmembrane Topology

Specific biotinylation of cell-surface proteins labels PEDF-R in ARPE-19 cells, demonstrating that PEDF-R is a plasma membrane protein in these cells (Notari et al. 2006). Immunocytochemistry of ARPE-19 cells using antibodies to specific peptides designed from presumptive extracellular (R^A) and intracellular (R^C) regions of the PEDF-R sequence (Fig. 4.1, bottom panel) provides information of the PEDF-R transmembrane topology. Only the anti-R^A antibody stains non-permeabilized cells, while both antibodies detect PEDF-R in permeabilized ARPE-19 cells (Notari et al. 2006). These results demonstrate that the R^A and R^C regions of PEDF-R are extracellular and intracellular, respectively, as predicted from the PEDF-R sequence.

4.6 Binding to PEDF Ligands

Epitope-tagged PEDF-R can be overexpressed using a cell-free system and the recombinant PEDF-R polypeptide can be purified by affinity column chromatography. Binding assays unequivocally show that the recombinant protein binds to PEDF when either one is immobilized or in solution. PEDF-R can rapidly and reversibly interact with PEDF sensor chips in a specific fashion by Surface Plasmon Resonance (Notari et al. 2006). The kinetic parameters reveal high binding affinity for the PEDF:PEDF-R interactions with a dissociation constant ($K_D = \sim 3$ nM) that is similar to the that of PEDF to intact cells. Furthermore, fluorescein-labeled human recombinant PEDF (Fl-PEDF) binds specifically to cell surfaces with a pattern similar to that observed with anti-R^A antibody (Notari et al. 2006). These results demonstrate that PEDF binds to PEDF-R at the plasma membrane interface.

4.7 Phospholipase Activity

The patatin-like phospholipase domain of PEDF-R has sequence homology to the catalytic domain of two well-known PLA enzymes, Patatin B2 and cytosolic PLA_2. The PLA active site of these enzymes is formed by a Ser-Asp catalytic dyad within the conserved motifs GXSXG and DXG/A (Hirschberg et al. 2001; Rydel et al. 2003). The sequence of human PEDF-R reveals structural homologies to these motifs, having a serine residue in position 47 (S^{47}) and aspartic acid residue in position 166 (D^{166}) (Fig. 4.1, bottom panel). Functional studies have demonstrated that the amino acids S^{47} and D^{166} are crucial for lipase activity of PEDF-R (Smirnova et al. 2006). These residues are located in the membrane interface by the second and third TM2 and TM3 domain of the transmembrane PEDF-R topology. The location of these critical residues suggests that the Ser-Asp catalytic dyad in PEDF-R is in the vicinity of potential phospholipid substrates.

PLA assays demonstrate that the recombinant PEDF-R exhibits PLA activity that liberates fatty acids from phospholipid substrates. The concentration response curve shows that the PLA specific activity of the recombinant PEDF-R is higher (>4-fold) than that of the commercial hog pancreas PLA_2 (Notari et al. 2006). Bromoenol lactone, a known inhibitor of triolein lipase activity for $iPLA_2s$, inhibits the PLA activity of PEDF-R. A pH curve reveals optimum enzymatic activity at pH 7.5 for recombinant PEDF-R protein. More interestingly, PEDF increased the PLA activity of PEDF-R, and, in contrast, PEDF did not affect commercial hog PLA_2 activity (Notari et al. 2006). These results demonstrate that PEDF stimulates the release of fatty acids and lysophosphatidic acid from phospholipids catalyzed by the PLA activity of PEDF-R.

4.8 PEDF-R Activity in Retinal Cells

Recent studies have demonstrated PEDF as a survival factor for R28 cells in response to serum starvation (Murakami et al.2008). R28 cells, rat retinal cells expressing neuronal genes, contain functional cell-surface PEDF-R, as detected by immunoblotting of R28 plasma membrane fractions (Fig. 4.2). Moreover, these fractions exhibit PLA activity (Fig. 4.3a) similar to human recombinant PEDF-R protein (Notari et al. 2006). Interestingly, the PLA activity of the R28 fractions further increases upon preincubation with PEDF ligand (Fig. 4.3b), similar to the activities of human recombinant PEDF-R and ARPE-19 plasma membrane fractions (Notari et al.2006).

The membrane PEDF-R protein is labile in solution upon extraction with detergents from the lipid environment of membranes. Extracted PEDF-R can readily lose activity upon storage. However the enzyme can be stabilized by adding 0.8 μM PEDF to the solubilization buffer used to extract proteins from membrane pellets obtained by high speed centrifugation. This approach increases protein solubility and the enzymatic activity of PEDF-R (Fig. 4.3c), which is further stimulated by preincubation of the fraction with PEDF ligand (Fig. 4.3c). These results suggest that binding of the membrane-embedded PEDF-R to PEDF ligands does not saturate its PLA activity and can provide structural stability to enhance activity. Thus, PEDF-R has a potential role to mediate the survival effect of PEDF on R28 cells.

4.9 Conclusions

PEDF-R is a newly-identified membrane-linked receptor with lipase activity and high binding affinity for PEDF present in the retina. The protein contains a functional phospholipase domain and a transmembrane topology for PEDF-R with extracellular loops available to interact with the PEDF ligand. The PEDF-mediated stimulation of the PLA activity of PEDF-R supports the idea that PEDF signaling is mediated by the released fatty acids and lysophospholipids from phospholipids at

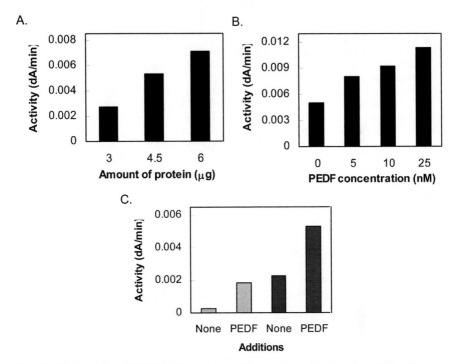

Fig. 4.3 PLA activity of PEDF-R. Detergent-soluble membrane fractions from R28 cells were assayed for PLA activity using (1,2-dilinoleoyl)-phosphatidylcholine as substrate and lipoxygenase as the coupling enzyme in reaction buffer (50 mM Tris-HCl, pH 7.5, 3 mM deoxycholate) as described (Jimenez-Atienzar et al. 2003). Formation of the product was measured spectrophotometrically by increase in the absorbance at 234 nm per min (dA/min; *y*-axis). (**a**) Dose response of PLA activity of R28-derived PEDF-R. Proteins from R28 cell membranes were solubilized with phosphate buffered saline pH 6.5 containing 0.1% NP-40, and the PLA activity was determined for increasing amounts of detergent-soluble protein fractions. (**b**) Effects of PEDF on the R28-derived PEDF-R activity. Extracts were preincubated with PEDF for 10 min and then assayed for PLA activity. Concentrations of PEDF used in each assay are indicated in the *x*-axis. (**c**) PEDF-R proteins were solubilized from ARPE-19 membrane protein precipitate with phosphate buffered saline pH 6.5 containing 0.5% CHAPS in the absence (*grey boxes*) or presence of 0.8 μM PEDF (*black boxes*). PLA activity was measured as in **Panel B** in the absence (*none*) or presence of 10 nM PEDF

the cell-surface interface. In the retina, DHA is one of the most abundant fatty acids in the membrane phospholipids, which in turn is the precursor of neuroprotectin D1, a neuroprotectant and antioxidant agent in the retina, RPE and CNS (Bazan 2005). The PEDF:PEDF-R interactions could participate in the generation of neuroprotectin D1 via its PLA activity to act as a bioactive signal mediator for the PEDF neurotrophic activity (Bazan et al. 2005). In summary, these findings suggest a molecular pathway by which PEDF ligand/receptor interactions on the cell-surface could generate a cellular signal.

References

Alberdi E, Aymerich MS, Becerra SP (1999) Binding of pigment epithelium-derived factor (PEDF) to retinoblastoma cells and cerebellar granule neurons. Evidence for a PEDF receptor. J Biol Chem 274:31605–31612

Aymerich MS, Alberdi EM, Martinez A et al (2001) Evidence for pigment epithelium-derived factor receptors in the neural retina. Invest Ophthalmol Vis Sci 42:3287–3293

Barnstable CJ, Tombran-Tink J (2004) Neuroprotective and antiangiogenic actions of PEDF in the eye: molecular targets and therapeutic potential. Prog Retin Eye Res 23:561–577

Bazan NG (2005) Neuroprotectin D1 (NPD1): a DHA-derived mediator that protects brain and retina against cell injury-induced oxidative stress. Brain Pathol 15:159–166

Bazan NG, Marcheselli VL, Hu J et al (2005) Pigment epithelium-derived growth factor (PEDF) selectively up-regulates NPD1 synthesis and release through the apical side of human RPE cells in primary cultures. Invest Ophthalmol Vis Sci 46:167

Becerra SP (2006) Focus on Molecules: pigment epithelium-derived factor (PEDF). Exp Eye Res 82:739–740

Becerra SP, Fariss RN, Wu YQ et al (2004) Pigment epithelium-derived factor in the monkey retinal pigment epithelium and interphotoreceptor matrix: apical secretion and distribution. Exp Eye Res 78:223–234

Bilak MM, Corse AM, Bilak SR et al (1999) Pigment epithelium-derived factor (PEDF) protects motor neurons from chronic glutamate-mediated neurodegeneration. J Neuropathol Exp Neurol 58:719–728

Bouck N (2002) PEDF: anti-angiogenic guardian of ocular function. Trends Mol Med 8:330–334

Cao W, Tombran-Tink J, Elias R et al (2001) In vivo protection of photoreceptors from light damage by pigment epithelium-derived factor. Invest Ophthalmol Vis Sci 42:1646–1652

Cayouette M, Smith SB, Becerra SP et al (1999) Pigment epithelium-derived factor delays the death of photoreceptors in mouse models of inherited retinal degenerations. Neurobiol Dis 6:523–532

Chader GJ (2005) Surmountable challenges in translating pigment epithelium-derived factor (PEDF) therapy from animal models to clinical trials for retinal degenerations. Retina (Philadelphia, PA) 25:S29–S30

Dawson DW, Volpert OV, Gillis P et al (1999) Pigment epithelium-derived factor: a potent inhibitor of angiogenesis. Science 285:245–248

Duh EJ, Yang HS, Haller JA et al (2004) Vitreous levels of pigment epithelium-derived factor and vascular endothelial growth factor: implications for ocular angiogenesis. Am J Ophthalmol 137:668–674

Duh EJ, Yang HS, Suzuma I et al (2002) Pigment epithelium-derived factor suppresses ischemia-induced retinal neovascularization and VEGF-induced migration and growth. Invest Ophthalmol Vis Sci 43:821–829

Hirschberg HJ, Simons JW, Dekker N et al (2001) Cloning, expression, purification and characterization of patatin, a novel phospholipase A. Eur J Biochem 268:5037–5044

Holekamp NM, Bouck N, Volpert O (2002) Pigment epithelium-derived factor is deficient in the vitreous of patients with choroidal neovascularization due to age-related macular degeneration. Am J Ophthalmol 134:220–227

Hubbard T, Andrews D, Caccamo M et al (2005) Ensembl 2005. Nucleic Acids Res 33:D447–D453

Jenkins CM, Mancuso DJ, Yan W et al (2004) Identification, cloning, expression, and purification of three novel human calcium-independent phospholipase A2 family members possessing triacylglycerol lipase and acylglycerol transacylase activities. J Biol Chem 279:48968–48975

Jimenez-Atienzar M, Cabanes J, Gandia-Herrero F et al (2003) Determination of the phospholipase activity of patatin by a continuous spectrophotometric assay. Lipids 38:677–682

Murakami Y, Ikeda Y, Yonemitsu Y et al (2008) Inhibition of nuclear translocation of apoptosis-inducing factor is an essential mechanism of the neuroprotective activity of pigment epithelium-derived factor in a rat model of retinal degeneration. Am J Pathol 173:1326–1338

Notari L, Baladron V, Aroca-Aguilar JD et al (2006) Identification of a lipase-linked cell membrane receptor for pigment epithelium-derived factor. J Biol Chem 281:38022–38037

Ogata N, Matsuoka M, Imaizumi M et al (2004) Decreased levels of pigment epithelium-derived factor in eyes with neuroretinal dystrophic diseases. Am J Ophthalmol 137: 1129–1130

Perez-Mediavilla LA, Chew C, Campochiaro PA et al (1998) Sequence and expression analysis of bovine pigment epithelium-derived factor. Biochim Biophys Acta 1398:203–214

Rydel TJ, Williams JM, Krieger E et al (2003) The crystal structure, mutagenesis, and activity studies reveal that patatin is a lipid acyl hydrolase with a Ser-Asp catalytic dyad. Biochemistry 42:6696–6708

Singh VK, Chader GJ, Rodriguez IR (1998) Structural and comparative analysis of the mouse gene for pigment epithelium-derived factor (PEDF). Mol Vis 4:7

Smirnova E, Goldberg EB, Makarova KS et al (2006) ATGL has a key role in lipid droplet/adiposome degradation in mammalian cells. EMBO Rep 7:106–113

Takita H, Yoneya S, Gehlbach PL et al (2003) Retinal neuroprotection against ischemic injury mediated by intraocular gene transfer of pigment epithelium-derived factor. Invest Ophthalmol Vis Sci 44:4497–4504

Tombran-Tink J, Chader GG, Johnson LV (1991) PEDF: a pigment epithelium-derived factor with potent neuronal differentiative activity. Exp Eye Res 53:411–414

Tombran-Tink J, Shivaram SM, Chader GJ et al (1995) Expression, secretion, and age-related downregulation of pigment epithelium-derived factor, a serpin with neurotrophic activity. J Neurosci 15:4992–5003

Wu YQ, Notario V, Chader GJ et al (1995) Identification of pigment epithelium-derived factor in the interphotoreceptor matrix of bovine eyes. Protein Expr Purif 6:447–456

Chapter 5
The Function of Oligomerization-Incompetent RDS in Rods

Dibyendu Chakraborty, Shannon M. Conley, Steven J. Fliesler, and Muna I. Naash

Abstract The photoreceptor-specific tetraspanin glycoprotein RDS (retinal degeneration slow) is associated with many forms of inherited retinal disease. RDS shares features in common with other tetraspanin proteins, including the existence of a large intradiscal D2 loop containing several cysteines. While these cysteines are used only for intramolecular disulfide bonds in most tetraspanins, RDS expresses a seventh, unpaired cysteine (C150) used for intermolecular disulfide bonding in the formation of large RDS oligomers. To study oligomerization-dependent *vs.* oligomerization-independent RDS functions in rods, we generated a transgenic mouse line harboring a point mutation that replaces this Cys with Ser (C150S), leading to the expression of an RDS protein that cannot form intermolecular disulfide bonds. The mouse opsin promoter (MOP) was used to direct C150S RDS expression specifically in rods in these transgenic mice (MOP-T). Here we report improvement in scotopic ERGs in MOP-T/$rds^{+/-}$ mice (compared to non-transgenic $rds^{+/-}$ controls) and the appearance of malformed outer segments (OSs) in MOP-T mice that do not express native RDS (MOP-T/$rds^{-/-}$). These results suggest that while normal OS structure and function require RDS oligomerization, some RDS function is retained in the absence of C150. Since one of the functions of other tetraspanin proteins is to promote assembly of a membrane microdomain known as the "tetraspanin web", future studies may investigate whether assembly of this web is one of RDS's oligomerization-independent functions.

The photoreceptor (PR)-specific glycoprotein RDS (retinal degeneration slow) is a member of the tetraspanin protein family. This family contains proteins that share a similar structural arrangement: four transmembrane domains containing some polar residues, a consistent loop arrangement, and the presence of cysteines in the so-called D2 loop. These proteins are expressed in almost every cell of the body and are involved in a diverse range of biological processes, including modulating the

M.I. Naash (✉)
Department of Cell Biology, University of Oklahoma Health Sciences Center, Oklahoma,
OK 73126-0901, USA
e-mail: muna-naash@ouhsc.edu

R.E. Anderson et al. (eds.), *Retinal Degenerative Diseases*, Advances in Experimental
Medicine and Biology 664, DOI 10.1007/978-1-4419-1399-9_5,
© Springer Science+Business Media, LLC 2010

immune system, enhancing fertilization, cell motility/adhesion, the formation of neuromuscular junctions, and, of course, retinal function (Hemler 2003). In spite of the variety of processes linked to tetraspanins, there are similarities in their roles in many tissues (Hemler 2003; Stipp et al. 2003). For example, RDS is a structural protein known to be required for the formation and maintenance of the PR outer segment (OS), a role with many parallels to that of the tetraspanin CD151, which has been shown to regulate cytoskeletal remodeling in epithelial and mesenchymal cells by interacting with integrins, protein kinase C, actin, and E-cadherin (Shigeta et al. 2003).

On the molecular level, tetraspanins are known to interact directly with themselves and other tetraspanins, with cell-matrix adhesion receptors, such as integrin $\alpha 3\beta 1$ and $\alpha 4\beta 1$ (Serru et al. 1999; Yauch et al. 1998), with other non-tetraspanin membrane proteins (Wu et al. 1995), and with cytoskeletal components (Delaguillaumie et al. 2002; Lagaudriere-Gesbert et al. 1998). Furthermore, via palmitoylation and other secondary interactions, tetraspanins form large functional complexes known as the "tetraspanin web". This typically contains a core of directly interacting tetraspanins linked covalently or non-covalently to other complex members and commonly defines a membrane microdomain similar to, but distinct from, lipid rafts (Hemler 2003; Levy and Shoham 2005; Stipp et al. 2003). Taken together, these findings support the notion that tetraspanins such as RDS may play a significant modulatory role in maintaining cell structure.

The *RDS* gene encodes a PR-specific glycoprotein found in both rods and cones (Connell and Molday 1990; Travis et al. 1991) that exhibits evolutionary conservation all the way from skates to humans (Li et al. 2003; Naash et al. 2003). RDS is restricted to the rims of PR discs, as well as the basal regions of rod and cone outer segments (OSs) adjacent to the cilia where disc morphogenesis occurs (Arikawa et al. 1992; Moritz et al. 2002). In the PR inner segment, RDS assembles into non-convalently bound tetramers, which are then trafficked to the OS where they are further assembled into disulfide bonded higher-order oligomers (Chakraborty et al. 2008b; Loewen and Molday 2000). RDS is necessary for disc assembly, orientation, and physical stability (Molday et al. 1987; Wrigley et al. 2000), and although most research on RDS has focused on its role in the PR and vision, recent insights into its other potential functions have come from research on other members of the tetraspanin family.

Over 80 mutations in the *RDS* gene have been identified in multiple forms of both rod- and cone-dominant hereditary retinal degeneration (Farjo and Naash 2006), http://www.retina-international.org/sci-news/rdsmut.htm. Both the phenotypic variability seen in patients with *RDS* mutations and animal/cell biological studies of RDS mutations support the hypothesis that RDS behaves differently in rod vs. cone PRs.

The vast majority of RDS disease-causing mutations reside within the large intradiscal polypeptide loop (D2) of RDS. The D2 loop is a common tetraspanin feature and contains the conserved cysteines that are involved in intramolecular disulfide bonding (Hemler 2001). In addition to these six Cys residues, RDS contains a seventh, unpaired cysteine (C150), which is involved in intermolecular disulfide bonding and is thought to be required for the formation of RDS oligomers (Chakraborty et al. 2008; Goldberg et al. 1998). Interestingly, the lack of this cysteine in other tetraspanins highlights one of the differences between the role of RDS in the PR vs. the biological functions of other tetraspanins. While it is likely that RDS forms a tetraspanin web within the OS disc membrane, it is also responsible for the formation of the OS disc rim region, a function which requires that RDS complexes help to bridge adjacent membranes. This bridging function is not one usually attributed to tetraspanins. Given that a large portion of the function of most tetraspanins is due to their role in the assembly of the tetraspanin web (a function that does not rely on intermolecular disulfide bonds, since other tetraspanins do not form them), we wanted to see what functions (if any) of RDS are retained when the ability to form these intermolecular disulfide bonds is disrupted.

The role of RDS intermolecular disulfide bonds in formation of the flattened OS disc was first highlighted in in vitro studies. When wildtype (WT) RDS is incorporated into microsomal vesicles under non-reducing conditions, an abnormal, flattened morphology is produced, whereas vesicles incorporating RDS under reducing conditions possess a characteristically rounded appearance (Wrigley et al. 2000). However, when mutant C150S RDS is expressed, vesicular flattening is abolished. Subsequent studies in which GFP-tagged C150S RDS was co-expressed in X. Laevis rods with WT RDS showed no dominant-negative effect on rod photoreceptors (Loewen et al. 2003). Studies in COS cells have confirmed the role of C150 in the formation of intermolecular disulfide bonds; C150S RDS expressed in COS cells folds properly and forms tetramers, but does not form higher-order oligomers (Goldberg et al. 1998). To further study the role of intermolecular disulfide bonding in the mammalian retina, we have generated two transgenic mouse models expressing C150S RDS in either rods (MOP-T) or cones (COP-T) by means of cell type-specific opsin promoters (Chakraborty et al. 2008). One of our goals is to differentiate between RDS functions that depend on intermolecular disulfide bonding (and, thus, higher-order oligomer formation) vs. those functions that do not, e.g., the formation of the RDS tetraspanin web.

Mice expressing C150S in cones exhibit a striking, dominant cone degeneration in which cone photoreceptors have extremely malformed OSs and die even in the presence of the WT RDS protein. Consistent with the structural defect, cone function is obliterated in these animals (Chakraborty et al. 2008). Interestingly, this dominant degenerative defect is not observed when C150S RDS is expressed in rods. While the different phenotype in the MOP-T vs. COP-T mice helps explain the differential role of RDS in rods and cones, the severity of the cone defect makes it difficult to study oligomerization-dependent vs. oligomerization-independent effects. Therefore, we have undertaken a further, more detailed examination of the milder rod phenotype of the MOP-T transgenic mice.

Previously, we showed that in rods and in the absence of native RDS, C150S RDS can form tetramers and retains the ability to bind ROM-1 (Chakraborty et al. 2008). However, velocity sedimentation studies showed that, as expected, C150S RDS does not form higher-order oligomers in the absence of WT RDS (Chakraborty et al. 2008). This observation is confirmed by the non-reducing Western blot shown

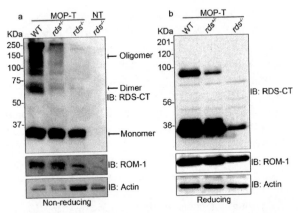

Fig. 5.1 Biochemical analysis of MOP-T; Retinas were harvested from transgenic (MOP-T) or non-transgenic (NT) animals at postnatal day (P) 30. Total retinal extracts were used for non-reducing (**a**) or reducing (**b**) SDS-PAGE followed by immunoblotting (IB) with the antibodies indicated (RDS-CT, ROM-1, rod outer segment membrane protein-1, an RDS homolog; and actin). Expression of C150S RDS does not interfere with the ability of WT RDS to form higher-order oligomers, but it cannot form oligomers alone

in (Fig. 5.1a). Higher-order oligomers can be seen when C150S RDS (MOP-T) is expressed in the presence of WT RDS, but in its absence no oligomers or disulfide linked dimers are observed. Under reducing conditions (Fig. 5.1b) oligomers are reduced to monomers and low levels of dimers. However, no dimers are detected in MOP-T/$rds^{-/-}$ retinas, although C150S monomer is stably expressed.

The results of functional full-field rod (scotopic a-wave) ERG studies undertaken at various ages are shown in (Fig. 5.2a). At early timepoints, there is no difference in retinal function between transgenic (MOP-T) and non-transgenic littermates (NT) in the WT RDS background confirming that there is no dominant negative effect on rods. Furthermore, although transgenic animals appear to lose rod function slightly faster than do non-transgenic controls, at 18 months of age both have similar rod function. This observation is confirmed on the structural level in (Fig. 5.2b). Light microscopic analysis undertaken at 18 months of age (Fig. 5.2b) shows that there is no structural difference in the retina between transgenic and non-transgenic mice on a WT background. These experiments clearly demonstrate that the presence of oligomerization-incompetent RDS (C150S RDS) is not harmful to rods in the presence of native RDS.

To further study the importance of RDS oligomerization for RDS function, ERG studies were undertaken at 2 months of age in multiple *RDS* backgrounds (Fig. 5.2c, *left panel*). In contrast to the situation in the WT background, when expressed in the $rds^{+/-}$ background, the presence of C150S RDS improves rod function (even though it cannot form oligomers). However, in the absence of native RDS ($rds^{-/-}$) no ERG signals were detected. As expected, since C150S RDS in MOP-T mice is not expressed in cones, no alterations in photopic (cone) amplitudes were detected (Fig. 5.2a, *right panel*). The lack of functional improvement in the $rds^{-/-}$ background confirms that RDS oligomerization is required for retinal function. However, the

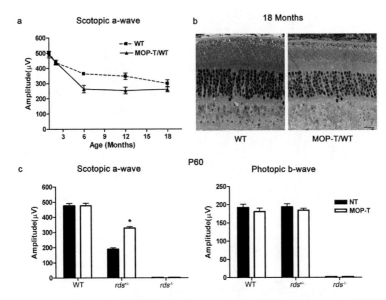

Fig. 5.2 Functional analysis of MOP-T; (**a**) Non-transgenic (WT) and transgenic (MOP-T/WT) animals in the WT background underwent full-field scotopic ERG. Shown are maximum scotopic a-wave amplitudes at various ages as indicated. At both early (1–2 months) and late (18 months) ages, there is no difference in maximum scotopic ERG amplitude between transgenic and non-transgenic mice. (**b**) Toluidine blue stained, plastic embedded sections were collected from eyes harvested from transgenic and non-transgenic animals at 18 months of age. Scale bar, 20 μm. The C150S transgene has no structural effect on the retina in the WT background. (**c**) At P60, transgenic and non-transgenic animals in multiple *RDS* backgrounds underwent full-field scotopic and photopic ERG. Shown are averages (+/– S.E.M.) from 5 to 7 animals/category. In the absence of WT RDS, no retinal function is detected, however, the presence of the C150S transgene improves the maximum scotopic a-wave amplitude in the heterozygous *rds*$^{+/-}$ mouse

functional improvement seen when oligomerization-incompetent RDS (C150S) is present in the heterozygous background (MOP-T/*rds*$^{+/-}$) suggests that complete retinal function may depend on other RDS functions that do not necessarily require intermolecular disulfide bonding.

To see whether there is any structural evidence to support this hypothesis, we undertook detailed ultrastructural (electron microscopic, EM) analyses. Previously we have shown that in the absence of native RDS (MOP-T/*rds*$^{-/-}$) the OS layer is virtually gone and looks similar to that of *rds*$^{-/-}$ retinas (Chakraborty et al. 2008). Consistent with the lack of function shown in Fig. 5.2c, the MOP-T/*rds*$^{-/-}$ retina had no properly formed OSs. The OS areas of *rds*$^{-/-}$ and MOP-T/*rds*$^{-/-}$ mice were not identical however; MOP-T/*rds*$^{-/-}$ mice had more membranous structures than their non-transgenic counterparts. To further study these structures, we performed EM immunogold analysis with monospecific antibodies against rhodopsin to determine whether these membranes are derived from the OS. In contrast to *rds*$^{-/-}$ retinas, where no opsin immunoreactivity is detected (due to complete absence of an OS layer), membranous material in the OS area of MOP-T/*rds*$^{-/-}$ did contain anti-opsin immunopositive staining. Furthermore, very rarely, rounded membranous

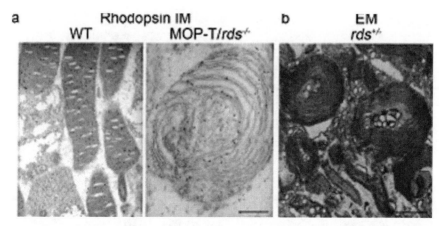

a   Rhodopsin IM   **b**   EM

    WT   MOP-T/*rds*$^{-/-}$ *rds*$^{+/-}$

Fig. 5.3 Ultrastructural analysis of MOP-T; Eyes were harvested from P30 transgenic and non-transgenic eyes and processed for immunogold/EM (**a**) or EM (**b**). (**a**) mAB 1D4 against rhodopsin was used to label OSs in MOP-T/*rds*$^{-/-}$ and WT (as a control) animals. No normal OSs were observed in MOP-T/*rds*$^{-/-}$ animals, only rounded whorl-like membranous structures reminiscent of those seen in the *rds*$^{+/-}$ (**b**), only larger. Scale bar, 2 μm

structures were observed in MOP-T/*rds*$^{-/-}$ retinas that were anti-opsin immunopositive (Fig. 5.3a). Interestingly, these structures are reminiscent of the malformed OSs seen in the *rds*$^{+/-}$ mouse (*cf*. Fig. 5.3b), although they are much more infrequent. The appearance of these structures suggests that MOP-T/*rds*$^{-/-}$ animals are trying, albeit unsuccessfully, to make OSs. Immunofluorescent labeling with anti- RDS antibody also was used to confirm that these attempted OSs contain the transgenic C150S RDS protein (data not shown).

Our structural and functional observations presented here support the idea that oligomerization-competent RDS is required for normal OS structure and function, but that RDS has some oligomerization-*independent* functions; hence, having a mutant (C150S) RDS is better than having no RDS at all. We hypothesize that one of these oligomerization-independent functions may be assembly of specialized membrane microdomains (i.e., the tetraspanin web); however, at present, there is no direct evidence to support this hypothesis. Current studies are underway to identify other RDS binding partners and determine the composition of the RDS tetraspanin web, while future studies may investigate the role of oligomerization-incompetent (C150S) RDS in that process.

Acknowledgments The monoclonal antibodies for this study (1D4) were generously shared with us by Dr. Robert Molday, University of British Columbia. The authors would like to thank Rasha Makkia for her excellent technical assistance with the transgenic animals. This study was supported by grants from the National Institutes of Health (EY10609 & EY018656 to MIN; EY007361 to SJF; Core Grant for Vision Research EY12190 to MIN), the Foundation Fighting Blindness (MIN), the Knights Templar Eye Research Foundation (DC) and a departmental Unrestricted Grant from Research to Prevent Blindness (SJF). Dr. Naash is the recipient of a Research to Prevent Blindness James S. Adams Scholar Award. Dr. Fliesler is the recipient of a Research to Prevent Blindness Senior Scientist Award.

References

Arikawa K, Molday LL, Molday RS et al (1992) Localization of peripherin/rds in the disk mem-
    branes of cone and rod photoreceptors: relationship to disk membrane morphogenesis and
    retinal degeneration. J Cell Biol 116:659–667
Chakraborty D, Ding XQ, Conley SM et al (2008a) Differential requirements for Rds intermolec-
    ular disulfide-linked oligomerization in rods versus cones. Hum Mol Genet 18:797–808
Chakraborty D, Ding XQ, Fliesler SJ et al (2008b) Outer segment oligomerization of Rds: evidence
    from mouse models and subcellular fractionation. Biochemistry 47:1144–1156
Connell GJ, Molday RS (1990) Molecular cloning, primary structure, and orientation of the
    vertebrate photoreceptor cell protein peripherin in the rod outer segment disk membrane.
    Biochemistry 29:4691–4698
Delaguillaumie A, Lagaudriere-Gesbert C, Popoff MR et al (2002) Rho GTPases link cytoskeletal
    rearrangements and activation processes induced via the tetraspanin CD82 in T lymphocytes. J
    Cell Sci 115:433–443
Farjo R, Naash MI (2006) The role of rds in outer segment morphogenesis and human retinal
    disease. Ophthalmic Genet 27:117–122
Goldberg AF, Loewen CJ, Molday RS (1998) Cysteine residues of photoreceptor peripherin/rds:
    role in subunit assembly and autosomal dominant retinitis pigmentosa. Biochemistry 37:
    680–685
Hemler ME (2001) Specific tetraspanin functions. J Cell Biol 155:1103–1107
Hemler ME (2003) Tetraspanin proteins mediate cellular penetration, invasion, and fusion events
    and define a novel type of membrane microdomain. Annu Rev Cell Dev Biol 19:397–422
Lagaudriere-Gesbert C, Lebel-Binay S, Hubeau C et al (1998) Signaling through the tetraspanin
    CD82 triggers its association with the cytoskeleton leading to sustained morphological changes
    and T cell activation. Eur J Immunol 28:4332–4344
Levy S, Shoham T (2005) Protein-protein interactions in the tetraspanin web. Physiology
    (Bethesda) 20:218–224
Li C, Ding XQ, O'Brien J et al (2003) Molecular characterization of the skate periph-
    erin/rds gene: relationship to its orthologues and paralogues. Invest Ophthalmol Vis Sci 44:
    2433–2441
Loewen CJ, Molday RS (2000) Disulfide-mediated oligomerization of Peripherin/Rds and Rom-1
    in photoreceptor disk membranes. Implications for photoreceptor outer segment morphogenesis
    and degeneration. J Biol Chem 275:5370–5378
Loewen CJ, Moritz OL, Tam BM et al (2003) The role of subunit assembly in peripherin-2 targeting
    to rod photoreceptor disk membranes and retinitis pigmentosa. Mol Biol Cell 14:3400–3413
Molday RS, Hicks D, Molday L (1987) Peripherin. A rim-specific membrane protein of rod outer
    segment discs. Invest Ophthalmol Vis Sci 28:50–61
Moritz OL, Peck A, Tam BM (2002) Xenopus laevis red cone opsin and Prph2 promoters allow
    transgene expression in amphibian cones, or both rods and cones. Gene 298:173–182
Naash MI, Ding XQ, Li C et al (2003) Peripherin/rds in skate retina. Adv Exp Med Biol 533:
    377–383
Serru V, Le Naour F, Billard M et al (1999) Selective tetraspan-integrin complexes
    (CD81/alpha4beta1, CD151/alpha3beta1, CD151/alpha6beta1) under conditions disrupting
    tetraspan interactions. Biochem J 340(Pt 1):103–111
Shigeta M, Sanzen N, Ozawa M et al (2003) CD151 regulates epithelial cell-cell adhesion through
    PKC- and Cdc42-dependent actin cytoskeletal reorganization. J Cell Biol 163:165–176
Stipp CS, Kolesnikova TV, Hemler ME (2003) Functional domains in tetraspanin proteins. Trends
    Biochem Sci 28:106–112
Travis GH, Sutcliffe JG, Bok D (1991) The retinal degeneration slow (rds) gene product is a
    photoreceptor disc membrane-associated glycoprotein. Neuron 6:61–70
Wrigley JD, Ahmed T, Nevett CL et al (2000) Peripherin/rds influences membrane vesicle
    morphology. Implications for retinopathies. J Biol Chem 275:13191–13194

Wu XR, Medina JJ, Sun TT (1995) Selective interactions of UPIa and UPIb, two members of the transmembrane 4 superfamily, with distinct single transmembrane-domained proteins in differentiated urothelial cells. J Biol Chem 270:29752–29759

Yauch RL, Berditchevski F, Harler MB et al (1998) Highly stoichiometric, stable, and specific association of integrin alpha3beta1 with CD151 provides a major link to phosphatidylinositol 4-kinase, and may regulate cell migration. Mol Biol Cell 9:2751–2765

Chapter 6
The Association Between Telomere Length and Sensitivity to Apoptosis of HUVEC

Ji Zhang, Chen Hui, Liu Su, Wu Xiaoyun, Huang Xi, and Fan Yingchuan

Abstract

Objectives: To study the association between the mean telomere length (MTL) of human umbilical endothelial cells (HUVEC) and their sensitivity to apoptosis.

Methods: Apoptosis of HUVEC was induced by using free hydroxyl radicals. The rate of apoptosis was determined and mean telomere length of HUVEC that were cultured for 1 or 3 months were measured by Southern Blot.

Results: At 0.2 mmol/l $FeSO_4$/0.0001 mmol/l H_2O_2 free radical concentration, the apoptosis rate was 8.0 and 17.5% and MTL was 4.66 ± 0.05 and 3.40 ± 0.46 kb for HUVEC cultured for 1 and 3 months, respectively. At 0.2 mmol/l $FeSO_4$/0.005 mmol/l H_2O_2, apoptosis rates were 17.4 and 36.0% and MTL were 3.67 ± 0.06 and 2.90 ± 0.20 kb for HUVEC cultured for 1 and for 3 months, respectively. Control HUVEC had apoptosis rates of 0.5 and 1.0% and MTL of 5.43 ± 0.45 and 4.57 ± 0.21 kb for 1 and 3 months, respectively. The MTL and the apoptosis rates in the treatment groups differed significantly from the controls ($p < 0.05$).

Conclusions: HUVEC with less culture time or short telomere were sensitive to oxidation stress. Oxidation stress also can enhance the shortening of telomere length.

6.1 Introduction

Since the telomere hypothesis, which states that more cell divisions in somatic cells result in shorter telomere lengths, while less cell divisions result longer telomere lengths, was raised (Harley et al. 1990), the relationship between the telomere

C. Hui (✉)
Department of Ophthalmology, Sichuan Provincial People's Hospital, Chengdu, Sichuan Province, 610072, China
e-mail: hui-chen@ouhsc.edu

Ji Zhang, Chen Hui, and Liu Su are co-first authors.

R.E. Anderson et al. (eds.), *Retinal Degenerative Diseases*, Advances in Experimental Medicine and Biology 664, DOI 10.1007/978-1-4419-1399-9_6,
© Springer Science+Business Media, LLC 2010

length and cell division or cell replicative senescence has been examined. Much effort has centered on whether the telomere can be used as a biologic timing device for ageing (Cawthon et al. 2003; Thomas et al. 2008). Evidence from kidneys, lens epithelium, and trabecular meshwork cells supporting this perspective has grown substantially in last few years (Melk et al. 2000; Pendergrass et al. 2001; Yamazaki et al. 2007). While others (Bodnar et al. 1998; van Steensel et al. 1998) found an association between telomere length and apoptosis; when the telomere length decreased to Hayflick limits, cells lost their ability to be susceptible to chromosomal fusion and their potential for division, going into replicative senescence and apoptosis or cancer.

Some researchers gradually realized that the ageing process is not simply a time problem, but is accompanied by or involves the accumulative effects from various environmental factors such as oxidation and radiation (Goytisolo et al. 2000). Hence research has been initiated to identify the bridge between the gene and the environment by using the telomere (Huda et al. 2007; Starr et al. 2008). The current study was initiated to examine the association among oxidation factors, telomeres, ageing, and apoptosis and to determine whether the sensitivity or susceptibility to apoptosis can be expressed by mean telomere length (MTL).

6.2 Methods

6.2.1 The Culture of HUVEC and the Construction of Cell Division Model

We used culture time to reflect both the amounts of cell division and telomere length according to our working hypothesis. For example HUVEC cultured for 1 month represented the less cell division group (long telomere length) and HUVEC cultured for 3 months represented the more cell division group (short telomere length).

6.2.2 Construction of an Apoptosis Model of HUVEC with Free Hydroxyl Radicals

The Fenton reaction ($Fe^{2+} + H_2O_2 = Fe^{3+} + OH^- + .OH$) was used to produce free hydroxyl radicals as the oxidative factor to induce apoptosis in HUVEC. The reaction system comprising 0.2 mmol/l $FeSO_4$ and 0.1, 0.05, 0.01, 0.005, or 0.0001 mmol/l H_2O_2 was tested to find the appropriate concentration of free radicals for inducing the apoptosis of HUVEC. Apoptosis was induced in HUVEC at 0.2 mmol/l $FeSO_4$/0.0001 mmol/l H_2O_2 and 0.2 mmol/l $FeSO_4$/0.005 mmol H_2O_2; and necrosis of HUVEC was found at the other concentrations. Thus, 0.2 mmol/l $FeSO_4$/0.0001 mmol/l H_2O_2 was added to 1-month-cultured HUVEC and 0.2 mmol/l $FeSO_4$/0.005 mmol H_2O_2 was added to 3-month-cultured HUVEC. Apoptosis of HUVEC was detected with HE stain, Hoechst 33,258 fluorescent stain, and apoptotic DNA ladder.

6.2.3 Measurement of Apoptosis Rates and Telomere Lengths

Fluorescent microscopy was used to determine apoptosis. The apoptosis rate of HUVEC with fluorescent stain was calculated by the amount of apoptotic HUVEC/(the amount of apoptosis HUVEC + the amount of normal HUVEC). MTL was measured by using Southern Blot.

6.2.4 Statistics Analysis

Chi-Square, random T test and Q test were performed using SAS software.

6.3 Results

6.3.1 Relationship Between the Time of Culture and the Telomere Length

HUVEC that were cultured for 1 month, which represented the group with less cell division, had significantly longer telomeres (5.43 ± 0.45 kb) than the telomeres (4.57 ± 0.21 kb) in HUVEC that were cultured for 3 months, which represented group with more cell division (p <0.05) (Table 6.1, Figs. 6.1 and 6.2).

Table 6.1 Mean telomere length of human umbilical endothelial cells that were cultured for 1 or 3 months

Groups	Mean telomere length (kb)	t	p
1 month	5.43 ± 0.45	3.022	0.0391
3 months	4.57 ± 0.21		

6.3.2 Relationship Among Apoptosis Rates, Culture Times and Oxidation

Apoptosis rates in the control group (without oxidation) were 0.5% at 1 month and 1.0% at 3 months (p >0.05), indicating that apoptosis rates of HUVEC without oxidation were not affected by culture time (Table 6.2). While the oxidation group exposed to 0.2 mmol/l $FeSO_4$/0.0001 mmol/l H_2O_2 had apoptosis rates of 8.0% at 1 and 17.5% at 3 months (p = 0.054) and the oxidation group exposed to 0.2 mmol/l $FeSO_4$/0.005 mmol H_2O_2 had rates of 17.4% at 1 and 36.0% at 3 months (p <0.05). These data indicate that the apoptosis rate was affected by the oxidation and as culture time increased (cell division amounts). Thus, HUVEC with shorter telomere length had a higher apoptosis rate than the apoptosis rate in HUVEC with shorter

Fig. 6.1 Southern Blot of
telomere lengths of HUVEC
that were cultured
1 month. 1: normal (control);
2: apoptosis group cultured in
0.2 mmol/l
FeSO$_4$/0.0001 mmol/l H$_2$O$_2$;
3: apoptosis group cultured in
0.2 mmol/l
FeSO$_4$/0.005 mmol/l H$_2$O$_2$

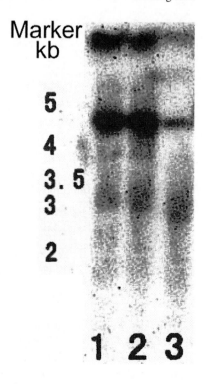

Table 6.2 The apoptosis rate of human umbilical endothelial cells that were cultured for 1 or 3 months and induced by free radicals

FeSO$_4$/H$_2$O$_2$ concentrations (mmol/l)	1 month (%)	3 months (%)	χ^2	p
Control	0.5	1.0	0.168	>0.05
0.2/0.0001	8.0	17.5	3.703	0.054 (<0.1)
0.2/0.005	17.4	36.0	8.733	<0.05

culture time and longer telomeres. We conclude that HUVEC with shorter telomeres are sensitive to free radicals.

6.3.3 Oxidation Enhances the Telomere Shortening

There are significant differences between the telomere lengths influenced by different oxidation concentrations (p <0.05) at which HUVEC were cultured for 1 or 3 months. As the free radical concentration increased, MTL decreased, indicating the increasing oxidation can enhance the telomere shortening (Table 6.3, Figs. 6.1 and 6.2).

Fig. 6.2 Southern Blot of telomere lengths of HUVEC that were cultured for 3 months. 1: normal (control); 2: apoptosis group cultured in 0.2 mmol/l FeSO$_4$/0.0001 mmol/l H$_2$O$_2$; 3: apoptosis group cultured in 0.2 mmol/l FeSO$_4$/0.005 mmol/l H$_2$O$_2$

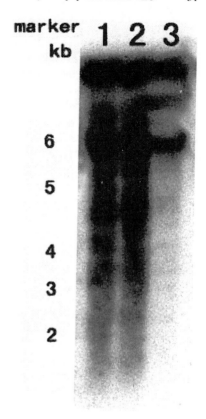

Table 6.3 Mean telomere length of human umbilical endothelial cells that were cultured for 1 or 3 months under different oxidation concentrations

Groups	Control (kb)	0.2 mmol/l FeSO$_4$/0.0001 mmol/l H$_2$O$_2$ (kb)	0.2 mmol/l FeSO$_4$/0.005 mmol/l H$_2$O$_2$ (kb)	F	p
1 month	5.43 ± 0.45	4.66 ± 0.05	3.67 ± 0.06	33.24	0.0006
3 months	4.57 ± 0.21	3.40 ± 0.46	2.90 ± 0.20	22.44	0.0016

6.4 Discussion

Over the past decades, scientists have found that the telomere shortening is present in Hutchinson-Gilford progeria and Down's syndrome (Vaziri et al. 1993). More recent reports show telomere shortening is associated with age-related diseases (Gilley et al. 2008), even cardiovascular diseases (Kurz et al. 2006; Brouilette et al. 2008), and diabetic nephropathy (Verzola et al. 2008). These studies attempted to elucidate the age-related mechanism between telomere length, age and the environment. We designed this experiment to simplify the detailed, complicated interactions among the environment and cell, gene-gene interactions, gene-protein interactions, and apoptosis and ageing. We show the environment-telomere-apoptosis interactions through the use of culture time to reflect the telomere age. As expected, telomeres of HUVEC shortened as culture time increased. Importantly, we found that the apoptosis rate was not only affected by oxidative concentrations, but also by the culture time and TML (as an indirect measure of the amount of cell division), indicating that the cells with more cell divisions or with short telomeres are sensitive or susceptible to oxidation. In other words, we hypothesize short-telomere cells are susceptible to apoptotic factors, while long-telomere cells are tolerant to apoptosis. Thus, we speculate the age-related diseases, degenerative diseases might occur at young ages in individuals who have short telomeres, and vice versa. This hypothesis can explain not only the variance of cells in an individual's organ to apoptosis, but also the differences between individuals. It can provide evidence for research on age-related diseases through the examination of telomere lengths.

Most importantly, this hypothesis also can be applied to non-dividing cells such as neurons or myocardial cells. Horvitz and Herskowitz (1992) and Morrison et al. (1997) elucidated the symmetric and asymmetric divisions for stem cells, especially the division of neuron stem cells. For symmetric division, cell division amounts are the same, while some cells experience more divisions and some have fewer divisions in asymmetric division. Translating this hypothesis to telomere length, asymmetric division in stem cells produces large amounts of cells with a significant variance in telomere lengths resulting from different division times. This is the reason that telomere length shows as a band or range on Southern blots, thus telomere length in non-dividing cells after birth are different, originating from asymmetric division of the stem cells. We have found this to be the case for telomere length variance in separated rabbit retinal ganglion cells (unpublished). Hence the telomere hypothesis may also be applied to age-related neuropathy such as glaucoma, retinal degeneration diseases to suggest an explanation for their sensitivity to apoptosis.

Furthermore, we found that oxidation can enhance the telomere shortening. This is consistent with the report by Toussaint et al. (2000), which showed telomeres are highly susceptible to oxidative stress. De Meyer et al. (2008) also showed that elevated levels of oxidative stress and inflammation further increase the rate of telomere attrition. These data show there is a relationship between telomere length and oxidation, suggesting that we can construct a "bridge" among genes and the environment, and ageing and apoptosis through the use of telomeres.

References

Bodnar AG, Ouellette M, Frolkis M et al (1998) Extension of life-span by introduction of telomerase into normal human cells. Science 279(5349):349–352

Brouilette SW, Whittaker A, Stevens SE et al (2008) Telomere length is shorter in healthy offspring of subjects with coronary artery disease: support for the telomere hypothesis. Heart 94(4): 422–425

Cawthon RM, Smith KR, O'Brien E et al (2003) Association between telomere length in blood and mortality in people aged 60 years or older. Lancet 361(9355):393–395

De Meyer T, Rietzschel ER, De Buyzere ML et al (2008) Studying telomeres in a population based study. Front Biosci 13:2960–2970

Gilley D, Herbert BS, Huda N et al (2008) Factors impacting human telomere homeostasis and age-related disease. Mech Ageing Dev 129(1–2):27–34

Goytisolo F-A, Samper E, Martin-Caballero J et al (2000) Short telomeres result in organismal hypersensitivity to ionizing radiation in mammals. J Exp Med 192(11):1625–1636

Harley CB, Futcher AB, Greider CW (1990) Telomeres shorten during ageing of human fibroblasts. Nature 345(6274):458–460

Horvitz HR, Herskowitz I (1992) Mechanisms of asymmetric cell division: two Bs or not two Bs, that is the question. Cell 68(2):237–255

Huda N, Tanaka H, Herbert BS (2007) Shared environmental factors associated with telomere length maintenance in elderly male twins. Aging Cell 6(5):709–713

Kurz DJ, Kloeckener-Gruissem B, Akhmedov A et al (2006) Degenerative aortic valve stenosis, but not coronary disease, is associated with shorter telomere length in the elderly. Arterioscler Thromb Vasc Biol 26(6):e114–e117

Melk A, Ramassar V, Helms LM et al (2000) Telomere shortening in kidneys with age. J Am Soc Nephrol 11(3):444–453

Morrison SJ, Shah NM, Anderson DJ et al (1997) Regulatory mechanisms in stem cell biology. Cell 88(3):287–298

Pendergrass WR, Penn PE, Li J et al (2001) Age-related telomere shortening occurs in lens epithelium from old rats and is slowed by caloric restriction. Exp Eye Res 73(2):221–228

Starr JM, Shiels PG, Harris SE et al (2008) Oxidative stress, telomere length and biomarkers of physical aging in a cohort aged 79 years from the 1932 Scottish Mental Survey. Mech Ageing 129(12):745–751

Thomas P, O'Callaghan NJ, Fenech M (2008) Telomere length in white blood cells, buccal cells and brain tissue and its variation with ageing and Alzheimer's disease. Mech Ageing Dev 129(4):183–190

Toussaint O, Medrano EE, von Zglinicki T (2000) Cellular and molecular mechanisms of stress-induced premature senescence (SIPS) of human diploidfibroblasts and melanocytes. Exp Gerontol 35(8):927–945

van Steensel B, Smogorzewska A, de Lange T (1998) TRF2 protects human telomeres from end-to-end fusions. Cell 92(3):401–413

Vaziri H, Schachter F, Uchida I et al (1993) Loss of telomeric DNA during aging of normal and trisomy 21 human lymphocytes. Am J Hum Genet 52:661–667

Verzola D, Gandolfo MT, Gaetani G et al (2008) Accelerated senescence in the kidneys of patients with type 2 diabetic nephropathy. Am J Physiol Renal Physiol 295(5):F1563–F1573

Yamazaki Y, Matsunaga H, Nishikawa M et al (2007) Senescence in cultured trabecular meshwork cells. Br J Ophthalmol 91(6):808–811

Chapter 7
Photoreceptor Guanylate Cyclases and cGMP Phosphodiesterases in Zebrafish

Ross F. Collery and Breandán N. Kennedy

Abstract Tightly regulated control of cGMP levels is critical for proper functioning of photoreceptors, and mutations in cGMP synthesis or degradation factors can lead to various forms of retinal disorder. Here we review heterogenous human retinal disorders associated with mutant retinal guanylate cyclases (RetGCs) and phosphodiesterase 6 (PDE6), and describe how zebrafish are being used to examine phototransduction components and their roles in these diseases. Though mutations in RetGCs and PDE6 lead to retinal disorders, there is a lack of molecular and biochemical data on routes of subsequent photoreceptor degeneration and visual impairment. Use of animal model systems provides important information to connect in vitro biochemical analyses of mutant genes with clinically observed pathologies of human retinal diseases. Zebrafish are an excellent in vivo system to generate animal models of human retinal disorders and study photoreceptor components, and have already provided valuable data on retinal diseases caused by phototransduction component mutations.

7.1 Regulation of cGMP Levels in Photoreceptor Outer Segments

Cyclic GMP (cGMP) is a key second messenger in photoreceptor outer segments (for review, see Kaupp and Seifert 2002), regulating intracellular calcium ion entry through cyclic nucleotide-gated (CNG) channels (Fig. 7.1). Depletion of cGMP causes these ion channels to close, while photoreceptors continue to efflux ions via other cGMP-independent ion channels. This leads to a drop in intracellular ionic

R.F. Collery (✉)
UCD School of Biomolecular and Biomedical Science, UCD Conway Institute of Biomolecular and Biomedical Research, University College Dublin, Dublin, Ireland
e-mail: rcollery@mcw.edu

R.E. Anderson et al. (eds.), *Retinal Degenerative Diseases*, Advances in Experimental Medicine and Biology 664, DOI 10.1007/978-1-4419-1399-9_7,
© Springer Science+Business Media, LLC 2010

concentration, hyperpolarisation of the photoreceptor plasma membrane and transmission to higher-order neurons in the retina. For photoreceptors to function, cGMP levels are tightly regulated at the levels of synthesis and degradation. In photoreceptor outer segments, cGMP is synthesised from GTP by membrane-bound retinal guanylate cyclases, (RetGC) (Fig. 7.1). Light stimulation of photoreceptor visual pigments activates a phosphodiesterase (PDE6) which hydrolyses cGMP to GTP (for reviews, see Arshavsky et al. 2002; Pugh et al. 1997). Inappropriate activity of either RetGC or PDE6 leads to an imbalance in cGMP levels, which is associated with multiple retinal disorders. Here, we outline human retinal diseases resulting from RetGC or PDE6 mutations, and describe the usefulness of the zebrafish to investigate these diseases.

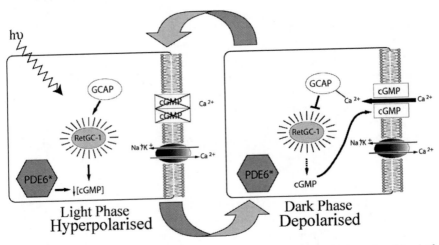

Fig. 7.1 The phototransduction cascade; during dark phase, RetGC synthesises a basal level of cGMP, which keeps some CNG channels in an open configuration, and allows the influx of calcium, while ion pumps efflux calcium. An incident photon (hυ) activates opsin, which (indirectly) derepresses phosphodiesterase 6, and breaks down cGMP. The CNG channels close as the cGMP level drops, and GCAP is derepressed, and stimulates RetGC-1. As the light impulse stops, the phosphodiesterase no longer breaks down cGMP, and RetGC-1 synthesises more cGMP, allowing some CNG channels to reopen, and the photoreceptor to depolarize

7.2 Retinal Disorders Associated with Mutations in RetGCs and PDE6

The central role played by RetGC-1 in phototransduction implies that its absence or incorrect function will have severe consequences for visual function. A lack of cGMP is thought to lead to the inability of photoreceptors to depolarise, and an overabundance of cGMP may lead to constitutive opening of the CNG channels, keeping photoreceptors constantly hyperpolarised and unable to respond to light impulses (for review, see Duda and Koch 2002). The human gene encoding RetGC-1 was the first gene implicated in Leber congenital amaurosis (LCA) (Perrault et al. 2000). LCA is an autosomal recessive, early-onset, retinal dystrophy and one of the most severe forms of inherited blindness in children. It is estimated that ~20% of LCA cases are caused by RetGC-1 mutations, which predominantly result in inactive RetGC-1 (Perrault et al. 2000). Tucker and colleagues observed that mutations in RetGC-1 could lead to LCA, or to other, less severe retinal disorders, depending on the position of the mutation (Tucker et al. 2004). This strengthened the proposal that mutations in different regions of RetGC-1 may contribute to a spectrum of retinal disorders that were previously segregated due to differing severity of symptoms (Perrault et al. 2000).

Another severe retinal degeneration, linked in this case with dominant RetGC-1 mutations, is cone-rod dystrophy 6 (CORD6). Kelsell and colleagues show that CORD6 symptoms, including loss of central vision, photophobia, and "bull's-eye" maculopathy are associated with mutations in the dimerisation domain of RetGC-1 (Kelsell et al. 1998). Despite the clinical analysis of the symptoms of CORD6, and a correlation between mutations in RetGC-1 and the severity of phenotype, there are few studies of the molecular effects associated with mutant RetGC-1 in the retina. It is not known whether dominant mutant RetGC-1 synthesises an excess of cGMP and is less easily inactivated in the retina as biochemical data suggest (Tucker et al. 1999; Ramamurthy et al. 2001), or if another cellular process leads to CORD6. There is a clear need to use in vivo models to better characterise the disease pathways induced by mutant RetGCs.

PDE6 is a holoenzyme composed of PDE6A, PDE6B and two PDE6G subunits in rods, and two PDE6C and two PDE6H subunits in cones (for review, see Ionita and Pittler 2007). Though the subunits work cooperatively, mutations in single subunits lead to distinct disease phenotypes. Rod-specific PDE6A mutations lead to autosomal recessive retinitis pigmentosa (arRP) (Huang et al. 1995), while mutations in PDE6B cause arRP or congenital stationary night blindness (Gao et al. 1996; Gal et al. 1994). Mutations in the cone-specific PDE6C are less well characterized, but are associated with cone photoreceptor loss and recessive achromatopsia (Chang et al. 2001; Chang et al. 2002). Mutations in the rod PDE6G subunit are associated with recessive retinitis pigmentosa (Tsang et al. 1996), while cone PDE6H subunit mutations lead to a recessive form of cone dystrophy (Piri et al. 2005). The heterogeneity of disease phenotypes reflects the spatial expression of different PDE6 subunits, and that disease-associated mutations are present in catalytic and inhibitory subunits of the PDE6 holoenzyme. As with retinal disorders associated with mutations in RetGC, the link between altered activity of PDE6 and photoreceptor degeneration is not well understood, and in vivo animal models will provide valuable data on these pathologies.

7.3 Analysis of Teleost RetGC and PDEs in Retinal Function and Disorders

The infraclass *Teleostei* are contained in the class *Actinopterygii*, the ray-finned fishes, and contains a number of discrete species of fishes that are extremely useful in genetic analyses, including visual function, development and disease (Collery et al. 2006). In particular, teleost models have abundant cone photoreceptors mediating color vision and thus are advantageous for analyzing cone retinopathies (for review, see Goldsmith and Harris 2003). In medaka (*Oryzias latipes*), four discrete guanylate cyclase mRNAs are expressed in the retina: *OlGC-R2 OlGC3, OlGC4* (*OlGC-R1*), and *OlGC-C* (*OlGC5*) (Hisatomi et al. 1999; Seimiya et al. 1997). In the retina, *OlGC-C* (*OlGC5*) is cone-exclusive whilst *OlGC4* (*OlGC-R1*) and *OlGC-R2*, are expressed only in rods; and all are expressed in the pineal (Hisatomi et al. 1999).

Recent data shows zebrafish to express three membrane-bound retinal GCs: zGC1, zGC2 and zGC3 (Rätscho et al. 2009) (Fig. 7.2a). zGC1 and zGC2 are expressed in rods, while zGC3 is expressed exclusively in cones. zGC1 and zGC2 are equivalent to human RetGC-2 both by sequence homology and rod localization, while zGC3 is equivalent to human cone RetGC-1. The zebrafish *zatoichi* mutant has no cone-driven visual response owing to a null mutation in zGC3, and was identified through a lack of optokinetic or optomotor visual function (Muto et al. 2005). As zGC3 corresponds to human RetGC-1, the *zatoichi* mutant may be considered an animal model of LCA. Although *zatoichi* zebrafish have no visual function, there is no observed abnormal retinal histology at 5 days post fertilization (Muto et al. 2005). This at least initial preservation of photoreceptors in *zatoichi* zebrafish allows testing of in vivo therapies such as gene therapy, cell transplantation and pharmacological modifiers to recover functionality of extant photoreceptors. In addition, *zatoichi* photoreceptors can be utilized to examine the effects of the absence of zGC3/RetGC-1, and to understand better the molecular mechanisms behind the progression of LCA.

Orthologues of human PDE6C, -A, -G and -H have also been identified in zebrafish (Vihtelic et al. 2005), and PDE6B can be found through database homology searches (zPDE6B, XM_679910). Similarly, PDE6 subunit orthologues can be found in medaka libraries (OlPDE6B, ENSORLG00000009868; OlPDE6C, ENSORLG00000005135; no PDE6A orthologue is currently discoverable in medaka). Phylogenetic comparisons indicate that PDE6A orthologues are most closely related between species, followed by PDE6B orthologues (Fig. 7.2b). Cone-specific PDE6C orthologues differ more between species, which may reflect comparison of diurnal and nocturnal animals.

Functional work already done in zebrafish has examined the effects on photoreceptors of mutations in the PDE6C subunit. Stearns and colleagues examined lines with a *pde6c* frameshift mutation that likely leads to a truncated protein or an mRNA targeted for degradation, where insufficient breakdown of cGMP leads to cone death, followed by localized rod death (Stearns et al. 2007). Similarly, Nishiwaki and colleagues examined lines with a *pde6* mutation that confers a single amino acid change within the cGMP-binding GAF domain, and found opsin mislocalization and cone death, though without accompanying rod death (Nishiwaki et al. 2008). It is currently unknown whether excess cGMP due to RetGC-1 mutations also leads to cone cell death. The death of cones associated with PDE6 components indicates the importance of the phototransduction cascade components in normal maintenance of photoreceptors, as well as visual signaling. The heterogeneity of disease phenotypes seen when comparing truncated and missense PDE6C zebrafish proteins illustrates how the zebrafish model system can be used to dissect how multiple mutations in a single gene can cause a range of symptoms. A loss of cones followed by rods when cone-specific PDE6C has a truncation mutation indicates that the rods die as a result of cone death; loss of cones without rod loss due to a single amino acid change in PDE6C indicates distinct mechanisms of degeneration. Work of this kind is useful to highlight potential routes for therapeutic intervention (e.g. cell death inhibitors *vs* cone cell transplantation).

In addition to using zebrafish to characterize altered visual function due to loss-of-function mutations in retGC or PDE6, transgenic zebrafish lines may be used to characterize gain-of-function disease phenotypes associated with dominant human visual diseases. We are currently assessing the pathology of expressing mutant human RetGC-1 in zebrafish cones to recapitulate CORD6, whose symptoms are well characterized (see Section 7.2), but where little is known about the in vivo effects of the mutant protein. Already, the misexpression of native GCs in the zebrafish has demonstrated the importance of correct levels and spatial expression of cGMP synthesis, as ectopic expression of zGC1 (*gucy2f*) leads to serious defects in the nervous system (Maddison et al. 2009).

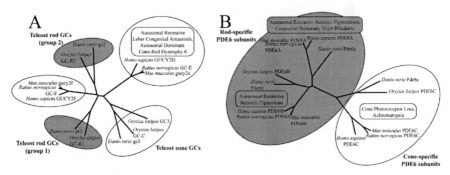

Fig. 7.2 (**a**) Phylogenetic tree showing retinal guanylate cyclases from human (*Homo sapiens*), Rat (*Rattus norvegicus*), Mouse (*Mus musculus*), Medaka (*Oryzias latipes*) and Zebrafish (*Danio rerio*). (**b**) Phylogenetic Tree showing PDE6 Subunits from the above species. Functionally related proteins are demarcated by *white* and *shaded ellipses*. Sequences were aligned using ClustalW. Disease phenotypes associated with mutations in these genes are inset in *rounded rectangles*

In summary, current zebrafish methods allow researchers to make transgenic lines expressing mutant proteins to study the effects of dominant heritable diseases, and to reduce or eliminate native proteins to study recessive and null mutation diseases. Identification of zebrafish genes orthologous to RetGCs and PDE6 subunits means that zebrafish can be used to generate models of recessive retinitis pigmentosa, congenital stationary night blindness, dominant cone-rod dystrophy, and achromatopsia. In parallel with furthering knowledge about the onset and progression of these diseases, zebrafish can be easily used to assay molecular and

pharmacological factors with potential to prevent retinal cell loss or malfunction-
ing, and to evaluate stem cell therapy or whole retinal transplantation to recover
visual function. In conclusion, teleosts are an important model to study inherited
human retinal disease.

References

Arshavsky VY, Lamb TD, Pugh EN Jr (2002) G proteins and phototransduction. Annu Rev Physiol
    64:153–187
Chang B, Hawes NL, Hurd RE et al (2001) A new mouse model of cone photoreceptor function
    loss (cpfl1). IOVS 42(Suppl.):S527 (Abstract)
Chang B, Hawes NL, Hurd RE et al (2002) Retinal degeneration mutants in the mouse. Vision Res
    42(4):517–525
Collery RM, Cederlund L, Smyth VA et al (2006) Applying transgenic zebrafish technology to
    study the retina. Adv Exp Med Biol 572:201–207
Duda T, Koch KW (2002) Retinal diseases linked with photoreceptor guanylate cyclase. Mol Cell
    Biochem 230(1–2):129–138
Gal A, Orth U, Baehr W et al (1994) Heterozygous missense mutation in the rod cGMP phos-
    phodiesterase beta-subunit gene in autosomal dominant stationary night blindness. Nat Genet
    7(4):551
Gao YQ, Danciger M, Zhao DY et al (1996) Screening of the PDE6B gene in patients with
    autosomal dominant retinitis pigmentosa. Exp Eye Res 62(2):149–154
Goldsmith P, Harris WA (2003) The zebrafish as a tool for understanding the biology of visual
    disorders. Semin Cell Dev Biol 14(1):11–18
Hisatomi O, Honkawa H, Imanishi Y et al (1999) Three kinds of guanylate cyclase expressed in
    medaka photoreceptor cells in both retina and pineal organ. Biochem Biophys Res Commun
    255(2):216–220
Huang SH, Pittler SJ, Huang X et al (1995) Autosomal recessive retinitis pigmentosa caused by
    mutations in the alpha subunit of rod cGMP phosphodiesterase. Nat Genet 11(4):468–471
Ionita MA, Pittler SJ (2007) Focus on molecules: rod cGMP phosphodiesterase type 6. Exp Eye
    Res 84(1):1–2
Kaupp UB, Seifert R (2002) Cyclic nucleotide-gated ion channels. Physiol Rev 82(3):769–824
Kelsell RE, Gregory-Evans K, Payne AM et al (1998) Mutations in the retinal guanylate cyclase
    (RETGC-1) gene in dominant cone-rod dystrophy. Hum Mol Genet 7(7):1179–1184
Maddison LA, Lu J, Victoroff T, Scott E, Baier H, Chen W (2009). A gain-of-function screen
    in zebrafish identifies a guanylate cyclase with a role in neuronal degeneration. Mol Genet
    Genomics 281(5):551–563
Muto A, Orger MB, Wehman AM et al (2005) Forward genetic analysis of visual behavior in
    zebrafish. PLoS Genet 1(5):e66
Nishiwaki Y, Komori A, Sagara H et al (2008) Mutation of cGMP phosphodiesterase 6α′-subunit
    gene causes progressive degeneration of cone photoreceptors in zebrafish. Mech Dev 125
    (11–12):932–946
Perrault I, Rozet JM, Gerber S et al (2000) Spectrum of retGC1 mutations in Leber's congenital
    amaurosis. Eur J Hum Genet 8(8):578–582
Piri N, Gao YQ, Danciger M et al (2005) A substitution of G to C in the cone cGMP-
    phosphodiesterase gamma subunit gene found in a distinctive form of cone dystrophy.
    Ophthalmology 112(1):159–166
Pugh EN Jr, Duda T, Sitaramayya A et al (1997) Photoreceptor guanylate cyclases: a review. Biosci
    Rep 17(5):429–473
Ramamurthy V, Tucker C, Wilkie SE et al (2001) Interactions within the coiled-coil domain of
    RetGC-1 guanylyl cyclase are optimized for regulation rather than for high affinity. J Biol
    Chem 276(28):26218–26229

Rätscho N, Scholten A, Scholten A et al (2009) Expression profiles of three novel sensory guany-
    late cyclases and guanylate cyclase-activating proteins in the zebrafish retina. Biochim Biophys
    Acta e-pub ahead of print
Seimiya M, Kusakabe T, Suzuki N (1997) Primary structure and differential gene expression of
    three membrane forms of guanylyl cyclase found in the eye of the teleost Oryzias latipes.
    J Biol Chem 272(37):23407–23417
Stearns G, Evangelista M, Fadool JM et al (2007) A mutation in the cone-specific pde6 gene causes
    rapid cone photoreceptor degeneration in zebrafish. J Neurosci 27(50):13866–13874
Tsang SH, Gouras P, Yamashita CK et al (1996) Retinal degeneration in mice lacking the gamma
    subunit of the rod cGMP phosphodiesterase. Science 272(5264):1026–1029
Tucker CL, Ramamurthy V, Pina AL et al (2004) Functional analyses of mutant recessive
    GUCY2D alleles identified in Leber congenital amaurosis patients: protein domain compar-
    isons and dominant negative effects. Mol Vis 10:297–303
Tucker CL, Woodcock SC, Kelsell RE et al (1999) Biochemical analysis of a dimerization domain
    mutation in RetGC-1 associated with dominant cone-rod dystrophy. Proc Natl Acad Sci U S A
    96(16):9039–9044
Vihtelic TS, Fadool JM, Gao J et al (2005) Expressed sequence tag analysis of zebrafish eye tissues
    for NEIBank. Mol Vis 11:1083–1100

Chapter 8
RDS in Cones Does Not Interact with the Beta Subunit of the Cyclic Nucleotide Gated Channel

Shannon M. Conley, Xi-Qin Ding, and Muna I. Naash

Abstract Retinal degeneration slow (RDS) is a photoreceptor specific tetraspanin membrane protein. It is expressed in the rim region of rod outer segment (OS) discs and cone OS lamellae. Mutations in RDS cause both rod and cone-dominant retinal degenerations. We have recently shown that RDS functions differently in rods vs. cones, and have used the cone-dominant $nrl^{-/-}$ and rod-dominant wild-type (WT) murine retinas to study these differences and help understand the mechanism of rod and cone OS biogenesis. We hypothesize that the differential role of RDS in rods vs. cones is in part related to differences in RDS binding partners. RDS has been shown to bind to the GARP portion of the β subunit of the rod-cyclic nucleotide gated (CNG) channel. This interaction has been hypothesized to play a role in anchoring the disc rim to the rod plasma membrane. In this study we show that RDS does not interact with the cone CNG. Given that cone lamellae are not entirely encased in plasma membrane and therefore may have different anchoring requirements compared with rods, this observation may help explain some of the differential behavior of RDS in rods vs. cones.

Over 70 different disease causing mutations in the photoreceptor specific protein retinal degeneration slow (RDS) have been identified. Usually, mutations in photoreceptor-specific genes cause predictable disease phenotypes, i.e. rod specific genes associate with forms of rod dominant diseases (such as retinitis pigmentosa, RP) while mutations in cone specific genes tend to cause cone-dominant diseases (such as macular degeneration, MD). In contrast, different mutations in RDS have been linked to both rod-dominant and cone-dominant disease. The spectrum of RDS-associated retinal disease phenotypes ranges from traditional RP to MD to butterfly macular dystrophy to cone-rod degeneration depending on the mutation (http://www.retina-international.com/sci-news/rdsmut.htm).

M.I. Naash (✉)
Department of Cell Biology, University of Oklahoma Health Sciences Center, 940 Stanton L. Young Blvd., BMSB 781, Oklahoma, OK 73126-0901, USA
e-mail: muna-naash@ouhsc.edu

R.E. Anderson et al. (eds.), *Retinal Degenerative Diseases*, Advances in Experimental Medicine and Biology 664, DOI 10.1007/978-1-4419-1399-9_8,
© Springer Science+Business Media, LLC 2010

The naturally occurring *retinal degeneration slow* ($rds^{-/-}$) mutant mouse has proved an excellent model for studying the phenotypic divergence in RDS-associated retinal degenerations. These mice do not form OSs and exhibit slow, progressive death of photoreceptors coupled with panretinal degeneration (Chaitin et al. 1988; Sanyal et al. 1980; Sanyal and Zeilmaker 1984). In the $rds^{+/-}$ mouse, OSs form but do not assemble into properly organized, stacked discs (Hawkins et al. 1985; Sanyal et al. 1986). This haploinsufficiency phenotype is characterized by an early onset slow rod degeneration followed by late onset slow cone degeneration (Cheng et al. 1997). The deformed discs are capable of subnormal levels of phototransduction, but the lack of a proper OS causes degeneration throughout the retina.

Unfortunately, the wild-type (WT) mouse retina is 95–97% rods rendering it difficult to study the mechanisms underlying cone degeneration associated with mutations in RDS. Even in cone only models such as the early ages of the rhodopsin knockout mouse ($rho^{-/-}$), the small number of cones makes analysis very difficult. The recent development of a cone-dominant mouse model containing a null mutation in the Neural Retinal Leucine Zipper (*NRL*) transcription factor gene (Daniele et al. 2005; Mears et al. 2001; Nikonov et al. 2005) has provided an elegant way to overcome the rod-bias problem. When retinal progenitor cells fail to receive the NRL regulatory cue, they divert from a developmental fate to rods and form blue-responsive cones instead (Farjo et al. 1997; Farjo et al. 1993; Mitton et al. 2000; Rehemtulla et al. 1996; Swaroop et al. 1992). The $nrl^{-/-}$ mouse is an ideal model for studying MD since it makes possible the examination of cones in the absence of rods. We have recently taken advantage of the $nrl^{-/-}$ mouse to study the behavior of RDS in cones. Unlike the WT rods, cones of the $nrl^{-/-}$ retina lacking RDS ($nrl^{-/-}/rds^{-/-}$) retain OS structures and the capacity for photopic visual function. The cone OSs of the $nrl^{-/-}/rds^{-/-}$ are severely malformed and have no lamellae, but continue to express OS proteins such as S-opsin. This situation is in marked contrast to the WT and underscores the different role of RDS in rods and cones.

The question remains though, what causes RDS to behave differently in rods vs. cones? Expression of RDS is limited to the OS rim region of both rod and cone photoreceptor disc rims/lamellae (Arikawa et al. 1992; Moritz et al. 2002). RDS forms tetramers in the photoreceptor inner segment which then traffic to the OS and further assemble via the second intracellular (D2) loop disulfide bonds into octamers and other higher order complexes. RDS is known to form non-covalent heterotetramers with its homologue, a protein called rod outer segment membrane protein 1 (ROM-1) in addition to homotetramers (Chakraborty et al. 2008; Goldberg and Molday 2000; Goldberg et al. 1995). However, differential interactions with ROM-1 are unlikely to be responsible for rod-cone differences in RDS behavior. Both rods and cones express ROM-1 and our biochemical studies on ROM-1 in the $nrl^{-/-}$ retina show that RDS/ROM-1 are biochemically similar in cones and rods (Chakraborty et al. 2008).

Little is known though about other potential RDS interacting partners in rods and cones. Tetraspanin proteins typically assemble with themselves and other proteins into a large functional protein complex known as the tetraspanin web which is similar to but distinct from lipid rafts (Hemler 2003; Levy and Shoham 2005; Stipp et al. 2003). This web consists of proteins that are covalently and non-covalently bound (similar to RDS and ROM-1) and of proteins that are more loosely associated. The function of tetraspanins is often dictated or modulated by the composition of this tetraspanin web, so it makes sense that differential behavior of RDS in rods vs. cones might result from different interacting partners in the two cell types.

In addition to ROM-1, RDS in the rod dominant retina is known to interact with at least two other proteins. The first protein, melanoregulin, is a protein associated with membrane fusion. Kathy Boesze Battaglia's group has shown that in concert with melanoregulin, RDS helps mediate membrane fusion and thus possibly OS disc sealing at the base of the OS (Boesze-Battaglia 2000; Boesze-Battaglia et al. 2007). The expression of melanoregulin and its potential interactions with RDS in cones have not been studied, but represent a particularly interesting area for future experimentation.

The second known RDS interacting protein is the β subunit of the rod cyclic nucleotide-gated (CNG) channel. The CNG channel functions as a heterotetramer comprised of α and β subunits (Kaupp et al. 1989). It is responsible for the resting dark current in rod photoreceptors and closes upon hydrolysis of cGMP by phosphodiesterase after light induced G-protein coupled receptor/second messenger signaling (Kaupp et al. 1989; Pugh 2000). The N-terminus of the β subunit has a large glutamic acid/proline rich domain called GARP (Colville and Molday 1996). There are also two free protein forms of this GARP domain, GARP-1 and the slightly longer GARP-2 (Colville and Molday 1996; Korschen et al. 1999).

These proteins are intrinsically disordered and have been known to act as scaffolding type proteins in other tissues (Batra-Safferling et al. 2006). Molday's group has shown that both free GARP and the GARP domain of the CNG channel β subunit can interact with RDS (Poetsch et al. 2001) in bovine rod OSs. They hypothesize that CNG-GARP-RDS interactions might be responsible for the anchoring filaments that have been observed between the disc rim and plasma membrane of rods (Poetsch et al. 2001; Roof and Heuser 1982). They further hypothesize that interactions between free GARP and RDS might serve to connect adjacent discs. Although there is no direct proof supporting this hypothesis, advanced structural analysis of GARP has shown that its size and shape are consistent with this role (Batra-Safferling et al. 2006).

Cones also have a cGMP gated channel responsible for maintenance of the dark, "off" current, but it is not the same channel as that expressed in rods. It is thought that differences in the regulation/kinetics of the cone vs. rod CNG channels help explain the differences in phototransduction kinetics between the two cell types. Cone channels have a ten-fold lower ligand sensitivity than rod channels and are between 30 and 100 times less sensitive to light (Picones and Korenbrot 1995; Pugh 2000). It has recently been shown that the cone channel also functions as a heterotetramers composed of α and β subunits (Matveev et al. 2008). The β subunit of the cone channel does not have a GARP domain, so we hypothesized that RDS would not interact with the cone channel thus partially explaining the differential role of RDS in rods vs. cones.

Our first step was to determine expression of the cone CNG channel in WT and $nrl^{-/-}$ retina using polyclonal antibodies against the cone CNG channel subunit CNGA3 and CNGB3 (Matveev et al. 2008). Immunohistochemical analysis of retinal sections taken from 1-month-old animals labeled with the CNGA3 and CNGB3 antibodies demonstrates that both subunits of the cone CNG channel are expressed in the cone OSs of WT and $nrl^{-/-}$ retinas (Fig. 8.1a). We do not detect any protein expression in other retinal cell types, or in other portions of the photoreceptor. The labeling pattern in the WT retina is consistent with cone-only expression, but to confirm this, co-labeling studies were undertaken with rod opsin (mAB 1D4, generously shared by Dr. Robert Molday) and CNGA3. The left panel of Fig. 8.1b shows CNGA3 labeling while the middle panel is rhodopsin (1D4) labeling. The labeling patterns are quite distinct and the two proteins do not co-localize (overlay, right) indicating that cone CNG is not expressed in rods. To confirm the size of the

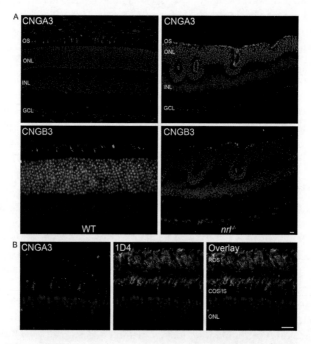

Fig. 8.1 CNGA3 and CNGB3 is expressed in cones OSs of WT and $nrl^{-/-}$ Retinas; (**a**) Paraffin embedded sections from P30 WT or $nrl^{-/-}$ mice were stained with CNGA3 and CNGB3 polyclonal antibodies and visualized using anti-rabbit Cy3 secondary antibody. Sections were counterstained with DAPI to label nuclei. Expression of cone channel subunits is limited to the OS layer in both WT and $nrl^{-/-}$ retina. Scale bar 20 μm. (**b**) P30 WT paraffin embedded sections were stained with CNGA3 (*left*) and mAB 1D4 (against rhodopsin-middle). The two proteins do not co-localize (*right*) indicating that cone CNG is not expressed in rods. Scale bar 10 μm. OS, *outer segment*; ONL, outer nuclear layer; INL, inner nuclear layer; GCL, ganglion cell layer

cone CNG subunits, whole retinal extracts from P30 retinas underwent reducing and non-reducing SDS-PAGE/Western blotting. Rod-dominant WT extracts were used as controls while $nrl^{-/-}$ was used as a cone-dominant model. Historically, the only available cone-dominant model has been the young rhodopsin knockout ($rho^{-/-}$) retina, so those retinas were also included as a control, although they express significantly lower quantities of cone proteins than the $nrl^{-/-}$ retina. Under reducing conditions, both the α and β subunits of cone CNG appear as monomers of approximately 75 kDa (Fig. 8.2a, b left) in all samples. This is consistent with the predicted peptide sizes of 72 kDa (A) and 79 kDa (B) and is in contrast to rod CNG channel subunits which have been shown to migrate abnormally on SDS-PAGE (Poetsch et al. 2001). The involvement of disulfide-linkages in multi-subunit channel assembly was examined by non-reducing SDS-PAGE. A significant amount of CNGB3 dimer was detected at ~170 kDa (Fig. 8.2b, right) although little dimerization of CNGA3 was noticed in these retinas (Fig. 8.2a, right).

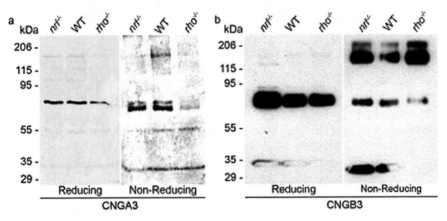

Fig. 8.2 CNGB3 is present as both a monomer and dimer, while CNGA3 is present only as a monomer; Retinal extracts from P30 WT (rod-dominant), $nrl^{-/-}$ and $rho^{-/-}$ (cone-dominant) mice underwent reducing (*left*) and non-reducing (*right*) SDS-PAGE and Western blotting. (**a**) CNGA3 is only present as the monomeric form (~75 kDa) while CNGB3 (**b**) exhibits a substantial quantity of both monomer and dimer

Since previous studies had shown that the bovine rod CNG channel associates with RDS (Poetsch et al. 2001) via the GARP portion of the CNG β-subunit, we wanted to confirm that we could detect this interaction in mice. Retinal extracts from one month old WT mice underwent immunoprecipitation (IP) with either the RDS antibody or the GARP monoclonal antibody 4B1 (generously shared by Dr. Robert Molday, University of British Columbia). Bovine rod OSs were used as a positive control while $nrl^{-/-}$ retinal extracts served as a negative control since they do not express the rod CNG-GARP. As shown in Fig. 8.3a (input), WT retinal extracts express both splice variants of free GARP while the rodless $nrl^{-/-}$ retinas do not. As demonstrated by reciprocal co-IP shown in the left two panels of Fig. 8.3a, in mouse rods, RDS does interact with GARP. To determine whether the cone CNG β-subunit

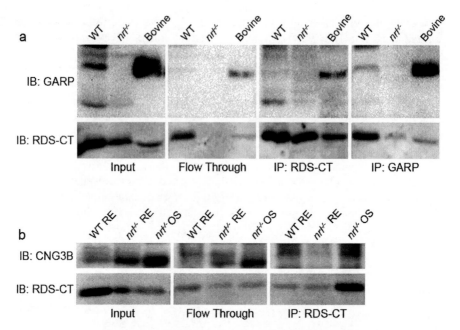

Fig. 8.3 The rod CNG β subunit interacts with RDS while the cone CNG β subunit does not; (a) Retinal extracts from WT and *nrl*[−/−] P30 mice and bovine OSs underwent IP using either RDS C-terminal antibody or monoclonal (4B1) GARP antibody. This reciprocal co-IP confirms that rod CNG does interact with RDS. (b) WT and *nrl*[−/−] retinal extracts and *nrl*[−/−] OSs underwent IP with RDS C-terminal antibody. Although CNGB3 was present in the samples, none was detected in the immunoprecipitants

interacts with RDS, similar experiments were undertaken. RDS complexes from WT and *nrl*[−/−] retinal extracts or *nrl*[−/−] OS preparations were immunoprecipitated using the RDS antibody. OS preparations (Chakraborty et al. 2008) were used as an enriched source of OS proteins such as CNG and RDS. The IP was successful as evidenced by detection of RDS in all three samples (Fig. 8.3b, bottom). However the β subunit of cone CNG was not detected in any of the immunoprecipitants although it was detected in the initial samples (Fig. 8.3b, top left).

These results confirm our hypothesis that the cone CNG β-subunit does not interact with RDS, most likely due to the lack of a GARP domain in the cone channel. Furthermore, they clearly identify the first difference in the RDS tetraspanin web in rods vs. cones. It is likely that additional study will identify further RDS interacting partners that are rod or cone specific and will further enhance our understanding of the role of RDS in OS biogenesis.

Acknowledgment The monoclonal antibodies for this study (4B1 and 1D4) were generously shared with us by Dr. Robert Molday, University of British Columbia. This study was supported by grants from the National Institutes of Health (EY10609 & EY018656), Core Grant for Vision Research EY12190, and the Foundation Fighting Blindness. Dr. Naash is the recipient of a Research to Prevent Blindness James S. Adams Scholar Award.

References

Arikawa K, Molday LL, Molday RS et al (1992) Localization of peripherin/rds in the disk membranes of cone and rod photoreceptors: relationship to disk membrane morphogenesis and retinal degeneration. J Cell Biol 116:659

Batra-Safferling R, Abarca-Heidemann K, Korschen HG et al (2006) Glutamic acid-rich proteins of rod photoreceptors are natively unfolded. J Biol Chem 281:1449

Boesze-Battaglia K (2000) Fusion between retinal rod outer segment membranes and model membranes: functional assays and role for peripherin/rds. Methods Enzymol 316:65

Boesze-Battaglia K, Song H, Sokolov M et al (2007) The tetraspanin protein peripherin-2 forms a complex with melanoregulin, a putative membrane fusion regulator. Biochemistry 46:1256

Chaitin MH, Carlsen RB, Samara GJ (1988) Immunogold localization of actin in developing photoreceptor cilia of normal and rds mutant mice. Exp Eye Res 47:437

Chakraborty D, Ding XQ, Fliesler SJ et al (2008) Outer segment oligomerization of rds: evidence from mouse models and subcellular fractionation. Biochemistry 47:1144

Cheng T, Peachey NS, Li S et al (1997) The effect of peripherin/rds haploinsufficiency on rod and cone photoreceptors. J Neurosci 17:8118

Colville CA, Molday RS (1996) Primary structure and expression of the human beta-subunit and related proteins of the rod photoreceptor cGMP-gated channel. J Biol Chem 271:32968

Daniele LL, Lillo C, Lyubarsky AL et al (2005) Cone-like morphological, molecular, and electrophysiological features of the photoreceptors of the Nrl knockout mouse. Invest Ophthalmol Vis Sci 46:2156

Farjo Q, Jackson A, Pieke-Dahl S et al (1997) Human bZIP transcription factor gene NRL: structure, genomic sequence, and fine linkage mapping at 14q11.2 and negative mutation analysis in patients with retinal degeneration. Genomics 45:395

Farjo Q, Jackson AU, Xu J et al (1993) Molecular characterization of the murine neural retina leucine zipper gene, Nrl. Genomics 18:216

Goldberg AF, Molday RS (2000) Expression and characterization of peripherin/rds-rom-1 complexes and mutants implicated in retinal degenerative diseases. Methods Enzymol 316:671

Goldberg AF, Moritz OL, Molday RS (1995) Heterologous expression of photoreceptor peripherin/rds and Rom-1 in COS-1 cells: assembly, interactions, and localization of multisubunit complexes. Biochemistry 34:14213

Hawkins RK, Jansen HG, Sanyal S (1985) Development and degeneration of retina in rds mutant mice: photoreceptor abnormalities in the heterozygotes. Exp Eye Res 41:701

Hemler ME (2003) Tetraspanin proteins mediate cellular penetration, invasion, and fusion events and define a novel type of membrane microdomain. Annu Rev Cell Dev Biol 19:397

Kaupp UB, Niidome T, Tanabe T et al (1989) Primary structure and functional expression from complementary DNA of the rod photoreceptor cyclic GMP-gated channel. Nature 342:762

Korschen HG, Beyermann M, Muller F et al (1999) Interaction of glutamic-acid-rich proteins with the cGMP signalling pathway in rod photoreceptors. Nature 400:761

Levy S, Shoham T (2005) Protein-protein interactions in the tetraspanin web. Physiology (Bethesda) 20:218

Matveev AV, Quiambao AB, Browning Fitzgerald J et al (2008) Native cone photoreceptor cyclic nucleotide-gated channel is a heterotetrameric complex comprising both CNGA3 and CNGB3: a study using the cone-dominant retina of Nrl–/– mice. J Neurochem 106:2042

Mears AJ, Kondo M, Swain PK et al (2001) Nrl is required for rod photoreceptor development. Nat Genet 29:447

Mitton KP, Swain PK, Chen S et al (2000) The leucine zipper of NRL interacts with the CRX homeodomain. A possible mechanism of transcriptional synergy in rhodopsin regulation. J Biol Chem 275:29794

Moritz OL, Peck A, Tam BM (2002) Xenopus laevis red cone opsin and Prph2 promoters allow transgene expression in amphibian cones, or both rods and cones. Gene 298:173

Nikonov SS, Daniele LL, Zhu X et al (2005) Photoreceptors of Nrl –/– mice coexpress functional S- and M-cone opsins having distinct inactivation mechanisms. J Gen Physiol 125:287

Picones A, Korenbrot JI (1995) Spontaneous, ligand-independent activity of the cGMP-gated ion channels in cone photoreceptors of fish. J Physiol 485 (Pt 3):699

Poetsch A, Molday LL, Molday RS (2001) The cGMP-gated channel and related glutamic acid-rich proteins interact with peripherin-2 at the rim region of rod photoreceptor disc membranes. J Biol Chem 276:48009

Pugh EN (2000) Handbook of biological physics. Elsevier/North-Holland, Amsterdam

Rehemtulla A, Warwar R, Kumar R et al (1996) The basic motif-leucine zipper transcription factor Nrl can positively regulate rhodopsin gene expression. Proc Natl Acad Sci USA 93:191

Roof DJ, Heuser JE (1982) Surfaces of rod photoreceptor disk membranes: integral membrane components. J Cell Biol 95:487

Sanyal S, De Ruiter A, Hawkins RK (1980) Development and degeneration of retina in rds mutant mice: light microscopy. J Comp Neurol 194:193

Sanyal S, Dees C, Zeilmaker GH (1986) Development and degeneration of retina in rds mutant mice: observations in chimaeras of heterozygous mutant and normal genotype. J Embryol Exp Morphol 98:111

Sanyal S, Zeilmaker GH (1984) Development and degeneration of retina in rds mutant mice: light and electron microscopic observations in experimental chimaeras. Exp Eye Res 39:231

Stipp CS, Kolesnikova TV, Hemler ME (2003) Functional domains in tetraspanin proteins. Trends Biochem Sci 28:106

Swaroop A, Xu JZ, Pawar H et al (1992) A conserved retina-specific gene encodes a basic motif/leucine zipper domain. Proc Natl Acad Sci USA 89:266

Chapter 9
Increased Expression of TGF-β1 and Smad 4 on Oxygen-Induced Retinopathy in Neonatal Mice

Fan Yingchuan, Lei Chuntao, Chen Hui, and Hu Jianbin

Abstract Retinal neovascularization (NV) is a major cause of the blindness associated with such ischemic retinal disorders as diabetic retinopathy, retinopathy of prematurity and retinal occlusion. Neovascularization is induced by complex interactions among growth factors and cytokines. Some studies confirm that VEGF play a central role in neovascularization, there remain some questions as to why VEGF antagonists are only partially effective. Transforming growth factor-β (TGF-β) has been implicated in the development of neovascularization (Gerard et al. 2000). Smad 4 plays the most important role in the TGF-β signal transduction (Zimowska 2006). In this study, we used the model of oxygen-induced retinopathy in neonatal mice to investigate the expression of TGF-β1 and Smad 4 mRNA in the retina, to explore their role in the development of retinal neovascularization.

9.1 Introduction

Retinal neovascularization (NV) is a major cause of the blindness associated with such ischemic retinal disorders as diabetic retinopathy, retinopathy of prematurity and retinal occlusion. Neovascularization is induced by complex interactions among growth factors and cytokines. Some studies confirm that VEGF play a central role in neovascularization, there remain some questions as to why VEGF antagonists are only partially effective. Transforming growth factor-β (TGF-β) has been implicated in the development of neovascularization (Gerard et al. 2000). Smad 4 plays the most important role in the TGF-β signal transduction (Zimowska 2006). In this study, we used the model of oxygen-induced retinopathy in neonatal mice to

L. Chuntao and C. Hui (✉)
Department of Ophthalmology, Sichuan Provincial People's Hospital, Chengdu, Sichuan, 610072, China
e-mail: hblct@163.com; chenhuicq@yahoo.com.cn

R.E. Anderson et al. (eds.), *Retinal Degenerative Diseases*, Advances in Experimental Medicine and Biology 664, DOI 10.1007/978-1-4419-1399-9_9,
© Springer Science+Business Media, LLC 2010

investigate the expression of TGF-β1 and Smad 4 mRNA in the retina, to explore their role in the development of retinal neovascularization.

9.2 Material and Methods

9.2.1 Animals

All experimental procedures were approved by the institutional committee for the use of Animals in Research and Education. Oxygen-induced retinopathy was induced in C57BL/6 newborn mice according to the protocol of Smith (Smith et al. 1994). Briefly, litters of 7-day-old mice, together with their mothers, were exposed to 75% ± 3% oxygen for 5 days and then returned to room air, followed by 5 days of room air recovery. Another natural sized litter was raised in room air as normal control. 17-day-old mice were killed by intraperitoneal injections of overdose of sodium pentobarbital. Both eyes were enucleated and placed in 4% Para formaldehyde in PBS, and embedded in paraffin. Serial 3-um axial sections of the retina were obtained. Sections were stained with hematoxylin and eosin. Numbers of nuclei on the internal limiting membrane at the vitreous side were counted.

9.2.2 Methods

9.2.2.1 TGF-β Immunohistochemistry (IH) and Smad-4 In Situ Hybridization (ISH)

Monoclonal TGF-β1 antibody was obtained from Santa Cruz Company. The reagents for streptavidin-biotin and DAB were obtained from Zymed Company. The dilution of the primary antibody was 1:100 and DAB was used for the detection. PBS replacing the primary antibody was used as control.

Expression of Smad-4 was detected by in situ hybridization (ISH). A biotin conjugated oligonucleotide probe of mouse Smad-4 was synthesized by Shanghai Shenneng Biological Company (5'-Biotin-GGT GGC GTT AGA CTC TGC CGG GGC TAA CAG-3'; 1035–1064 bp, GC% = 63.33). The secondary detection reagents were streptavidin-conjugated to HRP, and DAB, respectively. PBS replacing the probe was used as control.

The images were captures and analyzed with Image-pro Plus software system. The result of ISH was semi-quantified with optical density value (OD).

9.2.3 Statistical Analysis

The experimental data presented as mean ± standard deviation. SPSS software was used for t test to compare between two groups. $P<0.05$ was considered statistically significant.

9.3 Results

Extensive vitreous neovascularization was noted in oxygen-induced mice, in which the number of endothelial nuclei were 22 ± 3.5 (Fig. 9.1a). While the control mice showed lesser neovascularization, and we detected only a single endothelial cell nuclei each in 4 control sections (Fig. 9.1b; $P < 0.01$).

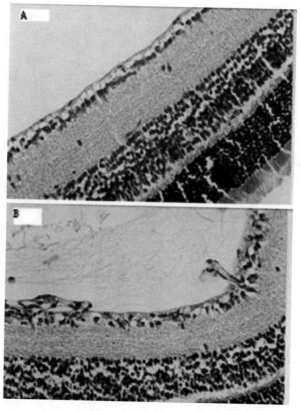

Fig. 9.1 HE strain, **a**: Normal control; **b**: Oxygen-induced group, which shows the endothelial cell entering into the internal limiting membrane

Positive brown signals in endothelial nuclei in the neovascularized region from IH and ISH were detected in the retina of all oxygen-induced group (Figs. 9.2a and 9.3a) and few in control group (Figs. 9.2b and 9.3b). The intensity of labeling recorded by Image-pro Plus software system were 0.214 ± 0.005 for IH and 0.209 ± 0.007 for ISH, while that in the control were 0.081 ± 0.007 for IH ($P < 0.01$) and 0.077 ± 0.005 for ISH ($P < 0.01$).

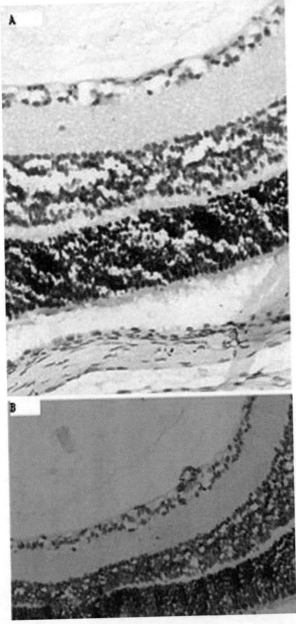

Fig. 9.2 IH, **a**: control group, in which few expression of TGF-β1 shown; **b**: Oxygen-induced group, marked expression of TGF-β1

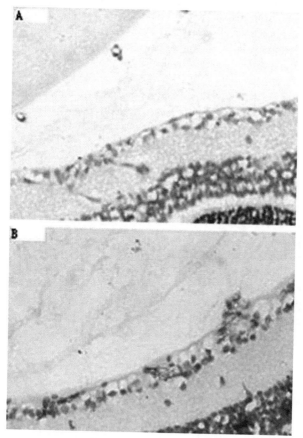

Fig. 9.3 ISH, **a**: control group, in which few expression of Smad 4 shown; **b**: Oxygen-induced group, marked expression of Smad 4

9.4 Discussion

TGF-β is a multifunctional cytokine with an array of biological effects such as cell growth, differentiation, and immunomodulation (Wakefield and Roberts 2002). In the experiment we found that expression of TGF-β1 and Smad-4 were increased in the retinal neovascular from oxygen-induced mice. But the roles of TGF-β1 and Smad 4 in the formation of neovascular are not clear.

Members of the transforming growth factor family (TGFb1, TGFb2, and TGFb3) are multifunctional proteins that regulate cell growth, differentiation, migration, and extracellular matrix production and also play important roles in embryonic development, wound healing, immune responses, and vascular development(Blobe et al. 2000; Behzadian et al. 2001). VEGF, on the other hand, shown to be play a critical role in the development of CNV and other retinal neovascularization disorders. There are some studies on the relationship between TGF-β and VEGF, which showed all three isoforms of TGF-β enhanced secretion of VEGF significantly. Increase in the mRNA levels of VEGF by TGF-β and blocking of its enhanced secretion by actinomycin-D, an inhibitor of transcription, suggested that TGF-β induced VEGF expression predominantly by transcriptional activation (Nagineni et al. 2003).

Current concept of TGFβ-Smad signaling pathway, which transfer the stimulating signal from outside into the affected cells by binding of the active form of TGF-β, to TGF-β receptor type II that initiates phosphorylation of TGF-β1 receptor type I, which is followed by the phosphorylation of receptor regulated Smad-2 and 3 proteins. These phosphorylated Smad proteins bind to costimulatory Smad protein (Smad-4) and are translocated to the nucleus for transmission of transcriptional signals (Mehra and Wrana 2000; Yamashita et al. 1997).

But on the contrary to the above findings, TGF-β has been shown to inhibit vascular tumor growth (Dong et al. 1996), in vitro studies have shown that TGF-β can inhibit proliferation of vascular endothelial cells and smooth muscle cells (Orlidge and D'Amore 1987). And also VEGF over expression in photoreceptors did not develop CNV in the transgenic mice. Therefore, the alternative hypothesis is that angiogenesis is stimulated by VEGF and other angiogenic factors released by the inflammatory cells and in cases where inflammatory reactions not observed, TGF-β does not induce angiogenesis. But in our experiment, we did not notice the inflammatory reaction, and therefore, we suggest that it may be related to the upregulated TGF-β (Zhao and Overbeek 2001).

In summary, our present study demonstrates the significant increase of TGF-β1 and Smad-4, which may play an important role in regulation of ocular vascular development. Further investigations are required to find out how TGF-β1 and Smad 4 signaling pathways act at molecular levels in regulation of vascular development. Understanding of the mechanism of TGF-β and Smad- mediated formation of neovascularization will provide new ideas to prevent or treat ocular neovascularization.

References

Behzadian MA, Wang XL, Windsor LJ et al (2001) TGF-beta increases retinal endothelial cell permeability by increasing MMP-9: possible role of glial cells in endothelial barrier function. Invest Ophthalmol Vis Sci 42:853–859

Blobe GC, Schiemann WP, Lodish HF (2000) Role of transforming growth factor b in human disease. N Engl J Med 342:1350–1358

Dong QG, Graziani A, Garlanda C et al (1996) Anti-tumor activity of cytokines against opportunistic vascular tumor in mice. Int J Cancer 65:700–708

Gerard C, William P, Harvey F (2000) Role of transforming growth factor ß in human disease. N Engl J Med 342:1350–1358

Mehra A, Wrana J (2000) TGF – beta and the Smad signal transduction pathway. Biochem Cell Biol 80:605–622

Nagineni CN, Samuel W, Nagineni S et al (2003) Transforming growth factor-beta induces expression of vascular endothelial growth factor in human retinal pigment epithelial cells: involvement of mitogen-activated protein kinases. J Cell Physiol 197:453–462

Orlidge A, D'Amore PA (1987) Inhibition of capillary endothelial cell growth by pericytes and smooth muscle cells. J Cell Biol 105:1455–1462

Smith LE, Wesolowski E, McLellan A et al (1994) Oxygen-induced retinopathy in the mouse. Invest Ophthalmol Vis Sci 35:101–111

Wakefield LM, Roberts AB (2002) TGF-b signaling: positive and negative effects on tumorigenesis. Curr Opinion Gen Dev 12:22–29

Yamashita H, Tobari I, Sawa M et al (1997) Functions of the transforming growth factor-beta super family in eyes. Nippon Ganka Gakkai Zasshi 101:927–947

Zhao S, Overbeek PA (2001) Elevated TGFbeta signaling inhibits ocular vascular development. Dev Biol 237:45–53

Zimowska M (2006) Signaling pathways of transforming growth factor beta family members. Postepy Biochem 52(4):360–366

Chapter 10
ZBED4, A Novel Retinal Protein Expressed in Cones and Müller Cells

Debora B. Farber, V.P. Theendakara, N.B. Akhmedov, and M. Saghizadeh

Abstract To identify genes expressed in cone photoreceptors, we previously carried out subtractive hybridization and microarrays of retinal mRNAs from normal and *cd* (cone degeneration) dogs. One of the isolated genes encoded ZBED4, a novel protein that in human retina is localized to cone photoreceptors and glial Müller cells. ZBED4 is distributed between nuclear and cytoplasmic fractions of the retina and it readily forms homodimers, probably as a consequence of its hATC dimerization domain. In addition, the ZBED4 sequence has several domains that suggest it may function as part of a co-activator complex facilitating the activation of nuclear receptors and other factors (BED finger domains) or as a co-activator/co-repressor of nuclear hormone receptors (LXXLL motifs). We have identified several putative ZBED4-interacting proteins and one of them is precisely a co-repressor of the estrogen receptor α.

10.1 Introduction

The most common types of inherited retinal degenerations in man and animals are those involving the specific demise of photoreceptor cells. The loss of rods occurs first in many of these disorders – usually as the result of mutated genes expressed selectively in rod photoreceptors – but it is followed by the demise of cones even when the defective gene is not expressed in these cells. In contrast, those retinal degenerations presenting first loss of cone photoreceptors caused by mutated genes expressed specifically in cones may or may not manifest subsequent loss of rods. Different hypotheses have been formulated as to why defective rod or cone-specific genes can lead to degeneration of the other type of photoreceptor. However, this is

D.B. Farber (✉)
Jules Stein Eye Institute, UCLA School of Medicine, 100 Stein Plaza, Los Angeles, CA 90095-7000, USA
e-mail: farber@jsei.ucla.edu

R.E. Anderson et al. (eds.), *Retinal Degenerative Diseases*, Advances in Experimental Medicine and Biology 664, DOI 10.1007/978-1-4419-1399-9_10,
© Springer Science+Business Media, LLC 2010

a subject that still needs to be studied much more, particularly because the relative paucity of cones in the mammalian retina has made their study difficult and has left behind the understanding of the molecular nature of our most used photoreceptors. In fact, very few cone genes have been characterized in detail and the functional significance of the majority of these genes remains unknown.

One of our goals has been precisely to isolate and characterize novel genes expressed in cones. We have already studied a few of these genes (i.e., Viczian et al. 1995; Ahkmedov et al. 1997; Ahkmedov et al. 1998; Reid et al. 1999; Akhmedov et al. 2002) and are currently involved in the characterization of *ZBED4*, a gene isolated by microarraying the output of the second round of Representational Difference Analysis using the mRNA from adult *cd* dog retina (that has lost a large number of its cones due to an autosomal recessive cone degeneration) and normal adult dog mRNA.

10.2 Methods and Results

The human ZBED4 gene contains two exons. The first exon (169 base pairs) is a part of the 5′ UTR; the second exon contains the rest of the 5′ UTR, the complete open reading frame and the 3′ UTR. After cloning and sequencing the complete *ZBED4* transcript, we confirmed that the generated sequence encodes a putative DNA-binding protein with several DNA binding domains and a dimerization domain (Fig. 10.1). In addition, human ZBED4 contains two LXXLL motifs, which are found in proteins that function as co-activators of nuclear hormone receptors. The presence of these motifs suggests a co-activator function for ZBED4. Overall, human, dog, mouse and rat ZBED4 proteins share 81–82% homology while chicken only exhibits 62% homology with the human counterpart.

10.2.1 ZBED4 mRNA is Expressed in Human Retina

Northern blots using human retinal RNA and a human 3′ UTR ZBED4 probe revealed two transcripts, 5.0 and 7.0 kb long. Both of these transcripts encode the same ZBED4 protein. The blot was also hybridized with a 5′ UTR/coding region probe. In this case, three transcripts were detected (5.0, 7.0 and 4.0 kb). All these mRNAs have been recently reported in the databases for ZBED4.

10.2.2 ZBED4 mRNA is Expressed in Mouse and Human Cones

Studies using real time PCR on mouse cone cells sorted by activated flow cytometry revealed the expression of *ZBED4* in cone photoreceptors. Dissociated mouse retinal cells were incubated with FITC-conjugated peanut agglutinin (PNA). PNA binds preferentially to galactosyl (ß-1, 3) N-acetylgalactosamine, which is present only in

A

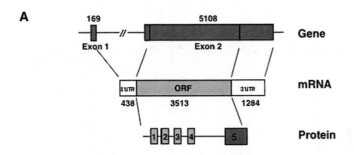

B

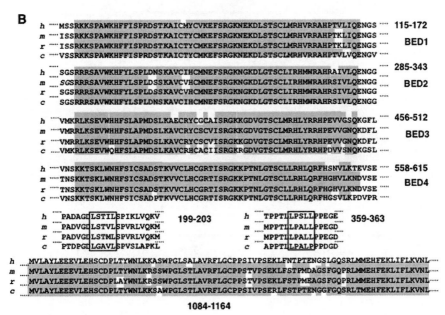

Fig. 10.1 (**a**) Diagrammatic representation of the genomic organization of human *ZBED4*, its corresponding mRNA and the conserved domains of the encoded protein; these domains are numbered: the zinc BED fingers (1–4) are shown as *light gray boxes* and the dimerization domain (5) as a *dark gray box*

the matrix surrounding cone photoreceptors, but not in that surrounding rods. FITC-labeled cone cells were then sorted by FACS (Fig. 10.2a) and their total RNA as well as that of the dissociated retinal cells was obtained. Figure 10.2b shows the results of the quantitative PCR experiments using these RNA samples and appropriate primers for *ZBED4*, cone *PDEα'*, and rod *PDEα* mRNAs. As we anticipated, the level of rod *PDEα* in the cone enriched cell fraction was barely detectable since PDEα is a rod-specific enzyme, whereas that of *PDEα'* mRNA was about 29-fold more abundant than *PDEα* in the cone enriched cell fraction. Accordingly, ZBED4 mRNA was also enriched by about 16-fold compared to *PDEα* mRNA.

A

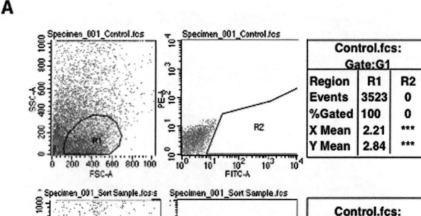

B

Genes	Fold expression of cone enriched/dissociated cells
PDEα'/ PDEα	29
ZBED4/PDEα	16

Fig. 10.2 FACS-sorted mouse cone cells and quantitative RT-PCR analysis of mRNA expression in sorted cones and non-sorted, dissociated cells; (**a**) A typical *dot* plot illustration of the cell suspension. *Upper panels*, control (not labeled cell suspension); *lower panels*, PNA-labeled cell suspension. Labeled cone cells from the R1 gated region were further sorted and found in the R2 region (*middle panels*). In these panels, the *x*-axis represents the relative fluorescence intensity, and the *y*-axis represents the relative granularity of cells. (**b**) cDNAs encoding rod *PDEα*, cone *PDEα'*, and *ZBED4* from cells before and after sorting were quantified by QPCR using β-actin cDNA as normalizer. Our results show the relative expression of cone *PDEα'* and ZBED4 mRNAs to rod PDEα mRNA in cone-enriched versus dissociated retinal cells

Sections of human retina used for in situ hybridization with a ZBED4 antisense riboprobe showed a positive signal in the inner segment of cone photoreceptor cells as expected. No signal was seen after hybridization with the control ZBED4 sense riboprobe (data not shown).

10.2.3 ZBED4 is Expressed Both in Nuclei and Cytoplasm of Human Cones

Immunohistochemistry studies were performed on sections of different donor human retinas and also on sections of cow retina using the polyclonal antibody generated against a ZBED4 N-terminus synthetic peptide. ZBED4 is present in the nucleus and in the inner segment of cones. The protein can also be observed in the pedicle of cones and in the innermost retinal layer (Fig. 10.3a). ZBED4 is not detectable in the outer segments. An oblique section of human retina (Fig. 10.3b) clearly shows the presence of ZBED4 in the cytoplasm of the inner segments. The same localization of ZBED4 can be seen in cow retina (Fig. 10.3c). Sections stained with pre-immune serum and with antibody against ZBED4 that had been pre-absorbed with the peptide used to generate it showed no positive signal.

10.2.3.1 Human ZBED4 is Also Expressed in Müller Cells Endfeet

In order to determine whether the anti-ZBED4 staining of the innermost retinal cell layer was specific for ganglion cells or the endfeet of Müller cells, we used markers for these cell types in double labeling experiments. Only the antibody against vimentin, a Müller glial cell marker, showed co-localization with ZBED4 at the Müller cell endfeet.

10.2.4 Human ZBED4 is Distributed Between Nuclear and Cytoplasmic Retinal Fractions

Cellular fractionation of human retinas was performed to separate nuclear and cytoplasmic extracts, followed by SDS-PAGE of the samples and immunoblotting. Anti ZBED4 polyclonal antibody specifically identified a protein with an apparent molecular mass of 135-kDa in both the nuclear and cytosolic extracts of human retina.

10.2.5 Subcellular Localization of ZBED4 in Stably Transfected Cells

To study the subcellular localization of ZBED4, its complete coding region was subcloned into the mammalian expression vector, pcDNA4/HisMax, tagged at the

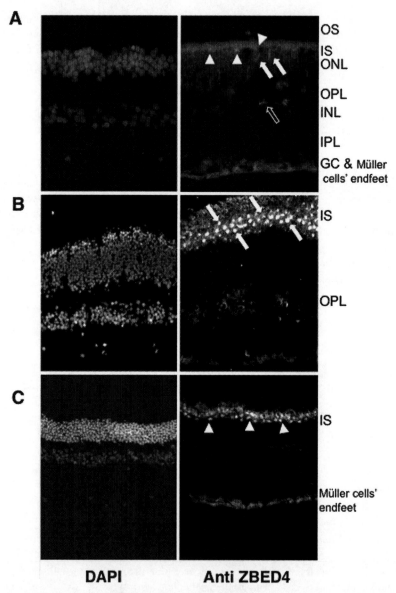

Fig. 10.3 Localization of the ZBED4 protein in human and bovine retinas; Human and bovine retinal sections were double-stained with N-terminus ZBED4 antibody followed by FITC-conjugated secondary antibody, rhodamine-conjugated PNA and DAPI. Individual images were obtained for the staining of nuclei (DAPI, *left panels*) and anti-ZBED4 (*right panels*) with the use of appropriate filters. (**a**) Human retinal section showing staining of cone nuclei (*arrows*) and cone *inner segments* (*arrowheads*). Note also the anti-ZBED4 staining of the *innermost layer* of the retina and of cone pedicles (*open arrowhead*). Magnification: 400X. (**b**) An obliquely cut retinal section shows the cone *inner segment* localization of ZBED4 (*arrows*). (**c**) Bovine retinal section, cone inner segment (*arrowheads*) are stained and to a lesser degree the endfeet of Müller cells. Magnification: 600X. *OS, outer segments*; *IS, inner segments*; *ONL*, outer nuclear layer; *OPL*, outer plexiform layer; *INL*, inner nuclear layer; *IPL*, inner plexiform layer; *GCL*, ganglion cell layer

N-terminus with both Xpress and poly-histidine (6-His) epitopes. HEK293 cells were stably transfected with this construct and the expressed fusion protein was double immunostained using an Anti-Xpress-FITC mouse monoclonal antibody and a rabbit polyclonal peptide antibody (aa 8–25) against ZBED4. Using fluorescence microscopy, the fusion protein was localized to the nuclei of transfected cells (Fig. 10.4) by both antibodies.

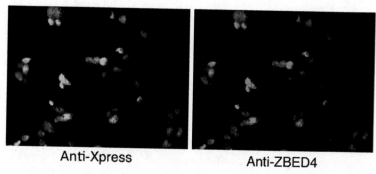

Anti-Xpress   Anti-ZBED4

Fig. 10.4 Intracellular distribution of the ZBED4 protein in HEK293 cells stably transfected with a ZBED4 expression vector; Cells were double stained with antibodies against ZBED4 and Xpress, and with DAPI for localization of nuclei. The images were obtained by fluorescence microscopy. Both antibodies detected nuclear localization of expressed ZBED4

10.2.6 Purification of His-Tagged ZBED4 and Its Dimerization In Vivo

A nickel column was used to purify the His-tagged ZBED4 from protein extracts corresponding to the nuclear fraction of the stably transfected HEK293 cells. Protein extracts from untransfected HEK 293 cells, stably transfected HEK 293 cells, and the purified His-tagged ZBED4 were then separated by SDS-PAGE on an inverted gradient gel. The presence of both the endogenous (135 kDa) and recombinant (139 kDa) ZBED4 proteins on the Western blot of the purified sample from the nickel column suggests self-association of these endogenous and recombinant ZBED4 proteins. The hATC domain of ZBED4 may be responsible for this dimerization. This is supported by studies that have shown that the conserved hydrophobic amino acids in the hATC domain of proteins function in self association, an essential feature required for nuclear accumulation (seen as puncta) and DNA binding (Yamashita et al. 2007).

10.2.7 Mass Spectrometry Identifies Putative Proteins Interacting with ZBED4

The enriched recombinant ZBED4 protein was subjected to SDS-PAGE on an inverted gradient gel and stained with SYPRO Ruby. The destained area of the gel that corresponded to the ZBED4 band on the Western blot was excised, trypsin-digested and subjected to MALDI-TOF-MS spectrometry. SAFB1 (scaffold attachment factor B1) is one of the proteins that were identified by mass spectrometry analysis. We are currently determining whether it interacts with ZBED4 (Table 10.1).

Table 10.1 Putative proteins interacting with ZBED4

Protein	Mr(expt)	Mr(calc)	Score	Peptide
SAFB1	1160.3943	1160.6111	69	K.ILDILGETCK.S
SF3B2	1231.3069	1231.6237	47	R.YGPPPSYPNLK.I
HNRPU	1646.9186	1646.8376	74	R.NFILDQTNVSAAAQR.R

10.3 Discussion

In the present study, we analyzed the expression of the novel ZBED4 mRNA and its encoded protein in human and mouse retinas, and in transfected HEK 293 cells. ZBED4 is an 1171 amino acid (~135 kDa) protein that has all the typical features of a nuclear regulatory protein. It contains four zinc finger BED domains with the characteristic $Cx_2Cx_nHx_{3-5}[H/C]$ signature in the amino-terminal-half, and a hATC dimerization domain in the carboxy-terminal end. In addition, two nuclear receptor-interacting modules (LXXLL) are present in the ZBED4 amino acid sequence.

Our in situ hybridization and FACS results indicated that the ZBED4 mRNA is expressed mostly in cone cells. Immunocytochemical localization of ZBED4 in human retinal sections using anti-ZBED4 antibodies showed a positive reaction in the inner segments of photoreceptors that were PNA-labeled, also indicating that the ZBED4 protein is expressed predominantly in cones. In addition, we demonstrated that the expression of this protein in the human retina is not only neuronal but, to a lesser degree, also glial, since we found it in the endfeet of Müller cells.

MALDI-TOF-MS spectrometry analysis of the ZBED4 protein band from the lane of the SDS-gel containing the enriched ZBED4 also identified another protein in the same band: the scaffold attachment factor B1. SAFB1 is known to be involved in chromatin organization, transcriptional regulation, RNA metabolism, stress response and can also function as a potent ERα co-repressor (Townson et al. 2003). Over-expression of SAFB1 inhibits ERα-mediated transcription, while its deletion from mouse embryo fibroblasts results in increased ERα activity (Oesterreich 2003). Since the sequence of ZBED4, just as that of SAFB1, indicates the presence of two nuclear receptor-interacting modules (LXXLL), ZBED4 may also be a co-activator/co-repressor of nuclear hormone receptors (NHRs). Therefore, we decided to characterize the interaction of ZBED4 and SAFB1 and to determine if they are part of the same activating or repressing complex. In addition to mediating effects of NHRs, some co-activators/co-repressors also seem to enhance the activity of other transcription factors such as c-Fos and c-Jun while others do not bind directly to NHRs but markedly enhance their ligand-dependent transcriptional activity in vivo by modulating another co-activator's activity (Clark et al. 1995). The characterization of ZBED4 and SAFB1 interaction will determine whether the complex binds to ERα and stimulates the transcription of cone-specific genes that have ERα response elements in their promoters. These studies may be of great significance as several epidemiological investigations have shown that changes in gene expression resulting from variations in hormonal regulation are associated with the incidence of ocular conditions such age-related macular degeneration (AMD) and idiopathic full thickness macular hole.

References

Akhmedov NB, Baldwin VJ, Zangerl B et al (2002) Cloning and characterization of the canine photoreceptor specific cone-rod homeobox (CRX) gene and evaluation as a candidate for early onset photoreceptor diseases in the dog. Mol Vis 8:79–84

Ahkmedov NB, Piriev NI, Pearce-Kelling S (1998) Canine cone transducin-γ gene and cone degeneration in the *cd* dog. Invest Ophthalmol Vis Sci 39:1775–1781

Ahkmedov NB, Piriev NI, Ray K et al (1997) Structure and analysis of the transducin β3-subunit gene, a candidate for inherited cone degeneration (*cd*) in the dog. Gene 194:47–56

Clark DV, Suleman DS, Beckenbach KA et al (1995) Molecular cloning and characterization of the dpy-20 gene of Caenorhabditis elegans. Mol Gen Genet 247:367–378

Oesterreich S (2003) Scaffold attachment factors SAFB1 and SAFB2: innocent bystanders or critical players in breast tumorigenesis? J Cell Biochem 90:653–661

Reid SNM, Akhmedov NB, Piriev NI (1999) The mouse X-linked juvenile retinoschisis cDNA: expression in photoreceptors. Gene 227:255–266

Townson SM, Dobrzycka KM, Lee AV et al (2003) SAFB2, a new scaffold attachment factor homolog and estrogen receptor corepressor. J Biol Chem 278:20059–20068

Viczian AS, Piriev NI, Farber DB (1995) Isolation and characterization of a cDNA encoding the α′ subunit of human cone cGMP-phosphodiesterase. Gene 166:205–211

Yamashita D, Komori H, Higuchi Y et al (2007) Human DNA replication-related element binding factor (hDREF) self-association via hATC domain is necessary for its nuclear accumulation and DNA binding. J Biol Chem 282:7563–7575

Chapter 11
Tubby-Like Protein 1 (Tulp1) Is Required for Normal Photoreceptor Synaptic Development

Gregory H. Grossman, Gayle J.T. Pauer, Umadevi Narendra, and Stephanie A. Hagstrom

Abstract Mutations in the photoreceptor-specific tubby-like protein 1 (*TULP1*) underlie a form of autosomal recessive retinitis pigmentosa in humans and photoreceptor degeneration in mice. In wild type (wt) mice, Tulp1 is localized to the photoreceptor inner segment, connecting cilium and synapse. To investigate the role of Tulp1 in the synapse, we examined the pre- and postsynaptic architecture in *tulp1–/–* mice. We used immunohistochemistry to examine *tulp1–/–* mice prior to retinal degeneration and made comparisons to wt littermates and rd10 mice. In the *tulp1–/–* synapse, the spatial relationship between the ribbon-associated proteins, Bassoon and Piccolo, are disrupted, and few intact ribbons are present. Furthermore, bipolar cell dendrites are stunted, most likely a direct consequence of the malformed photoreceptor synapses. Comparable abnormalities are not seen in rd10 mice. The association of early onset and severe photoreceptor degeneration, which is preceded by synaptic abnormalities, appears to represent a phenotype not previously described. Our new evidence indicates that Tulp1 is not only critical for photoreceptor function and survival, but is essential for the proper development of the photoreceptor synapse.

11.1 Introduction

Retinitis pigmentosa (RP) is a genetically and phenotypically heterogeneous disorder, affecting over 1 million individuals worldwide (Boughman et al. 1980; Bunker et al. 1984). Mutations in a gene named *TULP1* have been shown to cause a form of autosomal recessive RP (Hagstrom et al. 1998; Banerjee et al. 1998; Gu et al. 1998; Paloma et al. 2000). Tulp1 is expressed exclusively in photoreceptors, localizing to the inner segment (IS), connecting cilium (CC), perikarya and terminals,

S.A. Hagstrom (✉)
Department of Ophthalmic Research, Cole Eye Institute, Cleveland Clinic, 9500 Euclid Avenue; Department of Ophthalmology, Cleveland Clinic Lerner College of Medicine of Case Western Reserve University, Cleveland, OH 44195, USA
e-mail: hagstrs@ccf.org

R.E. Anderson et al. (eds.), *Retinal Degenerative Diseases*, Advances in Experimental Medicine and Biology 664, DOI 10.1007/978-1-4419-1399-9_11,
© Springer Science+Business Media, LLC 2010

which form synaptic contacts with dendrites of second order neurons in the outer plexiform layer (OPL) (Hagstrom et al. 1999; Ikeda et al. 2000; Hagstrom et al. 2001). Tulp1 is a cytoplasmic protein that associates with cellular membranes and the actin cytoskeleton (Xi et al. 2005). In *tulp1–/–* mice, there is an early-onset progressive photoreceptor degeneration, rod and cone opsins are mislocalized, and rhodopsin-bearing extracellular vesicles accumulate around the ellipsoid region of the IS (Hagstrom et al. 1999). These defects indicate that Tulp1 may be involved in actin cytoskeletal dynamics such as protein transport from the IS to the outer segment (OS) via the CC (Hagstrom et al. 1999; 2001; Xi et al. 2005; 2007). Additional evidence signifies that Tulp1 may also be involved in membrane dynamics at the highly active photoreceptor synapse. We have shown that Tulp1 co-localizes with and binds to the neuronal-specific protein Dynamin-1 at the IS and the photoreceptor terminals (Xi et al. 2007). Dynamin-1 is a GTPase that also binds actin and regulates vesicle movement at the trans-Golgi network, the plasma membrane and the synaptic membrane (van der Bliek 1999; McNiven et al. 2000; Xi et al. 2007). Furthermore, the b-wave component of the electroretinogram (ERG) generated by depolarizing bipolar cells (DBCs) is markedly reduced in young *tulp1–/–* mice, indicating an alteration in synaptic communication in the absence of Tulp1 (Xi et al. 2007). Based upon these findings, we hypothesize that Tulp1 plays a role in synaptic function.

In the present study, we examined the architecture of the *tulp1–/–* synapse at P16, an age at which synaptic development is complete in wild type (wt) mice (Dick et al. 2003), but precedes photoreceptor degeneration in *tulp1–/–* mice (Hagstrom et al. 1999). To test whether synaptic alterations are specific to the *tulp1–/–* retina and not a consequence of a generalized retinal degeneration, parallel studies were conducted in the retinal degeneration 10 (rd10) mouse, a mouse model of retinal degeneration due to a different molecular defect (Chang et al. 2002). These mice have a comparable rate of photoreceptor degeneration but do not exhibit early synaptic defects (Chang et al. 2007; Gargini et al. 2007). We show that at an early age, *tulp1–/–* mice lack the tight coupling between the ribbon-associated proteins, Bassoon and Piccolo, and few intact ribbons are present. In addition, dendrites of bipolar cells are attenuated at an early age. Similar defects are not seen in rd10 mice. Our results indicate that the absence of Tulp1 is associated with a synaptic malformation that precedes photoreceptor degeneration and most likely interferes with the proper development of post-receptoral dendrites. It is evident that Tulp1 plays an important role in photoreceptor synapse development as well as in photoreceptor function and survival.

11.2 Methods

11.2.1 Animals

The generation and genotyping of *tulp1–/–* mice has been described previously (Hagstrom et al. 1999). Homozygous rd10 breeders (B6.CXB1-*Pde6b*^{RD10}/J) were purchased from The Jackson Laboratory (Bar Harbor, Maine). Mice were euthanized by CO_2 inhalation followed by cervical dislocation. All experiments on animals were approved by the Institutional Animal Care and Use Committee of the Cleveland Clinic and were performed in compliance with the ARVO Statement for the Use of Animals in Ophthalmic and Visual Research.

11.2.2 Immunofluorescent Staining of Retinal Sections

Mouse eyes were prepared as previously described (Xi et al. 2007). Briefly, eyes were fixed in 4% paraformaldehyde, immersed through a graded series of sucrose solutions, embedded in OCT and flash frozen. The tissue was sectioned at 10 μm thickness using a cryostat. Retinal sections were blocked before incubation with primary antibodies overnight at 4°C. Primary antibodies and dilutions were as follows: Tulp1: rabbit polyclonal M-tulp1N 1:250 (Hagstrom et al. 2001); Piccolo: rabbit polyclonal 1:500 (ab20664: Abcam Inc); Bassoon: mouse monoclonal 1:500 (SAP7F407: Assay Designs Inc); Ribeye/CtBP2: mouse monoclonal 1:500 (612044: BD Biosciences); Protein Kinase C-α (PKC): rabbit polyclonal 1:1,000 (SC208: Santa Cruz Biotechnology Inc); Rhodopsin: mouse monoclonal 1:100 (B630N: P. Hargrave, Univ. of Florida). Sections were washed and incubated in fluorescent secondary antibodies at room temperature for 1 h. Secondary antibodies were: Alexa Fluor® 488 goat anti-rabbit IgG and goat anti-mouse IgG; Alexa Fluor® 594 goat anti-rabbit IgG and goat anti-mouse IgG (Invitrogen). The sections were then coverslipped in mounting media with DAPI (Vector Laboratories). Sections were imaged using an Olympus BX-60 fluorescent microscope equipped with a CCD monochrome camera (Hamamatsu Photonics, Bridgewater, NJ). For the imaging of ribbon-associated synaptic proteins (Bassoon, Piccolo and Ribeye), 2 μm Z-stacks were acquired using nearest neighbor deconvolution, followed by a maximum intensity Z-axis projection (SlideBook, Intelligent Imaging Innovations). For the co-localization of Bassoon and Piccolo, three-dimensional surface plots were generated from the Z-stacks.

11.3 Results

To describe the synaptic terminal architecture of tulp1–/– mice, we examined the distribution of synaptic proteins at ages prior to photoreceptor degeneration. Photoreceptor ribbon synapses are thought to be critical for the transport, release and recycling of synaptic vesicles (Morgans 2000; tom Dieck and Brandstätter 2006). Piccolo and Bassoon are proteins that have been associated with the organization of the photoreceptor synapse as well as the functioning of the ribbon (Dick et al. 2001; 2003). These proteins normally localize together at the presynaptic membrane with a crescent-like arrangement. We recently confirmed that Tulp1 is present in the photoreceptor synapse by its co-localization with Bassoon in the wt retina.

Figure 11.1a shows a surface plot of a wt mouse retinal section at P16, double-stained with antibodies to Piccolo (dark grey) and Bassoon (light grey). Arrows point to examples of the normal coupling between these two proteins. In contrast, the structure and distribution of both Piccolo and Bassoon staining appears abnormal in *tulp1–/–* mice at the same age (Fig. 11.1b). Their staining appears punctate, and normal ribbons are rarely seen. Furthermore, even though the two proteins are in close proximity, only a few terminals display any coupling between Piccolo and Bassoon (Fig. 11.1b; arrowheads indicate independent ribbon staining). Interestingly, Piccolo and Bassoon are correctly aligned in the terminals of rd10 mice at P16 (Fig. 11.1c). Moreover, this coupling is maintained at P21 (Fig. 11.1d), a time point at which photoreceptor cell death is maximal (Chang et al. 2007; Gargini et al. 2007), suggesting that the structural disturbance in the *tulp1–/–* photoreceptor synapse is not the result of an early degenerative process.

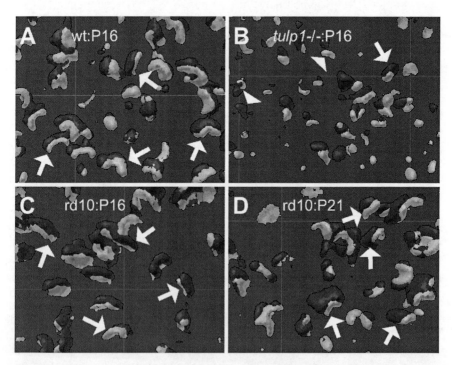

Fig. 11.1 Three-dimensional surface plots of Bassoon (*light grey*) and Piccolo (*dark grey*) immunofluorescence from the OPL of mouse retinal sections. In the wt OPL at P16 (**a**), rd10 at P16 (**c**) and P21 (**d**), photoreceptor synaptic ribbons are clearly visible. *Arrows* point to the coupling of Bassoon and Piccolo, forming individual crescent-shaped ribbons. In the *tulp1–/–* OPL at P16 (**b**), the ribbons appear to exhibit morphological anomalies, indicative of a structural defect. While both proteins are present and in close proximity, they are not united into the classic crescent-shaped ribbon formation (*arrowheads* highlight the separate ribbon staining of Bassoon and Piccolo). Gridlines, 10 μm

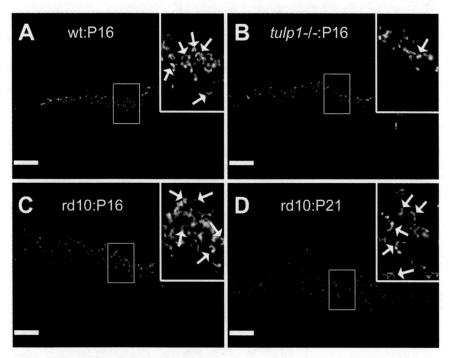

Fig. 11.2 Immunofluorescent staining of Ribeye in the OPL of mouse retinal sections. In the wt OPL at P16 (**a**), rd10 at P16 (**c**) and P21 (**d**), the synaptic ribbons decorated with Ribeye immunoreactivity display the classic crescent-like appearance (*arrows* highlight examples in magnified insets). In contrast, few intact ribbons are detectable in the *tulp1–/–* OPL at P16 (**b**). Scale bar, 10 μm

We further characterized the synaptic architecture using antibodies against Ribeye, a protein thought to constitute the core of the ribbon (Schmitz et al. 2000). Ribeye co-localizes and binds with Piccolo and Bassoon (tom Dieck et al. 2005; Heidelberger et al. 2005). Figure 11.2a shows that in the P16 wt OPL, numerous distinct crescent-shaped Ribeye-positive ribbons (see arrows) can be observed. This is also the case in rd10 retinas at P16 (Fig. 11.2c) and P21 (Fig. 11.2d), prior to and after the commencement of retinal degeneration. In contrast, the P16 *tulp1–/–* retina contains few normal ribbons (Fig. 11.2b), providing further evidence of a malformation of the ribbon synapse.

Next, we investigated the downstream consequences of the photoreceptor synaptic malformation on postsynaptic targets in *tulp1–/–* retinas using antibodies against Protein Kinase C-α (PKC), which labels rod DBCs and their dendrites (Greferath et al. 1990). At P16, wt DBC dendrites have elongated dendrites that penetrate the OPL, and each termination has a high degree of branching (Fig. 11.3a; vertical lines track a process of an individual DBC – indicated by an arrow). In contrast, DBC dendrites of P16 *tulp1–/–* mice are notably shorter and present far less branching (Fig. 11.3b). Interestingly, DBC terminals of the

Fig. 11.3 Immunofluorescent staining of DBC bodies (*arrows*) and dendrites (*vertical lines*) in the OPL of mouse retinal sections. In the wt OPL at P16 (**a**) and rd10 at P16 (**c**), long dendrites display ornate branching. In contrast, both the *tulp1–/–* OPL at P16 (**b**) and rd10 at P21 (**d**) have severely shortened dendrites. However, branching is still observed in the rd10 OPL at P16. Scale bar, 10 μm

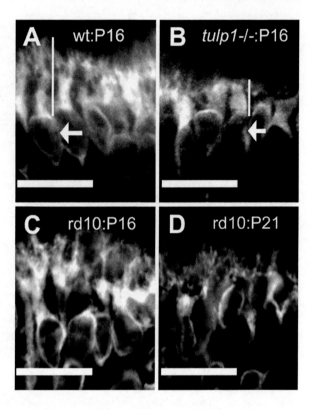

P16 rd10 retina resemble those of wt (Fig. 11.3c). DBC dendritic retraction was, however, noted in the P21 rd10 retina (Fig. 11.3d), which resembled the P16 *tulp1–/–* phenotype.

11.4 Discussion

In young *tulp1–/–* mice, two key ribbon-associated proteins, Piccolo and Bassoon, are rarely united into the horseshoe shape characteristic of the wt photoreceptor ribbon synaptic complex. These proteins are, however, situated in close proximity to one another and are both confined to the OPL. These observations indicate that in the absence of Tulp1, Piccolo and Bassoon are able to arrive at their correct destination, but are unable to coordinate into the normal synaptic architecture. In addition, immunostaining for Ribeye showed that in the *tulp1–/–* retina, few intact ribbons are present. We note that prior to and during the height of photoreceptor degeneration, normal synaptic architecture is readily seen in the rd10 retina. This does not necessarily indicate that the observed synaptic defects are unique to the *tulp1–/–* retina, but it does make clear that generalized photoreceptor degeneration is not sufficient to induce synaptic alterations. However, it may be the case that defects in ribbon-associated proteins are specific to mutants involving proteins that are critical for photoreceptor synapse formation.

Concomitant with a presynaptic malformation and prior to retinal degeneration, we show that mice lacking Tulp1 have a reduced dendritic composition. Due to the photoreceptor presynaptic structural defects in the *tulp1–/–* retina, we hypothesize that there should be a reduction in the signaling to second-order neurons. The attenuation of photoreceptor signaling has been associated with the consequent alterations in the downstream neural layers of the retina (Marc et al. 2003; Léveillard et al. 2004). Therefore, we hypothesize that the reduction of the DBC dendritic composition in *tulp1–/–* mice is a direct result of a decrease in neurotrophic and/or neurotransmitter release. It is important to note that in the rd10 retina, a reduction in length and branching of DBC dendrites is noted only during the height of photoreceptor cell death. The atrophy of postsynaptic dendritic processes has been observed in many models of retinal degeneration, and has been termed retraction to denote the negative remodeling from a prior developed state as a direct and downstream effect of photoreceptor cell death (Marc et al. 2003; Gargini et al. 2007). However, in the *tulp1–/–* retina, shortened dendrite lengths as well as reduced branching are detected prior to photoreceptor cell death.

In conclusion, the absence of Tulp1 results in abnormalities that affect structure and function in multiple retinal sites. The photoreceptor degeneration and OS defects of *tulp1–/–* mice have been described, providing evidence that Tulp1 may function in the polarized transport of proteins at the apical end of the photoreceptor (Hagstrom et al. 1999; 2001). We have shown that Tulp1 interacts with Actin and Dynamin-1, two proteins known to be critical in the cytoskeletal scaffold and involved in the molecular pathway of vesicular protein transport occurring from the IS to the OS and in vesicle cycling at photoreceptor terminals (Xi et al. 2005; 2007). Thus, Tulp1 may be functioning in intracellular protein trafficking throughout the photoreceptor cell, and in its absence, two distinct abnormalities at polar ends of the cell are highlighted. Here we provide evidence that photoreceptor ribbon synapses and DBC dendrites are also severely affected at an early age. These new findings indicate that Tulp1 is essential for photoreceptor cell survival, and is also required for the proper development of the photoreceptor synapse.

References

Banerjee P, Kleyn PW, Knowles JA et al (1998) TULP1 mutation in two extended Dominican kindreds with autosomal recessive retinitis pigmentosa. Nat Genet 18(2):177–179

Boughman JA, Conneally PM, Nance WE (1980) Population genetic studies of retinitis pigmentosa. Am J Hum Genet 32(2):223–235

Bunker CH, Berson EL, Bromley WC, Hayes RP, Roderick TH (1984) Prevalence of retinitis pigmentosa in Maine. Am J Ophthalmol 97(3):357–365

Chang B, Hawes NL, Hurd RE, Davisson MT, Nusinowitz S, Heckenlively JR (2002) Retinal degeneration mutants in the mouse. Vision Res 42(4):517–525

Chang B, Hawes NL, Pardue MT et al (2007) Two mouse retinal degenerations caused by missense mutations in the beta-subunit of rod cGMP phosphodiesterase gene. Vision Res 47(5):624–633

Dick O, Dieck S, Altrock WD et al (2003) The presynaptic active zone protein bassoon is essential for photoreceptor ribbon synapse formation in the retina. Neuron 37(5):775–786

Dick O, Hack I, Altrock WD, Garner CC, Gundelfinger ED, Brandstätter JH (2001) Localization of the presynaptic cytomatrix protein Piccolo at ribbon and conventional synapses in the rat retina: comparison with Bassoon. J Comp Neurol 439(2):224–234

Gargini C, Terzibasi E, Mazzoni F, Strettoi E (2007) Retinal organization in the retinal degeneration 10 (rd10) mutant mouse: a morphological and ERG study. J Comp Neurol 500(2):222–238

Greferath U, Grünert U, Wässle H (1990) Rod bipolar cells in the mammalian retina show protein kinase C-like immunoreactivity. J Comp Neurol 301(3):433–442

Gu S, Lennon A, Li Y et al (1998) Tubby-like protein-1 mutations in autosomal recessive retinitis pigmentosa. Lancet 351(9109):1103–1104

Hagstrom SA, Adamian M, Scimeca M, Pawlyk BS, Yue G, Li T (2001) A role for the Tubby-like protein 1 in rhodopsin transport. Invest Ophthalmol Vis Sci 42(9):1955–1962

Hagstrom SA, Duyao M, North MA, Li T (1999) Retinal degeneration in tulp1–/– mice: vesicular accumulation in the interphotoreceptor matrix. Invest Ophthalmol Vis Sci 40(12):2795–2802

Hagstrom SA, North MA, Nishina PM, Berson EL, Dryja TP (1998) Recessive mutations in the gene encoding the tubby-like protein TULP1 in patients with retinitis pigmentosa. Nat Genet 18(2):174–176

Heidelberger R, Thoreson WB, Witkovsky P (2005) Synaptic transmission at retinal ribbon synapses. Prog Retin Eye Res 24(6):682–720

Ikeda S, Shiva N, Ikeda A et al (2000) Retinal degeneration but not obesity is observed in null mutants of the tubby-like protein 1 gene. Hum Mol Genet 9(2):155–163

Léveillard T, Mohand-Saïd S, Lorentz O et al (2004) Identification and characterization of rod-derived cone viability factor. Nat Genet 36(7):755–759

Marc RE, Jones BW, Watt CB, Strettoi E (2003) Neural remodeling in retinal degeneration. Prog Retin Eye Res 22(5):607–655

McNiven MA, Cao H, Pitts KR, Yoon Y (2000) The dynamin family of mechanoenzymes: pinching in new places. Trends Biochem Sci 25(3):115–120

Morgans CW (2000) Presynaptic proteins of ribbon synapses in the retina. Microsc Res Tech 50(2):141–150

Paloma E, Hjelmqvist L, Bayés M et al (2000) Novel mutations in the TULP1 gene causing autosomal recessive retinitis pigmentosa. Invest Ophthalmol Vis Sci 41(3):656–659

Schmitz F, Königstorfer A, Südhof TC (2000) RIBEYE, a component of synaptic ribbons: a protein's journey through evolution provides insight into synaptic ribbon function. Neuron 28(3):857–872

tom Dieck S, Altrock WD, Kessels MM et al (2005) Molecular dissection of the photoreceptor ribbon synapse: physical interaction of Bassoon and RIBEYE is essential for the assembly of the ribbon complex. J Cell Biol 168(5):825–836

tom Dieck S, Brandstätter JH (2006) Ribbon synapses of the retina. Cell Tissue Res 326(2):339–346

van der Bliek AM (1999) Functional diversity in the dynamin family. Trends Cell Biol 9(3):96–102

Xi Q, Pauer GJ, Ball SL et al (2007) Interaction between the photoreceptor-specific tubby-like protein 1 and the neuronal-specific GTPase dynamin-1. Invest Ophthalmol Vis Sci 48(6):2837–2844

Xi Q, Pauer GJ, Marmorstein AD, Crabb JW, Hagstrom SA (2005) Tubby-like protein 1 (TULP1) interacts with F-actin in photoreceptor cells. Invest Ophthalmol Vis Sci 46(12):4754–4761

Chapter 12
Growth-Associated Protein43 (GAP43) Is a Biochemical Marker for the Whole Period of Fish Optic Nerve Regeneration

Manabu Kaneda, Mikiko Nagashima, Kazuhiro Mawatari, Tomoya Nunome, Kenichiro Muramoto, Kayo Sugitani, and Satoru Kato

Abstract In adult visual system, goldfish can regrow their axons and fully restore their visual function even after optic nerve transection. The optic nerve regeneration process in goldfish is very long and it takes about a half year to fully recover visual function via synaptic refinement. Therefore, we investigated time course of growth-associated protein 43 (GAP43) expression in the goldfish retina for over 6 months after axotomy. In the control retina, very weak immunoreactivity could be seen in the retinal ganglion cells (RGCs). The immunoreactivity of GAP43 started to increase in the RGCs at 5 days, peaked at 7–20 days and then gradually decreased at 30–40 days after axotomy. The weak but significant immunoreactivity of GAP43 in the RGCs continued during 50–90 days and slowly returned to the control level by 180 days after lesion. The levels of GAP43 mRNA showed a biphasic pattern; a short-peak increase (9-folds) at 1–3 weeks and a long plateau increase (5-folds) at 50–120 days after axotomy. Thereafter, the levels declined to the control value by 180 days after axotomy. The changes of chasing behavior of pair of goldfish with bilaterally axotomized optic nerve also showed a slow biphasic recovery pattern in time course. Although further experiment is needed to elucidate the role of GAP43 in the regrowing axon terminals, the GAP43 is a good biochemical marker for monitoring the whole period of optic nerve regeneration in fish.

12.1 Introduction

Unlike mammals, fish optic nerve regenerates and restores the visual function after optic nerve lesion (Sperry 1948). The optic nerve regeneration process in fish is a long-lasting one. We classified four periods of goldfish optic nerve regeneration after nerve lesion from morphological, biochemical and behavioral results (Kato et al. 1999, 2007). The first period is a preparation period within 5–6 days after nerve

S. Kato (✉)
Department of Molecular Neurobiology, University of Kanazawa, Kanazawa 920-8640, Japan
e-mail: satoru@med.kanazawa-u.ac.jp

R.E. Anderson et al. (eds.), *Retinal Degenerative Diseases*, Advances in Experimental Medicine and Biology 664, DOI 10.1007/978-1-4419-1399-9_12, © Springer Science+Business Media, LLC 2010

lesion. The second period is an axonal elongation period within 1–5 weeks after nerve lesion. The third period is a synaptic connection and refinement in the tectum within 1.5–4 months after nerve lesion. The fourth period is a recovery period of visual function within 5–6 months after nerve lesion.

In previous studies, many factors or substances involved in the axonal elongation process were identified (Ballestero et al. 1997; Liu et al. 2002; Sugitani et al. 2006). However, there are few studies as for the molecules involved in the processes of the first and third period mentioned above. There is nothing to involve in the whole periods of long optic never regeneration process in fish.

In the present study, we want to know a regeneration-associated molecule which involves in the whole period of optic nerve regeneration in goldfish. If we can find such a molecule, we can easily decide the start and end points of optic nerve regeneration. In a previous paper, we described the fast and slow phases of goldfish behavior during optic nerve regeneration after nerve lesion (Kato et al. 1999). In this study, we investigated two-point distance of pair of goldfish with bilaterally axotomized optic nerve. The visual-guided behavior could recover more than 4 months after nerve lesion. In this view point, we checked biochemical expressions in the goldfish retina for over 4 months. As a candidate molecule, we focused on growth-associated protein43 (GAP43), because it is a famous marker protein of growing axons in development and regeneration (Benowitz and Routenberg 1997). It is also well known that the localization of GAP43 is at the growth cone and presynaptic terminals (Benowitz and Routenberg 1997). The location of GAP43 at the growth cone is used to be a biochemical marker for growing axons. However, the location of GAP43 at the presynaptic terminals has been entirely neglected. The presynaptic terminals of goldfish visual regeneration system are the just site in which synaptic refinement of regrowing optic axons occurs in the tectum. Therefore, we investigate the expression of GAP43 mRNA and protein in the goldfish retina for over 4 months after optic nerve lesion.

12.2 Experimental Procedures

12.2.1 Animal

Goldfish (*Carassius auratus*) was used throughout the experiment. Goldfish after optic nerve transection were reared in a water tank at $22 \pm 1^\circ C$ with 12/12 h light and dark cycle. The eye was enucleated at appropriate time points under anesthesia.

12.2.2 Immunohistochemistry

The retina was isolated and fixed with 4% paraformaldehyde solution containing 0.1 M phosphate buffer (pH7.4) and 5% sucrose. The thin sections of the retina in 12 μm thickness were reacted with primary anti-GAP43 antibody (1:300) and further reacted with secondary anti-mouse IgG (1:500). The immunoreactivity was visualized with avidin-biotin immunoenzymatic method.

12.2.3 RT-PCR Analysis

Primers of forward and reverse forms of goldfish GAP43 cDNA were determined by referring to that of goldfish GAP43 cDNA (database No. emb: M26250). RT-PCR was performed in a linear range of product. GAPDH mRNA levels were used as a control under non-saturation level.

12.2.4 Behavioral Analysis

Images of moving two goldfish with bilateral optic nerve transection were captured by a computer image processing system (Kato et al. 2004). The positional coordinates of moving two fish were treated and analyzed at a frame rate of 30/s. The chasing ratio of two fish was counted as a percentage of chasing times/total observation time (Kaneda et al. 2008).

12.3 Results

12.3.1 Immunohistochemical Studies of GAP43 Protein in the Goldfish Retina After Optic Nerve Transection

We followed up the changes of GAP43 protein in the goldfish retina until 180 days after nerve injury with an immunohistochemical analysis. In the control retina, a faintly positive signal of GAP43 protein could be seen in the RGCs (Fig. 12.1a). The positive signals of GAP43 slightly increased in the RGCs 5 days (Fig. 12.1b) and peaked at 20 days (Fig. 12.1c) after axotomy. Thereafter, the positive signals gradually decreased in the RGCs 60 days (Fig. 12.1d) and 90 days (Fig. 12.1e), and finally returned to the control levels by 180 days (Fig. 12.1f) after nerve lesion.

12.3.2 Time Course of GAP43 mRNA Expression in the Goldfish Retina During Optic Nerve Regeneration

Next, we semi-quantitatively measured the level of GAP43 mRNA in the retina over 180 days after axotomy using RT-PCR method. After electrophoresis, a 639 bp single band was detected. The level of GAP43 mRNA rapidly increased at 3 days, peaked at 7–20 days (about 9-folds) and then rapidly decreased to 6-folds by 30 days after axotomy (Fig. 12.2a). The over control increase (5-folds) lasted for a long time (50–120 days), and then gradually returned to the basal level by 180

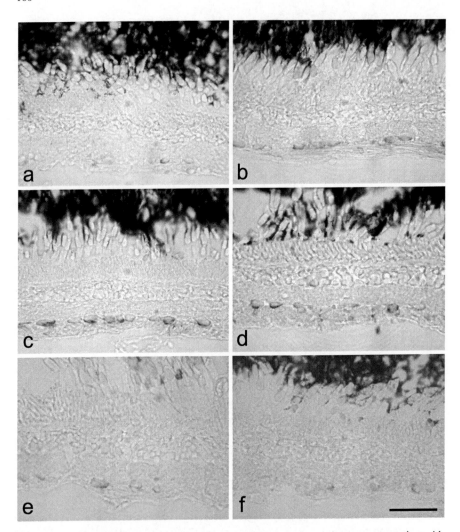

Fig. 12.1 Changes of GAP43 protein in the goldfish retina after optic nerve transection with immunohistochemical analysis. (**a**) In the control retina, weak immunoreactivity of GAP43 could be seen in the goldfish retinal ganglion cells (RGCs). (**b**) The immunoreactivity started to increase in the RGCs at 5 days (**b**), peaked at 20 days (**c**) and then gradually declined at 30–40 days after axotomy with a significant increase of immunoreactivity. Then the significant increase of immunoreactivity continued in the RGCs at 60 days (**d**) and gradually decreased at 90 days (**e**) and finally returned to the control value by 180 days after axotomy (**f**). Scale = 50 µm

days after axotomy (Fig. 12.2a). Thus, the time course of GAP43 mRNA levels in the retina after axotomy showed a biphasic pattern, a short peak increase and a long plateau increase (Fig. 12.2a). The PCR product was sequenced and the sequence was completely matched with that of goldfish cDNA fragment for GAP43. The levels of GAPDH mRNA did not change throughout the whole periods (data not shown).

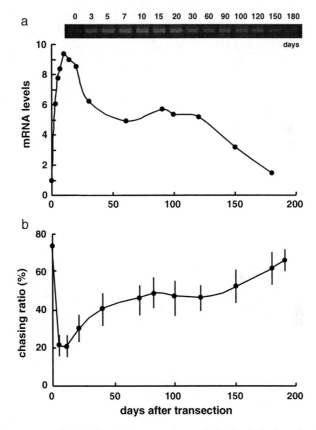

Fig. 12.2 Time course of GAP43 mRNA expression and chasing behavior of pair of goldfish with bilaterally axotomized optic nerve. (**a**) Changes of GAP43 mRNA levels during optic nerve regeneration. Levels of GAP43 mRNA rapidly increased at 3 days and peaked 9-folds at 7–20 days and then rapidly decreased 6-folds at 30 days after axotomy. The increase (5-folds) of GAP43 mRNA continued for a long time (50–120 days) after optic nerve lesion and then slowly returned to the control level by 180 days after axotomy. An *upper panel* shows a band amplified by RT-PCR for GAP43. The level of GAP43 mRNA shows a biphasic increase pattern in expression. (**b**) Changes of chasing behavior of pair of goldfish with optic nerve transection during optic nerve regeneration. Chasing ratio rapidly decreased just after optic nerve transection and then started to recover at 2–3 weeks after axotomy. The chasing ratio further increased a half value of control at 40 days and the recovery level continued for a long time (50–120 days). Thereafter the chasing behavior finally recovered by 180–200 days after axotomy. ($n = 15$–20 in each time point)

12.3.3 Chasing Behavior of Two Goldfish with Treatment of Optic Nerve Transection During Optic Nerve Regeneration

A pair of moving goldfish swims as a group with a short two-point distance (Kato et al. 1999). This habit of pair of goldfish is a schooling behavior of fish. In this behavioral analysis, we defined a chasing ratio with references to the two-point distance and accessing movement of two fish (Kato et al. 2004). We measured changes of chasing behavior for 30 min at various time points after optic nerve injury by using an image processing system. In control pair, the chasing ratio was 72% (Fig. 12.2b, 0 day). The bilateral optic nerve transection of two fish induced a significant reduction of this ratio to 20% just after axotomy. The low value was maintained for 1–2 weeks and then the chasing ratio gradually increased 40% at 40 days after axotomy. The value (40%) continued during 50–120 days and then was slowly recovered to control value by 180–200 days after injury (Fig. 12.2b).

12.4 Discussion

12.4.1 Termination of Optic Nerve Regeneration in Goldfish

The optic nerve regeneration in goldfish is a long process and therefore it is very difficult to decide the endpoint of this process. As for the fish optic nerve regeneration process, the excess number of ectopic optic axons initially reinnervate the tectum 3–6 weeks and then the optic axons are repulsed 2–4 months after axotomy. Finally exact topographic retinotectal connections are completed 5–6 months after axotomy (Edwards et al. 1985; Meyer and Kageyama 1999). In a previous paper, we followed up the time course of cell body response to nerve injury in the goldfish retina for over 4 months (Kato et al. 1999). We found that cell body of RGCs after optic nerve transection became hypertrophic 1 week and peaked 2-folds at 2 months after axotomy. Then the cell body returned to the normal size by 4 months after axotomy (Kato et al. 1999). Moreover, we described that two-point distance of pair of goldfish with axotomized optic nerve was initially very long and then gradually shortened 1.5–4 months and finally recovered the control value 5–6 months after axotomy (Kato et al. 1999). From these morphological and behavioral observations, the finish of optic nerve regeneration in goldfish is more than 5–6 months after axotomy. So far as we know, we have no biochemical marker expressing throughout the whole period of optic nerve regeneration. It is worthy to search such a maker for announcing the initial and terminal point of this long process, in basic and clinical neuroscience of nerve regeneration. In this view point, the present study was performed.

12.4.2 GAP43 Is a Good Marker for Monitoring the Long Process of Optic Nerve Regeneration in Fish

GAP43 protein was originally discovered as a rapidly transported acidic protein from cell bodies to the axons in the regenerating optic nerves after nerve crush (Skene and Willard 1981; Benowitz et al. 1981). Later, GAP43 was further localized at the major growth cone and presynaptic terminals (Deckker et al. 1989). In

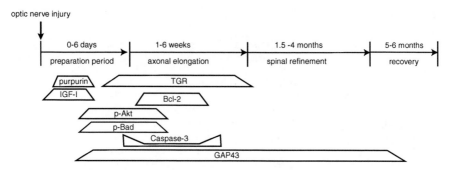

Fig. 12.3 Time course of regeneration-associated molecules in expression after optic nerve transection in goldfish. IGF-I, p-Akt and p-Bad expression increased 1–5 days (Koriyama et al. 2007) after axotomy. Purpurin expression increased 2–5 days (Matsukawa et al. 2004) after axotomy. Transglutaminase (TG_R) expression increased 10–30 days (Sugitani et al. 2006) after axotomy. Bcl-2 expression also increased 10–20 days and caspase-3 expression rather decreased in this period (Koriyama et al. 2007). In contrast, GAP43 expression increased for a long time 3–150 days after axotomy with a biphasic expression pattern

a previous paper (Bormann et al. 1998), changes of GAP43 mRNA were followed up in the zebrafish retina until 56 days after optic nerve transection. Their in situ hybridization studies showed that positive signals of GAP43 mRNA increased in the RGCs 1–2 weeks and then gradually decreased by 56 days after optic nerve injury. In the present study we investigated changes of GAP43 protein in the goldfish RGCs over 180 days after axotomy. The immunoreactivity of GAP43 started to significantly increase 5 days, peaked at 2–3 weeks and continued for near 150 days after axotomy (Fig. 12.1). Interestingly, the expression pattern of GAP43 mRNA was clearly biphasic, a short peak phase (9-folds) at 7–20 days and a long plateau phase (5-folds) at 50–120 days after axotomy (Fig. 12.2a). In the time course of schooling behavior of pair of goldfish with bilateral optic nerve transection was also biphasic, a rapid recover phase at 7–40 days and a long plateau phase at 50–120 days after axotomy. The similar time course between GAP43 expression and recovery phase of chasing behavior leads to a conclusion that changes in GAP43 expression in the fish retina during optic nerve regeneration well reflect the state of visual function after nerve injury. We have cloned many factors and enzymes as a regeneration-associated molecule during goldfish optic nerve injury (Liu et al. 2002; Matsukawa et al. 2004; Sugitani et al. 2006; Koriyama et al. 2007), they almost all worked as an axonal elongation factor in the goldfish optic nerve regeneration system (Fig. 12.3). GAP43 is an exceptional molecule which works throughout the whole period of optic nerve regeneration with a characteristic biphasic expression pattern. Further experiment is needed to elucidate the role of GAP43 on the short peak (7–20 days) and the long plateau (50–120 days) phases in the regrowing optic axons.

References

Ballestero RP, Wilmot GR, Agranoff BW et al (1997) gRICH68 and gRICH70 are 2′,3′-cyclic-nucleotide 3′-phosphodiesterases induced during goldfish optic nerve regeneration. J Biol Chem 272:11479–11486

Benowitz LI, Routenberg A (1997) GAP-43: an intrinsic determinant of neuronal development and plasticity. Trends Neurosci 20:84–91

Benowitz LI, Shashoua VE, Yoon MG (1981) Specific changes in rapidly transported proteins during regeneration of the goldfish optic nerve. J Neurosci 1:300–307

Bormann P, Zumsteg VM, Roth LW et al (1998) Target contact regulates GAP-43 and alpha-tubulin mRNA levels in regenerating retinal ganglion cells. J Neurosci Res 52:405–419

Deckker LV, De Graan PN, Versteeg DH et al (1989) Phosphorylation of B-50 (GAP43) is correlated with neurotransmitter release in rat hippocampal slices. J Neurochem 52:24–30

Edwards MA, Sharma SC, Murray M (1985) Selective retinal reinnervation of a surgically created tectal island in goldfish. I. Light microscopic analysis. J Comp Neurol 32:372–385

Kaneda N, Nagashima M, Nunome T et al (2008) Changes of phospho-growth-associated protein 43 (phospho-GAP43) in the zebrafish retina after optic nerve injury: A long-term observation. Neurosci Res 61:281–288

Kato S, Devadas M, Okada K et al (1999) Fast and slow recovery phases of goldfish behavior after transection of the optic nerve revealed by a computer image processing system. Neuroscience 93:907–914

Kato S, Koriyama Y, Matsukawa T et al (2007) Optic nerve regeneration in goldfish. In: Becker CG, Becker T (eds) Model organisms in spinal cord regeneration. Wiley-VCH, Weinheim

Kato S, Nakagawa T, Ohkawa M et al (2004) A computer image processing system for quantification of zebrafish behavior. J Neurosci Methods 134:1–7

Koriyama Y, Homma K, Sugitani K et al (2007) Upregulation of IGF-I in the goldfish retinal ganglion cells during the early stage of optic nerve regeneration. Neurochem Int 50:749–756

Liu ZW, Matsukawa T, Arai K et al (2002) Na,K-ATPase alpha 3 subunit in the goldfish retina during optic nerve regeneration. J Neurochem 80:763–770

Matsukawa T, Sugitani K, Mawatari K et al (2004) Role of purpurin as retinol-binding protein in goldfish retina during the early stage of optic nerve regeneration: its priming action on neurite outgrowth. J Neurosci 24:8346–8353

Meyer RL, Kageyama GH (1999) Large-scale synaptic errors during map formation by regeneration optic axons in the goldfish. J Comp Neurol 409:299–312

Skene JHP, Willard M (1981) Characteristics of growth-associated poly-peptides in regenerating toad retinal ganglion cell axons. J Neurosci 1:419–426

Sperry RW (1948) Patterning of central synapses in regeneration of the optic nerve in teleosts. Physiol Zool 21:351–361

Sugitani K, Matsukawa T, Koriyama Y et al (2006) Upregulation of retinal transglutaminase during the axonal elongation stage of goldfish optic nerve regeneration. Neuroscience 142:1081–1092

Chapter 13
Multiprotein Complexes of Retinitis Pigmentosa GTPase Regulator (RPGR), a Ciliary Protein Mutated in X-Linked Retinitis Pigmentosa (XLRP)

Carlos Murga-Zamalloa, Anand Swaroop, and Hemant Khanna

Abstract Mutations in Retinitis Pigmentosa GTPase Regulator (RPGR) are a frequent cause of X-linked Retinitis Pigmentosa (XLRP). The *RPGR* gene undergoes extensive alternative splicing and encodes for distinct protein isoforms in the retina. Extensive studies using isoform-specific antibodies and mouse mutants have revealed that RPGR predominantly localizes to the transition zone to primary cilia and associates with selected ciliary and microtubule-associated assemblies in photoreceptors. In this chapter, we have summarized recent advances on understanding the role of RPGR in photoreceptor protein trafficking. We also provide new evidence that suggests the existence of discrete RPGR multiprotein complexes in photoreceptors. Piecing together the RPGR-interactome in different subcellular compartments should provide critical insights into the role of alternative RPGR isoforms in associated orphan and syndromic retinal degenerative diseases.

13.1 X-Linked RP (XLRP)

XLRP is a relatively severe form of retinal degeneration, accounting for 10–20% of all RP (Bird 1975; Fishman 1978). Most affected males exhibit early-onset visual

H. Khanna (✉)
Department of Ophthalmology and Visual Sciences, Kellogg Eye Center, Ann Arbor, MI 48105, USA
e-mail: hkhanna@med.umich.edu

Retinitis Pigmentosa (RP: MIM 268000) is a leading cause of inherited blindness in developed countries. RP refers to a group of debilitating neurodegenerative diseases with clinically heterogeneous findings, which include bone spicule like pigmentary deposits in the retina, progressive loss of peripheral vision and eventually deterioration of central vision due to cone loss (Bird 1987; Fishman et al. 1988; Heckenlively et al. 1988; Sullivan and Daiger 1996). Over 30 RP genes have been identified so far (http://www.sph.uth.tmc.edu/Retnet) (Hartong et al. 2006). No effective approach exists for the management or treatment of RP.

R.E. Anderson et al. (eds.), *Retinal Degenerative Diseases*, Advances in Experimental Medicine and Biology 664, DOI 10.1007/978-1-4419-1399-9_13,
© Springer Science+Business Media, LLC 2010

symptoms with night-blindness in the first decade and rapid progression towards blindness by age 40 (Bird 1975; Fishman et al. 1988). Heterozygous carrier females can show electroretinographic (ERG) abnormalities and tapetal reflex (Fishman et al. 1986). Some XLRP patients have abnormal sperm phenotype (Hunter et al. 1988) or hearing defects (Iannaccone et al. 2004; Zito et al. 2003). To date, six genetic loci have been mapped: *RP2, RP3, RP6, RP23, RP24* and *RP34* (Fujita et al. 1996; Gieser et al. 1998; Hardcastle et al. 2000; McGuire et al. 1995; Melamud et al. 2006; Wright et al. 1991). The genes for two major forms of XLRP, *RP2* [Schwahn et al. 1998] and *RP3* [*RPGR* (Meindl et al. 1996; Roepman et al. 1996)], have been cloned.

Mutations in *RP2* account for approximately 10% of XLRP (Breuer et al. 2002; Hardcastle et al. 1999; Mears et al. 1999; Sharon et al. 2003). The *RP2* gene encodes a putative protein of 350 amino acids (Chapple et al. 2000; Schwahn et al. 1998). The crystal structure of the RP2 protein reveals an amino-terminal β-helix that is structurally and functionally homologous to the tubulin-specific chaperone, cofactor C (TBCC); most disease-causing missense mutations are present in this domain (Bartolini et al. 2002; Grayson et al. 2002; Kuhnel et al. 2006). RP2 interacts with ADP-ribosylation factor-like 3 (ARL3) (Kuhnel et al. 2006), a microtubule-associated small GTP-binding protein (Kahn et al. 2005) that localizes to the sensory cilium of photoreceptors (Grayson et al. 2002). However, the precise role of RP2 in photoreceptors has not been delineated.

13.2 Retinitis Pigmentosa GTPase Regulator (RPGR)

Mutations in the *RPGR* gene account for over 70% of XLRP and as much as 25% of simplex RP males (Breuer et al. 2002; Shu et al. 2007). Initial analysis of a ubiquitously-expressed $RPGR^{Ex1-19}$ transcript (derived from exons 1–19; 815 amino acids) identified mutations in only 10–20% of XLRP patients and families (Buraczynska et al. 1997; Fujita et al. 1997; Meindl et al. 1996; Roepman et al. 1996; Sharon et al. 2000). The discovery of an alternative transcript with a purine-rich terminal exon ORF15, which included a part of the original intron 15 (called $RPGR^{ORF15}$) revealed additional mutations in almost 50% of individuals with XLRP (Breuer et al. 2002; Sharon et al. 2003; Vervoort et al. 2000). Mutations in $RPGR^{ORF15}$ have also been identified in patients with cone-rod dystrophy, atrophic macular degeneration, and Coat's-like exudative vasculopathy (Ayyagari et al. 2002; Demirci et al. 2006; Demirci et al. 2002; Sharon et al. 2003; Yang et al. 2002). Some individuals with *RPGR* mutations are reported to show a syndromic phenotype that may include respiratory tract infections, hearing loss, and primary cilia dyskinesia (Iannaccone et al. 2004; Koenekoop et al. 2003; Moore et al. 2006; van Dorp et al. 1992; Zito et al. 2003). In addition, patients with mutations in RPGR exons 2–14 appear to display a more severe clinical phenotype than those with exon ORF15 mutations (Sharon et al. 2003). However, further genotype-phenotype studies are needed to elucidate the clinical heterogeneity associated with *RPGR* mutations.

13.3 RPGR Isoforms in the Retina

The N-terminal region of RPGR contains tandem repeats (termed RCC1-like domain; RLD) homologous to RCC1, which is a guanine nucleotide exchange factor (GEF) for Ran-GTPase that is involved in nucleo-cytoplasmic transport (Meindl et al. 1996; Renault et al. 2001). Complex splicing patterns are reported for *RPGR* though the physiological relevance of these transcripts is unclear (Hong and Li 2002; Kirschner et al. 1999; Vervoort et al. 2000; Yan et al. 1998). Multiple immunoreactive bands are observed using isoform-specific RPGR antibodies (Chang et al. 2006; He et al. 2008; Hong and Li 2002; Khanna et al. 2005; Mavlyutov et al. 2002; Otto et al. 2005; Shu et al. 2005; Yan et al. 1998).

Several different groups have reported the localization of RPGR in the retina. Initially RPGR was shown to localize to the photoreceptor cilium independent of the species tested (Hong et al. 2003); however, another study demonstrated species-specific differences in RPGR localization (Mavlyutov et al. 2002). By immunogold labeling, we demonstrated the $RPGR^{ORF15}$ protein in the transition zone and basal bodies of both mouse and human photoreceptor cilia though some additional labeling was detected in the inner and outer segments (Khanna et al. 2005; Shu et al. 2005). In proliferating cells, centrioles were labeled with anti-RPGR antibodies (He et al. 2008; Shu et al. 2005). It should be noted that primary cilia arise from mother centrioles in post-mitotic cells (Pedersen et al. 2008). Distinct localization of $RPGR^{ORF15}$ isoforms may reflect their relative abundance in distinct subcellular compartments of photoreceptors.

13.4 Animal Models of RPGR

A knockout (ko) mouse with deletion of exons 4–6 of *Rpgr* was reported to show late-onset cone-rod degeneration (Hong et al. 2000); however, this *Rpgr*-ko mouse is not a complete null and expresses some specific $RPGR^{ORF15}$ isoforms that localize to the transition zone of photoreceptor cilia (Khanna et al. 2005). Interestingly, ectopic expression of an ORF15 variant could partially rescue the *Rpgr*-ko phenotype (Hong et al. 2005), or behave as a dominant gain-of-function variant resulting in rapid disease progression (Hong et al. 2004). Attempts to generate a complete *Rpgr* null mutation in mouse have not been successful. Notably, frameshift mutations in $RPGR^{ORF15}$ have been identified in two naturally-occurring canine mutants; the XLPRA2 dog exhibits relatively rapid photoreceptor degeneration and severe ERG abnormalities, whereas the XLPRA1 mutant shows a milder phenotype (Beltran et al. 2006; Zhang et al. 2002). Aberrant behavior of the two mutant ORF15 proteins in cultured cells may reflect the phenotypic differences in the two canine models (Zhang et al. 2002).

13.5 Sensory Cilia

Photoreceptor outer segment (OS) membrane discs and inner segment (IS) are linked by a sensory cilium (CC), which is a modified primary cilium (Young 1968).

Ciliogenesis involves an evolutionarily conserved process, called Intraflagellar Transport (IFT) (Rosenbaum et al. 1999). In photoreceptors, components of the IFT complex and cargo proteins are synthesized in the IS, docked at the basal body, and transported distally by the anterograde heterotrimeric motor, Kinesin-II (Besharse et al. 2003). The IFT components are believed to be replenished by their transport back to the basal body by a presumptive retrograde motor cytoplasmic dynein 1b/2 (Besharse et al. 2003).

Vertebrate photoreceptors are highly metabolically active; approximately 10% of OS disks are turned over each day (Bok and Young 1972; Young 1968). It is estimated that ~2000 opsin molecules are transported to the OS per minute in an adult human retina (Besharse 1986; Williams 2002). The opsin molecules are synthesized in the IS and are targeted to the basal body, where they are fused with the ciliary membrane and trafficked distally to the OS (Deretic et al. 2005). Hence, it is not surprising that perturbations in ciliary transport of opsins or OS biogenesis are associated with severe retinal degeneration and blindness (Insinna and Besharse 2008).

13.6 Retinal Degeneration Caused by Mutations in Ciliary Proteins

IFT-mediated transport of rhodopsin and other signaling proteins is critical for photoreceptor survival and function. Conditional $Kif3a^{-/-}$ mice and $Tg737^{orpk}$, a hypomorphic allele of IFT88, result in opsin accumulation in the IS (Marszalek et al. 2000; Pazour et al. 2002). A number of retinal disease proteins CEP290/NPHP6, RPGRIP1 and RP1 are required for cilia-dependent OS transport, generation or maintenance (Chang et al. 2006; Liu et al. 2004; Zhao et al. 2003). Several pleiotropic disorders, such as Senior-Loken Syndrome, Joubert Syndrome, and Bardet-Biedl Syndrome, are also caused by mutations in ciliary proteins and share retinopathy as a common phenotype (Badano et al. 2006).

13.7 Macromolecular Complexes of RPGR^{ORF15}

RPGR exists in macromolecular complexes with other proteins in photoreceptors. Two proteins were initially identified by yeast two-hybrid analysis using the RPGR-RLD as bait: RPGRIP1, which is localized to the sensory cilium and mutated in retinopathy patients (Boylan and Wright 2000; Dryja et al. 2001; Hong et al. 2001); and delta subunit of rod cyclic guanosine monophosphate phosphodiesterase (PDE6D), a prenyl-binding protein involved in the retrieval of PDE from rod outer segment membranes by interacting with Rab13 (Linari et al. 1999; Zhang et al. 2004). Two chromosome-associated proteins SMC1 and SMC3 (Hirano 2006; Khanna et al. 2005; Liu et al. 2007) and two ciliary disease-associated proteins, NPHP5 (Otto et al. 2005) and CEP290/NPHP6 (Chang et al. 2006; Sayer et al. 2006) are also reported to be a part of the RPGR^{ORF15} macromolecular complexes.

In addition, RPGR can associate with Tg737/Polaris/IFT88 (Davenport and Yoder 2005; Pazour et al. 2002) and several microtubule transport proteins (Khanna et al. 2005).

13.8 Dissection of RPGR^{ORF15} Complexes

We hypothesize that RPGR isoforms are partitioned in distinct multiprotein complexes in photoreceptors. To evaluate this hypothesis, we have carried out sequential

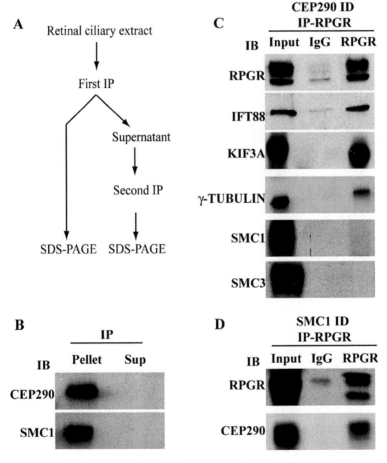

Fig. 13.1 (**a**) Schematic representation of the strategy to dissect distinct RPGR-containing multiprotein complexes in photoreceptor cilia. IP: Immunoprecipitation; Ab: antibody. (**b**) Protein extract (~150 μg) was subjected to immunoprecipitation using indicated antibodies. The precipitated beads (Pellet) and supernatant (Sup) were analyzed by SDS-PAGE and immunoblotting (IB) using same antibodies. No signal in the supernatant indicates sufficient immunodepletion of the respective proteins from the extract. (**c**) and (**d**) CEP290 – or SMC1 – immunodepleted (ID) extract was subjected to IP using RPGR antibody or rabbit IgG (immunoglobulin) followed by SDS-PAGE and immunoblotting (IB) using indicated antibodies

immunodepletion experiments. We initially used antibodies against two of the RPGR partners, CEP290/NPHP6 and SMC1, in order to immunodeplete RPGR that is part of these complexes from the retinal ciliary extract preparation. The remaining supernatant was subjected to immunoprecipitation (IP) with the anti-RPGR[ORF15] antibody, followed by immunoblotting to test for the presence or absence of remaining RPGR[ORF15]-interacting proteins (Fig. 13.1a). Even after immunodepletion of CEP290 from the retinal ciliary fraction (Fig. 13.1b), RPGR was still associated with IFT88, KIF3A, and γ-tubulin, but not with SMC1 and SMC3 (Fig. 13.1c). This data suggests that RPGR's complex with CEP290, SMC1, and SMC3 is distinct from that with IFT88, KIF3A, and γ-tubulin. On the other hand, after SMC1 immunodepletion, RPGR antibody could immunoprecipitate only a fraction of CEP290 from retinal ciliary extract. Similar results were obtained with SMC3 (data not shown).

These observations indicate that RPGR exists in at least three distinct complexes: first with IFT88, KIF3A, and γ-tubulin; second with CEP290, SMC1, and SMC3 and; third with CEP290 and probably other ciliary proteins (Fig. 13.2). Future detailed analysis of these and additional complexes should assist in dissecting the RPGR function in photoreceptors.

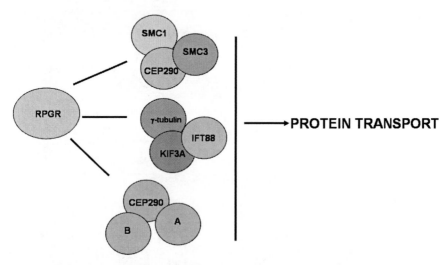

PUTATIVE RPGR COMPLEXES

Fig. 13.2 Schematic representation of the putative distinct RPGR complexes that can exist in photoreceptors. Proteins *A* and *B* represent as yet unidentified molecular partners that can be part of such complexes

13.9 Conclusion

Despite extensive investigations, the underlying mechanism of ciliary transport-associated photoreceptor dysfunction is poorly understood at this stage. We suggest that RPGR-defect could occur at multiple stages: (a) cargo loading onto the vesicles; (b) vesicular trafficking towards the basal body, (c) docking of the cargo-laden vesicles at the basal body, (d) selection of cargo and transfer to the IFT complex, or (e) anterograde transport towards the distal OS. We reckon that the different RPGR complexes may participate in some or all of these transport processes. Given the importance of these pathways in photoreceptor development and survival, mutations in RPGR may disrupt its interactome thereby leading to retinal degeneration.

Acknowledgments This work is supported by the grants from the National Eye Institute (RO1-EY007961), Midwest Eye Banks and Transplantation Center, and by NEI/NIH intramural program.

References

Ayyagari R, Demirci FY, Liu J et al (2002) X-linked recessive atrophic macular degeneration from RPGR mutation. Genomics 80(2):166–171

Badano JL, Mitsuma N, Beales PL et al (2006) The ciliopathies: an emerging class of human genetic disorders. Annu Rev Genomics Hum Genet 7:125–148

Bartolini F, Bhamidipati A, Thomas S et al (2002) Functional overlap between retinitis pigmentosa 2 protein and the tubulin-specific chaperone cofactor C. J Biol Chem 277(17):14629–14634

Beltran WA, Hammond P, Acland GM et al (2006) A frameshift mutation in RPGR exon ORF15 causes photoreceptor degeneration and inner retina remodeling in a model of X-linked retinitis pigmentosa. Invest Ophthalmol Vis Sci 47(4):1669–1681

Besharse JC (1986) The Retina: a model for cell biological studies Part I. Academic, New York, pp 297–352

Besharse JC, Baker SA, Luby-Phelps K et al (2003) Photoreceptor intersegmental transport and retinal degeneration: a conserved pathway common to motile and sensory cilia. Adv Exp Med Biol 533:157–164

Bird AC (1975) X-linked retinitis pigmentosa. Br J Ophthalmol 59(4):177–199

Bird AC (1987) Clinical investigation of retinitis pigmentosa. Prog Clin Biol Res 247:3–20

Bok D, Young RW (1972) The renewal of diffusely distributed protein in the outer segments of rods and cones. Vision Res 12(2):161–168

Boylan JP, Wright AF (2000) Identification of a novel protein interacting with RPGR. Hum Mol Genet 9(14):2085–2093

Breuer DK, Yashar BM, Filippova E et al (2002) A comprehensive mutation analysis of RP2 and RPGR in a North American cohort of families with X-linked retinitis pigmentosa. Am J Hum Genet 70(6):1545–1554

Buraczynska M, Wu W, Fujita R et al (1997) Spectrum of mutations in the RPGR gene that are identified in 20% of families with X-linked retinitis pigmentosa. Am J Hum Genet 61(6): 1287–1292

Chang B, Khanna H, Hawes N et al (2006) In-frame deletion in a novel centrosomal/ciliary protein CEP290/NPHP6 perturbs its interaction with RPGR and results in early-onset retinal degeneration in the rd16 mouse. Hum Mol Genet 15(11):1847–1857

Chapple JP, Hardcastle AJ, Grayson C et al (2000) Mutations in the N-terminus of the X-linked retinitis pigmentosa protein RP2 interfere with the normal targeting of the protein to the plasma membrane. Hum Mol Genet 9(13):1919–1926

Davenport JR, Yoder BK (2005) An incredible decade for the primary cilium: a look at a once-forgotten organelle. Am J Physiol Renal Physiol 289(6):F1159–F1169

Demirci FY, Rigatti BW, Mah TS et al (2006) A novel RPGR exon ORF15 mutation in a family with X-linked retinitis pigmentosa and Coats'-like exudative vasculopathy. Am J Ophthalmol 141(1):208–210

Demirci FY, Rigatti BW, Wen G et al (2002) X-linked cone-rod dystrophy (locus COD1): identification of mutations in RPGR exon ORF15. Am J Hum Genet 70(4): 1049–1053

Deretic D, Williams AH, Ransom N et al (2005) Rhodopsin C terminus, the site of mutations causing retinal disease, regulates trafficking by binding to ADP-ribosylation factor 4 (ARF4). Proc Natl Acad Sci USA 102(9):3301–3306

Dryja TP, Adams SM, Grimsby JL et al (2001) Null RPGRIP1 alleles in patients with Leber congenital amaurosis. Am J Hum Genet 68(5):1295–1298

Fishman GA (1978) Retinitis pigmentosa. Genetic percentages. Arch Ophthalmol 96(5): 822–826

Fishman GA, Farber MD, Derlacki DJ (1988) X-linked retinitis pigmentosa. Profile of clinical findings. Arch Ophthalmol 106(3):369–375

Fishman GA, Weinberg AB, McMahon TT (1986) X-linked recessive retinitis pigmentosa. Clinical characteristics of carriers. Arch Ophthalmol 104(9):1329–1335

Fujita R, Bingham E, Forsythe P et al (1996) A recombination outside the BB deletion refines the location of the X linked retinitis pigmentosa locus RP3. Am J Hum Genet 59(1):152–158

Fujita R, Buraczynska M, Gieser L et al (1997) Analysis of the RPGR gene in 11 pedigrees with the retinitis pigmentosa type 3 genotype: paucity of mutations in the coding region but splice defects in two families. Am J Hum Genet 61(3):571–580

Gieser L, Fujita R, Goring HH et al (1998) A novel locus (RP24) for X-linked retinitis pigmentosa maps to Xq26-27. Am J Hum Genet 63(5):1439–1447

Grayson C, Bartolini F, Chapple JP (2002) Localization in the human retina of the X-linked retinitis pigmentosa protein RP2, its homologue cofactor C and the RP2 interacting protein Arl3. Hum Mol Genet 11(24):3065–3074

Hardcastle AJ, Thiselton DL, Van Maldergem L et al (1999) Mutations in the RP2 gene cause disease in 10% of families with familial X-linked retinitis pigmentosa assessed in this study. Am J Hum Genet 64(4):1210–1215

Hardcastle AJ, Thiselton DL, Zito I et al (2000) Evidence for a new locus for X-linked retinitis pigmentosa (RP23). Invest Ophthalmol Vis Sci 41(8):2080–2086

Hartong DT, Berson EL, Dryja TP (2006) Retinitis pigmentosa. Lancet 368(9549):1795–1809

He S, Parapuram SK, Hurd TW et al (2008) Retinitis Pigmentosa GTPase Regulator (RPGR) protein isoforms in mammalian retina: insights into X-linked Retinitis Pigmentosa and associated ciliopathies. Vision Res 48(3):366–376

Heckenlively JR, Yoser SL, Friedman LH et al (1988) Clinical findings and common symptoms in retinitis pigmentosa. Am J Ophthalmol 105(5):504–511

Hirano T (2006) At the heart of the chromosome: SMC proteins in action. Nat Rev Mol Cell Biol 7(5):311–322

Hong DH, Li T (2002) Complex expression pattern of RPGR reveals a role for purine-rich exonic splicing enhancers. Invest Ophthalmol Vis Sci 43(11):3373–3382

Hong DH, Pawlyk BS, Adamian M et al (2004) Dominant, gain-of-function mutant produced by truncation of RPGR. Invest Ophthalmol Vis Sci 45(1):36–41

Hong DH, Pawlyk BS, Adamian M et al (2005) A single, abbreviated RPGR-ORF15 variant reconstitutes RPGR function in vivo. Invest Ophthalmol Vis Sci 46(2):435–441

Hong DH, Pawlyk BS, Shang J (2000) A retinitis pigmentosa GTPase regulator (RPGR)-deficient mouse model for X-linked retinitis pigmentosa (RP3). Proc Natl Acad Sci USA 97(7): 3649–3654

Hong DH, Pawlyk B, Sokolov M et al (2003) RPGR isoforms in photoreceptor connecting cilia and the transitional zone of motile cilia. Invest Ophthalmol Vis Sci 44(6):2413–2421

Hong DH, Yue G, Adamian M et al (2001) Retinitis pigmentosa GTPase regulator (RPGRr)-interacting protein is stably associated with the photoreceptor ciliary axoneme and anchors RPGR to the connecting cilium. J Biol Chem 276(15):12091–12099

Hunter DG, Fishman GA, Kretzer FL (1988) Abnormal axonemes in X-linked retinitis pigmentosa. Arch Ophthalmol 106(3):362–368

Iannaccone A, Wang X, Jablonski MM et al (2004) Increasing evidence for syndromic phenotypes associated with RPGR mutations. Am J Ophthalmol 137(4):785–786 author reply 786

Insinna C, Besharse JC (2008) Intraflagellar transport and the sensory outer segment of vertebrate photoreceptors. Dev Dyn 237(8):1982–1992

Kahn RA, Volpicelli-Daley L, Bowzard B et al (2005) Arf family GTPases: roles in membrane traffic and microtubule dynamics. Biochem Soc Trans 33(Pt 6):1269–1272

Khanna H, Hurd TW, Lillo C et al (2005) RPGR-ORF15, which is mutated in retinitis pigmentosa, associates with SMC1, SMC3, and microtubule transport proteins. J Biol Chem 280(39):33580–33587

Kirschner R, Rosenberg T, Schultz-Heienbrok R et al (1999) RPGR transcription studies in mouse and human tissues reveal a retina-specific isoform that is disrupted in a patient with X-linked retinitis pigmentosa. Hum Mol Genet 8(8):1571–1578

Koenekoop RK, Loyer M, Hand CK et al (2003) Novel RPGR mutations with distinct retinitis pigmentosa phenotypes in French-Canadian families. Am J Ophthalmol 136(4):678–687

Kuhnel K, Veltel S, Schlichting I et al (2006) Crystal structure of the human retinitis pigmentosa 2 protein and its interaction with Arl3. Structure 14(2):367–378

Linari M, Ueffing M, Manson F et al (1999) The retinitis pigmentosa GTPase regulator, RPGR, interacts with the delta subunit of rod cyclic GMP phosphodiesterase. Proc Natl Acad Sci USA 96(4):1315–1320

Liu Q, Tan G, Levenkova N et al (2007) The proteome of the mouse photoreceptor sensory cilium complex. Mol Cell Proteomics 6(8):1299–1317

Liu Q, Zuo J, Pierce EA (2004) The retinitis pigmentosa 1 protein is a photoreceptor microtubule-associated protein. J Neurosci 24(29):6427–6436

Marszalek JR, Liu X, Roberts EA et al (2000) Genetic evidence for selective transport of opsin and arrestin by kinesin-II in mammalian photoreceptors. Cell 102(2):175–187

Mavlyutov TA, Zhao H, Ferreira PA (2002) Species-specific subcellular localization of RPGR and RPGRIP isoforms: implications for the phenotypic variability of congenital retinopathies among species. Hum Mol Genet 11(16):1899–1907

McGuire RE, Sullivan LS, Blanton SH et al (1995) X-linked dominant cone-rod degeneration: linkage mapping of a new locus for retinitis pigmentosa (RP 15) to Xp22.13–p22.11. Am J Hum Genet 57(1):87–94

Mears AJ, Gieser L, Yan D et al (1999) Protein-truncation mutations in the RP2 gene in a North American cohort of families with X-linked retinitis pigmentosa. Am J Hum Genet 64(3): 897–900

Meindl A, Dry K, Herrmann K et al (1996) A gene (RPGR) with homology to the RCC1 guanine nucleotide exchange factor is mutated in X-linked retinitis pigmentosa (RP3). Nat Genet 13(1):35–42

Melamud A, Shen GQ, Chung D et al (2006) Mapping a new genetic locus for X linked retinitis pigmentosa to Xq28. J Med Genet 43(6):e27

Moore A, Escudier E, Roger G et al (2006) RPGR is mutated in patients with a complex X linked phenotype combining primary ciliary dyskinesia and retinitis pigmentosa. J Med Genet 43(4):326–333

Otto EA, Loeys B, Khanna H et al (2005) Nephrocystin-5, a ciliary IQ domain protein, is mutated in Senior-Loken syndrome and interacts with RPGR and calmodulin. Nat Genet 37(3):282–288

Pazour GJ, Baker SA, Deane JA et al (2002) The intraflagellar transport protein, IFT88, is essential for vertebrate photoreceptor assembly and maintenance. J Cell Biol 157(1):103–113

Pedersen LB, Veland IR, Schroder JM et al (2008) Assembly of primary cilia. Dev Dyn 237(8):1993–2006

Renault L, Kuhlmann J, Henkel A et al (2001) Structural basis for guanine nucleotide exchange on Ran by the regulator of chromosome condensation (RCC1). Cell 105(2):245–255

Roepman R, van Duijnhoven G, Rosenberg T et al (1996) Positional cloning of the gene for X-linked retinitis pigmentosa 3: homology with the guanine-nucleotide-exchange factor RCC1. Hum Mol Genet 5(7):1035–1041

Rosenbaum JL, Cole DG, Diener DR (1999) Intraflagellar transport: the eyes have it. J Cell Biol 144(3):385–388

Sayer JA, Otto EA, O'Toole J et al (2006) The centrosomal protein nephrocystin-6 is mutated in Joubert syndrome and activates transcription factor ATF4. Nat Genet 38(6):674–681

Schwahn U, Lenzner S, Dong J (1998) Positional cloning of the gene for X-linked retinitis pigmentosa 2. Nat Genet 19(4):327–332

Sharon D, Bruns GA, McGee TL et al (2000) X-linked retinitis pigmentosa: mutation spectrum of the RPGR and RP2 genes and correlation with visual function. Invest Ophthalmol Vis Sci 41(9):2712–2721

Sharon D, Sandberg MA, Rabe VW et al (2003) RP2 and RPGR mutations and clinical correlations in patients with X-linked retinitis pigmentosa. Am J Hum Genet 73(5):1131–1146

Shu X, Black GC, Rice JM et al (2007) RPGR mutation analysis and disease: an update. Hum Mutat 28(4):322–328

Shu X, Fry AM, Tulloch B et al (2005) RPGR ORF15 isoform co-localizes with RPGRIP1 at centrioles and basal bodies and interacts with nucleophosmin. Hum Mol Genet 14(9): 1183–1197

Sullivan LS, Daiger SP (1996) Inherited retinal degeneration: exceptional genetic and clinical heterogeneity. Mol Med Today 2(9):380–386

van Dorp DB, Wright AF, Carothers AD et al (1992) A family with RP3 type of X-linked retinitis pigmentosa: an association with ciliary abnormalities. Hum Genet 88(3):331–334

Vervoort R, Lennon A, Bird AC et al (2000) Mutational hot spot within a new RPGR exon in X-linked retinitis pigmentosa. Nat Genet 25(4):462–466

Williams DS (2002) Transport to the photoreceptor outer segment by myosin VIIa and kinesin II. Vision Res 42(4):455–462

Wright AF, Bhattacharya SS, Aldred MA et al (1991) Genetic localisation of the RP2 type of X linked retinitis pigmentosa in a large kindred. J Med Genet 28(7):453–457

Yan D, Swain PK, Breuer D et al (1998) Biochemical characterization and subcellular localization of the mouse retinitis pigmentosa GTPase regulator (mRpgr). J Biol Chem 273(31): 19656–19663

Yang Z, Peachey NS, Moshfeghi DM et al (2002) Mutations in the RPGR gene cause X-linked cone dystrophy. Hum Mol Genet 11(5):605–611

Young RW (1968) Passage of newly formed protein through the connecting cilium of retina rods in the frog. J Ultrastruct Res 23(5):462–473

Zhang Q, Acland GM, Wu WX et al (2002) Different RPGR exon ORF15 mutations in Canids provide insights into photoreceptor cell degeneration. Hum Mol Genet 11(9):993–1003

Zhang H, Liu XH, Zhang K et al (2004) Photoreceptor cGMP phosphodiesterase delta subunit (PDEdelta) functions as a prenyl-binding protein. J Biol Chem 279(1):407–413

Zhao Y, Hong DH, Pawlyk B et al (2003) The retinitis pigmentosa GTPase regulator (RPGR)-interacting protein: subserving RPGR function and participating in disk morphogenesis. Proc Natl Acad Sci USA 100(7):3965–3970

Zito I, Downes SM, Patel RJ et al (2003) RPGR mutation associated with retinitis pigmentosa, impaired hearing, and sinorespiratory infections. J Med Genet 40(8):609–615

Chapter 14
Misfolded Proteins and Retinal Dystrophies

Jonathan H. Lin and Matthew M. LaVail

Abstract Many mutations associated with retinal degeneration lead to the production of misfolded proteins by cells of the retina. Emerging evidence suggests that these abnormal proteins cause cell death by activating the Unfolded Protein Response, a set of conserved intracellular signaling pathways that detect protein misfolding within the endoplasmic reticulum and control protective and proapoptotic signal transduction pathways. Here, we review the misfolded proteins associated with select types of retinitis pigmentosa, Stargadt-like macular degeneration, and Doyne Honeycomb Retinal Dystrophy and discuss the role that endoplasmic reticulum stress and UPR signaling play in their pathogenesis. Last, we review new therapies for these diseases based on preventing protein misfolding in the retina.

14.1 Endoplasmic Reticulum Stress and Retinal Degeneration

The retina collects and transmits light information through an intricate network of highly specialized neural cells. To accomplish this unique sensory function, cells of the retina produce a specialized array of proteins such as rhodopsin. Transmission of accurate visual information depends on the continuous production of high-quality, functional proteins by cells of the retina. Cells have evolved elaborate mechanisms to ensure that membrane and secreted proteins are accurately folded and assembled before export or delivery to the cell surface. Stringent quality control is imposed by the endoplasmic reticulum (ER), a membrane-bound organelle, where virtually all plasma and secreted proteins begin their journey to the surface. Only properly folded proteins are allowed to exit the ER. Misfolded proteins are retained by the ER and degraded to prevent the generation of proteins that may be dysfunctional

J.H. Lin (✉)
Department of Pathology, University of California, San Diego, La Jolla, CA 92093-0612, USA
e-mail: matthew.lavail@ucsf.edu

R.E. Anderson et al. (eds.), *Retinal Degenerative Diseases*, Advances in Experimental Medicine and Biology 664, DOI 10.1007/978-1-4419-1399-9_14, © Springer Science+Business Media, LLC 2010

or potentially toxic. If ER protein quality control fails and chronic protein misfolding ensues, cell death occurs via apoptosis. Cells have evolved a set of intracellular signaling pathways termed the Unfolded Protein Response (UPR) that detect protein misfolding within the ER and direct protective and proapoptotic responses (Lin et al. 2008). The UPR provides an attractive molecular framework to investigate the molecular pathogenesis of retinal dystrophies arising from protein misfolding. Over 100 different heritable mutations have been identified that lead to death of retinal cells and loss of vision (www.sph.uth.tmc.edu/retnet/). Many of these genetic defects lead to the production of abnormal proteins by retinal cell types. Here we review some of the protein mutations linked to retinal degeneration and evidence that implicates UPR signaling in the cell death elicited by these mutations.

14.2 Misfolded Proteins in Photoreceptors

Rhodopsin is by far the predominant protein within photoreceptors, where it comprises ~30% of the entire proteome of photoreceptors and over 90% of all proteins in the outer segment region of photoreceptors (Hargrave 2001). Rhodopsin plays a critical role in phototransduction and is expressed solely by rod photoreceptors. Rhodopsin is the archetypal serpentine G-protein coupled receptor and consists of a 348 amino acid polypeptide organized into 7 transmembrane helices and a binding pocket for light-sensitive 11-cis-retinal (Hargrave 2001; Palczewski et al. 2000). Like virtually all membrane proteins, rhodopsin synthesis occurs at the ER, where the nascent rhodopsin polypeptide is co-translationally inserted into the membrane and undergoes multiple post-translational modifications including disulfide bond formation and glycosylation at asparagine residues (Fukuda et al. 1979; Kaushal et al. 1994; Krebs et al. 2004). Once properly folded, rhodopsin exits the ER and enters the Golgi apparatus where it undergoes additional sugar modifications and is eventually delivered to the rod photoreceptor outer segment (Liang et al. 1979). In the rod outer segment, the 11-cis-retinal vitamin A derivative is covalently linked to opsin (the apoprotein of rhodopsin) by a protonated Schiff base at a lysine residue to create the final rhodopsin chromophore. When light strikes rhodopsin, a photon is absorbed that causes the retinal to isomerize to the all-trans form which drives the rhodopsin protein through a series of transient photo-intermediates that bind and activate the G protein, transducin. A cascade of biochemical events ensues that result in a drop in cGMP concentration, the closing of the calcium conductance channels in the plasma membrane, and hyperpolarization of the cell, thereby generating an electrical signal and activating the neural circuitry underlying vision.

Mutations in the visual pigment, rhodopsin, are the most common cause of hereditary of RP and account for 25–30% of autosomal dominant RP (adRP) (Berson et al. 2001; Sohocki et al. 2001). Over 100 distinct missense mutations in rhodopsin have been identified that lead to retinal degeneration, including recessive and autosomal dominant forms of retinitis pigmentosa, and congenital stationary night blindness

(Retnet http://www.sph.uth.tmc.edu/RetNet). These mutations are found throughout the rhodopsin molecule. Seminal studies performed by the labs of Jeremy Nathans and Gobind Khorana in the 1990s demonstrated that the vast majority of adRP-linked rhodopsin mutations lead to misfolding of the rhodopsin protein.

Many of these studies have focused on the most common rhodopsin mutation leading to adRP in the United States, a missense mutation at amino acid position 23 of rhodopsin that replaces a proline with a histidine residue (P23H RHO) (Retnet http://www.sph.uth.tmc.edu/RetNet). P23H RHO fails to bind 11-cis-retinal (Kaushal and Khorana 1994; Kaushal et al. 1994; Liu et al. 1996). The crystal structure of rhodopsin indicates that the proline[23] residue is located in the N-terminal intradiscal tail within one of the β-strands that comprise the N-terminal plug of the molecule (Palczewski et al. 2000). The N-terminal plug normally positions and binds 11-cis-retinal to form fully functional rhodopsin. Mutations in this region, such as the P23H substitution, could lead to misfolding of the N-terminal plug and hence impair binding of the chromophore. Biochemical data support that the P23H mutation induces rhodopsin misfolding: mutant rhodopsins form oligomeric aggregates; P23H rhodopsin displays abnormal sensitivity to trypsin compared to wild-type rhodopsin when expressed in cell culture; P23H rhodopsin is not properly glycosylated compared to wild-type rhodopsin, and instead, is complexed with ER-resident chaperones such as BiP or Grp94 (Anukanth and Khorana 1994; Liu et al. 1996; Noorwez et al. 2004). Immunocytochemical and ultrastructural studies in cultured cells and retinas from transgenic mice and frogs also revealed that P23H rhodopsin is localized to the ER/Golgi, whereas wild-type rhodopsin translocates to the surface membrane (Frederick et al. 2001; Kaushal and Khorana 1994; Saliba et al. 2002; Sung et al. 1991; Tam and Moritz 2006). In sum, these findings provide biochemical, cellular, and genetic evidence that P23H rhodopsin is misfolded in the ER and set the foundation for investigating the molecular events downstream of rhodopsin misfolding and retention in the ER leading to photoreceptor cell death. Moreover, data established for P23H rhodopsin are likely to hold true for additional adRP-linked mutant rhodopsins; indeed, in Liu, Garriga, and Khorana PNAS 93:4554–4559, 1996, they state that: "We suggest that most, if not all, of the point mutations in the intradiscal domain identified in adRP cause partial or complete misfolding of rhodopsin (Liu et al. 1996)."

Recent studies indicate that the Unfolded Protein Response (UPR) signaling pathways link rhodopsin misfolding in the ER and cell fate. In a Drosophila model of retinal degeneration arising from rhodopsin misfolding, robust activation of the IRE1 signaling pathway of the UPR was observed in the fly and intriguingly, genetic down-regulation of this pathway accelerated retinal degeneration (Ryoo et al. 2007). In multiple rodent models of adRP that express different levels of P23H rhodopsin and undergo different rates of retinal degeneration, multiple distinct UPR signaling pathways were selectively activated in P23H animals compared to wild-type siblings. In these animals, proapoptotic UPR signaling molecules such as CHOP were markedly elevated in animals expressing misfolded rhodopsin at time points that preceded frank loss of photoreceptors, raising the possibility that activation of UPR signaling by misfolded rhodopsin directly drives photoreceptor cell death (Lin et al.

2007). Future studies will focus on determining causality between UPR activation and photoreceptor cell survival after rhodopsin misfolding.

Mutations in *ElovL4* have been identified in Stargadt-like macular degeneration, an autosomal dominant form of juvenile retinal degeneration (Zhang et al. 2001). *ElovL4* encodes an enzyme thought to be involved in the generation of long-chain fatty acids (Karan et al. 2004; Oh et al. 1997; Vasireddy et al. 2008). Consistent with its role in lipid biosynthesis, ELOVL4 is a membrane protein targeted to the ER (Karan et al. 2004; Vasireddy et al. 2005). Photoreceptors express high levels of ELOVL4, but in contrast to rhodopsin, its expression has also been reported in other cell types in the eye (Zhang et al. 2003). At the molecular level, mutations in *ElovL4* that trigger macular degeneration lead to premature truncations of the protein that all result in loss of an ER retention motif. In biochemical studies, mutant ELOVL4 is isolated as a higher-order complex, and in transfected cells, immunofluorescence reveals that mutant ELOVL4 is no longer distributed in a reticular manner but instead found as perinuclear aggregates (Karan et al. 2005; Vasireddy et al. 2005). These findings are consistent with misfolding of mutant ELOVL4. Intriguingly, in these in vitro studies, mutant ELOVL4 binds and sequesters wild-type ELOVL4 into higher order aggregates, perhaps accounting for its dominant phenotype (Karan et al. 2005; Vasireddy et al. 2005). Mutant ELOVL4 also activates the UPR in transfected cells, raising the possibility that these signaling pathways link ELOVL4 misfolding and aggregation in the ER and photoreceptor cell fate (Karan et al. 2005).

The *rd1* mutation results in the profound reduction of PDE6-β protein presumably through destabilization of the mutated mRNA or nascent protein. PDE6-β is a catalytic subunit of a phosphodiesterase that regulates cGMP levels in photoreceptors in response to light activation. Absence of the PDE6-β disrupts phosphodiesterase activity and accumulation of cGMP, which in turn, enhances cGMP-gated ion channels, leading to significant rises in intracellular calcium and ultimately photoreceptor cell death. Recent work demonstrates that multiple UPR signaling pathways are also activated in the *rd1* mouse at ages that precede frank photoreceptor cell death (Yang et al. 2007). These findings suggest that UPR signaling may also play a role in the pathogenesis of this type of retinal degeneration. However, PDE6-β is a cytosolic enzyme, whereas UPR signaling pathways are activated by perturbations in the ER. How would the *rd1* mutation then trigger the UPR? Besides protein folding, the ER also performs crucial cellular functions that include the synthesis of lipids and sterols and the storage of calcium. Defects in lipid/sterol metabolism and calcium homeostasis can also elicit endoplasmic reticulum stress (Lin et al. 2008). Calcium dysregulation in *rd1* and other retinal diseases could activate the UPR, though this remains to be investigated.

14.3 Misfolded Proteins in Retinal Pigment Epithelial Cells

A missense mutation in *fibulin-3* leading to an arginine-to-tryptophan substitution at amino acid 345 (R345W) has been found in an autosomal dominant maculopathy, malattia leventinese and Doyne Honeycomb Retinal Dystrophy (ML/DHRD) (Stone et al. 1999). *Fibulin-3* encodes an extracellular protein that is expressed and secreted by retinal pigment epithelial (RPE) cells (Marmorstein et al. 2002). In cell culture studies, mutant R345W Fibulin-3 is inefficiently secreted, and the majority is retained in the ER (Roybal et al. 2005). UPR signaling pathways are activated leading to increased BiP/grp78 and VEGF production (Blais et al. 2006; Roybal et al. 2005). These findings support a model whereby mutant fibulin-3 leads to macular degeneration through its misfolding in the ER and activation of UPR signaling pathways in RPE cells, followed by enhanced VEGF production and choroidal neovascularization. Enhanced VEGF levels and choroidal neovascularization are also key features of AMD (Campochiaro 2007), raising the possibility that abnormal ER stress and UPR activity in RPE may also be at play in sporadic types of macular dystrophy.

14.4 Pharmacologic Targeting of Protein Misfolding to Prevent Retinal Degeneration

Given the link between protein misfolding and retinal degeneration, most clearly established in the case of rhodopsin, pharmacologic prevention of protein misfolding has emerged as an exciting new strategy to treat these diseases. Chaperones are ubiquitous proteins dedicated to folding and stabilizing proteins, and recent studies by Noorwez and colleagues have demonstrated that retinoids and other related diffusible artificial chaperones can promote mutant rhodopsin binding of 11-cis-retinal such that it can function as a light chromophore (Noorwez et al. 2003, 2004, 2008). Mendes and colleagues have also recently demonstrated, in vitro, that retinoids and other agents that prevent protein aggregation can prevent cell death elicited by rhodopsin misfolding (Mendes and Cheetham 2008). These compounds suggest that preventing rhodopsin misfolding may be a new strategy to prevent retinal degeneration. This approach may also be efficacious in other retinal diseases arising from protein misfolding.

Acknowledgments We thank Victory Joseph for helpful comments. This work was funded by NIH grants EY01919, EY06842, EY02162, EY018313; the Foundation Fighting Blindness; and RPB.

References

Anukanth A, Khorana HG (1994) Structure and function in rhodopsin. Requirements of a specific structure for the intradiscal domain. J Biol Chem 269:19738–19744

Berson EL, Grimsby JL, Adams SM et al (2001) Clinical features and mutations in patients with dominant retinitis pigmentosa-1 (RP1). Invest Ophthalmol Vis Sci 42:2217–2224

Blais JD, Addison CL, Edge R et al (2006) Perk-dependent translational regulation promotes tumor cell adaptation and angiogenesis in response to hypoxic stress. Mol Cell Biol 26:9517–9532

Campochiaro PA (2007) Molecular targets for retinal vascular diseases. J Cell Physiol 210:575–581

Frederick JM, Krasnoperova NV, Hoffmann K et al (2001) Mutant rhodopsin transgene expression on a null background. Invest Ophthalmol Vis Sci 42:826–833

Fukuda MN, Papermaster DS, Hargrave PA (1979) Rhodopsin carbohydrate. Structure of small oligosaccharides attached at two sites near the NH2 terminus. J Biol Chem 254: 8201–8207

Hargrave PA (2001) Rhodopsin structure, function, and topography the Friedenwald lecture. Invest Ophthalmol Vis Sci 42:3–9

Karan G, Yang Z, Howes K et al (2005) Loss of ER retention and sequestration of the wild-type ELOVL4 by Stargardt disease dominant negative mutants. Mol Vis 11:657–664

Karan G, Yang Z, Zhang K (2004) Expression of wild type and mutant ELOVL4 in cell culture: subcellular localization and cell viability. Mol Vis 10:248–253

Kaushal S, Khorana HG (1994) Structure and function in rhodopsin. 7. Point mutations associated with autosomal dominant retinitis pigmentosa. Biochemistry 33:6121–6128

Kaushal S, Ridge KD, Khorana HG (1994) Structure and function in rhodopsin: the role of asparagine-linked glycosylation. Proc Natl Acad Sci USA 91:4024–4028

Krebs MP, Noorwez SM, Malhotra R et al (2004) Quality control of integral membrane proteins. Trends Biochem Sci 29:648–655

Liang CJ, Yamashita K, Muellenberg CG et al (1979) Structure of the carbohydrate moieties of bovine rhodopsin. J Biol Chem 254:6414–6418

Lin JH, Li H, Yasumura D et al (2007) IRE1 signaling affects cell fate during the unfolded protein response. Science 318:944–949

Lin JH, Walter P, Yen TS (2008) Endoplasmic reticulum stress in disease pathogenesis. Annu Rev Pathol 3:399–425

Liu X, Garriga P, Khorana HG (1996) Structure and function in rhodopsin: correct folding and misfolding in two point mutants in the intradiscal domain of rhodopsin identified in retinitis pigmentosa. Proc Natl Acad Sci USA 93:4554–4559

Marmorstein LY, Munier FL, Arsenijevic Y et al (2002) Aberrant accumulation of EFEMP1 underlies drusen formation in Malattia Leventinese and age-related macular degeneration. Proc Natl Acad Sci USA 99:13067–13072

Mendes HF, Cheetham ME (2008) Pharmacological manipulation of gain-of-function and dominant-negative mechanisms in rhodopsin retinitis pigmentosa. Hum Mol Genet 17: 3043–3054

Noorwez SM, Kuksa V, Imanishi Y et al (2003) Pharmacological chaperone-mediated in vivo folding and stabilization of the P23H-opsin mutant associated with autosomal dominant retinitis pigmentosa. J Biol Chem 278:14442–14450

Noorwez SM, Malhotra R, McDowell JH et al (2004) Retinoids assist the cellular folding of the autosomal dominant retinitis pigmentosa opsin mutant P23H. J Biol Chem 279: 16278–16284

Noorwez SM, Ostrov DA, McDowell JH et al (2008) A high-throughput screening method for small-molecule pharmacologic chaperones of misfolded rhodopsin. Invest Ophthalmol Vis Sci 49:3224–3230

Oh CS, Toke DA, Mandala S et al (1997) ELO2 and ELO3, homologues of the Saccharomyces cerevisiae ELO1 gene, function in fatty acid elongation and are required for sphingolipid formation. J Biol Chem 272:17376–17384

Palczewski K, Kumasaka T, Hori T et al (2000) Crystal structure of rhodopsin: a G protein-coupled receptor. Science 289:739–745

Roybal CN, Marmorstein LY, Vander Jagt DL et al (2005) Aberrant accumulation of fibulin-3 in the endoplasmic reticulum leads to activation of the unfolded protein response and VEGF expression. Invest Ophthalmol Vis Sci 46:3973–3979

Ryoo HD, Domingos PM, Kang MJ et al (2007) Unfolded protein response in a Drosophila model for retinal degeneration. Embo J 26:242–252

Saliba RS, Munro PM, Luthert PJ et al (2002) The cellular fate of mutant rhodopsin: quality control, degradation and aggresome formation. J Cell Sci 115:2907–2918

Sohocki MM, Daiger SP, Bowne SJ et al (2001) Prevalence of mutations causing retinitis pigmentosa and other inherited retinopathies. Hum Mutat 17:42–51

Stone EM, Lotery AJ, Munier FL et al (1999) A single EFEMP1 mutation associated with both Malattia Leventinese and Doyne honeycomb retinal dystrophy. Nat Genet 22:199–202

Sung CH, Schneider BG, Agarwal N et al (1991) Functional heterogeneity of mutant rhodopsins responsible for autosomal dominant retinitis pigmentosa. Proc Natl Acad Sci USA 88: 8840–8844

Tam BM, Moritz OL (2006) Characterization of rhodopsin P23H-induced retinal degeneration in a Xenopus laevis model of retinitis pigmentosa. Invest Ophthalmol Vis Sci 47:3234–3241

Vasireddy V, Sharon M, Salem N Jr et al (2008) Role of ELOVL4 in fatty acid metabolism. Adv Exp Med Biol 613:283–290

Vasireddy V, Vijayasarathy C, Huang J et al (2005) Stargardt-like macular dystrophy protein ELOVL4 exerts a dominant negative effect by recruiting wild-type protein into aggresomes. Mol Vis 11:665–676

Yang LP, Wu LM, Guo XJ et al (2007) Activation of endoplasmic reticulum stress in degenerating photoreceptors of the rd1 mouse. Invest Ophthalmol Vis Sci 48:5191–5198

Zhang K, Kniazeva M, Han M et al (2001) A 5-bp deletion in ELOVL4 is associated with two related forms of autosomal dominant macular dystrophy. Nat Genet 27:89–93

Zhang XM, Yang Z, Karan G et al (2003) Elovl4 mRNA distribution in the developing mouse retina and phylogenetic conservation of Elovl4 genes. Mol Vis 9:301–307

Chapter 15
Neural Retina and MerTK-Independent Apical Polarity of αvβ5 Integrin Receptors in the Retinal Pigment Epithelium

Mallika Mallavarapu and Silvia C. Finnemann

Abstract The apical plasma membrane domain of retinal pigment epithelial (RPE) cells in the eye faces the outer segment portions of rods and cones and the inter-photoreceptor matrix in the subretinal space. Two important receptor-mediated interactions between the apical surface of the retinal pigment epithelium (RPE) and adjacent photoreceptors are adhesion ensuring outer segment alignment and diurnal phagocytosis of shed outer segment fragments contributing to outer segment renewal. Both depend on the apical distribution of the integrin family adhesion receptor αvβ5 as lack of αvβ5 in mice causes weakened retinal adhesion and asynchronous phagocytosis. With age, lack of αvβ5 leads to accumulation of harmful lipofuscin in the RPE and to vision loss. Here, we discuss three different possible mechanisms that could generate the exclusive apical distribution of αvβ5 integrin receptors in the RPE. (1) αvβ5 could be apical in the RPE because RPE attachment to neural retina generally or αvβ5 ligands specifically in the subretinal space stabilize apical but not basolateral αvβ5 surface receptors. (2) αvβ5 could be apical in the RPE because it resides in a complex with other components of the phagocytic machinery that assembles at the apical, phagocytic surface of the RPE. (3) αvβ5 could be apical due to mechanisms intrinsic to this receptor protein and specifically to its β5 integrin subunit.

Abbreviations

POS   shed photoreceptor outer segment fragments
RPE   retinal pigment epithelium

S.C. Finnemann (✉)
Department of Biological Sciences, Fordham University, Bronx, NY 10458, USA
e-mail: finnemann@fordham.edu

R.E. Anderson et al. (eds.), *Retinal Degenerative Diseases*, Advances in Experimental Medicine and Biology 664, DOI 10.1007/978-1-4419-1399-9_15,
© Springer Science+Business Media, LLC 2010

15.1 Introduction

Post-mitotic retinal pigment epithelial cells (RPE) in the eye form a stationary monolayer epithelium whose lateral junctions seal off the neural retina from the underlying vascularized choroidal tissue forming the outer blood-retinal barrier. The plasma membrane of each RPE cell is strictly divided by a tight junction permeability barrier. The RPE's basolateral domain faces Bruch's membrane, a multi-layer basement membrane rich in adhesive glycoproteins such as laminin and collagen IV connecting to the vascularized choroid. The RPE's apical plasma membrane faces the avascular subretinal space where it adheres to components of the interphotoreceptor matrix and possibly the outer segment plasma membrane of photoreceptor rods and cones. These apical interactions are unusual compared to most other epithelial tissues that line fluid-filled lumina. Distinct protein distributions at its basolateral and apical surfaces are an obvious prerequisite for functions of the RPE associated with its control of molecular flux into and out of the neural retina, such as vectorial transport of ions, water, and metabolites. Moreover, other functions of RPE cells also take place exclusively at one of their surface domains. Diurnal phagocytosis of shed photoreceptor outer segment fragments and mechanically stable adhesion likely mostly to interphotoreceptor extracellular matrix components are two receptor protein-dependent functions that take place at the apical surface of the RPE in the eye (Finnemann and Chang 2008). To qualify for an essential role in the molecular machineries involved in these RPE functions membrane candidate proteins must therefore localize at least in part to the apical surface of the RPE in situ.

15.2 Functions of Apical αvβ5 Integrin Receptors in Retinal Phagocytosis and Adhesion

Diurnal synchronized phagocytosis of photoreceptor outer segment tips shed daily by photoreceptor cells is an essential task of the RPE deficiencies of which cause retinal degeneration in animal models and cause some forms of human retinitis pigmentosa. Prompted by the initial observation that onset of expression at the apical surface of the integrin family adhesion receptor αvβ5 correlates exactly with the begin of daily shedding and phagocytosis in maturing rat RPE (Finnemann and Bonilha 1997) we studied RPE phagocytosis in knockout mice lacking the β5 integrin subunit and thus αvβ5 integrin receptors (Nandrot and Kim 2004). As young adults, β5 integrin knockout mice had normal retinal morphology and function but we counted similar numbers of outer segment derived phagosomes in their RPE cells at all times of day. This was in sharp contrast to strain- and age-matched wild-type mice whose RPE contained phagosomes only within 3 h following light onset, similar to earlier observations by others. Furthermore, RPE cells of β5 knockout mice at old age contained excess numbers of autofluorescence inclusions resembling lipofuscin granules that increasingly accumulate in human RPE with age. At the same age, photoreceptor function measured by electroretinography was considerably impaired in β5 knockout mice suggesting that accumulation of debris accumulating with age in β5 knockout RPE is harmful for the retina. Finally, RPE cells isolated from young β5 knockout mice in culture demonstrated normal morphology but dramatically reduced binding activity towards isolated photoreceptor outer segment fragments. Notably, lack of αvβ5 in situ or in RPE in culture abolished the stimulation of tyrosine kinases focal adhesion kinase (FAK) and Mer tyrosine kinase (MerTK) both of which are essential for POS engulfment. Taken together, these results identified a critical function for αvβ5 receptors in synchronizing diurnal RPE phagocytosis likely by stimulating rhythmic downstream tyrosine kinase signaling.

Like diurnal phagocytosis, robust adhesion of the apical aspect of the RPE to the retina generally and the interphotoreceptor matrix and outer segments specifically is enormously important for retinal health. Its disruption in retinal detachment rapidly leads to a variety of well described stress responses in the neural retina (Fisher and Lewis 2005). If prolonged, retinal detachment will result in photoreceptor apoptotic cell death and hence vision loss (Cook and Lewis 1995). The receptor proteins on the RPE's apical surface that are responsible for retinal adhesion are only poorly characterized. Since αvβ5 integrin promotes adhesion to extracellular matrices in other tissues, we tested if apical αvβ5 receptors may contribute to retinal adhesion. β5 integrin knockout mice do not exhibit retinal detachment. However, using semi-quantitative detachment assays we demonstrated that resistance to shear forces is considerably reduced in these mice indicating weakened retinal adhesion (Nandrot et al. 2006). Since β5 knockout retinal adhesion differed to similar extent from wild-type retinal adhesion at all ages examined, we concluded that this impairment was not a consequence of asynchronous phagocytosis and lipofuscin accumulation. Instead, we concluded that αvβ5 integrin receptors fulfill two distinct functions at the apical surface of the RPE, retinal adhesion and phagocytosis.

15.3   Apical Polarity of αvβ5 Integrin Receptors is Independent of the Neural Retina

Integrin receptors that reside on cellular surfaces are likely engaged in receptor-ligand interactions. Unoccupied integrins may indicate lack of proper tissue context and have been demonstrate to be sufficient to induce apoptotic cell death (Frisch and Screaton 2001). Thus, it is generally thought that, at steady-state, integrins only localize to surfaces where appropriate ligands are available. Related to this, once ligand-bound, integrin receptors are more likely to persist at the cell surface for longer periods of time than unoccupied integrin receptors. Apical polarity of αvβ5 receptors in the RPE may thus be a consequence of unique availability of stabilizing ligands at the apical surface. This would imply that ligands for αvβ5 may be scarce or even absent at the basolateral surface of the RPE. However, this is an unlikely scenario.

First, RPE cells in the eye express numerous integrin receptors. All integrin receptors found to be expressed by the RPE in the retina besides $\alpha v \beta 5$ show a highly polarized basolateral distribution. This includes the integrin receptor, $\alpha v \beta 3$, which is most related to $\alpha v \beta 5$ sharing the αv subunit and with overlapping if not identical ligand binding preferences (Finnemann and Bonilha 1997). Our knowledge of integrin ligands available to RPE cells in the eye at either surface aspect are not fully characterized but the joint ligand for $\alpha v \beta 3$ and $\alpha v \beta 5$, vitronectin, localizes to Bruch's membrane. We have previously identified the extracellular RGD-domain glycoprotein MFG-E8 as sole ligand that activates $\alpha v \beta 5$ downstream signaling toward MerTK in the retina that is essential for diurnal phagocytosis (Nandrot and Anand 2007). Mice lacking MFG-E8 lack the diurnal rhythm of RPE phagocytosis exactly like mice lacking $\alpha v \beta 5$. This correlation is supported by RPE culture studies showing that recombinant MFG-E8 enhances wild-type phagocytosis and restores phagocytosis by MFG-E8 knockout RPE cells to wild-type levels but has no effect on uptake by $\beta 5$ knockout RPE cells. These data demonstrate that MFG-E8 is the only essential ligand for the phagocytic function of $\alpha v \beta 5$ in the retina. Notably, mice lacking MFG-E8 have only minimally reduced retinal adhesion in contrast to $\beta 5$ knockout mice. This implies that the retinal adhesive function of $\alpha v \beta 5$ uses ligands other than MFG-E8 in the subretinal space. At this time, these ligands remain unidentified. However, $\alpha v \beta 3$ can bind MFG-E8 like $\alpha v \beta 5$ but exclusively localizes to the basolateral and not the apical surface of the RPE in the retina. Taken together, these results suggest that ligands for $\alpha v \beta 5$ exist at both apical and basolateral surfaces of the RPE rendering selective retention at the apical surface unlikely.

Second, if specific apical ligands available to $\alpha v \beta 5$ generate the strict apical polarity observed for this receptor, disruption of the native apical interactions of RPE cells would likely promote $\alpha v \beta 5$ redistribution. Earlier studies aiming to identify molecular mechanisms involved in generating specific protein polarity in the RPE have shown that some transmembrane proteins that distribute apically in the RPE in the retina are non-polar or basolateral in RPE cell in culture. This has been particularly well studied for two type I transmembrane proteins, the Ig-CAM family cell adhesion receptor N-CAM and the matrix metalloproteinase protein EMMPRIN (Marmorstein and Gan 1998; Gundersen and Powell 1993). Both are commonly expressed by epithelial tissues and cell lines. Both are basolateral in kidney epithelium as well as in the best-characterized culture model for cell polarity, the kidney epithelium derived Madin Darby Kidney (MDCK) cell line. Both mostly distribute to the apical surface of RPE cells in the retina but rapidly relocalize in RPE in culture. N-CAM assumes a strictly lateral localization likely contributing to adhesive contacts between neighboring RPE cells in culture. EMMPRIN is non-polar in culture. While the precise interacting molecules remain to be identified, these data suggest that the steady-state apical distribution of both N-CAM and EMMPRIN in RPE in situ is a consequence of molecular interactions of the RPE's apical surface that take place in the subretinal space.

Yet, αvβ5 receptors maintain their apical steady-state polarity even in RPE cells in tissue culture. Indeed, immunofluorescence microscopy of αvβ5 surface receptors in primary, unpassaged mouse RPE, the immortalized rat RPE cell line RPE-J, the human spontaneously immortalized cell line ARPE-19 and the human RPE derived d407 cell line demonstrates that like RPE in the eye facing the interphotoreceptor matrix with its ligand MFG-E8 all these RPE model cells possess apical αvβ5 despite great species and phenotypical discrepancies among them otherwise (Fig. 15.1). These findings demonstrate that the apical polarity of αvβ5 is maintained

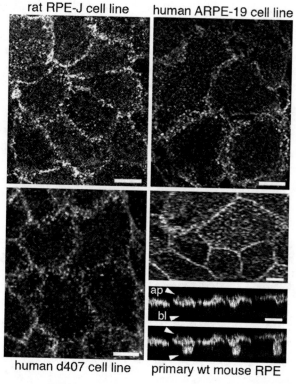

Fig. 15.1 Apical polarity of αvβ5 integrin receptors in RPE cells in culture. Rat RPE-J, human ARPE-19 and human d407 RPE cell lines, as indicated, were grown to confluence on glass coverslips and labeled live on ice with αvβ5 surface dimer-specific antibody P1F6. 3D projections representing the *upper* 2 μm of apical aspects of cells are shown. Wild-type 129 strain mouse RPE was isolated in patches from 10-day-old mouse eyes, cultured for 4 days before fixation and labeling with antibody recognizing the β5 integrin cytoplasmic domain. Images were acquired by laser scanning confocal microscopy. Representative whole cell maximal projections of the same field are shown in x–y plane and in x–z plane. x–z projection is shown with (*upper panel*) and without (*lower panel*) nuclei counterstaining. Approximate locations of apical (ap) and basolateral (bl) surfaces of cells are indicated by *arrowheads* in the *upper panel*. Scale bar is 10 μm for cell lines and 20 μm for primary RPE

by RPE cells autonomously independent of their apposition to and interactions with the neural retina and the MFG-E8-rich interphotoreceptor matrix.

15.4 Apical Polarity of αvβ5 Receptors is Independent of the Essential Engulfment Receptor MerTK

Phagocytic mechanisms involve the coordinated activities of numerous cell surface receptors, associated cytosolic proteins and the actin cytoskeleton. As outlined earlier, RPE phagocytosis in the eye and in culture involves αvβ5 integrin recognition of its ligand MFG-E8, which likely acts to bridge shed POS and αvβ5. In the mouse retina, this interaction is required for subsequent maximal stimulation of MerTK via FAK causing the burst of engulfment activity that characterizes the response to POS of wild-type RPE. Additional receptor proteins such as the receptor for modified lipids, CD36, likely contribute to RPE phagocytosis as well although their precise roles remain unresolved thus far. Given the close functional interaction of αvβ5 with MerTK we hence hypothesized that the apical polarity of αvβ5 may be a result of its integration into the complex phagocytic machinery of the RPE, which exists solely at the apical surface of the RPE in the eye. This would predict that αvβ5 apical polarity persists in RPE in culture as commonly studied primary and permanent RPE cell culture models (some of them mentioned above) retain specific phagocytic activity toward POS. We therefore studied whether αvβ5 was apical in mutant RPE cells that lack phagocytic function. Royal College of Surgeons (RCS) rats carry a

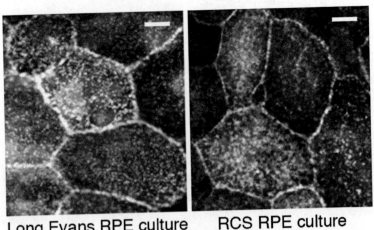

Long Evans RPE culture   RCS RPE culture

Fig. 15.2 Apical polarity of αvβ5 integrin receptors in MerTK-mutant RCS RPE cells. Wild-type Long Evans and mutant RCS rat RPE cells were isolated in patches from 10-day-old rat eyes and cultured for 4 days before live labeling on ice with αvβ5 surface dimer-specific antibody P1F6. Representative epifluorescence images are shown. Scale bar is 20 μm

mutation that eliminates MerTK protein expression. As a result, RCS RPE cells are unable to engulf POS in vivo and in vitro. Despite their phagocytic incompetence, RCS RPE cells in primary culture possess apical αvβ5 integrin receptors at equal levels as RPE cells isolated from wild-type rats (Fig. 15.2). This suggests that neither MerTK specifically nor a functional engulfment mechanism generally are required for the apical polarity of αvβ5 integrin receptors in RPE cells.

15.5   Motifs of the β5 Integrin Subunit Cytoplasmic Domain that May Promote Apical Polarity of αvβ5 Integrin Receptors

As discussed thus far, available data do not support a critical role for either neural retina apposition and specific ligands of the subretinal space, or for the essential phagocytic receptor MerTK and a functional phagocytic machinery in causing the unique apical polarity of αvβ5 integrin receptors in the RPE (Fig. 15.3). We therefore hypothesize that αvβ5 receptors traffic to or are specifically retained at the apical surface of the RPE as a result of specific motifs inherent to αvβ5 receptors. Because the αv subunit is not specific to αvβ5 but also forms basolateral αvβ3 receptors in the RPE, we will focus on possible contributions to receptor polarity of the β5 integrin protein subunit and particularly its cytoplasmic domain.

The β5 cytoplasmic domain consists of 60 amino acids (Legate and Fassler 2009). The β5 cytoplasmic tail is responsible for interaction with FAK in transfected cells (Eliceiri and Puente 2002) and FAK resides in the apical αvβ5 integrin complex in RPE cells where it is critical for stimulating MerTK and POS engulfment (Finnemann 2003). It contains an NPxY motif that is important for recruitment and binding of cytoplasmic proteins forming adhesive complexes in other proteins such as the actin binding protein talin (Horwitz and Duggan 1986; Calderwood 2004). Talin interacts with αvβ5 integrin receptors in transfected cells and this depends on the β5 subunit (Singh and D'Mello 2007). While this domain is thus likely important for αvβ5 function in RPE as well, it is also present in β1 and β3 integrin cytoplasmic domains and hence, does not explain the unique apical polarity of αvβ5. However, overall only 28 amino acids of the terminal 42 are identical between β5 and β3 tails. Single and di-leucine motifs contribute to trafficking mechanisms in other proteins (Deora and Gravotta 2004; Hunziker and Fumey 1994). Notably, in the β5 integrin the x position of the NPxY motif is leucine while in the β3 integrin the x position is isoleucine. Finally, The β5 integrin tail contains an inserted stretch of eight amino acids close to the carboxiterminus that has no homology to either β1 or β3 integrin and that effectively extends the β5 tails (Legate and Fassler 2009). Taken together, both β5 and β3 integrin subunits form phagocytic receptors with the αv subunit with very similar functions but in RPE cells only αvβ5 but not αvβ3 heterodimers localize to the apical plasma membrane. We therefore hypothesize that the unique residues and motifs of the β5 integrin cytoplasmic domain are responsible for the unique polarity of αvβ5 receptors.

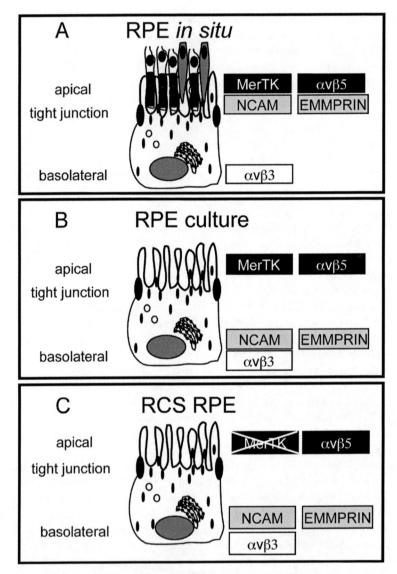

Fig. 15.3 Summary of steady-state polarity of selected transmembrane proteins in different RPE models as discussed in the text. **a.** Polarity in the RPE in the eye. **b.** Polarity in RPE cells in culture. **c.** Polarity in MerTK-deficient RCS RPE cells in culture

15.6 Perspective

αvβ5 integrin receptors fulfill two distinct and equally important functions at the apical surface of the RPE by contributing to retinal adhesion and by synchronizing diurnal POS phagocytosis. All evidence suggests that the unique apical polarity of αvβ5 receptors in the RPE is not merely a consequence of ligand-induced stabilization or of anchorage to the MerTK dependent engulfment machinery. Rather, we propose that RPE cells use a trafficking pathway to specifically sort αvβ5 to the apical surface. This pathway is likely to recognize motifs of the β5 cytoplasmic domain. Comparing trafficking and complex formation among αvβ5 receptors with cytoplasmic deletions and point mutations will be our future approach to identify trafficking-relevant residues and motifs of the β5 integrin cytoplasmic tail.

Acknowledgment   This work was supported by NIH grant R01-EY13295 to SCF.

References

Calderwood DA (2004) Talin controls integrin activation. Biochem Soc Trans 32(Pt3):434–437

Cook B, Lewis GP et al (1995) Apoptotic photoreceptor degeneration in experimental retinal detachment. Invest Ophthalmol Vis Sci 36(6):990–996

Deora AA, Gravotta D et al (2004) The basolateral targeting signal of CD147 (EMMPRIN) consists of a single leucine and is not recognized by retinal pigment epithelium. Mol Biol Cell 15(9):4148–4165

Eliceiri BP, Puente XS et al (2002) Src-mediated coupling of focal adhesion kinase to integrin alpha(v)beta5 in vascular endothelial growth factor signaling. J Cell Biol 157(1): 149–160

Finnemann SC (2003) Focal adhesion kinase signaling promotes phagocytosis of integrin-bound photoreceptors. EMBO J 22(16):4143–4154

Finnemann SC, Bonilha VL et al (1997) Phagocytosis of rod outer segments by retinal pigment epithelial cells requires alpha(v)beta5 integrin for binding but not for internalization. Proc Natl Acad Sci USA 94(24):12932–12937

Finnemann SC, Chang Y (2008) Photoreceptor-RPE interactions physiology and molecular mechanisms. In: Tombran-Tink J, Barnstable CJ (eds) From ophthalmology research: visual transduction and non-visual light perception. Humana Press, Totowa, NJ

Fisher SK, Lewis GP et al (2005) Cellular remodeling in mammalian retina: results from studies of experimental retinal detachment. Prog Retin Eye Res 24(3):395–431

Frisch SM, Screaton RA (2001) Anoikis mechanisms. Curr Opin Cell Biol 13(5):555–562

Gundersen D, Powell SK et al (1993) Apical polarization of N-CAM in retinal pigment epithelium is dependent on contact with the neural retina. J Cell Biol 121(2):335–343

Horwitz A, Duggan K et al (1986) Interaction of plasma membrane fibronectin receptor with talin – a transmembrane linkage. Nature 320(6062):531–533

Hunziker W, Fumey C (1994) A di-leucine motif mediates endocytosis and basolateral sorting of macrophage IgG Fc receptors in MDCK cells. EMBO J 13(13):2963–2969

Legate KR, Fassler R (2009) Mechanisms that regulate adaptor binding to beta-integrin cytoplasmic tails. J Cell Sci 122(Pt 2):187–198

Marmorstein AD, Gan YC et al (1998) Apical polarity of N-CAM and EMMPRIN in retinal pigment epithelium resulting from suppression of basolateral signal recognition. J Cell Biol 142(3):697–710

Nandrot EF, Anand M et al (2006) Novel role for alphavbeta5-integrin in retinal adhesion and its diurnal peak. Am J Physiol Cell Physiol 290(4):C1256–C1262

Nandrot EF, Anand M et al (2007) Essential role for MFG-E8 as ligand for alphavbeta5 integrin in diurnal retinal phagocytosis. Proc Natl Acad Sci USA 104(29):12005–12010

Nandrot EF, Kim Y et al (2004) Loss of synchronized retinal phagocytosis and age-related blindness in mice lacking alphavbeta5 integrin. J Exp Med 200(12):1539–1545

Singh S, D'Mello V et al (2007) A NPxY-independent beta5 integrin activation signal regulates phagocytosis of apoptotic cells. Biochem Biophys Res Commun 364(3):540–548

Chapter 16
Mertk in Daily Retinal Phagocytosis: A History in the Making

Emeline F. Nandrot and Eric M. Dufour

Abstract It took 62 years from the description of the retinal dystrophy in rats from the Royal College of Surgeons (RCS) strain to the discovery of the molecular defect underlying the phenotype. Phagocytosis of photoreceptor outer segments (POS) by retinal pigment epithelial (RPE) cells follows a daily rhythm with a peak of activity 1.5–2 h after light onset for rod photoreceptors. We identified a deletion in the Mer tyrosine kinase (MerTK) receptor in RCS rat that abolishes internalization of POS by RPE cells. Accumulation of debris in the subretinal space then leads to drastic photoreceptor degeneration and rapid loss of vision. Interestingly, in wild-type mice and rats, MerTK is phosphorylated at the time of the phagocytic peak. We also demonstrated that the couple αvβ5 integrin receptor and MFG-E8 ligand synchronizes daily retinal phagocytosis. Indeed, when either one is absent in knockout mice, phagocytosis follows steady-state levels, and peak activation of integrin-associated protein and of MerTK does not occur. We now have a more precise picture of the sequence of molecular events governing retinal phagocytosis. However, requirement of MerTK ligands in vivo and linked signaling pathways still remain elusive so far.

16.1 Introduction

The retina is constituted of post-mitotic cells organized in layers that differentiate during eye development. Among these, two adjacent cell types of the outer retina, photoreceptors (PR) and retinal pigment epithelial (RPE) cells, interact with each other functionally and are highly inter-dependant. RPE cells form a highly specialized monolayer endorsing many activities to ensure function and integrity of the neural retina and therefore vision (review: Strauss 2005). On their apical side, RPE cells extend microvilli that ensheath the outer segment of rod and cone PRs.

E.F. Nandrot (✉)
Centre de Recherche Institut de la Vision, UMR_S968, Inserm, UPMC University of Paris 06, 17 rue Moreau, 75012 Paris, France
e-mail: emeline.nandrot@inserm.fr

R.E. Anderson et al. (eds.), *Retinal Degenerative Diseases*, Advances in Experimental Medicine and Biology 664, DOI 10.1007/978-1-4419-1399-9_16,
© Springer Science+Business Media, LLC 2010

Photoreceptor outer segment (POS) structure consists of stacked membranous disks containing the phototransduction machinery. POS are subjected to sustained light exposure thus generating high levels of oxidative stress. In order to ensure life-long function, both photoreceptor rods and cones continuously replace their outer segments (Young 1967). New membranous disks are initiated in the connecting cilium, inserted at the base of the inner segment, and progressively move towards the distal end of the POS. As a counterpart regulatory mechanism, PRs shed their most distal tips every day to keep constant cell length. The daily shedding of POS tips is controlled by strong circadian rhythms influenced by the dark-light cycle (Goldman et al.1980). Animal studies in rod-dominant species revealed that rods mainly shed their outer segments within 2 h after the light onset (LaVail and Mullen 1976). Upon rhythmic shedding, RPE cells respond with a burst of synchronized phagocytosis that efficiently digests POS and recycles their components (Young and Bok 1969). In mammals, each RPE cell serves approximately 30 POS that shed 7% of their outer segment mass every day (Young 1967), thus rendering RPE cells the most active phagocytes in the body.

16.2 RCS Rat and MerTK Receptor: An Intimate Story

Over 70 years ago, Margherita C. Bourne described a retinal degeneration occurring in rats affected by cataracts (Bourne et al. 1938) (Fig. 16.1a). She started breeding affected rats together, and the following year, she showed that the defect was transmitted as an autosomic recessive trait (Bourne and Grüneberg 1939). This animal model would be known later as the Royal College of Surgeons (RCS) rat strain.

The first defect detected is the accumulation of POS disk-like structures observed at 12 days on electron micrographs and 18 days with light microscopy (Dowling and Sidman 1962). Electroretinogram (ERG) retinal responses begin to decrease at 18 days until no more response can be detected at 3 months (Dowling and Sidman 1962; Nandrot et al. 2000) (Fig. 16.1b). PR cell death starts around 3 weeks of age until the complete loss of PR cells at 3 months (Bourne et al. 1938; Dowling and Sidman 1962; Nandrot et al. 2000) (Fig. 16.1a). Then, further disruption of the whole retina structure and cell degeneration spreads to all the other cell layers.

Mullen and LaVail (1976) used chimeras of non-pigmented RCS and pigmented control rats and showed that RPE cells completely fail to engulf POS, which in turn causes the drastic accumulation of POS debris in the subretinal space. Consistently, Edwards and Szamier (1977) demonstrated in vitro that the RPE cells defect is POS-specific, RPE cells being able to phagocytose latex beads. The exact phagocytosis disruption was pinpointed by Chaitin and Hall (1983) and further confirmed by Hall and Abrams (1987): RCS RPE cells bound POS properly but were unable to subsequently internalize them.

It took almost 15 more years to identify the molecular defect underlying the RCS rat retinal dystrophy. The gene was first localized to chromosome 3 by MM LaVail (1981) using co-transmission of enzymatic markers with the retinal dystrophy. In

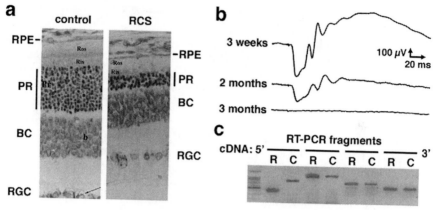

Fig. 16.1 Defective MerTK is responsible for the retinal degeneration in RCS rats. (**a**) Retinal sections of 2-month-old non-dystrophic (control) and dystrophic RCS (RCS) congenic rats were stained in order to visualize cell nuclei. Numbers of photoreceptor (PR) nuclei are greatly reduced in RCS rats, indicating an advanced stage of retinal degeneration. RPE: retinal pigment epithelium, BC: bipolar cells, RGC: retinal ganglion cells. (**b**) Scotopic electroretinogram (ERG) responses recorded from RCS rats during the retinal degeneration process. Already diminished at 3 weeks of age, they are completely absent at 3 months. (**c**) Rat *mertk* cDNA was amplified by RT-PCR from non-dystrophic control (C) and dystrophic RCS (R) retinas in 4 fragments spanning the full molecule (100 bp DNA ladder on the *left*). A deletion was detected in the 5' part of the cDNA, leading to a premature stop codon and a non-functional MerTK protein of 20 amino acids. Modified from Nandrot et al. (2000), with permission from Elsevier

2000, a single gene defect the Mer tyrosine kinase (MerTK) receptor was identified concomitantly by 2 research groups (D'Cruz et al. 2000; Nandrot et al. 2000). We used genetic mapping and biocomputing analysis to determine candidate genes. We identified a deletion in the MerTK cDNA (Nandrot et al. 2000) (Fig. 16.1c), which results from a large genomic deletion (D'Cruz et al. 2000). As a consequence, the 20-amino-acid MerTK protein is non-functional and RPE's ability to internalize POS is abolished. MerTK kinase dead (Mer^{KD}) transgenic mice develop the same phenotype as RCS rats (Duncan et al. 2003), resembling the symptoms of retinitis pigmentosa patients. In humans, MerTK mutations are associated with retinitis pigmentosa (Gal et al. 2000) and other pathologies such as rod-cone and cone-rod dystrophies (Tschernutter et al. 2006).

16.3 Changes Associated with Absence of MerTK in the Rat Retina

In order to study the effect of absence of MerTK and POS internalization on RPE cells function, we extensively analyzed differential expression of mRNAs and proteins during the peak of phagocytosis in non-dystrophic control and dystrophic RCS rats (Dufour et al. 2003). We choose to perform the study on 2- and 3-week-old rats, when phagocytosis already occurs in normal retina and degenerescence does not yet affect RCS rat retina.

Absence of MerTK and phagocytosis generate modulation of several genes expression. Some down-regulated genes are responsible for retinal pathologies, such as Sorsby's retinal dystrophy (*Timp3*) and retinitis pigmentosa (*RGRopsin*). Interestingly, one third of the genes down-regulated in RCS RPE cells were phagocytosis- or trafficking-related, and a large proportion of genes was related to modulations of metabolism. After ingestion of POS, membrane trafficking is required to compensate for membrane loss at the cell surface. Accordingly, abolition of MerTK entrained down-regulation of several genes involved in exocytosis, thus connecting RPE phagocytosis to the necessary local delivery of vesicles to the plasma membrane. Additionally, genes part of a same pathway, e.g. *Akt* and *mTor*, are both down-regulated in RCS rat RPE, confirming the consistency of the changes observed in our study. As well, we detected a down-regulation of genes related to oxygen metabolism associated with an up-regulation of genes linked to oxidative stress (mostly hypoxia). Taken together, these data show that loss of MerTK-associated phagocytosis decreases dramatically membranes biosynthesis and trafficking, and affects the global metabolic activity of RPE cells.

16.4 Daily Rhythmic Activation of Mertk: The Intracellular Way

RPE phagocytosis is a saturable receptor-mediated process divided in 2 independent steps, particle binding followed by internalization, which can be experimentally dissociated (Hall and Abrams 1987). $\alpha v\beta 5$ integrin receptors constitute the first molecular step of phagocytosis, by recognizing and binding POS (Finnemann et al. 1997; Finnemann 2003). $\alpha v\beta 5$ is the only integrin receptor that localizes to the apical, phagocytic surface of RPE in vitro and in vivo, and antibodies blocking $\alpha v\beta 5$ abolish POS binding by RPE but have no effect on internalization of POS prebound to the RPE surface (Finnemann et al. 1997). In contrast, the CD36 scavenger receptor seems to control the rate of internalization of bound POS (Finnemann and Silverstein 2001) and MerTK is absolutely required for POS internalization (Feng et al. 2002). MerTK receptors redistribute to the sites of internalized POS during phagocytosis assays (Feng et al. 2002; Finnemann 2003), and phosphorylation of tyrosine residues, thought to reflect MerTK activity, increases accordingly (Feng et al. 2002; Finnemann 2003).

Data on in vivo RPE phagocytosis regulation are more recent, and took advantage of the availability of other rodent models, the $\beta 5$ integrin knockout ($\beta 5^{-/-}$) and the MFG-E8 knockout (MFG-E8$^{-/-}$) mice. We were able to demonstrate that $\alpha v\beta 5$ integrin receptor and its ligand MFG-E8 are the proteins synchronizing the daily rhythm of POS phagocytosis by RPE cells (Nandrot et al. 2004; Nandrot et al. 2007). As expected, we detected a peak in the number of phagosomes present in RPE cells 2 h after light onset in wild-type mice (Fig. 16.2a). Furthermore, our data demonstrated a great increase in MerTK phosphorylation at the time of the phagocytosis peak

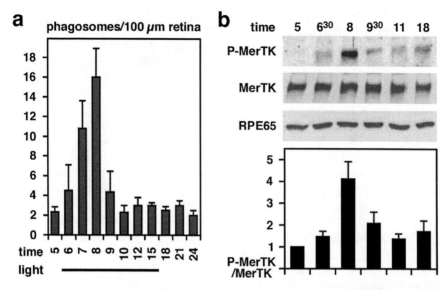

Fig. 16.2 MerTK activity peaks at the time of the retinal phagocytic burst. (**a, b**) We harvested eyecups from wild-type mice at different time-points of the 24-h phagocytic cycle. (**a**) Phagosomes present in RPE cells were counted on retinal sections. As previously described, phagocytosis peaks 2 h after the light onset (8 AM). (**b**) Protein lysates were analyzed by SDS-PAGE and immunoblotted for native and tyrosine-phosphorylated (P-MerTK) MerTK protein. RPE65 served as loading control. MerTK is activated at the time of the phagocytosis peak (8 AM). Band intensities were quantified to calculate relative levels of MerTK phosphorylation. Bars represent means ± standard deviation, $n = 3$. Modified from © Nandrot et al. 2004. Originally published in *The Journal of Experimental Medicine*. doi:10.1084/jem.20041447

(Fig. 16.2b), just after activation of the focal adhesion kinase (FAK) linked to $\alpha v \beta 5$ integrin receptors.

Strikingly, we showed that absence of $\alpha v \beta 5$ integrin ($\beta 5^{-/-}$) or of MFG-E8 (MFG-E8$^{-/-}$) abolished the morning phagocytosis peak and concomitant sequential FAK and MerTK phosphorylation. Interestingly, the loss of phagocytic rhythm is accompanied by age-dependent loss of vision and accumulation of autofluorescent oxidized deposits in the eye in $\beta 5^{-/-}$ mice only, features observed in age-related macular degeneration (AMD) patients.

16.5   The Debate About MerTK Ligands In Vivo

MerTK belongs to a family of three receptors called TAM for Tyro-3, Axl and MerTK sharing common vitamin K-dependent ligands, the related Gas6 and Protein S (Stitt et al. 1995). $\alpha v \beta 5$ integrin, CD36 and MerTK are common phagocyte receptors used by macrophages to phagocytose apoptotic bodies, suggesting that shed POS may be recognized as apoptotic bodies to be cleared (Finnemann and

Rodriguez-Boulan 1999; Scott et al. 2001). Apoptotic cells expose phosphatidylserine residues at their surface that are recognized via soluble bridge molecules such as the $\alpha v\beta 5$ integrin ligand MFG-E8 (Hanayama et al. 2002) or the MerTK ligands Gas6 and Protein S. Although our recent data demonstrate that MFG-E8 synchronizes $\alpha v\beta 5$ integrin-dependent phagocytosis of POS by RPE cells in vivo (Nandrot et al. 2007), MerTK ligands may also prove to be of importance for the proper fulfillment of POS phagocytosis.

Interestingly, stimulation of MerTK by the soluble ligand Gas6 enhances POS phagocytosis in vitro (Hall et al. 2001). However, mice knockout for Gas6 do not present any retinal phenotype, suggesting another ligand may be used for retinal phagocytosis. Moreover, MerTK ligands are expressed in the retina and may be relevant for POS phagocytosis. Indeed, Protein S is detected in the retina on eyecup sections (Prasad et al. 2006) and Gas6 and Protein S are present in retinal lysates (Hall et al. 2005). However, the precise function of MerTK ligands and their significance for RPE-photoreceptor in vivo have yet to be determined.

16.6 Perspectives

The continuous nature of POS renewal and shedding implies that deregulation or absence of this process could lead to drastic and devastating consequences for the retina: absence of RPE phagocytosis provokes rapid retinal degeneration (RCS rat model) as can be observed in retinitis pigmentosa, and alteration in the process will gradually cause the accumulation of PR-derived byproducts ($\beta 5^{-/-}$ knockout mouse model) leading to long term pathologies like AMD. Therefore strict timely regulation of the phagocytic function of RPE cells is of the highest importance to maintain retinal cell integrity and vision. Studies are underway to characterize MerTK activity during synchronized daily retinal phagocytosis.

Acknowledgments This work was supported by the following funding agencies, grants and awards: Ministère de l'Éducation Nationale, de la Recherche et de la Technologie, Université René Descartes, Faculté de Médecine Necker-Enfants Malades and Rétina France to the CERTO laboratory; Rétina France and Fondation pour la Recherche Médicale PhD grants, Fondation Bettencourt Schueller and Fondation Voir et Entendre Young Investigator grants to Emeline F. Nandrot; Rétina France and Fondation des Aveugles et Handicapés Visuels de France PhD grants to Eric M. Dufour; NIH grants EY13295, EY14184 and EY17173, Kirchgessner Research grant, William and Mary Greeve Scholarship by Research To Prevent Blindness, Inc., and Irma T. Hirschl Career Scientist Award to Silvia C. Finnemann.

References

Bourne MC, Campbell DA, Tansley K (1938) Hereditary degeneration of rat retina. Br J Ophthalmol 22:613–623
Bourne MC, Grüneberg H (1939) Degeneration of the retina and cataract, a new recessive gene in the rat (Rattus norvegicus). J Hered 30:130–136
Chaitin MH, Hall MO (1983) Defective ingestion of rod outer segments by cultured dystrophic rat pigment epithelial cells. Invest Ophthalmol Vis Sci 24:812–820

D'Cruz PM, Yasumura D, Weir J et al (2000) Mutation of the receptor tyrosine kinase gene mertk in the retinal dystrophic RCS rat. Hum Mol Genet 9(4):645–651

Dowling JE, Sidman RL (1962) Inherited retinal dystrophy in the rat. J Cell Biol 14:73–109

Dufour EM, Nandrot E, Marchant D et al (2003) Identification of novel genes and altered signaling pathways in the retinal pigment epithelium during the Royal College of Surgeons rat retinal degeneration. Neurobiol Dis 14(2):166–180

Duncan JL, LaVail MM, Yasumura D et al (2003) An RCS-like retinal dystrophy phenotype in mer knockout mice. Invest Ophthalmol Vis Sci 44:826–838

Edwards RB, Szamier RB (1977) Defective phagocytosis of isolated rod outer segments by RCS rat retinal pigment epithelium in culture. Science 197:1001–1003

Feng W, Yasumura D, Matthes MT et al (2002) Mertk triggers uptake of photoreceptor outer segments during phagocytosis by cultured retinal pigment epithelial cells. J Biol Chem 277:17016–17022

Finnemann SC (2003) Focal adhesion kinase signaling promotes phagocytosis of integrin-bound photoreceptors. EMBO J 22:4143–4154

Finnemann SC, Bonilha VL, Marmorstein AD, Rodriguez-Boulan E (1997) Phagocytosis of rod outer segments by retinal pigment epithelial cells requires αvβ5 integrin for binding but not for internalization. Proc Natl Acad Sci USA 94:12932–12937

Finnemann SC, Rodriguez-Boulan E (1999) Macrophage and retinal pigment epithelium phago- cytosis: apoptotic cells and photoreceptors compete for αvβ3 and αvβ5 integrins, and protein kinase C regulates αvβ5 binding and cytoskeletal linkage. J Exp Med 190:861–874

Finnemann SC, Silverstein RL (2001) Differential roles of CD36 and αvβ5 integrin in photorecep- tor phagocytosis by the retinal pigment epithelium. J Exp Med 194:1289–1298

Gal A, Li Y, Thompson DA et al (2000) Mutations in MERTK, the human orthologue of the RCS rat retinal dystrophy gene, cause retinitis pigmentosa. Nat Genet 26:270–271

Goldman AI, Teirstein PS, O'Brien PJ (1980) The role of ambient lighting in circadian disc shedding in the rod outer segment of the rat retina. Invest Ophthalmol Vis Sci 19: 1257–1267

Hall MO, Abrams TA (1987) Kinetic studies of rod outer segment binding and ingestion by cultured rat RPE cells. Exp Eye Res 45:907–922

Hall MO, Obin MS, Heeb MJ et al (2005) Both protein S and Gas6 stimulate outer segment phagocytosis by cultured rat retinal pigment epithelial cells. Exp Eye Res 81:581–591

Hall MO, Prieto AL, Obin MS et al (2001) Outer segment phagocytosis by cultured retinal pigment epithelial cells requires Gas6. Exp Eye Res 73:509–520

Hanayama R, Tanaka M, Miwa K et al (2002) Identification of a factor that links apoptotic cells to phagocytes. Nature 417:182–187

LaVail MM (1981) Assignment of retinal dystrophy (rdy) to linkage group IV of the rat. J Hered 72(4):294–296

LaVail MM, Mullen RJ (1976) Role of the pigment epithelium in inherited retinal degeneration analyzed with experimental mouse chimeras. Exp Eye Res 23:227–245

Mullen RJ, LaVail MM (1976) Inherited retinal dystrophy: primary defect in pigment epithelium determined with experimental rat chimeras. Science 192:799–801

Nandrot EF, Anand M, Almeida D et al (2007) Essential role for MFG-E8 as ligand for alphavbeta5 integrin in diurnal retinal phagocytosis. Proc Natl Acad Sci USA 104:12005–12010

Nandrot E, Dufour EM, Provost AC et al (2000) Homozygous deletion in the coding sequence of the c-mer gene in RCS rats unravels general mechanisms of physiological cell adhesion and apoptosis. Neurobiol Dis 7:586–599

Nandrot EF, Kim Y, Brodie SE et al (2004) Loss of synchronized retinal phagocytosis and age- related blindness in mice lacking αvβ5 integrin. J Exp Med 200:1539–1545

Prasad D, Rothlin CV, Burrola P et al (2006) TAM receptor function in the retinal pigment epithelium. Mol Cell Neurosci 33:96–108

Scott RS, McMahon EJ, Pop SM et al (2001) Phagocytosis and clearance of apoptotic cells is mediated by MER. Nature 411:207–211

Stitt TN, Conn G, Gore M et al (1995) The anticoagulation factor protein S and its relative, Gas6, are ligands for the Tyro 3/Axl family of receptor tyrosine kinases. Cell 80:661–670

Strauss O (2005) The retinal pigment epithelium in visual function. Physiol Rev 85(3):845–881

Tschernutter M, Jenkins SA, Waseem NH et al (2006) Clinical characterisation of a family with retinal dystrophy caused by mutation in the Mertk gene. Br J Ophthalmol 90:718–723

Young RW (1967) The renewal of photoreceptor cell outer segments. J Cell Biol 33:61–72

Young RW, Bok D (1969) Participation of the retinal pigment epithelium in the rod outer segment renewal process. J Cell Biol 42:392–403

Chapter 17
The Interphotoreceptor Retinoid Binding (IRBP) Is Essential for Normal Retinoid Processing in Cone Photoreceptors

Ryan O. Parker and Rosalie K. Crouch

Abstract 11-*cis* Retinal is the light-sensitive component in rod and cone photoreceptors, and its isomerization to all-*trans* retinal in the presence of light initiates the visual response. For photoreceptors to function normally, all-*trans* retinal must be converted back into 11-*cis* retinal through the visual cycle. While rods are primarily responsible for dim light vision, the ability of cones to function in constant light is essential to human vision and may be facilitated by cone-specific visual cycle pathways. The interphotoreceptor retinoid-binding protein (IRBP) is a proposed retinoid transporter in the visual cycle, but rods in $Irbp^{-/-}$ mice have a normal visual cycle. However, there is evidence that IRBP has cone-specific functions. Cone electroretinogram (ERG) responses are reduced, despite having cone densities and opsin levels similar to *C57Bl/6 (WT)* mice. Treatment with 9-*cis* retinal rescues the cone response in $Irbp^{-/-}$ mice and shows that retinoid deficiency underlies cone dysfunction. These data indicate that IRBP is essential to normal cone function and demonstrate that differences exist in the visual cycle of rods and cones.

17.1 Introduction

11-*cis* Retinal covalently binds opsin to form the light-sensitive visual pigments in rod and cone photoreceptors. In the dark, 11-*cis* retinal functions as an opsin inverse agonist, but when light strikes a visual pigment, 11-*cis* retinal is isomerized to all-*trans* retinal, an opsin agonist (Wald 1935, 1955). The photoisomerization of retinal triggers the photoresponse of rods and cones, but constant function requires that new 11-*cis* retinal continuously replace the all-*trans* retinal photoproduct. The retina and adjacent retinal pigment epithelium (RPE) accomplish this by efficiently converting all-*trans* retinal back to 11-*cis* retinal in a series of enzymatic steps known as the

R.O. Parker (✉)
Department of Neurosciences, Medical University of South Carolina, Charleston, SC, USA
e-mail: parkerry@musc.edu

R.E. Anderson et al. (eds.), *Retinal Degenerative Diseases*, Advances in Experimental Medicine and Biology 664, DOI 10.1007/978-1-4419-1399-9_17,
© Springer Science+Business Media, LLC 2010

visual cycle. While our understanding of the classical visual cycle is largely derived from the study of rods, cones are responsible for the bulk of human vision, and there is growing evidence that separate pathways generate a privileged supply of 11-*cis* retinal to facilitate cone function in constant light (Mata et al. 2002; Mata et al. 2005).

The classical visual cycle associated with rods is a compartmentalized cascade with steps occurring in both the photoreceptors and retinal pigment epithelium (RPE). all-*trans* Retinol is generated from all-*trans* retinal in the photoreceptors and passed to the RPE, where it is converted to 11-*cis* retinal for the photoreceptors (Fig. 17.1). While the compartmentalization of steps in the retina and RPE drives the

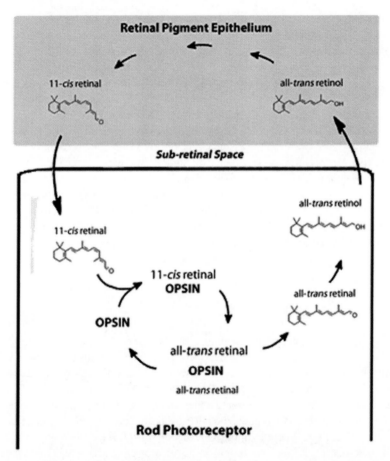

Fig. 17.1 The classical visual cycle; The visual cycle begins when all-*trans* retinal is released from the activated opsin and reduced to all-*trans* retinol in the photoreceptor outer segment. all-*trans* Retinol then exits the photoreceptor, crosses the sub-retinal space, and enters the retinal pigment epithelium (RPE). In the RPE, all-*trans* retinol is enzymatically converted to 11-*cis* retinal and returned back across the sub-retinal space to the photoreceptors. IRBP is thought to facilitate the delivery of all-*trans* retinol from the photoreceptors to the RPE and the return of 11-*cis* retinal from the RPE to the photoreceptors

flow specific retinoids in the appropriate direction, it requires that poorly soluble and potentially toxic retinoids traverse the aqueous sub-retinal space between the photoreceptors and the RPE. The Interphotoreceptor Retinoid Binding Protein (IRBP) is the most abundant soluble protein in the sub-retinal space (Loew and Gonzalez-Fernandez 2002) and is thought to facilitate this process (Bunt-Milam and Saari 1983; Fong et al. 1984).

In vitro studies have shown that IRBP promotes the release of all-*trans* retinol from photoreceptors (Ala-Laurila et al. 2006; Wu et al. 2007) and facilitates its delivery to the RPE (Okajima et al. 1994). Additionally, IRBP can also enhance 11-*cis* retinal release from the RPE (Edwards and Adler 2000), prevent its isomerization in the sub-retinal space (Crouch et al. 1992), and transfer 11-*cis* retinal to photoreceptors (Jones et al. 1989). Each of these steps would appear to be important for normal visual cycle function, and were IRBP essential for any of its proposed roles, an 11-*cis* retinal deficiency would inevitably occur in its absence. The $Irbp^{-/-}$ mouse was expected to confirm IRBP's importance to the visual cycle in vivo (Liou et al. 1998). Although rod function is diminished in $Irbp^{-/-}$ mice, the visual cycle in rods is surprisingly normal (Palczewski et al. 1999; Ripps et al. 2000), and rod dysfunction is thought to be secondary to degeneration (Liou et al. 1998). Cone function in $Irbp^{-/-}$ mice is also diminished (Ripps et al. 2000), but the underlying cause remains unclear.

17.2 The Cone Population in $Irbp^{-/-}$ Mice

Because the rod population in $Irbp^{-/-}$ mice is reported to degenerate (Liou et al. 1998), it is possible that cones are similarly affected, and ERGs and cone densities were used to look for cone degeneration. Cone ERGs from $Irbp^{-/-}$ mice were diminished as early as 1 month (Fig. 17.2a) but showed no evidence of decline through 9 months of age ($p = 0.28$) (Fig. 17.2a, b). Analysis of the cone densities of aging $Irbp^{-/-}$ mice produced similar results. Cone densities were calculated using retina flat-mounts stained with peanut agglutinin (PNA), a lectin that binds the glycoprotein sheath surrounding cones (Johnson et al. 1986). While a small drop in the cone densities was noted from 1 to 2 months (256 ± 4.3, $n = 4$; 222 ± 5.3, $n = 4$; $p = 0.03$), the population remained stable between 1 and 9 months ($p = 0.14$) (Fig. 17.2b). Cone densities were also similar in the dorsal and ventral retina, suggesting that neither the MWS nor SWS cones were uniquely affected. Thus, both ERGs and cone densities in aging $Irbp^{-/-}$ mice suggest that a significant degenerative process does not underlie cone dysfunction.

While a degenerative process does not appear to be present, IRBP has proposed developmental functions (Gonzalez-Fernandez and Healy 1990), and its absence could impair normal cone development. Thus, reduced cone densities could account for the attenuated cone response in $Irbp^{-/-}$ mice. Again, PNA-stained retina flat-mounts were used, and representative flat-mounts from $Irbp^{-/-}$ and WT mice at 1 and 8 months are shown in Fig. 17.3a. The similar densities found in $Irbp^{-/-}$ and

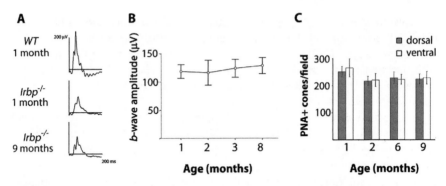

Fig. 17.2 A stable cone population in aging *Irbp*⁻/⁻ Mice; **a.** Single-flash photopic ERG responses from individual *WT* and *Irbp*⁻/⁻ mice to a 0.4 log cd*s/m² flash. **b.** Single flash photopic ERGs (0.4 log cd*s/m² stimulus) of *Irbp*⁻/⁻ mice at 1 ($n = 9$), 2 ($n = 12$), 3 ($n = 13$), and 8 ($n = 12$) months showed no significant change with age ($p = 0.28$, one-way ANOVA). Data points represent mean amplitudes ± S.D. **c.** Cone densities counted from PNA-stained retina flat-mounts of *Irbp*⁻/⁻ mice at 1 ($n = 4$), 2 ($n = 3$), 6 ($n = 4$), and 9 ($n = 4$) months showed a drop between 1 and 2 months ($p = 0.03$, Mann-Whitney test), but densities were stable between 2 and 9 months ($p = 0.14$, Kruskal-Wallis test). Densities were similar between the dorsal and ventral retina at all ages. All bars represent means ± S.D

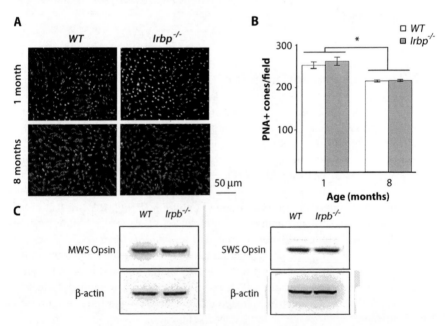

Fig. 17.3 a. Retina flat-mounts (400x) stained with PNA from *Irbp*⁻/⁻ and *WT* mice at 1 and 8 months. **b.** Cone densities were similar in *Irbp*⁻/⁻ and *WT* mice at 1 (*Irbp*⁻/⁻, $n = 4$; *WT*, $n = 4$; $p = 0.47$, Mann-Whitney test) and 8 (*Irbp*⁻/⁻, $n = 3$; *WT*, $n = 3$; $p = 1.00$, Mann-Whitney test) months. **c.** Western blots in *Irbp*⁻/⁻ and *WT* mice were used to identify MWS and SWS cone opsin levels from 20 μg of total retina protein. At 4 months of age, levels of both cone opsins were similar in *Irbp*⁻/⁻ and *WT* mice. After staining for either the MWS or SWS cone opsins, membranes were stripped and re-probed for β-actin as a loading control

WT mice at both 1 month ($Irbp^{-/-}$, 256 ± 4.3, $n = 4$; WT, 261 ± 11, $n = 4$; $p = 0.47$) and 8 months ($Irbp^{-/-}$, 218 ± 16, $n= 3$; WT, 216 ± 13, $n = 3$; $p = 1.0$) (Fig. 17.3b) suggests that cone development is normal in $Irbp^{-/-}$ mice. While PNA staining allows the rapid calculation of cone densities, PNA binds the sheath surrounding cones and not the cones, themselves. To account for this, western blots were used to compare cone opsin levels in $Irbp^{-/-}$ and WT mice. In agreement with the findings from flat-mounts, $Irbp^{-/-}$ and WT mice at 4 months of age had equivalent levels of MWS and SWS opsin (Fig. 17.3c). Retina cross-sections confirmed the correct localization of cone opsins to the outer segments (not shown). Together, the normal cone densities and opsin levels suggest that cone development is not impaired in $Irbp^{-/-}$ mice.

Neither degeneration nor development account for cone dysfunction in $Irbp^{-/-}$ mice, but an altered cone response could result from visual cycle deficits in IRBP's absence. We tested for 11-*cis* retinal deficiency in the cones of $Irbp^{-/-}$ mice by analyzing photopic ERGs before and after intraperitoneal (IP) injections of 9-*cis* retinal, a functional analogue of 11-*cis* retinal (Crouch and Katz 1980). Baseline responses from $Irbp^{-/-}$ mice were reduced relative to WT mice at all intensities but recovered dramatically after treatment with 9-*cis* retinal (0.375 mg, IP) (Fig. 17.4a). Intensity response plots from $Irbp^{-/-}$ mice ($n = 8$) show that cone responses increased significantly with 9-*cis* retinal treatment at intensities above –0.8 log cd*s/m^2 ($p = 0.005$) (Fig. 17.4b) and did not differ significantly from the responses of treated WT mice ($p = 0.25$) (Fig. 17.4c). 9-*cis* Retinal had no effect on rod function in $Irbp^{-/-}$ mice (*a*-wave, $p = 0.70$; *b*-wave, $p = 0.55$) and did not significantly alter the rod or cone responses in WT mice (not shown). Thus, the cones of $Irbp^{-/-}$ mice were uniquely

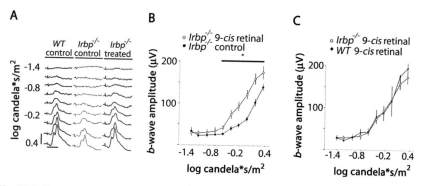

Fig. 17.4 Recovery of cone ERGs in $Irbp^{-/-}$ mice with exogenous 9-*cis* retinal; **a.** Representative ERG traces from 2 month old animals are shown. Control responses from the $Irbp^{-/-}$ mouse were reduced relative to WT at all intensities. After the intraperitoneal (IP) injection of 9-*cis* retinal (0.375 mg), responses from the same mouse recovered to WT levels. **b.** Intensity-response plots from ERG recordings of 2 month old $Irbp^{-/-}$ mice ($n = 8$) treated with 9-*cis* retinal (0.375 mg, IP) showed a significant recovery of cone responses at all intensities above –0.8 log cd*s/m^2 ($p = 0.005$, paired two-way ANOVA). **c.** Responses of WT ($n = 4$) and $Irbp^{-/-}$ mice after 9-*cis* retinal injections were not significantly different ($p = 0.25$, two-way ANOVA)

sensitive to exogenous 9-*cis* retinal, and the recovery of cone function to *WT* levels suggests that cone dysfunction in *Irbp*$^{-/-}$ mice results from an 11-*cis* retinal deficiency.

17.3 Implications for IRBP and Cone Function

IRBP is thought to link the photoreceptors and RPE in the classical visual cycle. While its absence does not alter retinoid metabolism in rods (Palczewski et al. 1999; Ripps et al. 2000), our findings show that IRBP is important to cone function. As IRBP is not essential to the rod visual cycle, rod dysfunction in the model is likely the result of a degenerative process. The accumulation of toxic photoproducts in the absence of IRBP's buffering abilities may be responsible (Ho et al. 1989; Crouch et al. 1992; Wu et al. 2007), but it is also likely that IRBP has important functions beyond retinoid transport. IRBP binds key outer segment components, such as docosahexaenoic acid (DHA), that are essential for normal outer segment formation (Chen et al. 1993; Shaw and Noy 2001). With disorganized outer segments common in the surviving rods of *Irbp*$^{-/-}$ mice (Liou et al. 1998), shortages of essential outer segment components could underlie rod dysfunction.

While both rod and cone responses are reduced in *Irbp*$^{-/-}$ mice, a unique mechanism underlies cone dysfunction. In the absence of significant degeneration or developmental abnormalities, reduced cone function in *Irbp*$^{-/-}$ mice resulted from cone-specific visual cycle deficits, and ERGs performed before and after 9-*cis* retinal injections confirmed that visual cycle deficits in *Irbp*$^{-/-}$ mice are cone-specific. 9-*cis* Retinal had no effect on the rod responses in *Irbp*$^{-/-}$ or *WT* mice, nor did it produce a significant change in *WT* cone responses. Only the cones of *Irbp*$^{-/-}$ mice responded to 9-*cis* retinal, and treatment resulted in increased responses that were similar to *WT*. Rescue of the cone response with 9-*cis* retinal shows that cones survive with high levels of unregenerated cone opsin and demonstrates that cones are uniquely dependent on IRBP for normal retinoid levels.

17.4 The Cone Visual Cycle

Despite identifying a cone-specific visual cycle disruption, a number of questions remain surrounding IRBP's contribution to cone function. In vitro studies suggest that IRBP can promote 11-*cis* retinal release from the RPE (Edwards and Adler 2000) and delivery to photoreceptors (Jones et al. 1989). While the flow of 11-*cis* retinal to rods is normal in *Irbp*$^{-/-}$ mice (Ripps et al. 2000), the flow to cones has not been analyzed, and it is possible that cones require IRBP to efficiently draw 11-*cis* retinal from the RPE. Another explanation is that IRBP functions as the retinoid transporter in the proposed cone visual cycle (Fig. 17.5). Cones are believed to have unique pathways for regenerating 11-*cis* retinal from 11-*cis* retinol generated in Müller cells (Das et al. 1992; Bustamante et al. 1995; Mata et al. 2002, 2005).

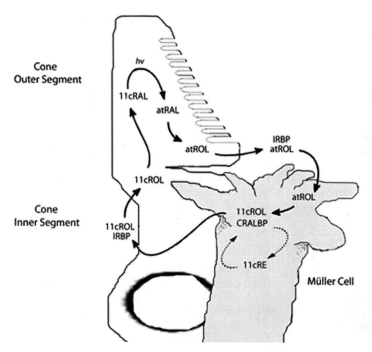

Fig. 17.5 The proposed cone visual cycle; Cones are thought to have unique access to retinoids from Müller cells in the inner retina. Like the classical visual cycle, the proposed cone pathway begins when all-*trans* retinal (atRAL) is reduced to all-*trans* retinol (atROL) in the cone outer segment. all-*trans* Retinol is transported to Müller cells located along the outer limiting membrane with the possible help of IRBP. Mller cells convert the all-*trans* retinol into 11-*cis* retinol (11cROL), which is released into the sub-retinal space and returned to the cones. Again, IRBP may facilitate this step, as one of its endogenous ligands is 11-*cis* retinol. Within the cones, 11-*cis* retinol converted to 11-*cis* retinal (11cRAL) and used to regenerate functional visual pigment

Central to this theory is the unique ability of cones to regenerate 11-*cis* retinal from 11-*cis* retinol supplied to the inner segment (Jones et al. 1989). Müller cells generate 11-*cis* retinol (Das et al. 1992) and contain CRALBP in microvilli located near the cone inner segments (Bunt-Milam and Saari 1983). IRBP co-localizes with the microvilli in a light-dependent manner (Uehara et al. 1990), is found in high concentration around cones (Carter-Dawson and Burroughs 1992a, Carter-Dawson and Burroughs 1992b), and binds 11-*cis* retinol endogenously (Saari et al. 1985). While a functional relationship between IRBP, Müller cells, and cone inner segments has not been proven, the presence of retinoid deficient cones in *Irbp*$^{-/-}$ mice provides additional evidence for this pathway.

In summary, IRBP is not essential to the rod visual cycle, but reduced cone function in *Irbp*$^{-/-}$ mice is due to 11-*cis* retinal deficiency and implies that IRBP is essential to the normal cycling of retinoids in cones. These findings represent the first in vivo evidence implicating IRBP as a retinoid transporter in the visual cycle, and indicate a critical role for IRBP in the cone function that is essential for human vision.

References

Adler A, Spencer S (1991) Effect of light on endogenous ligands carried by interphotoreceptor retinoid-binding protein. Exp Eye Res 53:337–346

Ala-Laurila P, Kolesnikov A, Crouch R et al (2006) Visual cycle: dependence of retinol production and removal on photoproduct decay and cell morphology. J Gen Physiol 128:153–169

Bunt-Milam A, Saari J (1983) Immunocytochemical localization of two retinoid-binding proteins in vertebrate retina. J Cell Biol 97:703–712

Bustamante J, Ziari S, Ramirez R, Tsin AT (1995) Retinyl ester hydrolase and the visual cycle in the chicken eye. Am J Physiol 269:R1346–R1350

Carter-Dawson L, Burroughs M (1992a) Interphotoreceptor retinoid-binding protein in the cone matrix sheath. Electron microscopic immunocytochemical localization. Invest Ophthalmol Vis Sci 33:1584–1588

Carter-Dawson L, Burroughs M (1992b) Interphotoreceptor retinoid-binding protein in the Golgi apparatus of monkey foveal cones. Electron microscopic immunocytochemical localization. Invest Ophthalmol Vis Sci 33:1589–1594

Chen Y, Saari J, Noy N (1993) Interactions of all-*trans*-retinol and long-chain fatty acids with interphotoreceptor retinoid-binding protein. Biochemistry 32:11311–11318

Crouch R, Katz S (1980) Effect of retinal Isomers on the VER and ERG of vitamin A-deprived rats. Vision Res 20:109–115

Crouch R, Hazard E, Lind T et al (1992) Interphotoreceptor retinoid-binding protein and alpha-tocopherol preserve the isomeric and oxidation state of retinol. Photochem Photobiol 56: 251–255

Das S, Bhardwaj N, Kjeldbye H et al (1992) Müller cells of chicken retina synthesize 11-*cis*-retinol. Biochem J 285(Pt 3):907–913

den Hollander A, McGee T, Ziviello C et al (2009) A homozygous missense mutation in the IRBP gene (RBP3) associated with autosomal recessive retinitis pigmentosa. Invest Ophthalmol Vis Sci 30(4):1864–1872

Edwards R, Adler A (2000) IRBP enhances removal of 11-*cis*-retinaldehyde from isolated RPE membranes. Exp Eye Res 70:235–245

Fong S, Liou G, Landers R et al (1984) Purification and characterization of a retinol-binding glycoprotein synthesized and secreted by bovine neural retina. J Biol Chem 259:6534–6542

Gonzalez-Fernandez F, Healy J (1990) Early expression of the gene for interphotoreceptor retinol-binding protein during photoreceptor differentiation suggests a critical role for the interphotoreceptor matrix in retinal development. J Cell Biol 111:2775–2784

Ho M, Massey J, Pownall H et al (1989) Mechanism of vitamin A movement between rod outer segments, interphotoreceptor retinoid-binding protein, and liposomes. J Biol Chem 264: 928–935

Hood D, Hock P (1973) Recovery of cone receptor activity in the frog's isolated retina. Vision Res 13:1943–1951

Johnson L, Hageman G, Blanks J (1986) Interphotoreceptor matrix domains ensheath vertebrate cone photoreceptor cells. Invest Ophthalmol Vis Sci 27:129–135

Jones G, Crouch R, Wiggert B et al (1989) Retinoid requirements for recovery of sensitivity after visual-pigment bleaching in isolated photoreceptors. Proc Natl Acad Sci USA 86:9606–9610

Liou G, Fei Y, Peachey N et al (1998) Early onset photoreceptor abnormalities induced by targeted disruption of the interphotoreceptor retinoid-binding protein gene. J Neurosci 18:4511–4520

Loew A, Gonzalez-Fernandez F (2002) Crystal structure of the functional unit of interphotoreceptor retinoid binding protein. Structure 10:43–49

Mata N, Radu R, Clemmons R et al (2002) Isomerization and oxidation of vitamin A in cone-dominant retinas: a novel pathway for visual-pigment regeneration in daylight. Neuron 36: 69–80

Mata N, Ruiz A, Radu R (2005) Chicken retinas contain a retinoid isomerase activity that catalyzes the direct conversion of all-*trans*-retinol to 11-*cis*-retinol. Biochemistry 44:11715–11721

Okajima T, Wiggert B, Chader G (1994) Retinoid processing in retinal pigment epithelium of toad (*Bufo marinus*). J Biol Chem 269:21983–21989

Palczewski K, Van Hooser J, Garwin G (1999) Kinetics of visual pigment regeneration in excised mouse eyes and in mice with a targeted disruption of the gene encoding interphotoreceptor retinoid-binding protein or arrestin. Biochemistry 38:12012–12019

Ripps H, Peachey N, Xu X (2000) The rhodopsin cycle is preserved in IRBP "knockout" mice despite abnormalities in retinal structure and function. Vis Neurosci 17:97–105

Saari J, Teller D, Crabb J (1985) Properties of an interphotoreceptor retinoid-binding protein from bovine retina. J Biol Chem 260:195–201

Shaw N, Noy N (2001) Interphotoreceptor retinoid-binding protein contains three retinoid binding sites. Exp Eye Res 72:183–190

Uehara F, Matthes M, Yasumura D et al (1990) Light-evoked changes in the interphotoreceptor matrix. Science 248:1633–1636

Wald G (1935) Carotenoids and the visual cycle. J Gen Physiol 19:351–371

Wald G (1955) The photoreceptor process in vision. Am J Ophthalmol 40:18–41

Wenzel A, Grimm C, Samardzija M et al (2005) Molecular mechanisms of light-induced photoreceptor apoptosis and neuroprotection for retinal degeneration. Prog Retin Eye Res 24:275–306

Wu Q, Blakeley L, Cornwall M et al (2007) Interphotoreceptor retinoid-binding protein is the physiologically relevant carrier that removes retinol from rod photoreceptor outer segments. Biochemistry 46:8669–8679

Chapter 18
Aseptic Injury to Epithelial Cells Alters Cell Surface Complement Regulation in a Tissue Specific Fashion

Joshua M. Thurman, Brandon Renner, Kannan Kunchithapautham, V. Michael Holers, and Bärbel Rohrer

Abstract We have recently shown that oxidative stress of ARPE-19 cells alters the expression of the cell surface complement regulatory proteins DAF and CD59, and permits increased activation of complement when the cells are subsequently exposed to serum. Based upon these results, we hypothesized that RPE cells respond to cellular stress as if it is infection, and reduce their surface expression of complement regulatory proteins to foster the local immune response. To test this hypothesis, we examined whether cellular hypoxia would produce a similar change in ARPE-19 cells. In addition, we asked whether this response to oxidative stress is universal in all epithelial cells, by examining the expression of complement regulatory proteins on the surface of the renal and pulmonary epithelial cells. We found that the expression of complement regulatory proteins is altered by aseptic cellular stressors such as hypoxia and oxidative stress, but the response to these conditions differs from tissue to tissue. In RPE cells oxidative stress reduces the expression of the cell surface complement regulators and sensitizes the cells to complement mediated injury. This specific response is not seen in epithelial cells from the lung or kidney, and is not induced by hypoxia. These studies help explain the unique mechanisms by which uncontrolled complement activation may contribute to the development of AMD.

18.1 Introduction

The complement proteins form an important part of the innate immune system, but uncontrolled activation of the alternative pathway of complement contributes to the development of age-related macular degeneration (AMD) (Gehrs and Anderson

B. Rohrer (✉)
Departments of Ophthalmology and Neurosciences, Division of Research, Medical University of South Carolina, Charleston, SC 29425, USA
e-mail: rohrer@musc.edu

R.E. Anderson et al. (eds.), *Retinal Degenerative Diseases*, Advances in Experimental Medicine and Biology 664, DOI 10.1007/978-1-4419-1399-9_18,
© Springer Science+Business Media, LLC 2010

2006). We recently reported that oxidative stress of ARPE cells alters the expression of cell surface complement regulatory proteins and permits increased activation of complement when the cells are subsequently exposed to complement-sufficient serum (Rohrer and Renner 2008). In a separate set of studies we have previously demonstrated that tissue ischemia alters complement regulation on the surface of renal epithelial cells (RPE) (Thurman et al. 2006). These findings suggest that epithelial cells from different organs may respond to cellular stressors by altering their expression of complement regulatory proteins, and that this response may contribute to autologous complement-mediated injury in diseases such as AMD.

Cells control complement activation on their surface through the expression of complement regulatory proteins. The three cell surface complement regulatory proteins are membrane cofactor protein (MCP; CD46), decay accelerating factor (DAF; CD55), and CD59. Crry is a rodent complement regulatory protein that is a homologue of MCP and DAF (Molina and Wong1992). Local complement activation is likely a result of the balance of complement proteins, activating molecules, and inhibitory molecules. As the interface of the internal milieu with the outside world, epithelial cells must be able to protect themselves from autologous complement-mediated injury while also fostering effective clearance of pathogens by complement proteins present in the serum. Retinal pigmented epithelial (RPE) cells likely perform surveillance functions, possibly triggering an inflammatory response when pathogens are detected.

We hypothesized that RPE cells respond to cellular stress as if it is infection, and reduce their surface expression of complement regulatory proteins to foster the local immune response. In addition to AMD, uncontrolled activation of the alternative pathway on barrier epithelial layers occurs in ischemic acute kidney injury (Thurman and Ljubanovic 2003) and in asthma (Taube and Thurman 2006); so we further hypothesized that the mechanisms of altered complement regulation that we have described for RPE cells might also be seen in epithelial cells derived from the kidney and lung. We have, therefore, examined whether oxidative stress induces changes in the expression of complement regulatory proteins on the surface of renal and pulmonary epithelial cells, similar to what we have observed in RPE cells.

18.2 Material and Methods

18.2.1 Reagents

The reagents used in these studies included pooled normal human serum (NHS; Quidel) as a source of complement proteins, or complement-sufficient mouse serum obtained by bleeding C57Bl/6 mice. Primary antibodies to DAF (Chemicon International), CD59 (Chemicon International), MCP (Monosan), Crry (BD Biosciences), and C3 (ICN Pharmaceuticals) were used. Species-specific secondary antibodies were from Jackson ImmunoResearch and MP Biomedicals, Inc.

18.2.2 Cell Culture

We used three different epithelial cell lines: the retinal pigment epithelial cell line, ARPE-19; the BUMPT, renal proximal tubular epithelial cell (PTEC) line; and the pulmonary epithelial cell line, A549. The ARPE-19, human RPE cell line (Dunn and Aotaki-Keen 1996; Dunn and Marmorstein 1998), was grown in DMEM-F12 (Gibco) with 10% fetal bovine serum (FBS) and penicillin-streptomycin (Pen-Strep). Upon reaching confluence, FBS was removed completely for 2 weeks for cells to form a monolayer with tight junctions. Monolayer barrier function was confirmed in parallel cultures grown on transwell inserts that allow for measurements of transepithelial resistance. The PTEC line was originally derived from the Immortmouse (Sinha and Wang 2003). These cells were grown in DMEM medium supplemented with 10% FBS, Pen-Strep, and 0.2 U/mL interferon-gamma (IFN-γ; Peprotech). The IFN-γ in this medium permits expression of the H-2Kb-tsA58 transgene in these cells (Sinha and Wang 2003). After the cells reached confluence they were changed to 1:1 DMEM/Ham's F12 supplemented with 5 mg/L transferrin (Invitrogen Life Technologies), 50 nM hydrocortisone (Sigma-Aldrich), and 5 mg/L insulin for 2 days to suppress expression of the transgene. Finally, the A549 cell line (Lieber and Smith 1976), was grown in DMEM (Gibco) with 10% FBS and Pen-Strep. To induce chemical hypoxia, cells were treated with 1 μM antimycin A (Sigma-Aldrich) for 1 h. In some experiments the cells were treated with 0.5 mM H_2O_2 for 1 h. This dose falls within the range also used by other investigators to induce oxidative stress in these cell types (Panayiotidis and Stabler 2008). For experiments in which complement activation on the surface of the cells was examined, the cells were subsequently incubated in 10% normal human serum (for the A549 and ARPE-19 cell lines), or complement-sufficient mouse serum (for the murine BUMPT cell line), at 37°C for 1 h

18.2.3 Flow Cytometry

The surface expression of the complement regulatory proteins DAF, MCP, and CD59, was examined by flow cytometry. Cells were released from the culture plates by treatment with Accutase (Innovative Cell Technologies, Inc.), and washed in PBS. The expression of surface proteins was examined by incubating the cells with primary antibody to the proteins, at 4°C for 1 h and washing the cells in PBS, and repeating this step with secondary antibodies when necessary. Cells were then washed and resuspended in 500 μL of PBS, run on a FACSCalibur machine (BD Biosciences), and analyzed with CellQuest Pro software (BD Biosciences). To measure complement activation on the cell surface, the cells were washed in PBS, incubated with a FITC-conjugated polyclonal antibody to C3 for 1 h at 4°C, and analyzed by FACS as described above.

18.3 Results

18.3.1 Oxidative Stress, but Not Chemical Hypoxia, Alters the Expression of Complement Regulatory Proteins on ARPE-19 Cells

We have previously found that antimycin A sensitizes renal epithelial cells to complement-mediated injury (Thurman et al. 2006). We have also previously reported that oxidative stress of ARPE-19 cells results in a decrease in levels of DAF and CD59 surface levels, whereas MCP remains unchanged (Rohrer and Renner 2008). To determine whether decreased expression of these complement regulatory proteins is a common response to many types of cellular stress, ARPE-19 cells were grown as monolayers and were treated with 1 μM antimycin A for 1 h. After treating the cells with antimycin A, cell surface expression of the complement regulatory proteins DAF, MCP, and CD59, was measured by FACS analysis (Fig. 18.1). Chemical hypoxia of the ARPE-19 cells resulted in a slight increase in surface

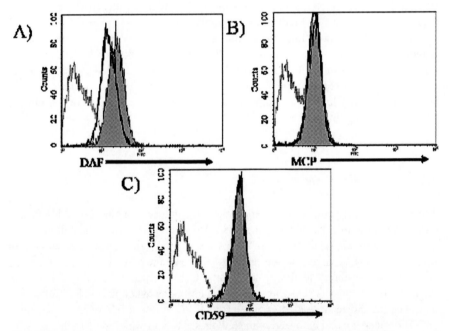

Fig. 18.1 Surface expression of endogenous complement inhibitors by ARPE-19 cells does not decrease in response to hypoxic stress; ARPE-19 cells were treated with 1 μM antimycin A for 1 h. The cells were stained for DAF, MCP, and CD59, and the surface expression of these proteins on experimental cells (*dark line*) was compared to controls (*shaded curve*) and isotype controls (*gray line*). (**a**) Surface expression of DAF increased in antimycin-A-treated cells; whereas (**b**) surface expression of MCP and (**c**) CD59 did not change after treatment with Antimycin A

levels of DAF, and the levels of MCP and CD59 were unchanged. Thus, the response of ARPE-19 cells to hypoxia and oxidative stress are distinct.

18.3.2 Oxidative Stress of Renal Tubular Epithelial Cells Does Not Alter Surface Expression of Crry by the Cells

Crry is the only membrane bound complement regulatory protein expressed by mouse renal PTECs (Thurman et al. 2006). To determine whether expression of Crry by PTECs is altered by oxidative stress, we treated PTECs with 0.5 mM H_2O_2 for 1 h and assessed surface levels of Crry by FACS analysis. Surface levels of Crry in the oxidatively stressed cells were not detectably different than levels in unmanipulated control cells (Fig. 18.2a). We also subjected PTECs to oxidative stress and then exposed them to 10% serum. Exposure of PTECs to 10% serum caused deposition of C3 onto the cell surface, but oxidative stress of the cells did not detectably alter the amount of C3 deposited on serum-exposed cells compared to unmanipulated control cells (Fig. 18.2b).

18.3.3 Expression of MCP, CD55 and CD59 on the Surface of Lung Epithelial Cells Increases After Oxidative Stress, but This Does Not Prevent Complement-Activation on the Cell Surface

We treated epithelial cells derived from human lung with the same dose of H_2O_2 and measured surface expression of the complement regulatory proteins MCP, CD55, and CD59 by FACS analysis. Cells treated with H_2O_2 demonstrated increased levels of all three proteins when compared to unmanipulated control cells (Fig. 18.2c–e). We also found that oxidative stress alone induced fixation of C3 to the cell surface even in the absence of exogenous serum (Fig. 18.2f). Based upon these results we suspect that oxidatively-stressed A549 cells secrete C3. Taken together, these data demonstrate that the A549 cells increase the surface expression of complement regulatory proteins in response to oxidative stress. This increased complement regulation may be offset by other cellular responses such as the release of C3 by the cells, however; and there is a net increase in complement deposition on the cell surface after treatment with H_2O_2.

18.4 Discussion

We have previously shown that oxidative stress of ARPE-19 cells alters the expression of complement regulatory proteins on the cell surface, resulting in greater deposition of C3 on the cell surface when they are subsequently exposed to complement sufficient serum (Rohrer and Renner 2008). In the current study we report

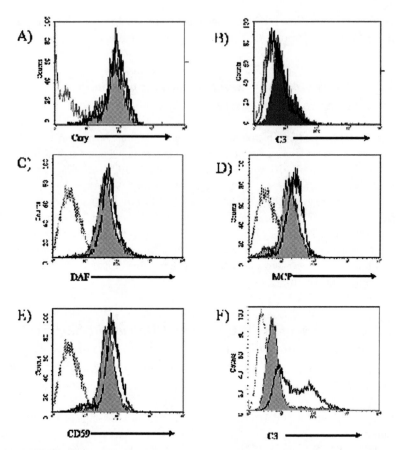

Fig. 18.2 Oxidative stress does not alter complement regulation on the surface of ptecs or A549 cells; Cells were grown to confluence and were treated with 0.5 mM H$_2$O$_2$ for 1 h. (**a**) PTECs were stained for Crry, and surface levels on oxidatively-stressed cells (*shaded curve*) were compared to unmanipulated controls (*solid line*) and an isotype control (*gray line*). (**b**) PTECs were treated with H$_2$O$_2$ and were then exposed to 10% mouse serum for 1 h. C3 deposition on the cells treated with H$_2$O$_2$ (*shaded curve*) was compared to that seen in unmanipulated controls (*solid line*) and an isotype control (*gray line*). Levels of (**c**) DAF, (**d**) MCP, and (**e**) CD59 on H$_2$O$_2$-treated A549 cells (*solid lines*) were compared with unmanipulated controls (*shaded curves*) and isotype controls (*gray lines*). (**f**) Levels of surface C3 were assessed from A549 cells treated with H$_2$O$_2$ (*solid line*) and were compared to unmanipulated cells (*shaded curve*) and isotype control antibody (*gray line*)

that chemical hypoxia of the ARPE-19 cells does not have a similar effect. Indeed, surface levels of DAF were increased after treatment of the cells with Antimycin A. We also tested the effects of oxidative stress on epithelial cells derived from kidney and lung. Treatment of PTECs with H$_2$O$_2$ did not alter the surface expression of the complement regulatory protein, Crry, and did not cause increased deposition of C3 on the cell surface after exposure to serum. Treatment of A549 cells with H$_2$O$_2$ increased the surface expression of MCP, CD55 and CD59. Thus, epithelial cells from different tissues have distinct responses to oxidative stress. Oxidative stress reduces the ability of RPE cells to regulate complement on the cell surface. PTEC cells were not significantly affected by the treatment. Pulmonary epithelial cells increased their expression of complement regulatory proteins, but were still more susceptible to complement activation, possibly due to increased production of complement-activating proteins by the cells.

Pathologic complement activation on epithelial barrier layers is characteristic of inflammatory diseases in several organs, including the eye (Gehrs and Anderson 2006), the kidney (Thurman et al. 2006), and the lung (Taube and Thurman 2006). We initially hypothesized that a reduction in cell surface complement-regulation might be a generalized response of epithelial cells to infection or cellular stress. Such a response might evolve to help protect the host from invasive infection. Our current results, however, suggest that epithelial cells from different organs respond to cellular stress in idiosyncratic ways. Oxidative stress markedly increases the susceptibility of RPE cells to complement activation, but chemical hypoxia did not have this effect. On the other hand, hypoxia increases the susceptibility of renal epithelial cells to complement-mediated injury, but oxidative stress had very little effect.

The unique response of RPE cells to oxidative stress may reflect the environment in which these cells reside. The eye must be kept absolutely free of invasive pathogens, but it is also an immunologically privileged location. Resident cells must therefore perform surveillance functions, and generate proinflammatory factors if they sense pathogens or tissue damage. In this context, modulated regulation of the complement system at the RPE cell layer could be a rapid and potent defense mechanism against ocular infection. Epithelial cells in organs such as the lung, in contrast, are regularly exposed to inhaled pathogens and may have a higher threshold for induction of proinflammatory signals. Renal epithelial cells should also maintain a sterile environment, so it is not immediately clear why RPEs are sensitive to oxidative stress, but the renal cells are sensitive to chemical hypoxia. These responses may relate to the pathogens these cells have evolved to detect. The important role of complement activation in the development of AMD (Hageman and Luthert 2001; Gehrs and Anderson 2006), however, underscores the delicate balance that must be maintained to protect the RPE cell layer from autologous injury while also preventing infectious injury.

In summary, we have found that epithelial cells derived from the eye and the lung express DAF, CD59, and MCP. Epithelial cells from the mouse kidney express Crry in an analogous distribution to MCP in human renal epithelial cells (Ichida and Yuzawa 1994; Thurman et al. 2006). The expression of these proteins is altered by aseptic cellular stressors such as hypoxia and oxidative stress, but the response to these conditions differs from tissue to tissue. In RPE cells, oxidative stress reduces the expression of the cell surface complement regulators and sensitizes the cells to complement-mediated injury. This specific response is not seen in epithelial cells from the lung or kidney, and is not induced by hypoxia. These studies help explain the unique mechanisms by which uncontrolled complement activation may contribute to the development of AMD. A greater understanding of the molecular events that cause AMD may help in the development of therapies to reduce tissue inflammation while minimizing the risk of infection.

Acknowledgments This work was supported in part by National Institutes of Health Grants DK077661 and DK076690 (JMT), DK035081 (MKP), EY13520 and EY017465 (BR) and HL082485 (ST), a vision core grant (EY014793), the Foundation Fighting Blindness, American Heart Association grant 0735101 N (VPF), a grant from the Sandler Program for Asthma Research (VMH), and an unrestricted grant to MUSC from Research to Prevent Blindness, Inc., New York, NY. BR is a Research to Prevent Blindness Olga Keith Weiss Scholar. The authors thank Luanna Bartholomew for editorial assistance. The authors declare the following disclosures. VMH is a co-founder of Taligen Therapeutics, Inc., which develops complement inhibitors for therapeutic use; JMT, VMH and BR are consultants for Taligen Therapeutics, Inc.

References

Dunn KC, Aotaki-Keen AE et al (1996) ARPE-19, a human retinal pigment epithelial cell line with differentiated properties. Exp Eye Res 62:155–169

Dunn KC, Marmorstein AD et al (1998) Use of the ARPE-19 cell line as a model of RPE polarity: basolateral secretion of FGF5. Invest Ophthalmol Vis Sci 39:2744–2749

Gehrs KM, Anderson DH et al (2006) Age-related macular degeneration – emerging pathogenetic and therapeutic concepts. Ann Med 38:450–471

Hageman GS, Luthert PJ et al (2001) An integrated hypothesis that considers drusen as biomarkers of immune-mediated processes at the RPE-Bruch's membrane interface in aging and age-related macular degeneration. Prog Retin Eye Res 20:705–732

Ichida S, Yuzawa Y et al (1994) Localization of the complement regulatory proteins in the normal human kidney. Kidney Int 46:89–96

Lieber M, Smith B et al (1976) A continuous tumor-cell line from a human lung carcinoma with properties of type II alveolar epithelial cells. Int J Cancer 17:62–70

Molina H, Wong W et al (1992) Distinct receptor and regulatory properties of recombinant mouse complement receptor 1 (CR1) and Crry, the two genetic homologues of human CR1. J Exp Med 175:121–129

Panayiotidis MI, Stabler SP et al (2008) Oxidative stress-induced regulation of the methionine metabolic pathway in human lung epithelial-like (A549) cells. Mutat Res doi:10.1016/j.mrgentox.2008.10.006

Rohrer B, Renner B et al (2008) Oxidative stress renders retinal epithelial cells susceptible to complement-mediated injury. XIIIth International Symposium on Retinal Degeneration, September 18–23, Emeishan, Sichuan, China

Sinha D, Wang Z et al (2003) Chemical anoxia of tubular cells induces activation of c-Src and its translocation to the zonula adherens. Am J Physiol Renal Physiol 284:F488–F497

Taube C, Thurman JM et al (2006) Factor B of the alternative complement pathway regulates development of airway hyperresponsiveness and inflammation. Proc Natl Acad Sci USA 103:8084–8089

Thurman JM, Ljubanovic D et al (2003) Lack of a functional alternative complement pathway ameliorates ischemic acute renal failure in mice. J Immunol 170:1517–1523

Thurman JM, Ljubanovic D et al (2006) Altered renal tubular expression of the complement inhibitor Crry permits complement activation after ischemia/reperfusion. J Clin Invest 116:357–368

Thurman JM, Royer PA et al (2006) Treatment with an inhibitory monoclonal antibody to mouse factor B protects mice from induction of apoptosis and renal ischemia/reperfusion injury. J Am Soc Nephrol 17:707–715

Chapter 19
Role of Metalloproteases in Retinal Degeneration Induced by Violet and Blue Light

C. Sanchez-Ramos, J.A. Vega, M.E. del Valle, A. Fernandez-Balbuena,
C. Bonnin-Arias, and J.M. Benitez-del Castillo

Abstract

Introduction: An essential role for metalloproteases (MMPs) has been described in blood vessel neoformation and the removal of cell debris. MMPs also play a key role in degenerative processes and in tumors. The participation of these enzymes in light-induced phototoxic processes is supported by both experimental and clinical data. Given that patients with age-related macular degeneration often show deposits, or drusen, these deposits could be the consequence of deficient MMP production by the pigment epithelium.

Objective: To gain insight into the regulation of metalloproteases in the pathogenia of retinal degeneration induced by light.

Materials and Methods: We examined the eyes of experimental rabbits exposed for 2 years to circadian cycles of white light, blue light and white light lacking short wavelengths. For the trial the animals had been implanted with a transparent intraocular lens (IOL) and a yellow AcrySof® IOL, one in each eye. After sacrificing the animals, the retinal layer was dissected from the eye and processed for gene expression analyses in which we examined the behavior of MMP-2, MMP-3 and MMP-9.

Results: MMP-2 expression was unaffected by the light received and type of IOL. However, animals exposed to white light devoid of short wavelengths or those fitted with a yellow IOL showed 2.9- and 3.6-fold increases in MMP-3 expression, respectively compared to controls. MMP-9 expression levels were also 3.1 times higher following exposure to blue light and 4.6 times higher following exposure to white light lacking short wavelengths or 4.2 times higher in eyes implanted with a yellow IOL.

C. Sanchez-Ramos (✉)
Optic II, Neurocomputing and Neurorobotic Group, University Complutense de Madrid, Madrid, Spain
e-mail: celiasr@opt.ucm.es

R.E. Anderson et al. (eds.), *Retinal Degenerative Diseases*, Advances in Experimental Medicine and Biology 664, DOI 10.1007/978-1-4419-1399-9_19,
© Springer Science+Business Media, LLC 2010

Conclusion: Exposure to long periods of light irrespective of its characteristics leads to the increased expression of some MMPs. This alteration could indicate damage to the extracellular matrix and have detrimental effects on the retina.

19.1 Introduction

The exposition to light radiation causes 3 types of damages on the retina: photomechanical, photothermal and photochemical damages. Light-induced damages mechanism is not exactly known, although there is a lot of references about the effects of light on the retina (Wenzel et al. 2001, Wu et al. 2006), also the mechanism to avoid these damages. In order to gain insight into the knowledge of the phototoxic damages causes by light radiation, it is necessary to focus the analysis in the level of the genetic expression of some possible mechanisms that are involved into the light-induced phototoxic processes. One of the possible mechanisms, which affects the degenerative processes, is the one in which are involved, a serial of proteins called metalloproteases (MMPs).

MMPs are a family of proteins that degraded, in a very selective way, the components of the basal layer and the extracellular matrix. An essential role for metalloproteases (MMPs) has been described in blood vessel neoformation and the removal of cell debris. MMPs also play a key role in degenerative processes and in tumors. MMPs are involved in every process that concerns the extracellular matrix restructuring and they act in a balanced way with their *endogenous inhibitors, the* TIMs (tissue inhibitor of MMPs).

Actually, 20 MMPs, grouped in 4 families: (1) colagenases (MMP-1, 8 and 13), which hydrolyze the interstitial collagen; (2) gelatinases (MMP-2 and 9), which hydrolyze the denatured collagen and some non-fibrilar proteins; (3) the family of stromelysin (MMP-3, 7, 10, 11 and 12) and 4) MMPs jointed to membranes (MMP-14, 15, 16 and 17). In this study 3 types of MMPs have been analyzed: MMP-2, MMP-3 y MMP-9.

These enzymes role in light-induced phototoxic processes is supported by both experimental and clinical data. Plantner (Plantner et al. 1991; Plantner 1992; Plantner and Drew, 1994) was the first on describing the presence of MMPs, specifically MMP-1, MMP-3 and MMP-9, on the matrix situated between the photoreceptors; later, the presence of MMP-2 was confirmed to increase due to light exposure (Plantner et al. 1998a). Light-induced retina's overstimulation causes an increase in the expression of the MMP-9 or gelatinase B, regardless of whether there's a lost of photoreceptors or not (Papp et al. 2007). In the other hand, laser's photocoagulation makes the pigment epithelium to produce MMP-2, MMP-3 and MMP-9 (Flaxel et al. 2007).

Given that patients with age-related macular degeneration (AMD) often show deposits, or drusen, these deposits could be the consequence of deficient MMP production by the pigment epithelium (Elliot et al. 2006). Also, there are many cases of patients with AMD and blood vessel neoformation, what suggests also the MMPs influence in the process.

In a general way, proteases from MMPs family are involved in every biological process that entails the extracellular matrix restructuring of basal layers and blood vessel neoformation. One of the characteristics of light-induced pathologies in humans, also in experimental models, is the appearance of not-well-characterized deposits, drusen. Because of this, these deposits could be a consequence of a reduction on the expression of MMPs, also this could shown the inability of the MMPS to degrade these deposits, that shape the drusen.

Because of and in order to contribute to a better knowledge of permanent and long-term (2 years) lighting effect on the retina, rabbit eyes (clear and yellow intraocular lenses, IOLs have been implanted) under different permanent lighting conditions have been studied: white light, blue light and white light without the blue-light part (called here yellow light).

19.2 Objective

To analyze the phototoxic effect of light on the retina and its prevention by using blue-light filtering IOLs. More specifically, to gain insight into the regulation of metalloproteases in the pathogenia of retinal degeneration induced by light.

19.3 Materials and Methods

Experimental rabbits eyes exposed for 2 years to circadian cycles of white light, blue light and white light lacking short wavelengths were examined. Also, animals had been implanted with a clear IOL (left eye) and a yellow AcrySof® IOL (right eye), one in each eye (Table 19.1). After sacrificing the animals, the retinal layer was dissected from the eye and processed for gene expression analyses in which we examined the behavior of MMP-2, MMP-3 and MMP-9 (Fig. 19.1 and Table 19.2).

Table 19.1 Lighting conditions diagram (yellow, white and blue) in combination with IOL's (clear/left eye, yellow/right eye) implanted in rabbits of the sample. IOL's and surgery used characteristics follows the protocol established for the Escuela de Óptica (UCM)

	Surgery (eye)			
ID	Left	Right	Light	Time (years)
13	Clear	Yellow	Yellow	2
G1	Clear	Clear	Non exposure	2
G3	Clear	Yellow	White	2
G5	Clear	Yellow	Yellow	2
G6	Clear	Yellow	Blue	2
E2	Clear	Yellow	Blue	2,5

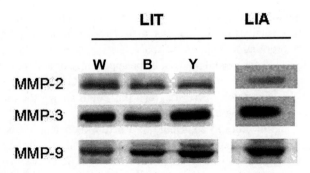

Fig. 19.1 Both eyes hemi-retinas of animals exposed to the same lighting levels were processed together. Total mRNA was extracted from the different experimental group's retinas by using the TRI reagent (Sigma; St. Louis, MO), also RNA integrity was quantified with agaroses gel electrophoresis. RNA extracted was processed for inverse transcription with the tampon solution provided by the laboratory Amersham Pharmacia Biotech (Little Chalfont, Buckinghamshire, UK). Primers sequences used are base on the sequences published for mouse (GenBank accession). Reaction was made on a cyclator (Hyband Th. Cycler). PCR final product was visualized by using a tinction of bromure ethidium under UV light follows by electrophoresis in agaroses gel (2%). Products were quantified in a PhosphorImager (Fuji)

Table 19.2 Primers used in the study, which have been manufactured following previous bibliography, concerning genetic sondas were made similar as mouse's genome. Every hybridation's results were satisfactory

Metalloproteases
• MMP-2: up: 5′-CCA CTG CCT TCG ATA CAC-3′, down: 5′-GAG CCA CTC TCT GGA ATC TTC AAA-3′
• MMP-3: up:5′-GCT TTG AAG GTC TGG GAG GAG GTG-3′,down: 5-CAG CTA TCT TCC TGG GAA ATC CTG-3′
• MMP-9: up: 5′-GTT CCC GGA GTG AGT TGA-3′, down: 5′-TTT ACA TGG CAC TGC AAA GC-3′

19.4 Results

These study findings indicate that exposure to long periods of light increases the expression of some MMPs and this could have harmful effects on the retina since it indicates damage to the extracellular matrix. Increased MMP expression could determine the faster turnover of the extracellular matrix to avoid the formation of matrix deposits.

Light exposure or the intraocular implant of a yellow lens does not modify MMP-2 expression. In animals exposed to light, lacking the blue portion of the spectrum, and in animals implanted with a yellow IOL, MMP-3 expression was 2.9 and 3.6 times higher than in controls, respectively. Similar behaviour was observed for MMP-9 expression which was upregulated in: animals exposed to blue light (3.1 times), animals exposed to white light lacking the blue portion of the spectrum (4.6 times) and animals fitted with a yellow intraocular lens (4.2 times). Light

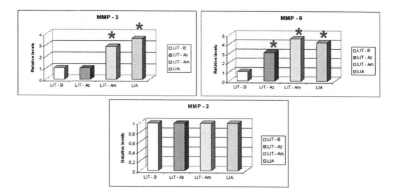

Fig. 19.2 Results obtained for MMP-2, MMP-3 and MMP-9. LIT-B: white IOL; LIT-Az: blue-light IOL; LIT-Am: yellow (white light without the blue-light part); LIO: yellow IOL

exposure results in no changes in the expression for MMP-2, whereas MM-3 and MMP-9 were up regulated, especially in the animals exposed to white-filtered light and carrying a yellow intraocular lens (Fig. 19.2).

These results agree partially with other animal model trials published before. There no modifications in MMP-2 expression, but Plantner (Plantner et al. 1998) found it increased in animals exposed to light. In the other hand, data concerning MMP-9 expression are coincident with the obtained for Papp (Papp et al. 2007). In general, these result can't support the hypothesis that drusen are a consequence of MMPs production drop in pigment epithelium (Elliot et al. 2006).

These results analysis can be made in 2 ways. First, long-term lighting exposure, irrespective of its characteristics, increases some MMPs expression and that could damage the retina, because this would indicate extracellular matrix injuries. In the other hand, the increase in the expression of the MMPs would be related with an accelerated turnover of the matrix to avoid the appearance of deposits that give rise to drusen.

19.5 Conclusion

Exposure to long periods of light irrespective of its characteristics leads to the increased expression of some MMPs. This alteration could indicate damage to the extracellular matrix and have detrimental effects on the retina.

References

Chen L, Wu W, Dentychev T et al (2004) Light damage induced changes in mouse retinal gene expression. Exp Eye Res 79:239–247
Curran T, Franza BR Jr. (1988) Fos and Jun: the AP-1 connection. Cell 55:395–397

Elliot S, Catanuto P, Stetler-Stevenson W et al (2006) Retinal pigment epithelium protection from oxidant-mediated loss of MMP-2 activation requires both MMP-14 and TIMP-2. Invest Ophthalmol Vis Sci 47:1696–1702

Flaxel C, Bradle J, Acott T et al (2007) Retinal pigment epithelium produces matrix metalloproteinases after laser treatment. Retina 27:629–634

Fujieda H, Sasaki H (2008) Expression of brain-derived neurotrophic factor in cholinergic and dopaminergic amacrine cells in the rat retina and the effects of constant light rearing. Exp Eye Res 86:335–343

Gauthier R, Joly S, Pernet V et al (2005) Brain-derived neurotrophic factor gene delivery to muller glia preserves structure and function of light-damaged photoreceptors. Invest Ophthalmol Vis Sci 46:3383–3392

Grimm C, Wenzel C, Hafezi F et al (2000) Gene expression in the mouse retina: effect of damaging light. Mol Vis 6:252–260

Llamosas MM, Cernuda-Cernuda R, Huerta JJ et al (1997) Neurotrophin receptors expression in the developing mouse retina: an immunohistochemical study. Anat Embryol (Berl) 195: 337–344

López-Otín C, Overall CM (2002) Protease degradomics: a new challenge for proteomics. Nat Rev Mol Cell Biol 3:509–519

Margrain TH, Boulton M, Marshall J et al (2004) Do blue light filters confer protection against age-related macular degeneration?. Prog Retin Eye Res 23:523–531

Meyers SM (2004) A model of spectral filtering to reduce photochemical damage in age-related macular degeneration. Trans Am Ophtalmol Soc 102:83–95

Papp AM, Nyilas R, Szepesi Z et al (2007) Visible light induces matrix metalloproteinase-9 expression in rat eye. J Neurochem 103:2224–2233

Plantner JJ (1992) The presence of neutral metalloproteolytic activity and metalloproteinase inhibitors in the interphotoreceptor matrix. Curr Eye Res 11:91–101

Plantner JJ, Drew TA (1994) Polarized distribution of metalloproteinases in the bovine interphotoreceptor matrix. Exp Eye Res 59:577–585

Plantner JJ, Le ML, Kean EL (1991) Enzymatic deglycosylation of bovine rhodopsin. Exp Eye Res 53:269–274

Plantner JJ, Jiang C, Smine A (1998) Increase in interphotoreceptor matrix gelatinase A (MMP-2) associated with age-related macular degeneration. Exp Eye Res 67:637–645

Plantner JJ, Smine A, Quinn TA (1998) Matrix metalloproteinases and metalloproteinase inhibitors in human interphotoreceptor matrix and vitreous. Curr Eye Res 17:132–140

Seiler MJ, Thomas BB, Chen Z, Arai S, Chadalavada S, Mahoney MJ, Sadda SR, Aramant RB (2008) BDNF-treated retinal progenitor sheets transplanted to degenerate rats – Improved restoration of visual function. Exp Eye Res 86:92–104

Thanos C, Emerich D (2005) Delivery of neurotrophic factors and therapeutic proteins for retinal diseases. Expert Opin Biol Ther 5:1443–1452

Wenzel A, Reme CE, Williams TP et al (2001) The Rpe65 Leu450Met variation increases retinal resistance against light-induced degeneration by slowing rhodopsin regeneration. J Neurosci 21:53–58

Wu J, Seregard S, Algvere PV (2006) Photochemical damage of the retina. Surv Ophthalmol 51:461–481

Chapter 20
Mitochondrial Decay and Impairment of Antioxidant Defenses in Aging RPE Cells

Yuan He and Joyce Tombran-Tink

Abstract In the eye, the retinal pigment epithelium (RPE) is exposed to a highly oxidative environment, partly due to elevated oxygen partial pressure from the choriocapillaris and to digestion of polyunsaturated fatty acid laden photoreceptor outer segments. Here we examined the vulnerability of RPE cells to stress and changes in their mitochondria with increased chronological aging and showed that there is greater sensitivity of the cells to oxidative stress, alterations in their mitochondrial number, size, shape, matrix density, cristae architecture, and membrane integrity as a function of age. These features correlate with reduced cellular levels of ATP, ROS, and $[Ca^{2+}]_c$, lower $\Delta\psi m$, increased $[Ca^{2+}]_m$ sequestration and decreased expression of mtHsp70, UCP2, and SOD3. Mitochondrial decay, bioenergetic deficiencies, and weakened antioxidant defenses in RPE cells occur as early as age 62. With increased severity, these conditions may significantly reduce RPE function in the retina and contribute to age related retinal anomalies.

20.1 Summary

In the eye, the retinal pigment epithelium (RPE) is exposed to a highly oxidative environment, partly due to elevated oxygen partial pressure from the choriocapillaris and to digestion of polyunsaturated fatty acid laden photoreceptor outer segments. Here we examined the vulnerability of RPE cells to stress and changes in their mitochondria with increased chronological aging and showed that there is greater sensitivity of the cells to oxidative stress, alterations in their mitochondrial number, size, shape, matrix density, cristae architecture, and membrane integrity as a function of age. These features correlate with reduced cellular levels of ATP, ROS, and $[Ca^{2+}]_c$, lower $\Delta\psi m$, increased $[Ca^{2+}]_m$ sequestration and decreased expression

J. Tombran-Tink (✉)

Department of Neural and Behavioral Sciences, Pennsylvania State University College of Medicine, Hershey, PA, USA

e-mail: jttink@aol.com

R.E. Anderson et al. (eds.), *Retinal Degenerative Diseases*, Advances in Experimental Medicine and Biology 664, DOI 10.1007/978-1-4419-1399-9_20,
© Springer Science+Business Media, LLC 2010

of mtHsp70, UCP2, and SOD3. Mitochondrial decay, bioenergetic deficiencies, and weakened antioxidant defenses in RPE cells occur as early as age 62. With increased severity, these conditions may significantly reduce RPE function in the retina and contribute to age related retinal anomalies.

20.2 Introduction

It is often argued that the metabolic rate of an organism determines its life span (Beckman and Ames 1998; Sohal et al. 2002; Pamplona et al. 2002) and that neurodegenerative diseases that occur with advanced aging have a common root in mitochondrial dysfunction. The mitochondria divide continuously throughout the life of a cell and their numbers in the cell varies according to organism, tissue type, and energy demands. They control a range of processes including cell signaling, differentiation, death, proliferation, and cell cycle. They produce most of the cells ATP, generate the bulk of ROS (Viña et al. 2006; Duchen 1999; Lane 2006), and are important to the organism's antioxidant defense systems (Mancuso 2007; Jezek and Hlavatá 2005; Czarna and Jarmuszkiewicz 2006; Inoue et al. 2003). These organelles are highly prone to oxidative damage, can accumulate mutations because they lack efficient mtDNA repair mechanisms, and can pass these mutations on to daughter cells (Passos et al. 2007; Chen et al. 2007; Stuart and Brown 2006). A shift in the balance of the number of normal and defective mitochondria in cells can influence senescence and apoptotic programs (Koopman et al. 2007; Chen et al. 2006; Hauptmann et al. 2008; Kwong et al. 2007).

There is compelling evidence that mitochondrial dysfunction is an early event in many neurodegenerative diseases including Alzheimer's disease (Lin and Beal 2006; Takuma et al. 2005; Beal 1998; Krieger and Duchen 2002; Eckert et al. 2008; Song et al. 2004; Schapira 1999; Valente et al. 2004) and that mitochondrial decay causes the cell's anti-stress pathways to operate with less efficiency (Wenzel et al. 2008; Hayakawa et al. 2008; Sasaki et al. 2008; Kimura et al. 2007). It is therefore conceivable that unchecked propagation and accumulation of dysfunctional mitochondria in aging RPE cells is also an underlying cause in the progression of age-related retinal diseases such as age AMD, a multifactorial disorder with etiology stemming, in part, from cumulative oxidative damage to the RPE (D'Cruz et al. 2000; Gal et al. 2000; Dorey et al. 1989; Green and Enger 1993; Beatty et al. 2000; Dunaief et al. 2002; Winkler et al. 1999). Histological changes are evident in the RPE and mitochondria of these cells at the earliest stages of AMD and precede vision loss, even though the disease has been primarily associated with photoreceptor damage (Green et al. 1985; Young 1987; Hageman et al. 2001; Penfold et al. 2001; Feher et al. 2006).

The RPE, a metabolically active epithelium crucial to maintaining the health of the retina, is continuously bombarded by high levels of oxidants (Weiter 1987; Zareba et al. 2006). Among its numerous responsibilities, this epithelium constitutes the blood retinal barrier, facilitates selective transport between the choroidal vasculature and outer retina, phagocytose and degrade shed photoreceptor outer segments, regenerate photopigments, secrete neurotrophic, adhesion, and vascular regulatory factors, and contributes to the integrity of Bruch's membrane and the choriocapillaris. Disruption in any of these high-energy requiring processes is detrimental to the health of the retina.

In the AMD retina there is abnormal regulation of several mitochondrial proteins including ATP synthase, cytochome C oxidase complex, and mtHsp70 (Nordgaard et al. 2008) and a link between mitochondrial dysfunction and RPE degeneration (Jin et al. 2005; Liang and Godley 2003; Jin et al. 2001; Wang et al. 2008; Suter et al. 2000). This is not surprising given the daily challenges the RPE faces. Here we provide evidence for structural and functional modifications in the mitochondria of RPE cells, attenuation of the cells antioxidant system, and increased sensitivity of the RPE to oxidative stress with increased chronological age. We propose that increased accumulation of defective mitochondria in RPE cells with aging contributes to reduced function of these cells and increased pathological consequences in the retina.

20.3 Materials and Methods

20.3.1 Primary Human RPE Cell Culture

Human RPE cells were isolated from non-diseased donors as previously described (McKay and Burke 1994) and cultures maintained in DMEM supplemented with 5% FBS. Cultures in third to sixth passages from normal human donors, ages 9, 52, 62, and 76 years, were used for the experiments below.

20.3.2 Hydrogen Peroxide Toxicity – PI Assays

Cells were seeded at a density of 1×10^5 for 24 h in serum free medium (SFM), then exposed to 320 μM H_2O_2 for 2 h. Cultures were washed and cell death estimated by propidium iodide (PI) (4 μg/ml) staining.

20.3.3 Mitochondrial Morphometrics

RPE cells were seeded onto fibronectin coated Thermanox cover slips, fixed and processed for electron microscopy (Pavlovic et al. 2008; Zagon et al. 2007). Twenty individual RPE cell EM micrographs were randomly taken along different planes of cells from each donor and for each group, a carbon grating replica was photographically recorded to calibrate the magnification of the cells (Laguens 1971). Micrographs were enlarged to 16,200X to count the mitochondria in three 49 μm^2 perinuclear areas of the cell (Fig. 20.3). The counting template consisted of

Area 1, placed closest to the nucleus in the mitochondrial dense region and Area 2 and 3 located at a 45° angle to area 1 and at the same distance of 10.5 μm from the nucleus. The mitochondria morphology was examined at 35,000x and morphometric analysis performed using the NIH Image J program. Data is presented at the mean for each individual area/20 cells and the mean of all three areas/20 cells.

RPE cell morphology was also examined using phase-contrast and confocal microscopy and cell size estimated by flow cytometry. Mitochondrial population was estimated by labeling detached cultures with 50 nM MitoTracker Red and analysis of 10,000 cells by flow cytometry (BD FACS AriaTM, Becton Dickinson, USA) at an excitation wavelength of 488 nm and emission of 590 nm.

20.3.4 Protein and Weight Estimation of RPE Cells and Mitochondria

RPE cells (1×10^6) for each donor age were harvested by centrifugation. Pellets were weighed, lysed, and protein concentrations estimated. Mitochondria were isolated using reagents from the Pierce mitochondria isolation kit for cultured cells (Pierce Chemical Co Rockford, Illinois, USA) (Hauptmann et al. 2008). Mitochondrial pellet weights were estimated, then the organelles were lysed, centrifuged, and concentration of protein in the supernatant estimated.

20.3.5 Measurement of ROS, ATP and Mitochondrial Membrane Potential ($\Delta\Psi m$)

Cellular oxidative stress was determined by the amount of ROS in the cytoplasm (Degli Esposti 2002; Amer et al. 2003) of the RPE cells essentially as we have described previously (He et al. 2008a). Cells were harvested by centrifugation, washed, and 2×10^6 cells/ml incubated at 37°C for 30 min with 0.4 μM ROS indicator H_2-DCF-DA. Excess H_2-DCF-DA was removed from the samples and cells analyzed by flow cytometry using 488 nm excitation and 530 nm emission wavelengths. ATP levels were determined using a luciferin/luciferase-based assay essentially as described (He et al. 2008a) and luminescence measured using a luminometer (Orion II Luminometer, Berthold Detection Systems, TN).

$\Delta\psi m$ measurements were carried out as we have previously described (He et al. 2008a) using the indicator JC-1, a lipophilic and cationic dye, which fluoresces red when it aggregates in the matrix of healthy, high-potential mitochondria and fluorescence green in cells with low $\Delta\Psi m$. JC-1 (1 μg/ml) was added to 2×10^6 cells/ml in suspension and samples incubated for 20 min at 37°C, washed, and analyzed by flow cytometry. Data were collected at an emission wavelength of 530 nm for green fluorescence and 590 nm for red fluorescence.

20.3.6 Measurement of ($[Ca^{2+}]_c$) and ($[Ca^{2+}]_m$)

Cytoplasmic calcium $[Ca^{2+}]_c$ levels were measured with the fluorescent probe fluo-3/AM and mitochondrial calcium $[Ca^{2+}]_m$ with Rhod-2/AM (K_d ~570 nM) as described (He et al. 2008b; Deng et al. 2006; Mironov et al. 2005) using 1×10^5 cells/well in SFM. The cells were loaded with either 1 μM fluo-3/AM for 30 min, or 1 μM rhod-2/AM for 1 h, trypsinized, washed twice, resuspended in 200 μl PBS, then analyzed by flow cytometry at excitation and emission wavelengths of 488 and 525 nm respectively, for fluo-3/AM, and 549 nm and 581 nm respectively, for Rhod-2/AM.

20.3.7 Expression of Mitochondrial Associated Genes

Total mRNA from RPE cultures was isolated, RT-PCR and real time-PCR performed at an annealing temperature of 58°C for 35 cycles for the mitochondria associated genes, mtHsp70, UCP2, ATPase-α, β, γ, SOD1, SOD2, SOD3, Bax, Bcl-2, COX1 and COX2 using their respective primers (Invitrogen, Carlsbad, CA). GAPDH was used as an internal RNA loading control and no reverse transcriptase (NRTs) reactions as negative controls to confirm that amplification was RNA dependent. For real-time PCR, the 2-step amplifying protocol was used with iQ SYBR green super-mix solution (BioRad). Both the melting curve and gel electrophoretic analyses were used to determine amplification homogeneity and quality of the reaction.

20.4 Results

20.4.1 Age Related Sensitivity of RPE Cells to Oxidative Stress

Phase-contrast micrographs of primary cultures of RPE cells show that RPE cells from the 9 yo donor grow as a monolayer of tightly packed cobblestone-like cells in culture whereas those from individuals >62 yo are larger and more fibroblastic in appearance (Fig. 20.1). The identity of the cells in the cultures was established by visual observation of the pigmented cells by phase contrast microscopy and using RPE65 as an expression marker. Visual observation and immunocytochmistry indicate that greater than 99% of the cells in the primary cultures were pigmented and expressed RPE65.

In Fig. 20.2, we show that there are age related differences in the susceptibility of RPE cells to oxidative stress. When treated with 160–320 uM H2O2, approximately 90% of cells were PI positive in cultures >62 yo compared to the 9 and 52 yo donors. Flow cytometry for PI fluorescence intensity also confirms greater cell death in the older cultures.

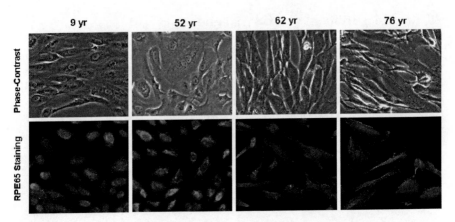

Fig. 20.1 Phase-contrast micrographs of primary cultures of RPE cells obtained from various donors ages (*upper*). Cells from donors >60 yo are larger and more fibroblastic in appearance compared to those obtained from 9 and 52 yo individuals. >99% of the cells in all cultures are pigmented and express RPE 65. Scale bar = 30 μm

20.4.2 Variation in Mitochondrial Number, Structure, and Size

We used a template that consisted of three identical counting areas to sample the number of mitochondria per unit area in the mitochondria polarized region of the RPE cells. RPE cells of all ages contain a mitochondrial-polarized region found in a crown-like shape in the perinuclear area although there is some distribution of these organelle throughout the cytoplasm of the cells (Fig. 20.3). In Table 20.1, we show that there are fewer mitochondria per unit area of the mitochondrial polarized cytoplasm of the RPE cells with increased donor age with >2 fold differences between cells from the youngest and oldest donors (p <0.05). The average number of mitochondria in all three areas/cell (mitochondria/147uM^2/cell) is 46.22 ± 12.86, 37.75 ± 13.78, 25.68 ± 8.69 and 20.15 ± 5.30 for the 9, 52, 62 and 76 yo RPE, respectively.

Electron microscopic comparison of the various RPE cultures shows very marked differences in the mitochondrial populations of the cells (Fig. 20.4). Those from the 9 and 52 yo individuals are numerous, more regular in size, and are either round or oval in shape. The cristae are distinctly visible and outer membranes intact. Cells from the 62 and 76 yo donors have mitochondria that are sparsely distributed in the cytoplasm, irregular in size, tubular in shape, have highly electron-dense matrices, less distinct cristae, and disrupted outer membranes. There is a higher density of mitochondria in the 9 and 52 yo cells compared to those from older individuals in the mitochondrial polarized perinuclear area of the cells.

These findings were also confirmed by confocal microscopy (Fig. 20.5) where we show that Mito Tracker Red (Hauptmann et al. 2008) labeling intensity decreases as a function of RPE age. Labeling was perinuclear and discrete in the 9 yo samples compared to the diffused, branching pattern of the 62 and 76 yo cells.

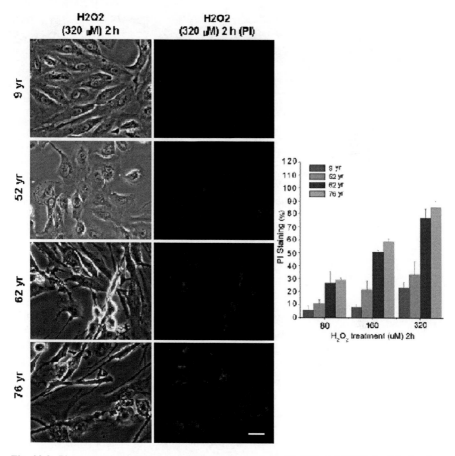

Fig. 20.2 Phase-contrast light micrographs of cells treated with 320 μM H2O2 for 2 h showing sensitivity to oxidative stress. Scale bar = 30 μm. PI staining indicates that there is ∼90% cell death in the 76 yo cultures compared to 26% in 9 yo after exposure the H2O2

Table 20.1 Results summarized from EM analyses indicate that mitochondria number decreases as a function of age in RPE cells

| Number of mitochondria/age | Cytoplasm area | | | |
	1(close to nucleus)	2	3	1 + 2 + 3
9 year	22.11 ± 3.62	13.78 ± 7.43	10.33 ± 5.55	46.22 ± 12.86
52 year	13.25 ± 5.22*	13.25 ± 6.51	11.25 ± 7.99	37.75 ± 13.78
62 year	10.00 ± 4.27*	7.63 ± 4.70*	8.05 ± 4.17	25.68 ± 8.69*
76 year	7.38 ± 2.93*	5.92 ± 4.82*	6.85 ± 3.48	20.15 ± 5.30*

$n = 20$ cells $\times$ 3 areas; area = 49 μm^2; $*p < 0.05$

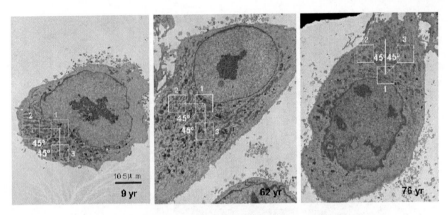

Fig. 20.3 EM micrographs showing mitochondria in perinuclear regions of cells from various donor ages and position of templates used for mitochondrial counting. Scale bar = 10.5 μm

In Table 20.2, we provide our results for cellular and mitochondrial weight and protein estimations for equal number of cells in each sample. There is a ∼1.6 fold increase in both wet weight and protein per 1×10^6 RPE cells from the 62 and 72 yo individuals compared to the 52 and 9 yo cultures. Although there are fewer mitochondria in the aging cells, there is a ∼2 fold increase in wet weight and amount of protein in mitochondrial samples isolated from the two older donor samples supporting the EM observations that mitochondria increase in size in the RPE with increased donor age.

20.4.3 ROS and ATP Production, and ΔΨm Decrease in RPE Cells with Aging

Data collected from flow cytometric acquisition/analyses indicate that the amount of ROS generated by the 62, and 76 yo RPE cultures decreases by 3.23-fold (± 0.18) and 4.76-fold (± 0.21) respectively, when compared to the 9 yo cultures (Fig. 20.6) (p <0.05) (Fig. 20.6). There is also an early and consistent decrease in ATP levels in 52, 62 and 76 yrs RPE cells by 31, 35 and 45%, respectively, compared to 9 yr old samples (p <0.05) (Fig. 20.7). The 31% deficiency in energy production at donor age 52 may account for the lower levels of ROS generation by the cells at later stages of aging. The bioenergetic profiles of the various aged RPE cells also correlate well with the Δψm in the cells. There is a 1.2-fold (±0.1), 1.52-fold (±0.2) and 2.1-fold (±0.3) decrease in Δψm in the 52, 62 and 76 yo cells, respectively compared to the 9 yo cultures (Fig. 20.8). Together, these analyses suggest increased impairment in mitochondrial function with chronological aging of RPE cells.

Fig. 20.4 Electron micrographs (magnification 35,000× and 12,500×) of primary RPE cultures. Mitochondria in 9 yo RPE cells are *oval* and *regular* in shape and contain intact membranes with visibly distinct *inner* and *outer* *membranes* and cristae. Those in 62 and 76 yo are fewer, larger, irregular in size, *tubular* in shape, have highly electron dense matrices, and disruption in membranes and cristae. Scale bar = 1.5 μm

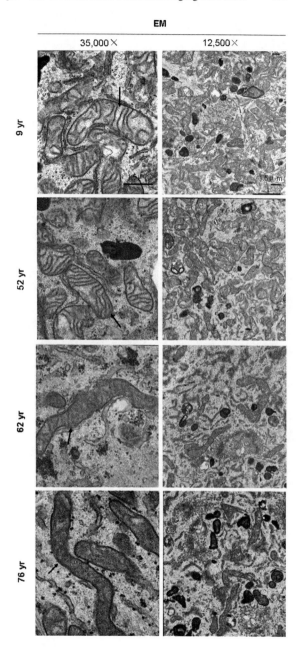

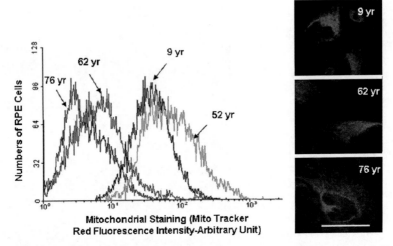

Fig. 20.5 Fluorescence intensity of Mito Tracker Red is decreased with aging of the RPE cells seen here by flow cytometry and confocal microscopy. Scale bar $= 30\,\mu$m

Table 20.2 Mitochondria weight and protein concentration/1×10^6 RPE cells from each donor age

	9	52	62	76
Cell weight/10^6 cells(mg)	14.34 ± 0.62	13.81 ± 0.33	$24.11 \pm 1.27^*$	$22.33 \pm 1.81^*$
Cytoplasmic protein/10^6 cells(mg)	0.41 ± 0.08	0.39 ± 0.15	$0.64 \pm 0.09^*$	$0.61 \pm 0.05^*$
Mitochondria weight/10^6 cells(mg)	1.73 ± 0.14	1.51 ± 0.11	$2.87 \pm 0.18^*$	$2.95 \pm 0.35^*$
Mitochondria protein/10^6 cells(mg)	0.08 ± 0.01	0.08 ± 0.01	$0.14 \pm 0.02^*$	$0.13 \pm 0.01^*$

$^*p < 0.05$

20.4.4 Age-Related Variations in ($[Ca^{2+}]_c$) and ($[Ca^{2+}]_m$) in RPE Cells

There is abundant evidence of altered calcium dynamics in cells with increased aging, a condition that renders the cells more vulnerable to degenerative events (Toescu et al. 2004). We noted a correlation between lower $[Ca^{2+}]_c$ levels and increased mitochondrial sequestration of Ca^{2+} in RPE cells with aging (Fig. 20.9). The relative amounts of fluo-3AM and Rhod-2 fluorescence intensity in the cultures reflect a 1.52-fold ($\pm$ 0.33) and 1.85-fold ($\pm$ 0.28) decrease in $[Ca^{2+}]_c$ and a 2.32-fold ($\pm$ 1.49) and 2.75-fold ($\pm$ 1.88) increase in $[Ca^{2+}]_m$ levels in the 62 and 76

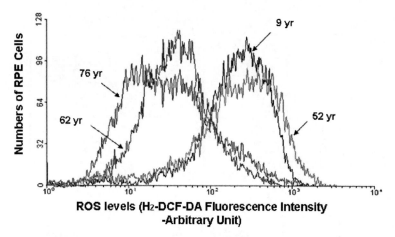

Fig. 20.6 Distribution of the fluorescent intensity for the ROS indicator, H_2-DCF-DA, in RPE cultures using flow cytometry. A decrease in ROS levels is seen with increased aging

Fig. 20.7 ATP levels are decreased in RPE cells with increased donor age

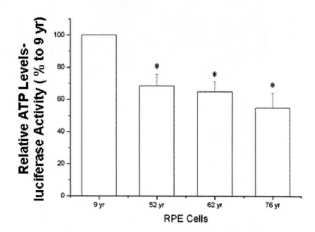

yo cells, respectively compared to the youngest counterpart (Fig. 20.9) ($p < 0.05$). Disruption in calcium homeostatic mechanisms together with lower energy levels in the aging RPE cells may certainly impose limits on these cells in their response to environmental stress.

20.4.5 Expression of Genes Associated with Mitochondrial Function

Given the structural, biochemical, and functional changes in the mitochondria with increased donor age, we examined the expression of several genes important to mitochondrial health and function to ascertain if any may have a mechanistic link with

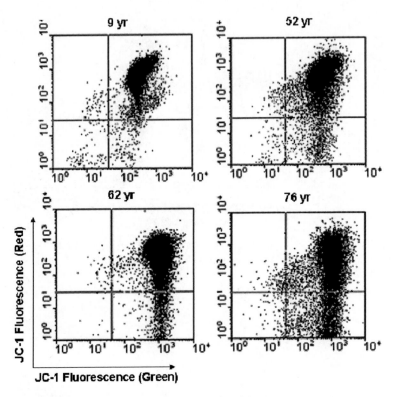

Fig. 20.8 ΔΨm are decreased in RPE cells with increased donor age

the changes observed above. In our studies we found a consistent decrease in the mRNA levels of mtHsp70, UCP2, SOD3, Bcl-2 and Bax and increase in SOD2 expression with increased aging of the RPE cells (Fig. 20.10) but no significant differences in the expression of ATPase-α, b, γ, SOD1, COX1 and COX2 between cells of the various donor ages (data not show). This data suggest that there are variations in expression of genes important to mitochondrial function that may alter the threshold level of the cells to environmental hazards.

Although, we recognize that a limitation of this study is the size of the RPE donor samples used, we showed a longitudinal decrease in structural and functional integrity of the mitochondria in RPE cells with aging. Since this presentation was made at the XIIIth International Symposium on Retinal Degeneration in China (September 2008), we have analyzed RPE samples from 4 other individuals >60 year old and have confirmed these findings. There is still the difficulty in obtaining samples from younger donors, but the human ARPE19 cell line derived from a 19 year old male showed features of cell growth, morphology, and mitochondrial structure and function that were similar to primary cultures from the 9 yo donor (data not shown).

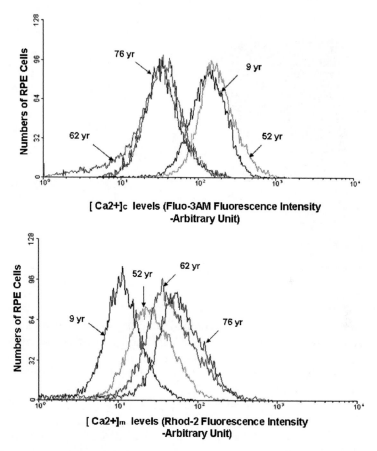

Fig. 20.9 Flow cytometry showing that RPE cells sequester more $[Ca^{2+}]_m$ and have lower levels of $[Ca^{2+}]_c$ with increased aging

20.5 Discussion

The RPE is in a location in the retina where it is constantly bombarded by reactive oxygen species. Cumulative oxidative damage can cause this tissue to degenerate (Beatty et al. 2000; Dunaief et al. 2002; Winkler et al. 1999). We examined the function of these organelles in RPE cells and the susceptibility of these cells to oxidative stress with increased chronological aging. Our study showed that with increased aging there are numerous structural abnormalities in the mitochondria of RPE cells which correlate with decreased bioenergetic levels of the cells, attenuation of the cell's antioxidant system, and increased sensitivity to oxidative stress. Our work is supported by the findings of Feher et al (Feher et al. 2006) who showed, in a larger sampling of individuals, that there are structural abnormalities in the mitochondria of the RPE with advancing age and that these abnormalities increase in severity in individuals with AMD.

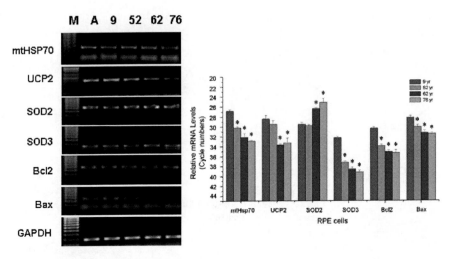

Fig. 20.10 Expression of antioxidant and apoptotic genes in RPE cells of various donor ages

It is well known that the numbers of mitochondria vary between cells in a tissue (Knott et al. 2008) and that this organelle can undergo ultrastructural remodelling to tailor energy output to meet environmental demands on the cell (Bereiter-Hahn and Vöth 1994; Bertoni-Freddari et al. 1993, 2001). mtDNA are highly susceptible to oxidative stress and unlike nuclear DNA, mutations in mtDNA are not repaired and can be inherited or acquired by individual cells (Sastre et al. 2000; Barja 2004; Melov 2004). A cell can have several populations of mtDNA (Kmiec et al. 2006). Over 80% of mtDNA codes for functional proteins, thus most mtDNA mutations lead to functional problems (Knott et al. 2008; Reeve et al. 2008). For example, Leber's hereditary optic neuropathy is associated with mutation in NADH-COQ reductase, ragged muscle fibers with mutation in mt lysine tRNA, and Kaerns-Sayre syndrome with several large deletions in mtDNA (Pätsi et al. 2008; Finsterer 2007). Diabetes, stroke, Alzheimer's and Parkinson's diseases, lactic acidosis, myopathy, osteoporosis, cancer, cardiovascular diseases, and aging, all show strong associations with mitochondrial dysfunction (Knott et al. 2008; Beal 2007; Lin and Beal 2006). The oxidative stress theory of aging, an expansion of the mitochondrial theory of aging, is based on the idea that somatic mutations in mtDNA provoke respiratory chain dysfunction, which leads to enhanced ROS production which, in turn, promotes further mtDNA mutations and cell function collapse (Passos et al. 2007; Ishikawa et al. 2008). This vicious cycle is amplified in mitochondrial biogenesis, which occurs in a cell cycle-independent manner. It is, therefore, not surprising that aging cells accumulate a subpopulation of dysfunctional mitochondria which, in excess, may weaken the cell's response to environmental hazards and promote cellular aging and untimely degeneration of the cell.

A general trend in mitochondria structure is seen with aging: in older organisms, there are studies showing a decrease in mitochondrial numbers but an increase in the organelle's size due to fusion with other mitochondria or lack of fission (Bertoni-Freddari et al. 1993, 2008). This is seen at the synaptic terminals of old rats where there is a marked increase in the percentage of oversized organelles, often referred to as megamitochondria (Melov 2004). These are found in some adverse conditions as well, such as in cells exposed to large amounts of free radicals over an extended period (Karbowski et al. 1999; Wakabayashi 2002). The speculation is that numeric loss of mitochondria is due to impaired duplicative capacity of these organelles and that a shift in size compensates for numbers (Bertoni-Freddari et al. 1993; Solmi et al. 1994; Bertoni-Freddari et al. 2003, 2005). Our ultrastructural studies indicate that there are 'megamitochondria' in the aging RPE cells and that these are abnormal in appearance and have disruptions in the cristae architecture, a condition previously reported with cross-linking ATP synthase complexes (Ko et al. 2003; Gavin et al. 2004).

To cope with toxic oxygen intermediates, the RPE evolved effective defenses against oxidative damage and is particularly rich in anti-oxidants. However, several antioxidant enzymes, including mtHsp70, UCP2, and SOD3 have reduced expression in the RPE with aging. This may be one explanation why the primary cultures of RPE cells from older donors are more susceptible to oxidative stress. Strangely, however, there is a decrease in ROS production in the RPE from donor samples >60 yo which contradicts popular findings that ROS increases in aging tissues. One explanation is that the increase in SOD2 expression that we noted in these cells with aging may have a compensatory effect on attenuating ROS production with life span extension as a primary goal. Our finding of significantly lower ATP levels in the aging RPE cells underscores the 'low metabolic rate – high life expectancy' principle. However, one can argue that these in vitro studies do not predict organismal ageing or disease progression.

Some mitochondrial-specific actions leading to apoptosis include loss of $\Delta\Psi m$, induction of MPT opening, increased mitochondrial calcium levels, and cytosolic translocation of apoptogenic factors, such as cytochrome c (Armstrong 2006; Green and Kroemer 2004). Although the aging RPE cells have decreased $\Delta\Psi m$, as would be expected from the lower ATP levels they generate, there was no cytochrome c released by the cells or increased expression of the proapoptotic Bax gene. It is known that mitochondria Ca^{2+} overload triggers mitochondrial permeability transition pore (MPTP) opening, which lowers $\Delta\Psi m$ (Jackson and Thayer 2006; Dahlem et al. 2006). The high $[Ca^{2+}]_m$ in the aging RPE cells may, therefore, account for the lower $\Delta\Psi m$ in the cells.

Reduction in mitochondrial function and increased susceptibility of RPE cells to oxidative stress is likely to be part of the normal aging process in the retina. While accumulation of a relatively small number of defective mitochondria by these cells may compromise epithelial function but not trigger apoptosis, acute degeneration signals may be propagated when there is an excess in number of these dysfunctional organelles in any RPE cell of the epithelium.

In conclusion, we present strong evidence for structural and biochemical abnormalities in the mitochondria of RPE cells as a function of normal aging. We propose that impairment of mitochondrial function makes RPE cells more vulnerable to oxidative damage and that excess accumulation of dysfunctional mitochondria in some RPE cells may trigger a degeneration cascade in a focal region of the epithelium that could be an underlying event in the onset of some retinal pathologies.

Acknowledgments This work was supported by grants from the Ben Franklin Foundation, PA, USA, the National Basic Research Program of China (No. 2007CB512200), and the National Natural Science Foundation of China (No.30672275, No.30400486), NEI Core Grant P30 EY01931 (PI, Janice M Burke), and by an unrestricted grant from Research to Prevent Blindness, Inc. to the Medical College of Wisconsin. The first author received support from the China Scholarship Council.

References

Amer J, Goldfarb A, Fibach E (2003) Flow cytometric measurement of reactive oxygen species production by normal and thalassaemic red blood cells. Eur J Haematol 70:84–90

Armstrong JS (2006) Mitochondrial membrane permeabilization: the sine qua non for cell death. Bioessays 28:253–260

Barja G (2004) Free radicals and aging. Trends Neurosci 27:595–600

Beal MF (1998) Mitochondrial dysfunction in neurodegenerative diseases. Biochim Biophys Acta 1366:211–223

Beal MF (2007) Mitochondria and neurodegeneration. Novartis Found Symp 287:183–192 discussion 192–196

Beatty S, Koh H, Phil M et al (2000) The role of oxidative stress in the pathogenesis of age-related macular degeneration. Surv Ophthalmol 45:115–134

Beckman KB, Ames BN (1998) Mitochondrial aging: open questions. Ann NY Acad Sci 854: 118–127

Bereiter-Hahn J, Vöth M (1994) Dynamics of mitochondria in living cells: shape changes, dislocations, fusion, and fission of mitochondria. Microsc Res Tech 27:198–219

Bertoni-Freddari C, Balietti M, Giorgetti B et al (2008) Selective decline of the metabolic competence of oversized synaptic mitochondria in the old monkey cerebellum. Rejuvenation Res 11:387–391

Bertoni-Freddari C, Fattoretti P, Casoli T (1993) Morphological plasticity of synaptic mitochondria during aging. Brain Res 628:193–200

Bertoni-Freddari C, Fattoretti P, Casoli T et al (2001) Quantitative cytochemical mapping of mitochondrial enzymes in rat cerebella. Micron 32:405–410

Bertoni-Freddari C, Fattoretti P, Giorgetti B et al (2005) Age-related decline in metabolic competence of small and medium-sized synaptic mitochondria. Naturwissenschaften 92:82–85

Bertoni-Freddari C, Fattoretti P, Paoloni R et al (2003) Inverse correlation between mitochondrial size and metabolic competence: a quantitative cytochemical study of cytochrome oxidase activity. Naturwissenschaften 90:68–71

Chen JH, Hales CN, Ozanne SE (2007) DNA damage, cellular senescence and organismal ageing: causal or correlative? Nucleic Acids Res 35:7417–7428

Chen X, Stern D, Yan SD (2006) Mitochondrial dysfunction and Alzheimer's disease. Curr Alzheimer Res 3:515–520

Czarna M, Jarmuszkiewicz W (2006) Role of mitochondria in reactive oxygen species generation and removal; relevance to signaling and programmed cell death. Postepy Biochem 52: 145–156

Dahlem YA, Wolf G, Siemen D et al (2006) Combined modulation of the mitochondrial ATP-dependent potassium channel and the permeability transition pore causes prolongation of the biphasic calcium dynamics. Cell Calcium 39:387–400

D'Cruz PM, Yasumura D, Weir J et al (2000) Mutation of the receptor tyrosine kinase gene Mertk in the retinal dystrophic RCS rat. Hum Mol Genet 9:645–651

Degli Esposti M (2002) Measuring mitochondrial reactive oxygen species. Methods 26:335–340

Deng X, Yin F, Lu X et al (2006) The apoptotic effect of brucine from the seed of Strychnos nux-vomica on human hepatoma cells is mediated via Bcl-2 and Ca2+ involved mitochondrial pathway. Toxicol Sci 91:59–69

Dorey CK, Wu G, Ebenstein D (1989) Cell loss in the aging retina. Relationship to lipofuscin accumulation and macular degeneration. Invest Ophthalmol Vis Sci 30:1691–1699

Duchen MR (1999) Contributions of mitochondria to animal physiology: from homeostatic sensor to calcium signaling and cell death. J Physiol 16:1–17

Dunaief JL, Dentchev T, Ying GS et al (2002) The role of apoptosis in age-related macular degeneration. Arch Ophthalmol 120:1435–1442

Eckert A, Hauptmann S, Scherping I et al (2008) Soluble beta-amyloid leads to mitochondrial defects in amyloid precursor protein and tau transgenic mice. Neurodegener Dis 5:157–159

Feher J, Kovacs I, Artico M et al (2006) Mitochondrial alterations of retinal pigment epithelium in age-related macular degeneration. Neurobiol Aging 27:983–993

Finsterer J (2007) Genetic, pathogenetic, and phenotypic implications of the mitochondrial A3243G tRNALeu (UUR) mutation. Acta Neurol Scand 116:1–14

Gal A, Li Y, Thompson DA (2000) Mutations in MERTK, the human orthologue of the RCS rat retinal dystrophy gene, cause retinitis pigmentosa. Nat Genet 26:270–271

Gavin PD, Prescott M, Luff SE et al (2004) Cross-linking ATP synthase complexes in vivo eliminates mitochondrial cristae. J Cell Sci 117:2333–2343

Green WR, Enger C (1993) Age-related macular degeneration histopathologic studies. The 1992 Lorenz E. Zimmerman Lecture. Ophthalmology 100:1519–1535

Green DR, Kroemer G (2004) The pathophysiology of mitochondrial cell death. Science 305: 626–629

Green WR, McDonnell PJ, Yeo JH (1985) Pathologic features of senile macular degeneration. Ophthalmology 92:615–627

Hageman GS, Luthert PJ, Victor Chong NH et al (2001) An integrated hypothesis that considers drusen as biomarkers of immune-mediated processes at the RPE-Bruch's membrane interface in aging and age related macular degeneration. Prog Retin Eye Res 20:705–732

Hauptmann S, Scherping I, Dröse S et al (2008) Mitochondrial dysfunction: an early event in Alzheimer pathology accumulates with age in AD transgenic mice. Neurobiol Aging Feb 21 30(10):1574–1586

Hayakawa N, Yokoyama H, Kato H et al (2008) Age-related alterations of oxidative stress markers in campal CA1 sector. Exp Mol Pathol May 20

He Y, Ge J, Tombran-Tink J (2008b) Mitochondrial defects and dysfunction in calcium regulation in glaucomatous trabecular meshwork cells. Invest Ophthalmol Vis Sci 49:4912–4922

He Y, Tombran-Tink J, Ge J et al (2008a) Mitochondrial complex I defect induces ROS release and degeneration in trabecular meshwork cells of POAG patients: protection by antioxidants. Invest Ophthalmol Vis Sci 49:1447–1458

Inoue M, Sato EF, Nishikawa M (2003) Mitochondrial generation of reactive oxygen species and its role in aerobic life. Curr Med Chem 10:2495–2505

Ishikawa K, Takenaga K, Akimoto M et al (2008) ROS-generating mitochondrial DNA mutations can regulate tumor cell metastasis. Science 320:661–664

Jackson JG, Thayer SA (2006) Mitochondrial modulation of Ca2+-induced Ca2+-release in rat sensory neurons. J Neurophysiol 96:1093–1104

Jezek P, Hlavatá L (2005) Mitochondria in homeostasis of reactive oxygen species in cell, tissues, and organism. Int J Biochem Cell Biol 37:2478–2503

Jin GF, Hurst JS, Godley BF (2001) Rod outer segments mediate mitochondrial DNA damage and apoptosis in human retinal pigment epithelium. Curr Eye Res 23:11–19

Jin M, Yaung J, Kannan R et al (2005) Hepatocyte growth factor protects RPE cells from apoptosis induced by glutathione depletion. Invest Ophthalmol Vis Sci 46:4311–4319

Karbowski M, Kurono C, Wozniak M et al (1999) Free radical-induced megamitochondria formation and apoptosis. Free Radic Biol Med 26:396–409

Kimura K, Tanaka N, Nakamura N et al (2007) Knockdown of mitochondrial heat shock protein 70 promotes progeria-like phenotypes in caenorhabditis elegans. J Biol Chem 282:5910–5918

Kirkwood TB (2005) Understanding the odd science of aging. Cell 120:437–447

Kmiec B, Woloszynska M, Janska H (2006) Heteroplasmy as a common state of mitochondrial genetic information in plants and animals. Curr Genet 50:149–159

Knott AB, Perkins G, Schwarzenbacher R et al (2008) Mitochondrial fragmentation in neurodegeneration. Nat Rev Neurosci 9:505–518

Ko YH, Delannoy M, Hullihen J et al (2003) Mitochondrial ATP synthasome. Cristae-enriched membranes and a multiwell detergent screening assay yield dispersed single complexes containing the ATP synthase and carriers for Pi and ADP/ATP. J Biol Chem 278: 12305–12309

Koopman WJ, Verkaart S, Visch HJ et al (2007) Human NADH:ubiquinone oxidoreductase deficiency: radical changes in mitochondrial morphology? Am J Physiol Cell Physiol 293: C22–C29

Krieger C, Duchen MR (2002) Mitochondria, Ca2+ and neurodegenerative disease. Eur J Pharm. 447:177–188

Kwong JQ, Henning MS, Starkov AA et al (2007) The mitochondrial respiratory chain is a modulator of apoptosis. J Cell Biol 179:1163–1177

Laguens R (1971) Morphometric study of myocardial mitochondria in the rat. J Cell Biol 48: 673–676

Lane N (2006) Mitochondrial disease: powerhouse of disease. Nature 440:600–602

Liang FQ, Godley BF (2003) Oxidative stress-induced mitochondrial DNA damage in human retinal pigment epithelial cells: a possible mechanism for RPE aging and age-related macular degeneration. Exp Eye Res 76:397–403

Lin MT, Beal MF (2006) Mitochondrial dysfunction and oxidative stress in neurodegenerative diseases. Nature 443:787–795

Mancuso C, Scapagini G, Currò D et al (2007) Mitochondrial dysfunction, free radical generation and cellular stress response in neurodegenerative disorders. Front Biosci 12:1107–1123

McKay BS, Burke JM (1994) Separation of phenotypically distinct subpopulations of cultured human retinal pigment epithelial cells. Exp Cell Res 213:85–92

Melov S (2004) Modeling mitochondrial function in aging neurons. Trends Neurosci 27:601–606

Mironov SL, Ivannikov MV, Johansson M (2005) [Ca2+]i signaling between mitochondria and endoplasmic reticulum in neurons is regulated by microtubules. From mitochondrial permeability transition pore to Ca2+-induced Ca2+ release. J Biol Chem 280:715–721

Nordgaard CL, Karunadharma PP, Feng X et al (2008) Mitochondrial proteomics of the retinal pigment epithelium at progressive stages of age-related macular degeneration. Invest Ophthalmol Vis Sci 49:2848–2855

Pamplona R, Barja G, Portero-Otín M (2002) Membrane fatty acid unsaturation, protection against oxidative stress, and maximum life span: a homeoviscous-longevity adaptation? Ann N Y Acad Sci 959:475–490

Passos JF, Saretzki G, von Zglinicki T (2007) DNA damage in telomeres and mitochondria during cellular senescence: is there a connection? Nucleic Acids Res 35:7505–7513

Pavlovic J, Floros J, Phelps DS et al (2008) Differentiation of xenografted human fetal lung parenchyma. Early Hum Dev 84:181–193

Penfold PL, Madigan MC, Gillies MC et al (2001) Immunological and aetiological aspects of macular degeneration. Prog Retin Eye Res 20:385–414

Pätsi J, Kervinen M, Finel M et al (2008) Leber hereditary optic neuropathy mutations in the ND6 subunit of mitochondrial complex I affect ubiquinone reduction kinetics in a bacterial model of the enzyme. Biochem J 409:129–137

Reeve AK, Krishnan KJ, Turnbull DM (2008) Age related mitochondrial degenerative disorders in humans. Biotechnol J 3:750–756

Sasaki T, Unno K, Tahara S et al (2008) Age-related increase of superoxide generation in the brains of mammals and birds. Aging Cell 7:459–469

Sastre J, Pallardó FV, García de la Asunción J et al (2000) Mitochondria, oxidative stress and aging. Free Radic Res 32:189–198

Schapira AH (1999) Mitochondria in the aetiology and pathogenesis of Parkinson's disease. Parkinsonism Relat Disord 5:139–143

Sohal RS, Mockett RJ, Orr WC (2002) Mechanisms of aging: an appraisal of the oxidative stress hypothesis. Free Radic Biol Med 33:575–586

Solmi R, Pallotti F, Rugolo M et al (1994) Lack of major mitochondrial bioenergetic changes in cultured skin fibroblasts from aged individuals. Biochem Mol Biol Int 33:477–484

Song DD, Shults CW, Sisk A et al (2004) Enhanced substantia nigra mitochondrial pathology in human alpha-synuclein transgenic mice after treatment with MPTP. Exp Neurol 186:158–172

Stuart JA, Brown MF (2006) Mitochondrial DNA maintenance and bioenergetics. Biochim Biophys Acta 1757:79–89

Suter M, Remé C, Grimm C et al (2000) Age-related macular degeneration. The lipofusion component N-retinyl-N-retinylidene ethanolamine detaches proapoptotic proteins from mitochondria and induces apoptosis in mammalian retinal pigment epithelial cells. J Biol Chem 275:39625–39630

Takuma K, Yao J, Huang J et al (2005) ABAD enhances Abeta-induced cell stress via mitochondrial dysfunction. FASEB J 19:597–598

Toescu EC, Verkhratsky A, Landfield PW (2004) Ca2+ regulation and gene expression in normal brain aging. Trends Neurosci Oct 27(10):614–620

Valente EM, Abou-Sleiman PM, Caputo V et al (2004) Hereditary early-onset Parkinson's disease caused by mutations in PINK1. Science 304:1158–1160

Viña J, Sastre J, Pallardó FV et al (2006) Role of mitochondrial oxidative stress to explain the different longevity between genders: protective effect of estrogens. Free Radic Res 40:1359–1365

Wakabayashi T (2002) Megamitochondria formation - physiology and pathology. J Cell Mol Med 6:497–538

Wang AL, Lukas TJ, Yuan M et al (2008) Increased mitochondrial DNA damage and down-regulation of DNA repair enzymes in aged rodent retinal pigment epithelium and choroid. Mol Vis 14:644–651

Weiter JJ (1987) Phototoxic changes in the retina. In: Miller, D (ed) Clinical light damage to the eye. Springer-Verlag, New York

Wenzel P, Schuhmacher S, Kienhöfer J et al (2008) Manganese superoxide dismutase and aldehyde dehydrogenase deficiency increase mitochondrial oxidative stress and aggravate age-dependent vascular dysfunction. Cardiovasc Res July 22 80:280–289

Winkler BS, Boulton ME, Gottsch JD et al (1999) Oxidative damage and age-related macular degeneration. Mol Vis 5:32

Young RW (1987) Pathophysiology of age-related macular degeneration. Surv Ophthalmol 31:291–306

Zagon IS, Sassani JW, Myers RL et al (2007) Naltrexone accelerates healing without compromise of adhesion complexes in normal and diabetic corneal epithelium. Brain Res Bull 72:18–24

Zareba M, Raciti MW, Henry MM (2006) Oxidative stress in ARPE-19 cultures: do melanosomes confer cytoprotection? Free Radic Biol Med 40:87–100

Chapter 21
Ciliary Transport of Opsin

Deepti Trivedi and David S. Williams

Abstract As part of the renewal of photoreceptor outer segment disk membranes, membrane proteins are transported along the region of the cilium, connecting the inner and outer segments. Genetics studies have indicated the role of motor proteins in this transport. Direct analysis of live cells is needed to increase our understanding of the transport mechanisms further. Here, we show that transfection of hTERT-RPE1 cells with constructs encoding RHO-EGFP, but not RHO-mCherry, results in the distribution of fluorescently-tagged opsin in the plasma membrane. When the cells have differentiated and possess cilia, a portion of the RHO-EGFP was observed along the cilia. Due to the remarkable conservation of ciliary protein function, this system of Rho-Egfp transfected hTERT-RPE1 cells provides a valid model with which to study the ciliary transport of opsin directly in live cells.

21.1 Introduction

For the renewal of the disk membranes of photoreceptor outer segments, membrane proteins are delivered to the base of the outer segment from the inner segment (Young 1967). Early EM autoradiography studies demonstrated labeled protein in the connecting cilium (the region of the photoreceptor cilium between the basal body and the most basal disk membrane of the outer segment), indicating that the protein traveled along this conduit to the outer segment (Young 1968). However, subsequent immunocytochemistry analyses failed to detect opsin in this structure (e.g. Nir and Papermaster 1983; Besharse et al. 1985), suggesting the notion that delivery of opsin-containing membrane might follow an extraciliary route (Besharse and Wetzel 1995), as proposed originally by Richardson (1969). Later studies showed immunogold labeling of opsin in the connecting cilia of mice that were

D. Trivedi (✉)
Jules Stein Eye Institute, University of California, 200 Stein Plaza, Los Angeles, CA 90095, USA
e-mail: dtrivedi@ucla.edu

R.E. Anderson et al. (eds.), *Retinal Degenerative Diseases*, Advances in Experimental Medicine and Biology 664, DOI 10.1007/978-1-4419-1399-9_21,
© Springer Science+Business Media, LLC 2010

mutant for the molecular motor, myosin VIIa, thus not only supporting the ciliary route, but suggesting the involvement of a molecular motor in the transport of opsin along the cilium (Liu et al. 1999). Evidence for the participation in ciliary opsin transport by the microtubule motor, kinesin-2 (Marszalek et al. 2000), which is significantly faster than unconventional myosins, led to the realization that the rapid transport of opsin along the connecting cilium likely resulted in a relatively low concentration of the protein in this structure (Williams 2002). Only following extensive etching of sections, was significant immunogold labeling of opsin detected in the connecting cilia of wild-type retinas (Wolfrum and Schmitt 2000).

With the acceptance of the delivery of opsin (and other membrane proteins) to the outer segment occurring via the connecting cilium, attention has turned to understanding the mechanisms of its delivery. Molecular motors appear to be involved, based on genetics studies. While these in vivo studies indicate a physiological requirement for a given motor, it is not clear how direct that role is, and the relative functions of different motors. In addition to kinesin-2 (Marszalek et al. 2000; Jimeno et al. 2006) and myosin VIIa (Liu et al. 1999), the requirement of another kinesin, based on a homodimer of KIF17, has been indicated from zebrafish studies (Insinna et al. 2008). Motor associated proteins, such as intraflagellar transport proteins (IFTs), are also required (Pazour et al. 2002). To gain a better understanding of the molecular mechanisms underlying opsin transport along the connecting cilium, the transport process needs to be studied directly, rather than inferred from endpoint studies. Imaging of live cells provides such an approach.

Since procedures to maintain photoreceptor cells in cell culture conditions are not well established, we have used lines of polarized ciliated cells as a starting point. Use of these cells is justified based on the extensive conservation of ciliary protein function. For example, from algae to mammals, kinesin-2 and intraflagellar transport (IFT) proteins function in the movement of proteins along the axonemes of cilia and flagella (Rosenbaum and Witman 2002). Conservation of ciliary organization is also manifest by several syndromic diseases that are based on ciliopathies (Fliegauf et al. 2007).

In the present paper, we describe our initial studies in establishing hTERT-RPE1 cells, expressing fluorescently-tagged opsin, and show that the tagged opsin is present in the cilia of these cells.

21.2 Methods

Cell culture: hTERT-RPE1 cells were grown in DMEM/F12 culture medium with 5% PBS and 1% penicillin/streptomycin, as suggested by ATCC. Cells were incubated at 37°C with 5% CO2. To induce the growth of cilia in confluent cultures, the complete medium was replaced with the medium containing 0.5% FBS, one day after transfection. They were kept in the low serum condition for 48 h before imaging.

Transfection: Transfection was achieved using lipofectamine 2000 (Invitrogen). After 4–6 h, normal growth medium was replaced.

Immunocytochemistry: Cells were fixed in 4% paraformaldehyde for 10 min and subsequently washed with PBS. They were then blocked with 5% goat serum and incubated for 1 h in primary antibody. After subsequent washes with PBS, the cells were incubated with the secondary antibody, washed and mounted in mowiol. Acetylated tubulin (Cat# T7451, Sigma) and KAP3 (Cat# SC-8877, Santa Cruz) antibodies were used.

Microscopy: Both live and fixed cell confocal microscopy was performed using a spinning disk confocal microscope (Perkin Elmer). Images were processed using Velocity software.

21.3 Results

Opsin has been shown to be targeted to the apical surface of MDCK cells (Chuang and Sung 1998). Here, we have used another epithelial cell line, hTERT-RPE1 cells, to test whether, following transfection, opsin is targeted not only to the apical surface, but to the cilium protruding from the apical surface of each of these cells.

An exposed C-terminus is necessary for the correct localization of rhodopsin; the placement of a protein tag at the C terminus of opsin interferes with its ability to localize properly to the plasma membrane in cell culture as well as in vivo (e.g. Moritz et al. 2001). However, a fusion protein, containing RHO-EGFP, with the last 8 amino acids of opsin repeated after the EGFP, was found to function and localize normally in Xenopus (Moritz et al. 2001; Jin et al. 2003). We followed the same design, using bovine rod opsin cDNA, fused with either EGFP or mCherry (Fig. 21.1a). Both these constructs were used for transfection of hTERT-RPE1 cells. Although the RHO-EGFP localized to the plasma membrane in these cells, RHO-mCherry did not; it aggregated in inner compartments of the cells (Fig. 21.1b). This observation indicated that only the Rho-Egfp construct was useful for our studies.

In order to induce the hTERT-RPE1 cells to grow cilia, confluent cells growing in normal serum conditions were 'starved' of serum (0.5% serum). Under these conditions, they generated cilia within 48 h (Fig. 21.2). As expected, the cilia were found to contain KAP3, a component of the heterotrimeric kinesin-2 (Fig. 21.2b). To test whether opsin was located in the cilia, cells were cotransfected cells with Rho-Egfp and a construct that generated the protein, Smoothened (SMO), with a CFP tag. Smoothened, when overexpressed, can completely suppress Patched activity and is localized to the cilium (Taipale et al. 2000), and is thus an effective cilium marker. We observed that RHO-EGFP was present with SMO-CFP in the cilia (Fig. 21.3).

21.4 Discussion

In this preliminary study, we report that a portion of EGFP-tagged opsin (but not RHO-mCherrry) is delivered to the cilia of transfected hTERT-RPE1 cells. Given the conservation among cilia, analysis of opsin transport in the hTERT-RPE1 cell

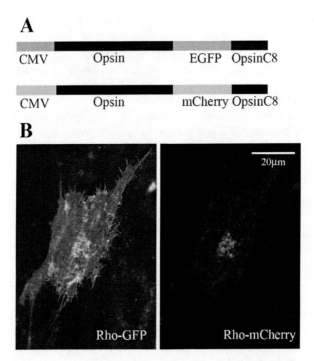

Fig. 21.1 Rho-Egfp and Rho-mCherry constructs. **a,** Schematic of Rho-Egfp and Rho-mCherry constructs. Bovine Rho cDNA was placed under the CMV promoter and tagged with either Egfp or mCherry at the C terminus. The 3′ 24 base pairs of Rho were added to the 3′ of the Egfp or mCherry tag. **b,** Comparison of the localization of RHO-EGFP and RHO-mCherry, following cotransfection of the same cell. RHO-EGFP (*left*) localizes to the plasma membrane while RHO-mCherry (*right*) forms internal aggregates

cilia should provide insight into mechanisms underlying the transport of opsin from the inner segment to the outer segment.

The conservation of protein function in cilia is remarkable. Heterotrimeric kinesin-2 has been detected in photoreceptor cilia (Beech et al. 1996), and we have demonstrated its presence in the primary cilia of hTERT-RPE1, in the present study (Fig. 21.2b). However, much further afield, the FLA-10 protein of Chlamydomonas flagella was identified as a subunit of kinesin-2 (Kozminski et al. 1995). In some of the first studies on axonemal transport, FLA-10 was found to be required for the transport of 'rafts' of IFT protein complexes to the tip of the flagellum, where growth occurs (Cole et al. 1998). Similarly, KIN1 and KIN2, which are genes for motor subunits of kinesin-2 in Tetrahymena, are required for the assembly of new cilia and the maintenance of preexisting cilia (Brown 1999). In C. elegans, a kinesin-2 has been identified in immotile chemosensory cilia, together with the IFT proteins, osm-1 and osm-6. GFP-tagged kinesin-2 and osm-6 have been observed moving in a distal direction together along the sensory cilia of live worms (Orozco et al. 1999).

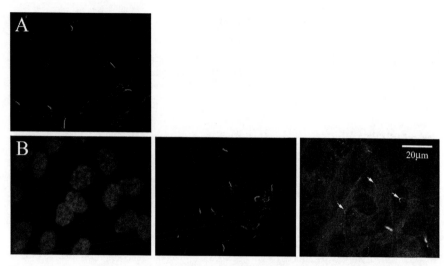

Fig. 21.2 Cilia of hTERT-RPE1 cells. **a**, Serum starvation for 48 h leads to cell differentiation and the production of cilia. Cells are labeled with acetylated tubulin antibodies to indicate the cilia. **b**, KAP3 antibody localizes to the cilia. *Left panel*: DAPI staining of the cells to indicate the nuclei. *Middle panel*: Acetylated tubulin antibody labeling, showing the cilia of the cells. *Right panel*: KAP3 antibody labeling shows localization in the cilia (*arrowheads*)

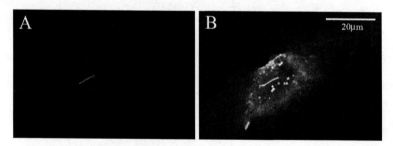

Fig. 21.3 RHO-EGFP localization in cilia, as indicated by the prsence of SMO-CFP, in hTERT-RPE1 cells, transfected with both Rho-Egfp and Smo-Cfp. **a**, Overexpressed SMO-CFP localized to cilia. **b**, RHO-EGFP in the same cell

While the presence of kinesin-2 appears to be of particular importance with respect to opsin transport, as shown by genetics studies (Marszalek et al. 2000; Pazour et al. 2002; Jimeno et al. 2006), a number of other ciliary proteins are linked to syndromic ciliopathies that include photoreceptor degeneration, thus adding further support to the conservation of protein function in cilia. Examples include NPHP5, which underlies a form of Senior-Loken syndrome (Otto et al. 2005), CEP290 (or NPHP6), which has been linked to Joubert syndrome (Sayer et al. 2006), and the Bardet-Biedl syndrome (BBS) proteins (Blacque and Leroux 2006).

Together, the conservation of protein function in cilia, and the delivery of opsin along the cilia of hTERT-RPE1 cells, indicate that polarized epithelial cells, such as hTERT-RPE1 cells, that are transfected with tagged opsin provide a valid model system in which to study the ciliary transport of opsin.

Acknowledgments We thank Dr Zhaohuai Yang, UCSD, for providing with the Rho-Gfp and Rho-mCherry constructs, and Dr Carolyn Ott, NIH, for providing with the Smo-CFP construct. We also thank Dr Vanda Lopes for providing the hTERT-RPE1 cell line.

References

Beech PL, Pagh Roehl K, Noda Y et al (1996) Localization of kinesin superfamily proteins to the connecting cilium of fish photoreceptors. J Cell Sci 109:889–897

Besharse JC, Forestner DM, Defoe DM (1985) Membrane assembly in retinal photoreceptors. III. Distinct membrane domains of the connecting cilium of developing rods. J Neurosci 5: 1035–1048

Besharse JC, Wetzel MG (1995) Immunocytochemical localization of opsin in rod photoreceptors during periods of rapid disc assembly. J Neurocytol 24:371–388

Blacque OE, Leroux MR (2006) Bardet-Biedl syndrome: an emerging pathomechanism of intracellular transport. Cell Mol Life Sci 63:2145–2161

Brown SS (1999) Cooperation between microtubule- and actin-based motor proteins. Ann Rev Cell Dev Biol 8:1751–1755

Chuang JZ, Sung CH (1998) The cytoplasmic tail of rhodopsin acts as a novel apical sorting signal in polarized MDCK cells. J Cell Biol 142:1245–1256

Cole DG, Diener DR, Himelblau AL et al (1998) Chlamydomonas kinesin-II-dependent intraflagellar transport (IFT): IFT particles contain proteins required for ciliary assembly in Caenorhabditis elegans sensory neurons. J Cell Biol 141:993–1008

Fliegauf M, Benzing T, Omran H (2007) When cilia go bad: cilia defects and ciliopathies. Nat Rev Mol Cell Biol 8:880–893

Insinna C, Pathak N, Perkins B et al (2008) The homodimeric kinesin, Kif17, is essential for vertebrate photoreceptor sensory outer segment development. Dev Biol 316:160–170

Jimeno D, Feiner L, Lillo C et al (2006) Analysis of kinesin-2 function in photoreceptor cells using synchronous Cre-loxP knockout of Kif3a with RHO-Cre. Invest Ophthalmol Vis Sci 47: 5039–5046

Jin S, McKee TD, Oprian DD (2003) An improved rhodopsin/EGFP fusion protein for use in the generation of transgenic Xenopus laevis. FEBS Lett 542:142–146

Kozminski KG, Beech PL, Rosenbaum JL (1995) The Chlamydomonas kinesin-like protein FLA10 is involved in motility associated with the flagellar membrane. J Cell Biol 131: 1517–1527

Liu X, Udovichenko IP, Brown SDM et al (1999) Myosin VIIa participates in opsin transport through the photoreceptor cilium. J. Neurosci 19:6267–6274

Marszalek JR, Liu X, Roberts EA et al (2000) Genetic evidence for selective transport of opsin and arrestin by kinesin-II in mammalian photoreceptors. Cell 102:175–187

Moritz OL, Tam BM, Papermaster DS et al (2001) A functional rhodopsin-green fluorescent protein fusion protein localizes correctly in transgenic Xenopus laevis retinal rods and is expressed in a time-dependent pattern. J Biol Chem 276:28242–28251

Nir I, Papermaster DS (1983) Differential distribution of opsin in the plasma membrane of frog photoreceptors: an immunocytochemical study. Invest Ophthalmol Vis Sci 24:868–878

Orozco JT, Wedaman KP, Signor D et al (1999) Movement of motor and cargo along cilia [letter]. Nature 398:674

Otto EA, Loeys B, Khanna H et al (2005) Nephrocystin-5, a ciliary IQ domain protein, is mutated in Senior-Loken syndrome and interacts with RPGR and calmodulin. Nat Genet 37:282–288

Pazour GJ, Baker SA, Deane JA et al (2002) The intraflagellar transport protein, IFT88, is essential for vertebrate photoreceptor assembly and maintenance. J Cell Biol 157:103–113

Richardson TM (1969) Cytoplasmic and ciliary connections between the inner and outer segments of mammalian visual receptors. Vision Res 9:727–731

Rosenbaum JL, Witman GB (2002) Intraflagellar transport. Nat Rev Mol Cell Biol 3:813–825

Sayer JA, Otto EA, O'Toole JF et al (2006) The centrosomal protein nephrocystin-6 is mutated in Joubert syndrome and activates transcription factor ATF4. Nat Genet 38:674–681

Taipale J, Chen JK, Cooper MK et al (2000) Effects of oncogenic mutations in Smoothened and Patched can be reversed by cyclopamine. Nature 406:1005–1009

Williams DS (2002) Transport to the photoreceptor outer segment by myosin VIIa and kinesin II. Vision Res 42:455–462

Wolfrum U, Schmitt A (2000) Rhodopsin transport in the membrane of the connecting cilium of mammalian photoreceptor cells. Cell Motil Cytoskeleton 46:95–107

Young RW (1967) The renewal of photoreceptor cell outer segments. J. Cell Biol 33:61–72

Young RW (1968) Passage of newly formed protein through the connecting cilium of retina rods in the frog. J Ultrastruct Res 23:462–473

Chapter 22
Effect of Hesperidin on Expression of Inducible Nitric Oxide Synthase in Cultured Rabbit Retinal Pigment Epithelial Cells

Luo Xiaoting, Zeng Xiangyun, Li Shumei, Dong Minghua, and Xiong Liang

Abstract

Objective: To study the effect of hesperidin on expression of inducible nitric oxide synthase (iNOS) in cultured rabbit retinal pigment epithelial (RPE) cells under the condition of high glucose in vitro.

Method: Hesperidin was extracted from Pericarpium Citri Reticulatae by ultrasound and ethanol precipitation and was detected qualitatively by high performance liquid chromatogram. The third to fifth primary cultured rabbit RPE were selected. The cells were divided into 6 groups including the control group cultured in DMEM, the model group cultured in DMEM containing 33 mmol/L glucose without any drug and four experimental groups which were exposed to hesperidin at the concentration of 10, 20, 40 and 80 mg/L at 37°C under 5% CO_2 for 2 h and then cultured in DMEM containing 33 mmol/L glucose. The proliferation of RPE was measured by the MTT assay. The levels of NO produced were measured by spectrophotometry. The changes of iNOS expressed in RPE cells were determined with immunohistochemistry.

Results: The growth rate of RPE cells was associated with the concentration of hesperidin. NO production induced by high glucose was significantly inhibited by hesperidin. iNOS expression in hesperidin-treated group was decreased compared with the control group ($p < 0.001$).

Conclusion: Hesperidin can increase the proliferation of rabbit RPE cells, and inhibit the level of NO and iNOS expression, so hesperidin can protect rabbit RPE cells.

L. Shumei (✉)

Department of Preventive Medicine, Gannan Medical College, Ganzhou, China

e-mail: gnyxylsm@163.com

Supplied by: Department of Education of Jiangxi Province (NO.GJJ08401) and Gannan Medical College (NO.2006070). Brief introduction of author: Luo Xiaoting, female, born in 1976, is an associate professor. Her research field is mainly in molecular pharmacology. Tel: 0797-8657990; Fax: 0797-8200037; E-mail: xtluo76@yahoo.com.cn

22.1 Introduction

Diabetic retinopathy (DR), a principal cause of blindness, is characterized by increased retinal vascular permeability and progressive retinal vascular closure, resulting in tissue hypoxia and neovascularization, but the precise mechanisms are not fully understood. Glucose concentration, per se, is the critical risk factor in the pathogenesis of diabetic complications (Civan et al. 1994). Recently, those pathogenetic factors have been reported to be associated with the renin-angiotensin system and vascular endothelial growth factor, probably via nitric oxide (NO). NO may be associated with the onset and development of DR (Izumi et al. 2006). Moreover, increasing evidence suggests that the inducible nitric-oxide synthase (iNOS) is associated with DR (Leal et al. 2007; Toda and Nakanishi-Toda 2007).

The retinal pigment epithelium (RPE) is a monolayer of cells that lies in the back of the vertebrate eye and transports metabolites, ions, and fluid between the neural retina and the choroidal blood supply. RPE, which forms a blood–retinal barrier between the neural retina and choriocapillaris, plays an important role in maintaining ocular homeostasis. High glucose can injury the RPE, influence the retinal function and have important effect on the development of DR (Roufail et al. 1998). High glucose could inhibit RPE cells proliferation. RPE cells cultured with high glucose could enhance expression of iNOS of the cells in vitro, at least in part, by activation of p38 MAPK pathway which suggested that RPE cells under the effecting of high glucose might participate in the pathological reaction of diabetic retinopathy (Hong et al. 2007). iNOS isoform plays a predominant role in leukostasis and blood-retinal barrier breakdown in DR and its mechanism involves ICAM-1 upregulation and tight junction protein down regulation.

Citrus fruit holds a unique place in plant kingdom and occupies a resulting solitary position in the human diet. However, most people always throw away Pericarpium Citri Reticulatae, the rind of citrus, after enjoying this fruit, which is a huge waste. In fact there are many uses for Pericarpium Citri Reticulatae. It is important for the preparation of traditional Chinese herbal medicines and foods in China. For instance, it has been used in the treatment of indigestion, cough and detoxification in China for thousands of years. Now Pericarpium Citri Reticulatae is acknowledged in the People's Republic of China pharmacopoeia. The major components in Pericarpium Citri Reticulatae are flavonoids. Hesperidin (5,7,3′-trihydroxy-4′-methoxy-flavanone7-rhamnoglucoside) (Fig. 22.1), a flavanone-type flavonoid, is abundant in Pericarpium Citri Reticulatae and has been reported to exert a wide range of pharmacological effects (Tommasini et al. 2005). Hesperidin has a wide range of biological effects, such as inhibition of key enzymes in mitochondrial respiration, protection against coronary heart disease, and anti-spasmolytic, anti-inflammatory, antioxidative, vascular, estrogenic, cytotoxic antitumor, and antimicrobial activities (Luo and Li 2008). Hesperidin can improve venous tone, enhance microcirculation, assist healing of

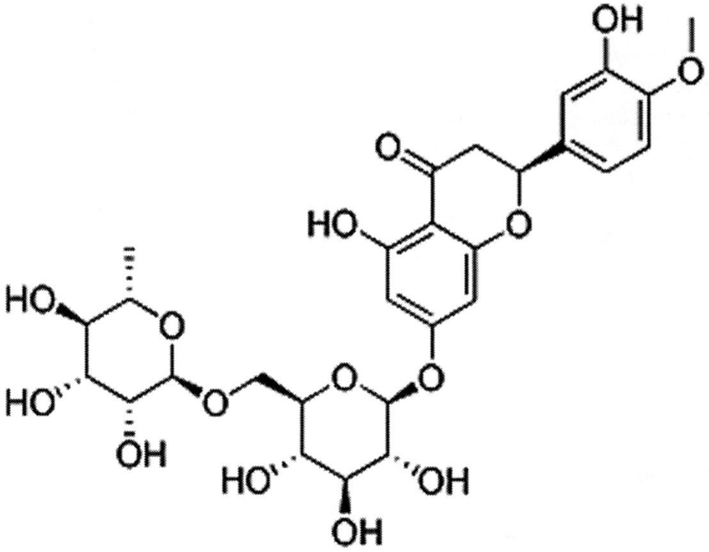

Fig. 22.1 Chemical structure of hesperidin isolated from Pericarpium Citri Reticulatae

venous ulcers and it is used for the treatment of chronic venous insufficiency, hemorrhoids and the prevention of postoperative thromboembolism (Kanaze et al. 2003).

We tested the hypothesis that hesperidin might affect development of DR through the regulation of NO or iNOS. To assess this, in this study, hesperidin was isolated from Pericarpium Citri Reticulatae of Newhall Citrus reticulata Blanco in order to explore the effect of hesperidin on expression of iNOS in cultured rabbit retinal pigment epithelial (RPE) cells under the condition of high glucose in vitro.

22.2 Materials and Methods

22.2.1 Preparing Hesperidin Extract of Pericarpium Citri Reticulatae

Pericarpium Citri Reticulatae was cut into pieces, dried at 30–40°C, and crushed into 1–2 mm particles by Chinese herbal medical pulverizer. The particles (100 mg) were weighted accurately and soaked by 500 ml distilled water for 30–45 min. After the particles absorbed water sufficiently, they were washed by distilled water to make them colorless and then filtered. They were carried out with 400 ml saturated calcareous water in the ultrasonic cleaning bath (Sonoc, PRC) which worked at

25 kHZ frequency at 25°C for 30 min. After that, the liquid was adjusted to pH 13.0 by 5 mol/L NaOH and removed of dregs of Pericarpium Citri Reticulatae through the vacuum filtration. The filtrate was neutralized into pH 4.5 by 1 mol/L. When the crystals were separated from the filtrate, the crystals were obtained by the filtration and changed into the crude hesperidin at 70°C by vacuum dehydration. The crude hesperidin was dissolved with 500 ml 50% ethanol containing 1% NaOH and filtered to remove the insoluble. The filtrate was shifted into pH 5.0 by 1 mol/L HCl in order to get the sediment. The sediment was washing by 50% ethanol and then by diluted water to approach the neutrality. Finally, the refined hesperidin was extracted after the sediment was arescent at 70°C by vacuum dehydration.

22.2.2 Identification of Hesperidin by High Performance Liquid Chromatogram (HPLC)

Identification of hesperidin was carried out on HPLC system (Agilent HP1100, USA), consisting of the G1311A pump and G1311A UV spectrophotometric detector. Data collection and integration were accomplished using a Chromato-Solution. The analytes were determined at room temperature on an analytical column (Hypersil C18, 4.6 × 250 mm, 5 μm). The mobile phase consisted of a mixture of acetonitrile, water, and methanol (20:79.6:0.4, v/v). The mobile phase was passed under vacuum through a 0.45 μm membrane filter and degassed before use. The analysis was carried out at a flow rate of 1.5 ml/min with the detection wavelength set at 283 nm.

22.2.3 Cell Culture

For the isolation of RPE cells, rabbit eyes were cut circumferentially through the sclera approximately 1 mm posterior to the ora serrata; after the vitreous was aspirated and the retina gently separated from the RPE cell layer, the eye cup was washed with Dulbecco's minimum essential medium (DMEM; Gibco, USA) and incubated at 37°C with 0.05% trypsin and 0.02% ethylenediaminetetraacetic acid (EDTA; Sigma, USA). After 1 h the trypsin solution was aspirated from the eye cup and replaced with DMEM supplemented with 20% fetal bovine serum (FBS; Sijiqing, PRC). The RPE cells, released by gentle pipetting, were transferred to a 75 cm^2 tissue culture flask containing DMEM supplemented with 20% FBS without antibiotics. The cells were cultured at 37°C in a humidified atmosphere of 5% CO$_2$ and 95% air; the medium was changed every 4 days thereafter. After 4–5 weeks, when the cells had reached confluence, they were passaged by trypsinization. The third to fifth passage cells were used for all experiments.

22.2.4 MTT Cell Viability Assay

Rabbit RPE cells were plated at a density of 5×10^4 cells/well in a 96 well plate to determine the protection of hesperidin. The cells were divided into 6 groups including the control group cultured in DMEM, the model group cultured in DMEM containing 33 mmol/L glucose without any drug and four experimental groups which were exposed to hesperidin at the concentration of 10, 20, 40 and 80 mg/L at 37°C under 5% CO_2 for 2 h and then cultured in DMEM containing 33 mmol/L glucose. After incubated cells in the presence of hesperidin for 48 h, viable cells were stained with MTT [3-(4, 5-dimethylthiazol-2-yl)-2, 5-diphenyl-tetrazolium bromide] (0.5 mg/ml) for 4 h. The medium was then removed and the formazan crystals produced were dissolved by adding dimethylsulfoxide (200 μl). The optical density (A value) at 490 nm was measured by the microplate reader (Thermo, USA).

22.2.5 Assay of NO Production

The levels of NO produced were monitored by determining nitrite levels in culture medium. This was performed by mixing medium with Griess reagent (1% sulfanilamide, 0.1% N-1-naphthylenediamine dihydrochloride, and 2.5% phosphoric acid). 100 μl of medium was collected at the indicated time points for the determination of nitrite level. Absorbance was measured at 540 nm after incubation for 10 min using the 721 spectrophotometer (Tuopu, PRC).

22.2.6 Cellular Immunohistochemistry of iNOS

The glutaraldehyde-fixed RPE cells were reduced with sodium borohydride (0–1%) for 10 min. They were incubated in 0.3% hydrogen peroxide (H_2O_2) in 90% methanol for 30 min to inactivate the endogenous peroxidase activity. After washing in 0.01 M PBS, sections were blocked for 4 h in 10% goat normal serum and then incubated in the primary antiserum for iNOS (1:500 dilution, rabbit polyclonal, Zhongshan Goldenbridge, PRC). The secondary antibody used was biotinylated goat anti-rabbit IgG (1:200 dilution, Zhongshan Goldenbridge, PRC) for 6 h at 4°C. The antigen-antibody complex was localized employing an avidin-biotin-peroxidase system (ABC kit, Zhongshan Goldenbridge, PRC) according to the manufacturer's instructions. Peroxidase staining was developed using 3,3′-diaminobenzidine tetrahydrochloride (0.06%) as chromogen, in 0.1 M acetate-imidazole buffer (pH 7.4) together with H_2O_2 (0.06%) and nickel sulphate (0.5%). To demonstrate the specificity of the antibody, negative control was incubated and processed similarly but with theomission of the primary antiserum. The results of iNOS expressed in RPE cells were present of integral optical density (IOD) using the semiquantitative analysis by computer image analytical system (Leica, Germany).

22.2.7 Statistical Analysis

Results are presented as mean ± SEM. The RPE cells viability (A value), NO level, IOD value of iNOS expressed in RPE cells were analyzed by one-way analysis of variance (ANOVA) using SPSS14.0 software. Difference was compared between the groups. When p <0.05, difference had remarkably statistical significance.

22.3 Results

22.3.1 Identification of Hesperidin by HPLC

The purity of hesperidin extracted from the Pericarpium Citri Reticulatae was 98.7% indentitified by HPLC.

22.3.2 RPE Cells Morphology

RPE cells in the control group were in the presence of applanation and polygon. Intracytoplasm of RPE cells had few pigment granules and the cell body was impellucidus. The RPE cells in the model group had multiple and irregular shapes. The cell body thinningzed in the model group compared with in the model group. Cellular shape of the RPE cells in the experimental groups was less obvious change than in the control group compared with in the model group.

22.3.3 Influence of Hesperin on RPE Cell Proliferation Under the Condition of High Glucose

As shown in Table 22.1, A value in the model group (0.284 ± 0.004) was markedly lower than in the control group (0.456 ± 0.007). It indicated that the treatment of RPE cells with 33 mmol/L glucose caused an obviously decrease of cellular viability. After pretreated with hesperidin, cell viability was elevated compared with the model group (p <0.0001). The growth rate of RPE cells was associated with the concentration of hesperidin.

22.3.4 Assay of NO and iNOS

To determine the NO-blocking effect of hesperidin, we monitored nitrite levels in culture media after stimulating cells with high glucose in the presence or absence of hesperidin for 24 h. Nitrite concentrations in medium were increased by high glucose compared with control cells (Table 22.1), and had remarkably statistical significance (p < 0.0001). This NO production induced by high glucose was significantly inhibited by hesperidin at 10–80 mg/L.

Table 22.1 The one-way ANOVA results of RPE cells viability (A), NO level, IOD value of iNOS expressed in RPE cells of each group ($\bar{x} \pm s$)

Groups	n	A Value	NO (μmol/L)	iNOS
Control	6	0.456 ± 0.007	11.36 ± 0.01	0.0742 ± 0.0008
Model	6	0.284 ± 0.004	29.35 ± 0.01	0.1936 ± 0.0010
Hesperidin (10 mg/L)	6	0.318 ± 0.001	21.34 ± 0.12	0.1177 ± 0.0018
Hesperidin (20 mg/L)	6	0.343 ± 0.003	19.46 ± 0.07	0.1057 ± 0.0022
Hesperidin (40 mg/L)	6	0.377 ± 0.004	16.56 ± 0.09	0.0926 ± 0.0009
Hesperidin (80 mg/L)	6	0.410 ± 0.003	14.56 ± 0.01	0.0810 ± 0.0005
F		205.2	5637	1038
p		<0.0001	<0.0001	<0.0001

To examine whether the blocking of NO production by hesperidin is mediated by the process of iNOS expression, iNOS protein levels were measured by immunohistochemistry. Hesperidin significantly inhibited high glucose induced iNOS protein in RPE cells (Table 22.1). These results suggest that iNOS is suppressed by hesperidin in high glucose activated RPE cells.

22.4 Discussion

NO is a free radical gas that is synthesized from l-arginine by three different isoforms of NO synthase (NOS). NO plays an important role in homeostatic vasodilatation and regulation of blood flow, but excess release induces tissue disorders because of increased oxidative stress, especially caused by the production of peroxynitrite. More and more physiological studies have indicated the involvement of NO in impulse transduction in the outer retina and in the modulation of visual signal during retinal information processing. The increased plasma NO levels in patients with type 2 diabetes indicate that NO may be associated with the pathogenesis of DR (Izumi et al. 2006). Ocular blood flow is regulated by NO derived from the endothelium and efferent nitrergic neurons. Endothelial dysfunction impairs ocular hemodynamics by reducing the bioavailability of NO and increasing the production of reactive oxygen species (ROS). On the other hand, NO formed by inducible NOS (iNOS) expressed under influences of inflammatory mediators evokes neurodegeneration and cell apoptosis, leading to serious ocular diseases (Toda and Nakanishi-Toda 2007). While not typically expressed in the central nervous system (CNS) under physiological conditions, iNOS is transcriptionally induced by various stimuli associated with pathologic insults including, hypoxia, bacterial components, viral proteins, and cytokines. Once expressed, iNOS catalyzes the nicotinamide adenine dinucleotide phosphate-dependent oxidation of L-arginine to nitric oxide (NO) and citrulline. Unlike other NOS isoforms, iNOS has continuously high and longlasting activity and, depending on the temporal expression and cellular context, can either be toxic or protective. Continued presence of NOS-immunoreactivity in the photoreceptors from 16–17 weeks of fetal life to adulthood indicates other functions besides their definitive involvement in the photoreceptor function of transduction and information processing (Shashi and Tapas 1999).

Retinopathy is one of the most severe ocular complications of diabetes and is a leading cause of acquired blindness in young adults. Sustained hyperglycemia plays a central role in the development of diabetic retinopathy; prolonged exposure of the cells to high glucose is shown to cause both acute and reversible changes in cellular metabolism, and long term irreversible changes in stable macromolecules (Madsen-Bouterse and Kowluru 2008).

Hesperidin is a kind of ubiquitous plant component and has a variety of biological effects. Moreover, it has also been reported that hesperidin reduced by around 10–30% the synthesis of NO by macrophages when inducible NO synthase was already expressed with LPS/IFN-gamma for 24 h (Rao et al. 2008). Sakata et al. (2003) indicated hesperidin as a COX-2 and iNOS inhibitor, might be related to the anti-inflammatory and anti-tumorigenic efficacies. Treatment with hesperidin suppressed production of PGE2, nitrogen dioxide (NO_2), and expression of iNOS protein (Sakata et al. 2003).

In this study, hesperidin was isolated from Pericarpium Citri Reticulatae of Newhall Citrus reticulata Blanco and its inhibitory activity on iNOS induction in RPE cells treated by high glucose was determined. MTT assay discovered that the cell viability in high glucose model group was obvious lower than in the normal control group and the difference had statistical significance, which indicated high glucose had resulted in the injury of RPE cells; however, the cell viability in the experimental groups, which had been pretreated by hesperidin, was higher than in the high glucose model group. It was found that hesperidin potently inhibits highglucose-inducible NO production by suppressing iNOS expression in RPE cells. It showed that the injury of RPE cells induced by high glucose might be associated with the activation of iNOS and mass production of NO. Further studies will have to elucidate the molecular mechanisms of protection of hesperidin on RPE cells.

References

Civan MM, Marano CW, Matschinsky FW et al (1994) Prolonged incubation with elevated glucose inhibits the regulatory response to shrinkage of cultured human retinal pigment epithelial cells. J Membr Biol 139(1):1–13

Hong J, Yuan Z, Shuai J et al (2007) High glucose induce production of iNOS by human retinal pigment epithelium cells through activation of the p38 signal pathway. Acta Universitatis Medicinalis Nanjing (Natural Science) 27(9):970–973

Izumi N, Nagaoka T, Mori F et al (2006) Relation between plasma nitric oxide levels and diabetic retinopathy. Jpn J Ophthalmol 50(5):465–468

Kanaze FI, Gabrieli C, Kokkalou E et al (2003) Simultaneous reversed-phase high-performance liquid chromatographic method for the determination of diosmin, hesperidin and naringin in different citrus fruit juices and pharmaceutical formulations. J Pharm Biomed Anal 33(2): 243–249

Leal EC, Manivannan A, Hosoya K et al (2007) Inducible nitric oxide synthase isoform is a key mediator of leukostasis and blood-retinal barrier breakdown in diabetic retinopathy. Invest Ophthalmol Vis Sci 48(11):5257–5265

Luo X, Li S (2008) Progress in Biologic Activity Effects of Hesperidin. J Gannan Med Univ 28(2):301–304

Madsen-Bouterse SA, Kowluru RA (2008) Oxidative stress and diabetic retinopathy: pathophysiological mechanisms and treatment perspectives. Rev Endocr Metab Disord 9(4): 315–327

Rao YK, Fang SH, Tzeng YM (2008) Antiinflammatory activities of flavonoids and a triterpene caffeate isolated from Bauhinia variegata. Phytother Res 22(7):957–962

Roufail E, Soulis T, Boel E et al (1998) Depletion of nitric oxide synthase-containing neurons in the diabetic retina: reversal by aminoguanidine. Diabetologia 41(12):1419–1425

Sakata K, Hirose Y, Qiao Z et al (2003) Inhibition of inducible isoforms of cyclooxygenase and nitric oxide synthase by flavonoid hesperidin in mouse macrophage cell line. Cancer Lett 199(2):139–145

Shashi W, Tapas CN (1999) Nitric oxide synthase immunoreactivity in the developing and adult human retina. J Biosci 24(4):483–490

Toda N, Nakanishi-Toda M (2007) Nitric oxide: ocular blood flow, glaucoma, and diabetic retinopathy. Prog Retin Eye Res 26(3):205–238

Tommasini S, Calabrò ML, Stancanelli R et al (2005) The inclusion complexes of hesperetin and its 7-rhamnoglucoside with (2-hydroxypropyl)-beta-cyclodextrin. J Pharm Biomed Anal 39 (3–4):572–580

Chapter 23
Profiling MicroRNAs Differentially Expressed in Rabbit Retina

Naihong Yan, Ke Ma, Jia Ma, Wei Chen, Yun Wang, Guiqun Cao,
Dominic Man-Kit Lam, and Xuyang Liu

Abstract MicroRNAs (miRNAs) are small non-coding RNAs, which regulate gene expression at the post-transcriptional level. Recent studies indicate that miRNAs may constitute a major mechanism underlying mammal's retinal development. The overall objective of this study is to compare and contrast retinal miRNAs expression between newborn and adult rabbits, and to identify some of the genes possibly associated with retinal development. Retinas were isolated from 3-day-old and 2-month-old rabbits. A miRNA microarray designed to detect 924 miRNAs was used to determine the expression profile of miRNAs from newborn and adult rabbits. The expression of twenty-eight miRNAs was found to differ significantly between newborn and adult rabbit retina. Among these, 17 appear to be up-regulated and the other 11 miRNAs down-regulated, suggesting a role of differential miRNA expression in retinal development. Computer prediction tools indicate that some of the target genes might be directly associated with signal pathways relevant to visual development.

23.1 Introduction

MicroRNAs (miRNAs) are an abundant class of non-coding RNAs (typically 19 ~ 23 nucleotides) playing an important role in regulation of post-transcriptional gene expression. The first discovered miRNA, lin-4, is involved in developmental timing in the nematode *Caenorhabditis elegans* (Lee et al. 1993). After that, thousands of miRNAs have since been identified in various organisms through random cloning and sequencing or computational prediction. Recent advances have led to a more detailed understanding of miRNA biogenesis and function. Primary miRNA transcripts are processed by the RNaseIII nuclease Drosha, into pre-miRNAs. The

X. Liu (✉)

Department of Ophthalmology, Torsten Wiesel Research Institute, West China Hospital, Sichuan University, Chengdu, China
e-mail: xliu1213@yahoo.com.cn

R.E. Anderson et al. (eds.), *Retinal Degenerative Diseases*, Advances in Experimental Medicine and Biology 664, DOI 10.1007/978-1-4419-1399-9_23, © Springer Science+Business Media, LLC 2010

pre-miRNAs are exported from the nucleus into the cytoplasm by Exportin-5 and further processed by Dicer to yield the mature forms (Lee et al. 2003; Yi et al. 2003). The 5'-seed region of a miRNA (the 5' end of miRNA with conserved 8mer and 7mer sites) interacts with the 3' untranslated region (3'-UTR) of a target mRNA by partial sequence complementarities, resulting in the degradation of the target mRNA and thus translational inhibition (Gregory et al. 2004). Many miRNAs are conserved and those may regulate up to 30% of gene expression (Lewis et al. 2005). In general, miRNAs are expressed in a highly tissue-specific manner and controlled major cellular processes, including metabolism, apoptosis, differentiation and development, but most of their biological functions remain unknown (Wienholds et al. 2005).

Recent studies showed that miRNAs have a major function in translational regulation of mammalian retinal development. Retina converts light into neural signals that can be relayed to the brain. It contains only seven cell types but performs very sophisticated visual signal processing. As a part of forebrain ectoderm, the retina regulates gene expression through intrinsic and extrinsic factors ensuring a tightly controlled temporal and spatial developmental sequence (Cepko et al. 1996). It is likely that miRNAs play important roles in the normal development and function of the retina. Xu et al. compared miRNA expression profiles among retina, brain, and heart by microarray analysis in adult mouse and found that 21 of 78 miRNAs expressed in adult mouse retina are potentially retina-specific (Xu et al. 2007). Ryan et al. isolated miRNAs specifically expressed in different ocular tissues including retina indicating that those miRNAs play a role in differentiation and development (Ryan et al. 2006). Arora et al. analysed six independent retinal microarray gene expression datasets and showed that many miRNAs capable of regulating genes important for retinal function are present in the retina. Conservation of miRNA expression patterns from rat to human retinas supports the evidence from other tissues that disruption of miRNAs might be a cause of certain visual abnormalities (Arora, McKay and Simpson 2007).

These studies greatly enhance our understanding of the role of miRNA expression in retinal development. However, to identify the entire set of miRNAs and their target genes from retinal tissues at different developing stages is also of momentously physiological and pathological significance to understand regulatory networks and molecular mechanism of retinal development. In this study, we analyzed the expression pattern of miRNAs in the rabbit retina at different development stages using miRNA microarray.

23.2 Materials and Methods

23.2.1 Rabbit Retina Tissues

Rabbits were obtained from the Experimental Animal Center of Sichuan University (Chengdu, China). Retinas were obtained from 3-day-old newborn rabbits (Marker I) and 6-month-old adult rabbits (Marked M). Each group consists of

3 individual samples. After euthanizing the rabbits with a sodium pentobarbital overdose, retinal tissues were collected and frozen in liquid nitrogen immediately. All studies were conducted in accordance with the ARVO Statement for the Use of Animals in Ophthalmic and Vision Research.

23.2.2 RNA Extraction

The frozen retinal tissues were ground to fine powder in a liquid nitrogen-cooled mortar, and the homogenized samples total RNA was extracted with Trizol reagent (Invitrogen, Carlsbad, CA, USA) according to manufacturer's protocol. RNA integrity was evaluated by 1% formaldehyde agarose gel electrophoresis.

23.2.3 miRNA Microarray Analysis

miRNAs were enriched from extracted total RNA using mirVana miRNA Isolation Kit (Ambion, Foster City, CA, USA) and labeled with mirVana Array Labeling Kit (Ambion). miRNA microarray assay was performed by CapitalBio Corporation (Beijing, China) based on Sanger miRNAs database miRBase 10.0 (http://microrna.sanger.ac.uk, August, 2007). The microarray contained 924 degenerated oligonucleotide probes from human, rat and mouse. The individual oligonucleotide probe was printed in triplicate on chemical modification glass slides and includes eight subarrays.

The miRNA microarray was double channel fluorescence chip; all oligonucleotide probes were labeled with Cy3 (green color) and Cy5 (red color) fluorescent dyes. Fluorescence scanning used a double-channel laser scanner (LuxScan 10 K/A, CapitalBio, Beijing, China). Then the figure signal was transformed to digital signal using image analysis software (LuxScan3.0, CapitalBio, Beijing, China). Labeled miRNAs were used for hybridization to determine differential expression between I and M samples, and the procedure was repeated with switched fluorescent labeling.

23.2.4 Data Analysis

Microarray data were normalized and analyzed using Significance Analysis of Microarrays software program (SAM, Stanford University, CA, USA). SAM identifies genes with statistically significant changes in expression by assimilating a set of gene-specific t-tests. Hierarchical clustering analysis of miRNA expression was performed using CLUSTER 3.0/TreeView software (Chiang et al. 2001).

23.2.5 Bioinformatics Analysis of the Selected Mirnas

Target genes were predicted using two target prediction programs: PicTar (http://pictar.bio.nyu.edu/) and TargetScan (http://www.targetscan.org/) and analyzed for their information and function using NCBI (http://www.ncbi.nlm.nih.gov/)

and UCSC (http://genome.ucsc.edu/) database (Lall et al. 2006; Lewis et al. 2003). Genes directly correlated with retinal development were selected for analysis.

23.3 Results and Discussion

23.3.1 miRNA Microarray Analysis

Microarray assay provides a powerful tool for analyzing both miRNA expression patterns and quantitative expression levels, the fluorescence scanning map was shown in Fig. 23.1. Class comparison and SAM were performed to identify differences in miRNA expression of retinal tissues. Twenty-eight miRNAs were detected as differential expression between newborn and adult rabbit retina. Among these, 17 appear to be up-regulated and the other 11 miRNAs down-regulated, suggesting that these miRNAs might play a role in retinal development (Table 23.1).

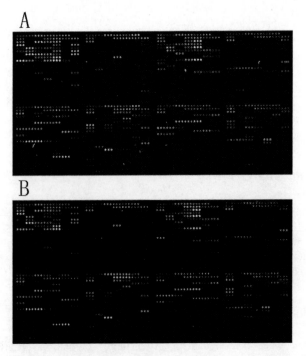

Fig. 23.1 Fluorescence scanning map of miRNA microarray. **a**: pseudocolor image I Cy3, pseudocolor image M Cy5; **b**: pseudocolor image I Cy5; D: pseudocolor image M Cy3

Table 23.1 miRNAs microarray SAM results of I and M samples

Up-regulated miRNA	Newborn/adult	Down-regulated miRNA	Newborn/adult
hsa-miR-18a	4.1486	hsa-miR-30c	−3.9409
hsa-miR-130b	5.8852	hsa-miR-125b	−5.6260
hsa-miR-20a	12.9398	hsa-miR-204	−4.0983
mmu-miR-34b-5p	10.1031	hsa-miR-192	−4.6176
hsa-miR-216a	8.0302	hsa-miR-185	−3.7080
hsa-miR-20b	6.9742	hsa-miR-29a	−4.7579
hsa-miR-17	6.7509	hsa-miR-22	−4.5589
hsa-miR-18b	14.4449	hsa-miR-29c	−3.3060
hsa-miR-106a	8.1018	hsa-miR-422a	−16.4091
hsa-miR-19a	5.5511	hsa-miR-29b	−5.1833
hsa-miR-106b	5.4884	hsa-miR-129-3p	−6.8226
hsa-miR-93	5.1490		
hsa-miR-15b	3.8734		
hsa-miR-19b	4.5873		
hsa-miR-16	6.3309		
hsa-miR-92b	9.5928		
hsa-miR-181c	5.6769		

23.3.2 Putative miRNA Target Gene Prediction

PicTar and TargetScan 4.0 prediction programs were used to predict changes in the miRNAs, and the putative targets related to miRNA were screened using the UCSC and NCBI databases. Our studies shown that some screened genes appear to be directly correlated with retinal development, and might be involve in signal pathways for cell growth, apoptosis, transcription factor binding, enzyme activator activity, cell proliferation, regulation of cell cycle, neurogenesis, or cell cycle. Some of the target genes might also be directly associated with signal pathways relevant to visual development including sensory perception of light, visual perception, Hs_GPCRDB_Class_A_Rhodopsin-like (Human G-Protein Coupled Receptors DataBase Class A Rhodopsin-like) and rhodopsin-like receptor activity, etc (Table 23.2).

For this study, we chose the rabbit retina because it is amenable to pre- and post-natal manipulation and because the developments of many neuron-specific properties have been investigated using this retina as a model system (Lam et al. 1980; Fung et al. 1982; Lam 1987). By comparing the miRNA expression profile in newborn and adult-rabbit retina using miRNA array technology, we have identified a number of putative miRNA and target genes that might contribute to retinal development and maturation. Further investigations, including miRNA analyses at different developmental stages and comparison with other relevant studies might shed light on the molecular mechanisms regulating neural development.

Table 23.2 Signals pathways relevant to visual development, miRNAs and predicted target genes

Putative pathway	miRNA	Putative gene
Sensory perception of light	hsa-miR-20a;hsa-miR-106a;hsa-miR-29c hsa-miR-106b;hsa-miR-20b;hsa-miR-18a hsa-miR-22;hsa-miR-18b	VSX1, PHYH, PROM1, FBN1 PRPF3, COL11A1, ABCA4, VAX2, GUCA1A, CDS1
Visual perception	hsa-miR-422a, hsa-miR-29a;hsa-miR-29c hsa-miR-22;hsa-miR-18a;hsa-miR-18b hsa-miR-106b;hsa-miR-20b;hsa-miR-19a	PPEF2, VSX1, PHYH, PROM1 EML2, BBS2, GUCA1A, CDS1 FBN1, PRPF3, GNAT1
Hs_GPCRDB_Class_A_ Rhodopsin-like activity	hsa-miR-29a;hsa-miR-29c;hsa-miR-18a hsa-miR-18b;hsa-miR-22;hsa-miR-20a hsa-miR-106a;hsa-miR-106b	PRLHR, GPR161, CMKOR1, OR10H1, MTNR1A, ADRB2, HRH2, NPFFR2, GPR37
Rhodopsin-like receptor activity	hsa-miR-93hsa-miR-20a;hsa-miR-106a hsa-miR-29a;hsa-miR-29chsa-miR-18a hsa-miR-106b;hsa-miR-20b;hsa-miR-18b	GPR146, PRLHR, GPR161, CMKOR1, OPRL1, HRH1, UTS2R, HTR2C, ADRB2

References

Arora A, McKay GJ, Simpson DAC (2007) Prediction and verification of miRNA expression in human and rat retinas. Invest Ophthalmol Vis Sci 48:3962–3967

Cepko CL, Austin CP, Yang X et al (1996) Cell fate determination in the vertebrate retina. Proc Natl Acad Sci 93:589–595

Chiang DY, Brown PO, Eisen MB (2001) Visualizing associations between genome sequences and gene expression data using genome-mean expression profiles. Bioinformatics 17:49–55

Fung SC, Kong YC, Lam DMK (1982) Prenatal development of GABAergic, glycinergic and dopaminergic neurons in the rabbit retina. J Neuroscience 2:1623–1632

Gregory RI, Yan KP, Amuthan G et al (2004) The Microprocessor complex mediates the genesis of microRNAs. Nature 432:235–240

Lall S, Grün D, Krek A et al (2006) A genome-wide map of conserved microRNA targets in C. elegans. Curr Biol 16:460–471

Lam DMK (1987) Development of neurotransmitter systems in the retina: biochemical, anatomical, and physiological correlates. In: Tso MO (ed) Retinal diseases. Lippincott Co, Philadelphia, pp 103–120

Lam DMK, Fung SC, Kong YC (1980) Post-natal development of GABAergic neurons in the rabbit retina. J Comp Neurol 193:89–102

Lee Y, Ahn C, Han J et al (2003) The nuclear RNase III Drosha initiates microRNA processing. Nature 425:415–419

Lee RC, Feinbaum RL, Ambros V (1993) The C. elegans heterochronic gene lin-4 encodes small RNAs with antisense complementarity to lin-14. Cell 75:843–854

Lewis BP, Burge CB, Bartel DP (2005) Conserved seed pairing, often flanked by adenosines, indicates that thousands of human genes are microRNA targets. Cell 120:15−20

Lewis BP, Shih I H, Jones-Rhoades MW et al (2003) Prediction of mammalian microRNA targets. Cell 115:787−798

Ryan DG, Oliveira-Fernandes M, Lavker RM (2006) MicroRNAs of the mammalian eye display distinct and overlapping tissue specificity. Mol Vis 12:1175−1184

Wienholds E, Kloosterman WP, Miska E et al (2005) MicroRNA expression in zebrafish embryonic development. Science 309:310−311

Xu S, Witmer PD, Lumayag S et al (2007) MicroRNA (miRNA) transcriptome of mouse retina and identification of a sensory organ-specific miRNA cluster. J Biol Chem 282:25053−25066

Yi R, Qin Y, Macara IG et al (2003) Exportin-5 mediates the nuclear export of pre-microRNAs and short hairpin RNAs. Genes Dev 17:3011−3016

Chapter 24
Unexpected Transcriptional Activity of the Human *VMD2* Promoter in Retinal Development

Meili Zhu, Lixin Zheng, Yumi Ueki, John D. Ash, and Yun-Zheng Le

Abstract Vitelliform macular dystrophy (VMD) is associated with mutations in the *VMD2* gene, which encodes a chloride channel protein and is thought to be preferentially expressed in the retinal pigmented epithelium (RPE). In an effort to establish an inducible gene knockout system for the RPE, we recently used a 3.0-kb human *VMD2* promoter to direct the expression of a reverse tetracycline-inducible system controlled Cre recombinase in transgenic mice. Although Cre function was localized to the RPE in most *VMD2-cre* mouse lines, Cre activity was also identified in neural retina in approximately half of the transgenic lines. In two *VMD2-cre* mouse lines, Cre activity was predominately localized to retinal Müller cells. This surprising expression pattern is likely caused by the transcriptional activity of our transgene system during retinal development. Therefore, our results suggest that transcription of *VMD2* gene may occur in progenitors of Müller cells. The two *VMD2-cre* mouse lines that demonstrated Cre activity specifically in the RPE or predominantly in the Müller cells were fully characterized. These *VMD2-cre* mice are potentially useful for dissecting cellular mechanisms of age-related macular degeneration or diabetic retinopathy, two leading causes of blindness with high relevance to gene expression in the RPE or Müller cells.

24.1 Introduction

Vitelliform macular dystrophy (VMD), also called Best disease, is associated with mutations in the *VMD2* gene, which encodes a chloride channel protein and is thought to be preferentially expressed in the retinal pigmented epithelium (RPE) (Marquardt et al. 1998; Petrukhin et al. 1998; Tsunenari et al. 2003). In an effort to establish an inducible gene knockout system for the RPE, we recently used a 3.0-kb

Y.-Z. Le (✉)
Departments of Medicine, Cell Biology and Ophthalmology; Harold Hamm Oklahoma Diabetes Center; Dean A. McGee Eye Institute, University of Oklahoma Health Sciences Center, Oklahoma, OK 73104, USA
e-mail: yun-le@ouhsc.edu

R.E. Anderson et al. (eds.), *Retinal Degenerative Diseases*, Advances in Experimental Medicine and Biology 664, DOI 10.1007/978-1-4419-1399-9_24,
© Springer Science+Business Media, LLC 2010

human *VMD2* promoter to direct the expression of a reverse tetracycline-inducible system controlled Cre recombinase in transgenic mice. However, functional analysis of these transgenic mice demonstrated that Cre activity was not exclusively present in the RPE. In addition to the RPE, Cre function was also identified in other retinal cells, including Müller cells. In this report we summarize the expression pattern of two *VMD2-cre* mouse lines that demonstrated Cre activity specifically in the RPE or predominantly in the Müller cells.

24.2 Materials and Methods

24.2.1 Experiment with Animals

Transgenic mice were generated as described previously (Le et al. 2008). All animal procedures were performed according to the guidelines of the ARVO statement for the 'Use of Animals in Ophthalmic and Vision Research' and were approved by the Institutional Animal Care and Use Committees at the University of Oklahoma Health Sciences Center, the Dean A. McGee Eye Institute, and the Oklahoma Medical Research Foundation. PCR analysis diagnostic for *cre*, *rtTA* and Cre-activatable *lacZ* genes was carried out, as described previously (Le et al. 2008). Doxycycline was administered through the drinking water of pregnant mothers at a concentration of 0.5 mg/mL in 5% sucrose.

24.2.2 β-Galactosidase Assay

β-Galactosidase assay was carried out using cryprotected retinal sections. Briefly, eyes were fixed in 2% paraformaldehyde and 0.25% glutaraldehyde in phosphate-buffered saline (PBS) at 4°C for 1 h. The lens was then removed and the posterior part of the eye was cryoprotected in 30% sucrose, frozen in OCT medium, and sectioned. Retinal sections (10 μm) were briefly fixed in 0.5% glutaraldehyde for 5 min, washed with PBS 3 times, and incubated in X-gal (5-bromo-4-chloro-3-indolyl-β-D-galactoside) staining solution (1 mg/ml X-gal, 6 mM potassium ferricyanide, 6 mM potassium ferrocyanide, 2 mM MgCl2, 0.02% NP-40, and 0.01% sodium deoxycholate in 1X PBS) at room temperature for 3–12 h, depending on experimental requirements. Sections were then cover-slipped and observed under a microscope.

24.3 Results

24.3.1 Generation of Transgenic Mice

Human *VMD2* gene is thought to be expressed preferentially in the RPE (Marquardt et al. 1998; Petrukhin et al. 1998) and has been used to direct transgene expression in the RPE (Esumi et al. 2004). To generate tetracycline-inducible RPE-specific Cre mice (Le et al. 2008), we used a 3.0-kb human *VMD2* promoter to direct the expression of the tetracycline inducible transactivator *rtTA*, which in turn, should drive the expression of the tetracycline-responsive element (*TRE*) controlled *cre* gene in the presence of doxycycline. The *VMD2-cre* transgenic mice were generated by co-injection of linearized and purified *VMD2-rtTA* and *TRE-cre* DNA (see Le et al. for detail 2008). Analyzing segregation patterns of all transgenic founders and their progenies by PCR indicated that both transgenes were co-integrated to a single chromosome in all transgenic animals (data not shown). All germline-transmitted mice were normal in size, morphology, and behavior, and were characterized further.

24.3.2 Localization of Cre Function in Transgenic Mice

To localize Cre expression, all *cre*-positive mice were bred with *R26R* mice. *R26R* mice were genetically modified so that *lacZ* gene could be activated after Cre-mediated excision of a *loxP*-flanked transcriptional 'STOP' DNA segment (Soriano 1999). β-Galactosidase staining from double transgenic F1 *VMD2-cre/R26R* mice was used to localize Cre activity. Of the ten *VMD2-cre* transgenic lines identified in our initial screening for Cre function, four lines were selected for further characterization, based on the levels and locations of Cre expression. Two lines demonstrated homogeneous Cre activity in the RPE. Figure 24.1b, d shows Cre activated β-galactosidase reporter was expressed in the RPE of a *VMD2-cre* transgenic line (Le et al. 2008). Two lines demonstrated predominant Cre activity in Müller cells. Figure 24.1a, c shows Cre-activated β-galactosidase reporter was expressed in the Müller cells of another *VMD2-cre* mouse line (Ueki et al. 2009).

The transgenic line with Cre activity in Müller cells (Fig. 24.1c) also demonstrated some Cre activity in photoreceptor inner segment and what appeared to be bipolar and horizontal cells (Ueki et al. 2009). However, we were not able to detect Cre protein with Western blot and immunohistochemistry. To determine the initiation of Cre activity, this line of *VMD2-cre* mice were bred with floxed *gp130* (*gp130^{ff}*) mice (Betz et al. 1998). In *VMD2-cre+/gp130^{ff}* mice, Cre-mediated recombination occurred as early as embryonic day 15 (Fig. 24.2). Therefore, it is most likely that Cre was expressed through a brief transcription from the *VMD2* promoter during embryonic development in retinal progenitor cells. The efficiency of Cre-mediated recombination at *gp130* locus was 52% in Müller cells in this transgenic line (Ueki et al. 2009), a reasonable frequency for cell-specific gene knockout studies. Despite our efforts to generate mice with inducible Cre expression, this mouse line demonstrated limited inducibility in respect to Cre expression.

24.4 Discussion

In this study, we used a 3.0-kb human *VMD2* promoter to direct tetracycline-inducible system controlled Cre expression in transgenic mice. Most transgenic lines demonstrated Cre function in the RPE. The fact that approximately half of the

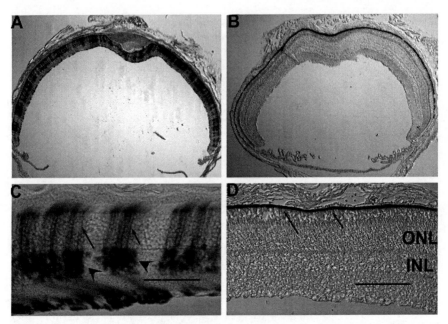

Fig. 24.1 Localization and functional analysis of Cre expression with β-galactosidase staining in F1 double transgenic *VMD2-cre/R26R mice*. **a, c**: Representative result of β-galactosidase staining (*dark staining*) in retinal sections of a *VMD2-cre* mouse line showing identifiable staining in retinal Müller cells (*Arrows* in **c**) and unidentifiable staining in neurons in inner nuclear layer (*arrowheads*). **b, d**: Representative result of β-galactosidase staining in the RPE (*arrows* in **d**) of a *VMD2-cre* mouse line. Scale bar equals to 100 μm. Outer nuclear layer (ONL) and inner nuclear layer (INL) are labeled. Cre function was localized to photoreceptor inner segment, Müller cells, and unknown INL neurons in one *VMD2-cre* mouse line (**a, c**) and the RPE in another *VMD2-cre* mouse line (**b, d**)

transgenic lines demonstrated Cre activated reporter expression in retinal Müller cells (data not shown) suggest that this unanticipated Cre expression is likely an intrinsic characteristic of the *VMD2* promoter. However, more studies are needed to confirm this point. As the 3.0-kb *VMD2* promoter used in this study may not contain all control elements necessary for identical expression patterns of the endogenous gene and genetic elements in our two gene system may affect transcription, we can not completely rule out that the unanticipated Cre function in Müller cells may be caused by the interaction between the tetracycline-inducible gene expression system and the *VMD2* promoter during transcription. Although Esumi et al. demonstrated that a 585-bp *VMD2* promoter was capable of targeting β-galactosidase reporter expression to the RPE exclusively in transgenic mice (Esumi et al. 2004), we need to point out that there is a fundamental difference between a *VMD2* promoter directly controlled reporter expression and our study. In their study, the β-galactosidase activity reflects the cellular location of constitutive *VMD2* promoter activity and any transient activity during embryonic development may not be detected in the assay. Since Cre-mediated excision is usually permanent in vivo, a transient Cre

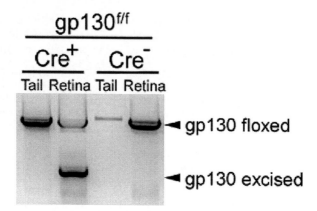

Fig. 24.2 PCR analysis of Cre-mediated recombination in the retina of a *VMD2-cre* +/*gp130*^ff^ mouse using retinal and tail DNA. A *VMD2-cre* −/*gp130*^ff^ mouse was used as a control. By embryonic day 15, Cre function was detected in the retina of *VMD2-cre* +/*gp130*^ff^ mice

expression at any developmental stage will permit the expression of Cre-activated β-galactosidase reporter permanently, under the control of a generalized promoter (*ROSA26*) (Fig. 24.1). Therefore, the effect of transient *VMD2* promoter activity is likely 'amplified' in our study. As Cre-mediated recombination was detectable in the retina at embryonic day 15 in cells that ultimately became Müller cells (Ueki et al. 2009), it is reasonable to conclude that *VMD2* promoter is transcriptionally active in progenitors of Müller cells. Due to a lack of information about the expression pattern of β-galactosidase reporter under the direct control of 3.0-kb *VMD2* promoter in transgenic mice, we are not in a position to conclude if the 3.0-kb *VMD2* promoter confers transcriptional activity outside the RPE. Since we were not able to detect Cre expression in postnatal retina by Western blots or immunohistochemistry, it is very unlikely that the 3.0-kb *VMD2* promoter is active in mature Müller cells. At this time, it is unclear if the *VMD2* protein is made in non-RPE lineage during development. If so, the physiological significance of *VMD2* protein in these cells remains to be determined. Nevertheless, our study indicates a possibility that transcription of *VMD2* gene occurs in non-RPE lineage during retinal development.

In summary, we use the *VMD2* promoter to generate inducible RPE-specific Cre mice for conditional gene activation and inactivation. In the process, we obtained transgenic mouse line with additional utility, i.e. transgenic mice expressing Cre in Müller cells with a reasonable efficiency (Ueki et al. 2009). Since the retinal integrity is essential to the usefulness of retinal cell-specific *cre* mice, classical parameters used in characterizing this type of mice (Le et al. 2004; Le et al. 2006), we also investigated the retinal integrity of the two *VMD2-cre* mouse lines (discussed here) for up to 10 months. We did not detect any abnormality in the retinal integrity in these mice, as documented in our original descriptions (Le et al. 2008; Ueki et al. 2009). The 10-month window provides crucial time required for most conditional gene knockout studies. Therefore, these two *VMD2-cre* mouse lines will be useful tools for dissecting cellular mechanisms of retinal diseases, particularly for age-related macular degeneration and diabetic retinopathy, two leading causes of blindness with high relevance to gene expression in the RPE and Müller cells.

Acknowledgments We thank W. Zheng and Y. W. Le for technical assistance and Drs. N. Esumi and D. Zack for providing human *VMD2* promoter DNA. This study was supported by NIH grants RR17703, EY16459, and EY12190, ADA grant 1-06-RA-76, AHAF grant M2008-059, FFB grant BR-CMM-0808-0453-UOK and unrestricted grants from Hope for Vision and Research to Prevent Blindness.

References

Betz UA, Bloch W, van den Broek M et al (1998) Postnatally induced inactivation of gp130 in mice results in neurological, cardiac, hematopoietic, immunological, hepatic, and pulmonary defects. J Exp Med 188:1955–1965

Esumi N, Oshima Y, Li Y et al (2004) Analysis of the VMD2 promoter and implication of E-box binding factors in its regulation. J Biol Chem 279:19064–19073

Le Y, Ash JD, Al-Ubaidi MR et al (2004) Targeted expression of Cre recombinase to cone photoreceptors in transgenic mice. Mol Vis 10:1011–1018

Le YZ, Zheng W, Rao PC et al (2008) Inducible expression of cre recombinase in the retinal pigmented epithelium. Invest Ophthalmol Vis Sci 49:1248–1253

Le Y, Zheng L, Zheng W et al (2006) Mouse opsin promoter controlled expression of Cre recombinase in transgenic mice. Mol Vis 12:389–398

Marquardt A, Stohr H, Passmore LA et al (1998) Mutations in a novel gene, VMD2, encoding a protein of unknown properties cause juvenile-onset vitelliform macular dystrophy (Best's disease). Hum Mol Genet 7:1517–1525

Petrukhin K, Koisti MJ, Bakall B et al (1998) Identification of the gene responsible for best macular dystrophy. Nat Genet 19:241–247

Soriano P (1999) Generalized lacZ expression with the ROSA26 Cre reporter strain. Nat Genet 21:70–71

Tsunenari T, Sun H, Williams J et al (2003) Structure-function analysis of the bestrophin family of anion channels. J Biol Chem 278:41114–41125

Ueki Y, Ash JD, Zhu M, Zheng L, Le Y-Z (2009) Expression of Cre recombinase in the retinal Müller cells. Vis Res 49:615–621

Chapter 25
Microarray Analysis of Hyperoxia Stressed Mouse Retina: Differential Gene Expression in the Inferior and Superior Region

Yuan Zhu, Riccardo Natoli, Krisztina Valter, and Jonathan Stone

Abstract

Aim: Hyperoxia-induced photoreceptor degeneration occurs preferentially in the inferior retina of C57BL/6J mice. This study investigates differential gene expression in the inferior and superior retina of C57BL/6J mouse, before and after hyperoxic stress.

Methods: At the age of P (postnatal day) 83–90, mice were placed in constant normoxia or hyperoxia (75% O_2) for 2 weeks. Retinas from control and exposed mice were removed and RNA was extracted from superior and inferior regions. The RNA from 2 animals (1 male and 1 female) at each condition was extracted, purified and hybridized to an Affymetrix MouseGene 1.0 ST Array to elucidate gene expression. Experiments were run in triplicate and analysis of the expression patterns was performed using GeneSpring and Partek Genomics Suite softwares.

Results: Over 400 genes showed significant differential expression by location and treatment using 2-way ANOVA analysis. In the control material, no genes showed a differential expression greater than twofold between inferior and superior retina. After hyperoxic stress, 154 genes in the inferior and 30 genes in the superior retina showed a greater than twofold change in expression. Among those, genes such as *Edn2*, *GFAP*, *Bcl3* and *C1qb* showed expression differences of greater than three fold between inferior and superior retina. Real time PCR was used to verify gene expression of control genes as well as genes of interest.

Conclusion: These microarray data may provide clues for identifying previously unknown factors and pathways responsible for the vulnerability of inferior retina to hyperoxic stress and for the eventual identification of therapeutic targets.

Y. Zhu (✉)
School of Biology and ARC Centre of Excellence in Vision Science, The Australian National University, RSBS, Bldg 46, Biology Place, Canberra, ACT2601, Australia
e-mail: yuan.zhu@anu.edu.au

R.E. Anderson et al. (eds.), *Retinal Degenerative Diseases*, Advances in Experimental Medicine and Biology 664, DOI 10.1007/978-1-4419-1399-9_25,
© Springer Science+Business Media, LLC 2010

25.1 Introduction

Hyperoxia has been shown to be specifically toxic to photoreceptors in the retina of the rabbit and rodents (Noell 1955; Yamada et al. 1999; Yamada et al. 2001; Walsh et al. 2004; Geller et al. 2006; Natoli et al. 2008a, Natoli et al. 2008b), and may be an important factor in the later stages of photoreceptor degenerations, as the photoreceptor population is depleted (Stone et al. 1999). This study investigates a regional variation in the susceptibility of the mouse to hyperoxia, in which photoreceptor degeneration reliably begins in retina close to (0.5 mm from) and inferior to the optic disc (Smit-McBride et al. 2007; Natoli et al. 2008a). The source of this regional variation is not known, although factors such as rhodopsin content and oxygen delivery have been discussed (Rapp and Williams 1977; Chung et al. 1999). In a recent study, we have examined global changes in gene expression induced in the C57BL/6 J mouse retina by hyperoxic exposure for up to 14d (Natoli et al. 2008b). Here we have examined differences in gene expression between inferior and superior retina of C57BL/6 J mouse, before and after hyperoxic exposure.

25.2 Methods

C57BL/6 J mice, a hyperoxia-vulnerable strain, were raised in dim cyclic illumination (12 h 5 lux, 12 h dark) and maintained in this level of lighting during the experiment. At the age of P (postnatal day) 83–90, some mice were exposed to constant hyperoxia (75% O_2) for 14 days. The mice were housed, with free access to food and water, in plexiglass chambers in which the oxygen level was controlled by a feedback device (OXYCYCLER, Reming Bioinstruments, NY).

Retinas from control (normoxic) and hyperoxia-challenged mice were removed and divided into superior and inferior halves, and RNA was extracted. The RNA from 2 animals (1 male and 1 female) at each condition was pooled, purified and hybridized to an Affymetrix GeneChip® Mouse Gene 1.0 ST Array. This array is comprised of more than 750,000 unique oligonucleotide features constituting more than 28,000 genes. Labelling, hybridization and scanning of the microarray were performed at the ACRF Biomolecular Resource Facility at the John Curtin School of Medical Research, Australian National University.

Experiments were run in duplicate and analysis of the expression patterns was performed using GeneSpring (Agilent Technologies, Santa Clara, CA) and Partek Genomics Suite (Partek Inc., St. Louis, MO) software. Analyses of gene ontology and molecular pathways were performed using Ingenuity Pathway Analysis (Ingenuity® Systems, www.ingenuity.com) for the most highly variable genes in inferior and superior retina after hyperoxia.

Quantitative PCR (qPCR) was used to validate the expression changes of nine genes identified in the microarray experiment. Three biologic groups were used and RNA extraction was carried out as for microarray experiments. Taqman® probes were obtained (Applied Biosystems, Foster City, CA) and qPCR performed on a Rotor-Gene 3,000 (Corbett Robotics, Mortlake, NSW, Australia). *GAPDH* was included as a reference gene and cycle threshold means were used to calculate fold change using the Pfaffl Equation (Pfaffl, 2001).

25.3 Result

The array quality was assessed by pseudocolour imaging and a sample graph of probe intensities (Fig. 25.1). All eight samples showed consistent pattern of labelling and distribution, indicating that there were no major hybridization defects.

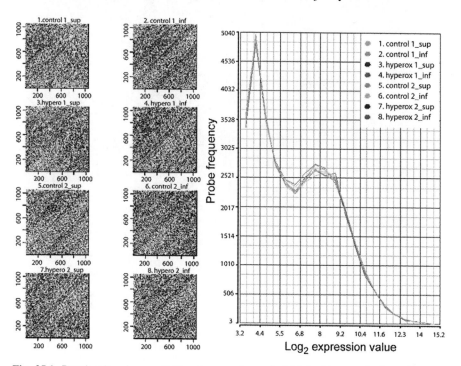

Fig. 25.1 Pseudocolour images (*left*) and a sample graph (*right*) of $\log_2$ probe intensities for each of the 8 samples. Each pseudocolour image (shown here in *black* and *white*) was created from the logged CEL file data to display signal intensities for the whole of the microarray. The graph provides another comparison of the distributions of gene expression as a function of fold change. The pseudocolour images were examined at high resolution (not illustrated), for evidence of discontinuities in hybridisation. These diagrams indicate that there were no major technical flaws in any of the 8 hybridizations involved

Hierarchical clustering was performed using the heat map function in Partek Genomics Suite (Fig. 25.2). The replicates of one group should cluster more closely to each other, than to other samples. The analysis showed strong replicate clustering for three groups (1 with 5; 3 with 7; 4 with 8) but not sample 2 with sample 6. The distance between these two samples suggest some biological variability of

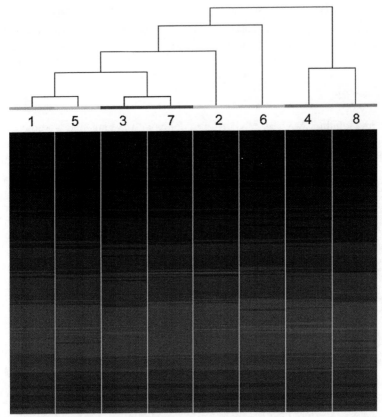

1.Control Sup #1; 2. Control Inf #1; 3. Hyperoxia Sup #1; 4. Hyperoxia Inf #1;
5.Control Sup #2; 6. Control Inf #2; 7. Hyperoxia Sup #2; 8. Hyperoxia Inf #2.

Fig. 25.2 Hierarchical clustering diagram of genes (rows) and samples (columns). The genes are organised vertically in each sample by the level of their expression, with lowest expression genes at the *top* of the column and highest expression genes at the *bottom*. The columns are clustered according to the similarity of expression of individual genes. Samples 1 and 5 are replicates of superior regions of control retinas; samples 2 and 6 are replicates of inferior regions of control retinas; samples 3 and 7 are replicates of superior regions of hyperoxia-exposed retinas; samples 4 and 8 are replicates of inferior regions of hyperoxia-exposed retinas

gene expression in inferior control retina. Overall, superior retina samples prior to and after hyperoxia clustered more closely to each other than to other groups. Gene expression in the inferior retina diverged from superior retina, with hyperoxia increasing the separation.

Data were then analysed by two-way ANOVA (analysis of variance) using a 2 fold change as the criterion for significant differences (increases and decreases) in expression (Table 25.1). There are significantly more genes differentially expressed in the inferior than superior retina (e.g. 392 genes changed significantly in the superior retina while 849 genes changed in the inferior at $p \leq 0.01$). When the criteria

Table 25.1 Numbers of genes changing expression with hyperoxia, in superior and inferior retina, assessed with different levels of probability

	Gene expression change after hyperoxia	
	Superior	Inferior
p-value ≤0.01	392	849
p-value ≤0.001	40	142
p-value ≤0.05, >2 fold	30 (19 ↑+ 11↓)	154 (69 ↑+ 85 ↓)
p-value ≤0.01, >2 fold	14 (10 ↑+ 4 ↓)	78 (63 ↑+ 15 ↓)

↑, up-regulation, ↓ down-regulation

combined the p-value ≤ 0.01 with fold change > 2, the number of genes differentially expressed was 5.5 times greater in the inferior than in the superior retina (78 vs 14). The genes showing the largest fold difference between inferior and superior retina after hyperoxia include *Edn2* (endothelin 2), *C1qb* (complement component 1, q subcomponent, beta polypeptide), *Gfap* (glial fibrillary acidic protein) and *Bcl-3* (B-cell leukemia/lymphoma 3).

Expression changes of 9 genes chosen using the combined criteria of p-value ≤ 0.01 with fold change > 2 were tested by qPCR, to verify changes found in the gene array, including *Edn2*, *Gfap*, *Bcl-3*, nuclear receptor subfamily 2, group E, member 3 (*Nr2e3*), wingless-related MMTV integration site 8A (*Wnt8a*), cyclic nucleotide gated channel alpha 2 (*Cnga2*), exportin 6 (*Xpo6*), medium-wave-sensitive cone opsin 1 (*Opn1mw*) and hypoxia inducible factor 1, alpha subunit (*Hif1a*). With the exception of *Xpo6*, the regulation changes of all these genes were confirmed by qPCR (Table 25.2).

Table 25.2 Validation of microarray data using quantitative PCR

Gene	Fold change of signal microarray		Fold change of signal qPCR		Validate	
	Sup	Inf	Sup	Inf	Sup	Inf
Edn2	1.714	8.411	6.041	17.336	Yes	Yes
Gfap	2.596	6.347	4.977	9.434	Yes	Yes
Bcl3	1.47	4.716	7.717	22.299	Yes	Yes
Nr2e3	1.049	−1.193	1.623	−1.005	Yes	Yes
Wnt8a	1.039	−1.159	1.459	−1.195	Yes	Yes
Cnga2	1.096	−1.044	1.338	−1.129	Yes	Yes
Xpo6	1.022	−1.071	−1.185	1.208	No	No
L-M opsin	1.098	1.092	1.327	1.496	Yes	Yes
Hif1a	−1.012	1.001	1.445	1.493	No	Yes

The results of quantitative PCR were from three independent experiments; Sup, superior; Inf, inferior

Ingenuity Pathway Analysis was used to characterize functional groups of genes of interest. Using the combined criteria above, 317 genes were selected for pathway analysis. From these, 266 genes were modelled into identified mechanisms, functions, and pathways of relevance. The strongest associated functional networks were 'cell death', 'neurological disease', 'cell growth and proliferation', 'cancer' and 'organismal development'.

25.4 Conclusions

These microarray data provided clues to previously unknown factors and pathways responsible for the vulnerability of inferior retina to hyperoxic stress. Understanding gene expression changes of such genes as *Edn2, Bcl3* can contribute to the eventual identification of therapeutic targets.

Acknowledgments This research was supported by grants from the National Health and Medical Research Council (NHMRC) and Australian Research Council (ARC). The authors thank Dr. Stephem Ohms for his assistance in using Partek Genomics software and providing suggestions in statistics.

References

Chung HS, Harris A, Halter PJ et al (1999) Regional differences in retinal vascular reactivity. Invest Ophthalmol Vis Sci 40:2448–2453

Geller S, Krowka R, Valter K et al (2006) Toxicity of hyperoxia to the retina: evidence from the mouse. Adv Exp Med Biol 572:425–437

Natoli R, Provis J, Valter K et al (2008a) Expression and role of the early-response gene Oxr1 in the hyperoxia-challenged mouse retina. Invest Ophthalmol Vis Sci 49:4561–4567

Natoli R, Provis J, Valter K et al (2008b) Gene regulation induced in the C57BL/6 J mouse retina by hyperoxia: a temporal microarray study. Mol Vis 14:1983–1994

Noell WK (1955) Visual cell effects of high oxygen pressures. Am Physiol Soc Fed Proc 14: 107–108

Pfaffl MW (2001) A new mathematical model for relative quantification in real-time RT-PCR. Nucleic Acids Res 29:e45

Rapp LM, Williams TP (1977) Rhodopsin content and electroretinographic sensitivity in light-damaged rat retina. Nature 267:835–836

Smit-McBride Z, Oltjen SL, LaVail MM et al (2007) A strong genetic determinant of hyperoxia-related retinal degeneration on mouse chromosome 6. Invest Ophthalmol Visual Sci 48: 405–411

Stone J, Maslim J, Valter-Kocsi K et al (1999) Mechanisms of photoreceptor death and survival in mammalian retina. Prog Ret Eye Res 18:689–735

Walsh N, Bravo-Nuevo A, Geller S et al (2004) Resistance of photoreceptors in the C57BL/6-c2J, C57BL/6 J, and BALB/cJ mouse strains to oxygen stress: evidence of an oxygen phenotype. Curr Eye Res 29:441–447

Yamada H, Yamada E, Hackett SF et al (1999) Hyperoxia causes decreased expression of vascular endothelial growth factor and endothelial cell apoptosis in adult retina. J Cell Physiol 179: 149–156

Yamada H, Yamada E, Ando A et al (2001) Fibroblast growth factor-2 decreases hyperoxia-induced photoreceptor cell death in mice. Am J Pathol 159:1113–1120

Chapter 26
Photoreceptor Sensory Cilia and Inherited Retinal Degeneration

Qin Liu, Qi Zhang, and Eric A. Pierce

Abstract The outer segments of photoreceptor cells are specialized sensory cilia, and share many features with other primary and sensory cilia. Like other cilia, photoreceptor sensory cilium (PSC) comprises a membrane domain of outer segment and its cytoskeleton. We have recently identified the protein components of mouse PSCs, and found that the list of PSC proteins, called the PSC proteome, contains many novel cilia proteins. Studies have shown that many of the identified retinal degeneration disease genes encode proteins which are part of the PSC. Furthermore, mutations in genes encoding proteins expressed both in photoreceptors and other cilia result in systemic diseases, such as Usher syndrome, Bardet-Biedl syndrome (BBS), and Senior-Loken syndrome that involve retinal degeneration along with other disorders consequent to cilia dysfunction such as deafness and polycystic kidney disease. Based on these findings, we hypothesize that genes that encode proteins required for formation of PSCs are good candidate retinal degeneration disease genes. This chapter will summarize our studies on identifying novel PSC proteins from the PSC proteome. As an example of these studies, we demonstrated that tetratricopeptide the repeat domain 21B (TTC21B) protein is a novel PSC protein and is required for normal cilia formation in primary and photoreceptor sensory cilia.

26.1 PSC Proteins Involved in Inherited Retinal Degenerations

Inherited retinal degenerations (IRDs) are characterized by progressive dysfunction and death of photoreceptor cells, and are genetically heterogeneous, with over 140 disease genes identified to date (RetNet 2008). IRDs occur in non-syndromic and syndromic forms. It is estimated that 65% of retinitis pigmentosa (RP) cases

Q. Liu (✉)
F.M. Kirby Center for Molecular Ophthalmology, University of Pennsylvania School of Medicine, Philadelphia, PA, USA
e-mail: qinliu3@mail.med.upenn.edu

R.E. Anderson et al. (eds.), *Retinal Degenerative Diseases*, Advances in Experimental Medicine and Biology 664, DOI 10.1007/978-1-4419-1399-9_26,
© Springer Science+Business Media, LLC 2010

are non-syndromic, and 30–35% of individuals with RP have associated a broad set of non-ocular disease, including Alstrom, Bardet-Biedl, Joubert, Meckel, Senior Loken/nephronophthisis and Usher syndromes (Hartong et al. 2006; Badano et al. 2006; Daiger et al. 2007; Hildebrandt and Zhou 2007). Recent evidence indicates that dysfunction of sensory cilia is the underlying cause of these multisystemic disorders (Badano et al. 2006). This highlights the importance of recognition of photoreceptor outer segments as specialized sensory cilia, and also explains the connection of IRDs at a mechanistic level to a larger class of systemic cilia disorders, in which retinal degeneration is found in association with multiple cilia-related diseases, including cystic renal disease, polydactyly, mental retardation, obesity and gonadal malformations, diabetes, and situs inversus (Badano et al. 2006). The inclusion of IRDs in the larger class of cilia disorders allows information from investigations of other types of cilia to be applied to PSCs and inherited retinal disorders. The synergy also operates in reverse, so that findings from studies of photoreceptor biology have the potential to be relevant to understanding cilia function and diseases in general.

While significant progress has been made in identifying IRD disease genes, the genes which harbor mutations that cause disease in approximately 50% of IRD patients remain to be identified (Hartong et al. 2006; Badano et al. 2006; Daiger et al. 2007; Hildebrandt and Zhou 2007). Finding the genetic cause of IRDs has become increasingly important, as the recent reports of early successes with gene therapy for LCA2 indicate that we are entering an era of genetic therapies for IRDs (Maguire et al. 2008). Notably, the majority of the IRD disease genes identified over the past 3 years encode proteins that were first identified to be part of photoreceptor sensory cilia in the PSC complex proteome (see below) (Chang et al. 2006; Valente et al. 2006; Sayer et al. 2006; den Hollander et al. 2006). Based on these observations, we propose that novel cilia proteins detected in the PSC proteome are important for PSC structure and function, and genes that encode these novel cilia proteins are thus good candidate disease genes for IRDs. As described below, we have been testing these hypotheses by identifying novel PSC proteins that are required for correct cilia formation and/or function, and then screening the genes that encode functionally validated PSC proteins for mutations that cause IRDs and related ciliopathies.

26.2 Structure of Photoreceptor Sensory Cilium Complex

Photoreceptor outer segments are specialized sensory cilia. This is not a new idea, but rather a new appreciation of a concept that has been in the literature for many years (De Robertis 1956; Allen 1965; Matsusaka 1974). Until recently, the importance of primary and sensory cilia in biology and disease is being more broadly recognized (Singla and Reiter 2006; Christensen et al. 2007; Slough et al. 2008; Breunig et al. 2008; Simons and Mlodzik 2008). Primary cilia are present on most vertebrate cell types. These structures are typically sensory organelles, and are involved in many critical aspects of cell biology. For example, sensation of flow by primary cilia is required for maintenance of renal nephron structure and body axis determination. Primary cilia play important roles in various aspects of development, such as planar cell polarity as regulated by hedgehog and wnt signaling (Singla and Reiter 2006; Davis et al. 2006; Gerdes et al. 2007).

The sensory cilia elaborated rod and cone photoreceptors are among the largest of mammalian cilia (Pan et al. 2005; Yang et al. 2005). Like other cilia, photoreceptor sensory cilium comprises a membrane domain of outer segment and its cytoskeleton. The membrane domain of outer segments is highly specialized, in this case for light detection, with the proteins required for phototransduction located in or associated with the membrane discs stacked in tight order at ~30 per micron along the axoneme. The cytoskeleton of PSCs includes a basal body, transition zone (also called the 'connecting cilium'), axoneme and rootlet. The axoneme begins at the basal body, passes through a transition zone and into the outer segment. The basal bodies also nucleate the ciliary rootlet, which extends into the inner segment (Yang et al. 2005). The transition zone in photoreceptor sensory cilia is analogous to transition zones in other cilia, and is the region where the triplet microtubule structure of the basal bodies converts to the doublet microtubule structure of the axoneme (Horst et al. 1990). This region was first called the 'connecting cilium' by DeRobertis in 1956, when he was studying some of the first electron micrographs of photoreceptor cells (De Robertis 1956). This name was applied before the structure of cilia was completely defined, and it was understood that the axoneme of photoreceptor outer segments extends through the transition zone, and for up to 2/3rds of the length of the outer segment (De Robertis 1956; Kaplan et al. 1987). In recognition of the homology between PSCs and other cilia, this region will be called the transition zone below.

26.3 Protein Components of Photoreceptor Sensory Cilium: PSC Proteome

The recognition of photoreceptor outer segments as cilia allows for consideration of the whole photoreceptor sensory cilium as a biologic structure, which is valuable for the study of photoreceptor cell biology and disease pathogenesis. A number of proteins have been identified to be components of the cytoskeletons of PSCs, primarily through study of proteins produced by retinal degeneration disease genes. These include BBS2, BBS4, BBS7, BBS8, CEP290, CIP98(DFNB31), GPR98, IQCB1, LCA5, MYO7A, Nephrocystin-1 (NPHP1), Nephroretinin (NPHP4), PCDH15, RP1, RPGR, RPGRIP1, TTC8, USH1G, Usherin (USH2A) (Liu et al. 1997; Hong et al. 2000; Liu et al. 2002; Zhao et al. 2003; Ansley et al. 2003; Liu et al. 2004; Otto et al. 2005; Roepman et al. 2005; Reiners et al. 2005a; Reiners et al. 2005b; Chang et al. 2006; Fliegauf et al. 2006; Liu et al. 2007; den Hollander et al. 2007; Maerker et al. 2008). This list presents only a small portion of PSC cytoskeleton proteins. To initiate studies of PSCs from a broader perspective, we reported a complete proteome of mouse PSCs (Liu et al. 2007).

The PSC proteome identified by ≥3 unique peptides contains 1968 proteins, including ~1,500 proteins not detected in cilia from lower organisms. This includes 105 hypothetical proteins, and many cilia proteins not previously identified in photoreceptors. Several measures show that the proteome is highly accurate, and includes the majority of proteins (95%) in PSCs. Analyses of PSC complexes from rootletin knockout mice, which lack ciliary rootlets and separate from the inner segments of photoreceptor cells easily without the major inner segment component of the PSC complex cytoskeleton, confirm that 1,185 of the identified PSC complex proteins are derived from the outer segment (Yang et al. 2005; Liu et al. 2007). The PSC complex proteome accelerates greatly the progress toward improved understanding of how photoreceptor cilia are built and maintained, and how these processes are disrupted in disease.

26.4 Novel Photoreceptor Cilia Proteins in PSC Proteome

The PSC complex proteome contains many cilia proteins not previously identified in photoreceptors, including 13 proteins produced by genes which harbor mutations that cause cilia diseases. We have selected a subset of ~200 novel proteins from the PSC complex proteome for initial evaluation. These novel proteins were selected based on having features that are shared with known PSC and other cilia proteins. This includes: 1. proteins with WD repeat, and tetratricopeptide (TPR) domains, which are common in IFT proteins (Jekely and Arendt 2006); 2. proteins with other domains shared with IRD disease proteins, such as coiled-coil and GTP-binding domains (Fan et al. 2004; Cantagrel et al. 2008); 3. hypothetical proteins that are especially abundant in the PSC based on the mass spectrometry data; and 4. proteins that are shared with the Ciliaproteome, a meta-analysis of cilia datasets from other organisms (Gherman et al. 2006). In this section, we will describe briefly the approaches that have been used to study the novel PSC proteins in our laboratory.

26.4.1 Subcellular Locations of Candidate Novel PSC Proteins

The proteins selected were either hypothetical or not previously identified in cilia. In hopes of gaining insights into the function of these proteins, we first determined their location in PSCs or renal cilia by expressing epitope-tagged versions of the proteins from a pCAG-V5-cDNA-IRES-EGFP Gateway expression vector. The cDNA clones were obtained from the Invitrogen Ultimate ORF clone collection, or the MGC and IMAGE cDNA clone collections, or amplified by RT-PCR from mouse retinal cDNA. The V5-tagged PSC cDNA plasmids were expressed in a ciliated mouse inner medullary collecting duct (mIMCD3) cell line, which stably expresses somatostatin receptor 3 (Sstr3)-EGFP in the primary cilia (Berbari et al. 2008), as well as in the photoreceptor cells of neonatal rats by using in vivo electroporation technique (Matsuda and Cepko 2004). The location of the V5-tagged proteins were assessed by immunostaining with anti-V5 antibodies in the mIMCD3 cells 48 h after transfection or in the photoreceptor cells 4 weeks following transfection via in vivo electroporation.

Observations from our initial studies showed that a clear V5 signal was found for the majority of the novel proteins evaluated to date. This includes 15 proteins specifically in PSC cytoskeletons, 13 proteins in PSCs, 32 proteins in the PSC plus other parts of the cell, and 26 proteins in the inner segment. Four proteins localized to the basal bodies and/or cilia of the mIMCD3 cells. The reliability of the location of the recombinant proteins were confirmed by anti-peptide antibodies we generated for 4 of the novel PSC proteins. The 28 proteins novel identified to be part of PSCs and their cytoskeleton are of particular interest, and are being studied further in the functional analyses as described below.

26.4.2 Functional Analysis of Novel PSC Proteins in Photoreceptor and Renal Cilia

26.4.2.1 shRNAs Against Novel PSC Genes

To investigate the function of validated novel PSC in cilia, shRNA-mediated knock-down techniques were used in renal cells in culture and photoreceptor cells in vivo. Three to four oligonucleotides encoding the identified shRNA sequences were cloned into the pCAG-mir30-puro vector. The activity of the cloned and sequence verified shRNAs were quantified following transfection into mIMCD3 cells using quantitative RT-PCR assays with TaqMan probes (Giulietti et al. 2001). For genes that are not expressed in mIMCD3 cells, the shRNA plasmids were co-transfected with pCAG-V5-*cDNA*-IRES-EGFP plasmids containing the cDNAs of interest, and the loss of the EGFP signal taken as evidence of successful knockdown (Matsuda and Cepko 2004). shRNA sequences that are verified to provide significant knockdown of the target gene ($\geq 70\%$) were used for the phenotypic analyses described below. Non-targeted shRNAs (shRNA-NT) and shRNAs for luciferase (shRNA-Luc) were used as controls for these and all other shRNA experiments.

26.4.2.2 Evaluation of Phenotypes of shRNA Knockdown in mIMCD3 Cells and PSCs

We used Sstr3-EGFP mIMCD3 cells to assess the function of the novel PSC proteins in renal primary cilia. Cells transfected with the validated pCAG-mir30-puro-shRNA plasmids were subjected to selection with puromycin for 72 h, and then serum starved for 24 h to stimulate cilia formation (Tucker et al. 1979). The cells were labeled with acetylated α-tubulin antibody to mark axonemes, and then were scored for the presence and length of the axonemes and cilia, as indicated by the acetylated α-tubulin signal and Sstr3-EGFP signal, respectively.

To assess the function of novel PSC proteins in photoreceptor cilia, we used in vivo electroporation to transfect rat photoreceptor cells with a combination of two plasmids: the pCAG-mir30-puro-shRNA plasmid with a validated shRNA against the PSC gene of interest and the pCAG-Flag-Prph2-IRES-EGFP plasmid. The IRES-EGFP marks the transfected cells, and the Flag-Prph2 allows for evaluation of their outer segment structure. Vibratome sections with EGFP signal and good morphology were stained with anti-Flag antibodies followed by three-dimensional volume reconstructions of the confocal images using Volocity 3D imaging software (Improvision, Waltham, MA). The structures of the outer segments of transfected photoreceptor cells will be compared with those of the control shRNA-NT transfected retinas.

26.5 TTC21B Protein in Photoreceptor Sensory Cilia and Renal Primary Cilia

So far, we have identified dozens of novel cilia proteins using the approaches described above. In collaboration with other investigators, we are screening several of the validated PSC genes for mutations in patients with IRDs and related ciliopathies. As one example of these studies, we have identified TTC21B as a novel cilia protein. Functional studies showed that Ttc21b was required for normal PSC structure and renal primary cilia formation. *TTC21B* was initially selected for analyses for several reasons. TTC21B protein contains TPR domains, which are common to IFT proteins; Ttc21b was relatively abundant in the PSC complex proteome (14 unique peptides); and Ttc21b was shared with the Ciliaproteome dataset (Jekely and Arendt 2006; Gherman et al. 2006; Liu et al. 2007). Other investigators have recently reported that TTC21B is a retrograde IFT protein (Tran et al. 2008).

26.5.1 TTC21B Localizes to the Basal Bodies and Transition Zone of Primary and Photoreceptor Sensory Cilia

To identify the location of the TTC21B protein in renal and photoreceptor cilia, we expressed V5-tagged human TTC21B in renal IMCD3 cells and photoreceptor cells, and developed antibodies against mouse Ttc21b. Staining of the transfected mIMCD3 cells with anti-V5 antibodies shows that TTC21B is located at the base of the primary cilia (Fig. 26.1a). In addition, there is a portion of the TTC21B signal that extends beyond the basal body. Results from the transfected photoreceptor cells shows that the V5 tagged TTC21B protein is mainly located at the transition zones of PSCs, with a small portion of signal extending into the axonemes (Fig. 26.1b). This result was confirmed by anti-Ttc21b antibody staining in mouse retina. As shown in Fig. 26.1c, Ttc21b is located in the transition zones of PSCs.

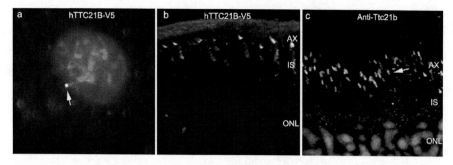

Fig. 26.1 Ttc21b in mIMCD3 cells and retina. **a.** V5-tagged TTC21b (*arrow*) is located at the base of cilia in transfected mIMCD3 that stably express the cilium marker Sstr3-EGFP. **b.** V5-tagged TTC21b is located at the transition zones in transfected photoreceptor cells with pCAG-V5-TTC21B-IRES-EGFP, with a small portion of signal extending into the axonemes. **c.** Antibodies to mouse Ttc21b (*arrow*) show that the protein is located in the transition zone of photoreceptor cilia. Ax, axoneme; IS, inner segment; ONL, outer nuclear layer

26.5.2 *TTC21B is Required for Primary Cilia and Photoreceptor Sensory Cilia Formation*

To determine if Ttc21b is required for cilia formation, we generated two shRNAs against *Ttc21b*, and cloned them into the pCAG-mir30-puro vector. Both shRNAs provide 70–80% knockdown of *Ttc21b* mRNA levels following transfection into mIMCD3 cells. We then evaluated the effects of *Ttc21b* shRNA-mediated knockdown on the structures of primary cilia and PSCs. In cultured mIMCD3 cells, transfection of either of the shRNA-Ttc21b plasmids resulted in notable shortening of primary cilia (1.6 ± 1.1 μm), as demonstrated by shorter axonemes and lack of the Sstr3-EGFP signal. In contrast, cilia in cells transfected with a control non-targeted shRNA (shRNA-NT) are long (6.4 ± 1.3 μm). Co-transfection of shRNA-resistant human *TTC21B* cDNA with the shRNA-*Ttc21b* restored cilia to almost full length (4.8 ± 1.1 μm; $p < 0.0001$) (data not shown). These data suggest that TTC21B is required for formation of normal primary cilia.

In a similar fashion, we also used the in vivo electroporation technique to assess the effect of shRNA-mediated knockdown of novel PSC proteins on photoreceptor outer segment structure. The 3D volume reconstructions of the confocal images demonstrate that *Ttc21b* knockdown results in abnormal PSC structure, with 'bulbs' in place of or at the distal end of the outer segments of most transfected photoreceptor cells. In contrast, the outer segments of control shRNA-NT transfected photoreceptors are slender rods (data not shown). A recent publication suggests that TTC21B is a retrograde IFT protein, and demonstrated similar bulbs at the distal ends of renal cilia following *Ttc21b* knockdown, which are thought to be caused by loss of the retrograde IFT activity (Tran et al. 2008).

26.6 Future Direction: Screening Novel PSC Genes
for Mutations that Cause IRDs

As mentioned above, many IRDs and related ciliopathies are caused by mutations in genes that encode components of PSCs and other cilia (Badano et al. 2006; Liu et al. 2007; Hildebrandt and Zhou 2007). While significant progress has been made in identifying IRD disease genes, the genes which harbor mutations that cause disease in approximately half of IRD patients remain to be identified (Hartong et al. 2006; Badano et al. 2006; Daiger et al. 2007; Hildebrandt and Zhou 2007). To identify the candidate disease genes for IRDs, we have initiated the screening for mutations in validated PSC genes in patients with cilia related disorders, including recessive and dominant RP, LCA, and other syndromic cilia disorders such as BBS. This work of mutation screening is being performed in collaboration with several other investigators. For future studies, we will continue testing the hypothesis that genes that encode novel PSC proteins are good candidate disease genes for IRDs and related ciliopathies. We are optimistic that continued screening of validated PSC genes for mutations in patients with ciliopathies will lead to the identification of additional disease genes.

References

Allen RA (1965) Isolated cilia in inner retinal neurons and in retinal pigment epithelium. J Ultrastruct Res 12:730–747

Ansley SJ, Badano JL, Blacque OE et al (2003) Basal body dysfunction is a likely cause of pleiotropic Bardet-Biedl syndrome. Nature 425:628–633

Badano JL, Mitsuma N, Beales PL et al (2006) The ciliopathies: an emerging class of human genetic disorders. Annu Rev Genomics Hum Genet 7:125–148

Berbari NF, Johnson AD, Lewis JS et al (2008) Identification of ciliary localization sequences within the third intracellular loop of G protein-coupled receptors. Mol Biol Cell 19:1540–1547

Breunig JJ, Sarkisian MR, Arellano JI et al (2008) Primary cilia regulate hippocampal neurogenesis by mediating sonic hedgehog signaling. Proc Natl Acad Sci USA 105:13127–13132

Cantagrel V, Silhavy JL, Bielas SL et al (2008) Mutations in the cilia gene ARL13B lead to the classical form of Joubert syndrome. Am J Hum Genet 83:170–179

Chang B, Khanna H, Hawes N et al (2006) In-frame deletion in a novel centrosomal/ciliary protein CEP290/NPHP6 perturbs its interaction with RPGR and results in early-onset retinal degeneration in the rd16 mouse. Hum Mol Genet 15:1847–1857

Christensen ST, Pedersen LB, Schneider L et al (2007) Sensory cilia and integration of signal transduction in human health and disease. Traffic 8:97–109

Daiger SP, Bowne SJ, Sullivan LS (2007) Perspective on genes and mutations causing retinitis pigmentosa. Arch Ophthalmol 125:151–158

Davis EE, Brueckner M, Katsanis N (2006) The emerging complexity of the vertebrate cilium: new functional roles for an ancient organelle. Dev Cell 11:9–19

De Robertis E (1956) Electron microscope observations on the submicroscopic organization of the retinal rods. J Biophys Biochem Cytol 2:319–330

den Hollander AI, Koenekoop RK, Yzer S et al (2006) Mutations in the CEP290 (NPHP6) gene are a frequent cause of leber congenital amaurosis. Am J Hum Genet 79:556–561 den Hollander AI, Koenekoop RK, Mohamed MD et al (2007) Mutations in LCA5, encoding the ciliary protein lebercilin, cause Leber congenital amaurosis. Nat Genet 39: 889–895

Fan Y, Esmail MA, Ansley SJ et al (2004) Mutations in a member of the Ras superfamily of small GTP-binding proteins causes Bardet-Biedl syndrome. Nat Genet 36:989–993

Fliegauf M, Horvath J, von SC et al (2006) Nephrocystin specifically localizes to the transition zone of renal and respiratory cilia and photoreceptor connecting cilia. J Am Soc Nephrol 17: 2424–2433

Gerdes JM, Liu Y, Zaghloul NA et al (2007) Disruption of the basal body compromises proteasomal function and perturbs intracellular Wnt response. Nat Genet 39:1350–1360

Gherman A, Davis EE, Katsanis N (2006) The ciliary proteome database: an integrated community resource for the genetic and functional dissection of cilia. Nat Genet 38:961–962

Giulietti A, Overbergh L, Valckx D et al (2001) An overview of real-time quantitative PCR: applications to quantify cytokine gene expression. Methods 25:386–401

Hartong DT, Berson EL, Dryja TP (2006) Retinitis pigmentosa. Lancet 368:1795–1809

Hildebrandt F, Zhou W (2007) Nephronophthisis-associated ciliopathies. J Am Soc Nephrol 18:1855–1871

Hong DH, Pawlyk BS, Shang J et al (2000) A retinitis pigmentosa GTPase regulator (RPGR)-deficient mouse model for X-linked retinitis pigmentosa (RP3). Proc Natl Acad Sci USA 97:3649–3654

Horst CJ, Johnson LV, Besharse JC (1990) Transmembrane assemblage of the photoreceptor connecting cilium and motile cilium transition zone contain a common immunologic epitope. Cell Motil Cytoskeleton 17:329–344

Jekely G, Arendt D (2006) Evolution of intraflagellar transport from coated vesicles and autogenous origin of the eukaryotic cilium. Bioessays 28:191–198

Kaplan MW, Iwata RT, Sears RC (1987) Lengths of immunolabeled ciliary microtubules in frog photoreceptor outer segments. Exp Eye Res 44:623–632

Liu Q, Zhou J, Daiger SP et al (2002) Identification and Subcellular Localization of the RP1 Protein in Human and Mouse Photoreceptors. Invest Ophthalmol Vis Sci 43:22–32

Liu Q, Zuo J, Pierce EA (2004) The retinitis pigmentosa 1 protein is a photoreceptor microtubule-associated protein. J Neurosci 24:6427–6436

Liu Q, Tan G, Levenkova N et al (2007) The proteome of the mouse photoreceptor sensory cilium complex. Mol Cell Proteomics 6:1299–1317

Liu X, Vansant G, Udovichenko IP et al (1997) Myosin VIIa, the product of the Usher 1B syndrome gene, is concentrated in the connecting cilia of photoreceptor cells. Cell Motil Cytoskeleton 37:240–252

Maerker T, van WE, Overlack N et al (2008) A novel Usher protein network at the periciliary reloading point between molecular transport machineries in vertebrate photoreceptor cells. Hum Mol Genet 17:71–86

Maguire AM, Simonelli F, Pierce EA et al (2008) Safety and efficacy of gene transfer for Leber's congenital amaurosis. N Engl J Med 358:2240–2248

Matsuda T, Cepko CL (2004) Electroporation and RNA interference in the rodent retina in vivo and in vitro. Proc Natl Acad Sci USA 101:16–22

Matsusaka T (1974) Membrane Particles of the Connecting Cilium. J Ultrastruct Res 48: 305–312

Otto EA, Loeys B, Khanna H et al (2005) Nephrocystin-5, a ciliary IQ domain protein, is mutated in Senior-Loken syndrome and interacts with RPGR and calmodulin. Nat Genet 37: 282–288

Pan J, Wang Q, Snell WJ (2005) Cilium-generated signaling and cilia-related disorders. Lab Invest 85:452–463

Reiners J, Marker T, Jurgens K et al (2005a) Photoreceptor expression of the Usher syndrome type 1 protein protocadherin 15 (USH1F) and its interaction with the scaffold protein harmonin (USH1C). Mol Vis 11:347–355

Reiners J, van Wijk E, Marker T et al (2005b) Scaffold protein harmonin (USH1C) provides molecular links between Usher syndrome type 1 and type 2. Hum Mol Genet 14:3933–3943

RetNet (2008) RetNet Web site address.

Roepman R, Letteboer SJ, Arts HH et al (2005) Interaction of nephrocystin-4 and RPGRIP1 is disrupted by nephronophthisis or Leber congenital amaurosis-associated mutations. Proc Natl Acad Sci USA 102:18520–18525

Sayer JA, Otto EA, O'Toole JF et al (2006) The centrosomal protein nephrocystin-6 is mutated in Joubert syndrome and activates transcription factor ATF4. Nat Genet 38:674–681

Simons M, Mlodzik M (2008) Planar cell polarity signaling: from fly development to human disease. Annu Rev Genet 42:517–540

Singla V, Reiter JF (2006) The primary cilium as the cell's antenna: signaling at a sensory organelle. Science 313:629–633

Slough J, Cooney L, Brueckner M (2008) Monocilia in the embryonic mouse heart suggest a direct role for cilia in cardiac morphogenesis. Dev Dyn 237:2304–2314

Tran PV, Haycraft CJ, Besschetnova TY et al (2008) THM1 negatively modulates mouse sonic hedgehog signal transduction and affects retrograde intraflagellar transport in cilia. Nat Genet 40:403–410

Tucker RW, Pardee AB, Fujiwara K (1979) Centriole ciliation is related to quiescence and DNA synthesis in 3T3 cells. Cell 17:527–535

Valente EM, Silhavy JL, Brancati F et al (2006) Mutations in CEP290, which encodes a centrosomal protein, cause pleiotropic forms of Joubert syndrome. Nat Genet 38:623–625

Yang J, Gao J, Adamian M et al (2005) The ciliary rootlet maintains long-term stability of sensory cilia. Mol Cell Biol 25:4129–4137

Zhao Y, Hong DH, Pawlyk B et al (2003) The retinitis pigmentosa GTPase regulator (RPGR)-interacting protein: subserving RPGR function and participating in disk morphogenesis. Proc Natl Acad Sci USA 100:3965–3970

Chapter 27
Role of Elovl4 Protein in the Biosynthesis of Docosahexaenoic Acid

Martin-Paul Agbaga, Richard S. Brush, Md Nawajes A. Mandal, Michael H. Elliott, Muayyad R. Al-Ubaidi, and Robert E. Anderson

Abstract The disk membranes of retinal photoreceptor outer segments and other neuronal and reproductive tissues are enriched in docosahexaenoic acid (DHA, 22:6n3), which is essential for their normal function and development. The fatty acid condensing enzyme Elongation of Very Long chain fatty acids-4 (ELOVL4) is highly expressed in retina photoreceptors as well as other tissues with high 22:6n3 content. Mutations in the *ELOVL4* gene are associated with autosomal dominant Stargardt-like macular dystrophy (STGD3) and results in synthesis of a truncated protein that cannot be targeted to the endoplasmic reticulum (ER), the site of fatty acid biosynthesis. Considering the abundance and essential roles of 22:6n3 in ELOVL4-expressing tissues (except the skin), it was proposed that the ELOVL4 protein may be involved in 22:6n3 biosynthesis. We tested the hypothesis that the ELOVL4 protein is involved in 22:6n3 biosynthesis by selectively silencing expression of the protein in the cone photoreceptors derived cell line 661W and showed that the ELOVL4 protein is not involved in DHA biosynthesis from the short chain fatty acid precursors 18:3n3 and 22:5n3.

27.1 Introduction

Mammalian fatty acid elongases are a group of condensing enzymes that mediate elongation of fatty acids by the addition of two carbon units of malonyl-CoA. Currently seven members of these condensing enzymes named ELOngation of Very Long chain fatty acids (ELOVL) have been reported. Their roles in fatty acid chain elongation, their fatty acid specificity, as well as the steps within the carbon chain they act on, have been studied and reviewed (Leonard et al., 2004; Meyer et al.,

M.-P. Agbaga (✉)
Department of Cell Biology, Dean McGee Eye Institute, University of Oklahoma Health Sciences Center, 608 Stanton L.Young Blvd, DMEI 409, Oklahoma, OK 73104, USA
e-mail: martin-paul-agbaga@ouhsc.edu

R.E. Anderson et al. (eds.), *Retinal Degenerative Diseases*, Advances in Experimental Medicine and Biology 664, DOI 10.1007/978-1-4419-1399-9_27,
© Springer Science+Business Media, LLC 2010

2004; Tvrdik et al., 2000; Westerberg et al., 2004). The fourth member of this group, ELOVL4, was first discovered and reported in 2001 as a truncated protein associated with autosomal dominant Stargardt-like macular dystrophy (STGD3), an inherited juvenile form of macular degeneration (Bernstein et al., 2001; Edwards et al., 2001; Zhang et al., 2001). On the basis of features of the ELOVL4 protein, which are characteristic of fatty acid elongases, and its tissue distribution, the ELOVL4 protein was proposed by Zhang et al. (2001) to be involved in biosynthesis of docosahexaenoic acid (DHA, 22:6n3), the most abundant fatty acid in the retina, other neural tissues, and the testis.

We used an immortalized cell line derived from mouse cones (661W) (Al-Ubaidi et al., 1992) that expresses ELOVL4 and possesses the machinery for fatty acid elongation and desaturation. These cells were able to elongate short chain polyunsaturated fatty acids (PUFA) of the n3 and n6 family to longer chain fatty acids up to C24 when they were incubated with 18:3n3, 20:5n3 or 22:5n3. We tested the hypothesis that the ELOVL4 protein is involved in the elongation of PUFA to 22:6n3 by selectively silencing the expression of endogenous ELOVL4 in 661W cells and determined that the ELOVL4 protein is not involved in the biosynthesis of 22:6n3 from short chain PUFA precursors.

27.2 Materials and Methods

27.2.1 RNA Interference

A pool of siRNA designed for the silencing of the mouse *Elovl4* gene (genome smartpool reagent M-054863-00-0005) was purchased from Dharmacon, Inc. (Lafayette, CO). 661W cells (2×10^5 cells in 2 ml of medium/well using a 24-well plate or 2×10^4 cells in 200 µl of medium/well using a 96-well plate) were transfected with the *Elovl4* siRNA or the control siRNA using I-fect transfection reagent (Neuromics, Edina, MN), according to the manufacturer's instructions. All transfections were performed in a mixture of Opti-MEM (Invitrogen, Carlsbad, CA) and complete medium without antibiotics. Transfections were optimized by varying the doses of the transfection reagents and the siRNA. Cells were incubated with the transfection siRNA/I-fect complexes for 12 h in Opti-MEM and then switched to complete DMEM. Cell lysis and protein isolation were done 72 h post transfection. The efficacy of gene silencing was assessed by RT-PCR and Western blotting using a rabbit polyclonal antibody against mouse ELOVL4 described previously (Agbaga et al., 2008).

27.2.2 Construction of Mouse Anti Elovl4 Gene shRNA

From the four siRNA pools, two individual siRNAs that efficiently silenced the *Elovl4* expression in 661W cells were selected and converted to short-hairpin oligonucleotides that were synthesized by Integrated DNA Technologies (IDTDNA, Coralville, IA). The short hairpin oligonucleotides were annealed and cloned into the *Hind*III/*Sfi*I site under the U6 promoter of pSilencer U6 AR1 CMV IRES-EGFP vector (Ambion Inc, Austin, TX) or into Genscript pRNAT-U6.2/Lenti (Piscataway, NJ) vector to generate shRNA vectors. A scrambled sequence, which does not target mouse *Elovl4* expression, was used as a control. The shRNAs were individually transfected into 661W cells and green fluorescent protein (GFP) positive cells were sorted by flow cytometry, cultured, and used for fatty acid supplementation experiments.

27.2.3 Tissue Culture

661W cells were plated at a density of 2×10^6 cells/ml in DMEM supplemented with 10% calf serum and antibiotics, and treated for 72 h with 5–30 μg/ml of the sodium salts of either 18:3n3 or 22:5n3. After 72 h, the cells were collected and washed once in 0.1 M phosphate buffer containing 50 μM of fraction V fatty acid-free BSA (Sigma, St Louis MO) and then in 0.1 M phosphate buffer. Finally, cells were pelleted and stored at –80°C until used. For radioactive tracer studies, the cells were plated as above and then incubated with 2–4 μCi/ml of fraction V fatty acid-free BSA conjugated [1-^{14}C]-18:3n3 for 48–72 h. The cells were collected and stored as before.

27.2.4 Fatty Acid Analysis

Total lipids were extracted from fatty acid supplemented and control cells by the method of Bligh and Dyer (Bligh and Dyer 1959) and converted to fatty acid methyl esters (FAMEs) by the procedure of Morrison and Smith (1964). FAMEs were analyzed by gas-liquid chromatography as described (Tanito et al., 2008). Fatty acid phenacyl esters (FAPES) were prepared from total lipid extracts for high performance liquid chromatography (HPLC) analysis as previously described (DeMar and Anderson 1997; DeMar et al., 1996).

27.3 Results

27.3.1 661W Cells Express Elovl4 and Can Elongate 18:3n3 and 22:5n3 to Longer Chain Fatty Acids

To determine the specific step(s) in fatty acid elongation that the ELOVL4 protein catalyses, we determined that an immortalized retinal cell line (661W) expresses *Elovl4* mRNA and protein (Fig. 27.1). Addition of 18:3n3 and 22:5n3 to the culture media showed that 661W cells possess the metabolic machinery necessary for elongation of these PUFA to C-24 PUFA. 18:3n3 was efficiently elongated to C20 and C24 PUFA (Fig. 27.2a) and 22:5n3 was elongated to 24:5n3 with some retro-conversion to 20:5n3 (Fig. 27.2b). Since formation of 22:6n3 involves desaturation of 24:5n3 to 24:6n3, which is then metabolized in the peroxisome by β-oxidation to 22:6n3 (Voss et al., 1991), we conclude that 661W cells have the biochemical machinery necessary for elongation of n3 PUFA.

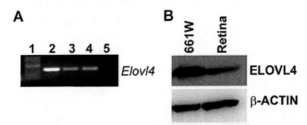

Fig. 27.1 Endogenous expression of Elovl4 in 661W cells; (**a**) RT-PCR of *Elovl4* cDNA from 661W cells. Complementary DNA from the 661W cells was used as a template to amplify the *Elovl4* transcript with actin used as a control (data not shown). Representative results are presented. Lanes: 1, 100-bp markers; 2, mouse retina cDNA; 3–4, 661W cDNA; 5, no reverse transcriptase control. (**b**) A representative Western blot analysis of 30 μg protein from 661W cells and mouse retina confirmed the expression of ELOVL4 in 661W cells. Bottom panel is β-actin loading control

27.3.2 Knock-Down of Endogenous Elovl4 Does Not Affect C18–C24 PUFA Synthesis

siRNA and shRNA mediated silencing of the *Elovl4* message in 661W cells resulted in knock-down of the ELOVL4 protein as determined by Western blot analysis (Fig. 27.3). As shRNA-D2 was efficient at silencing ELOVL4 protein expression (Fig. 27.3d), we chose cells transfected with this construct and sorted for fatty acid biosynthesis studies. As shown in Fig. 27.4, ELOVL4 knock-down did not affect the ability of the 661W cells to elongate 18:3n3 to 20:5n3, 22:5n3, and 24:5n3 as determined by HPLC (Fig. 27.4a) and GC-FID (Fig. 27.4b). If ELOVL4 catalyzed any particular one of these elongation steps, there would have been an increase in the radioactivity (or mass) in the precursor fatty acid and a decrease in radioactivity (or mass) of the product of the accumulated precursor in the silenced condition.

27.4 Discussion

The highest expression of ELOVL4 is found in the retina, followed by testis, skin and brain. Except for the skin, all of these tissues have high contents of 22:6n3, which is required for their normal development and function (Benolken et al., 1973; Salem et al., 2001). This fatty acid must either be obtained from diet or be syn-thesized through sequential desaturation and elongation of dietary n3 PUFA such

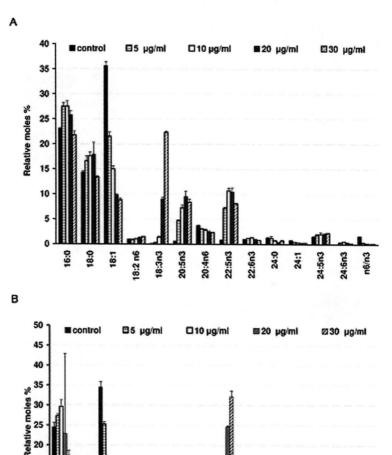

Fig. 27.2 Elongation of 18:3n3 and 22:5n3 in 661W cells; (**a**) 661W cells were cultured in medium supplemented with increasing concentrations of 18:3n3 or (**b**) 22:5n3 and grown for 72 h. Total cellular lipids were extracted, converted to fatty acid methyl esters (FAMEs), and analyzed by gas-liquid chromatography. 18:3n3 was elongated and desaturated to 20:5n3, 22:5n3, and 24:5n3. However, there was negligible conversion to 24:6n3 and 22:6n-3. Similarly, 22:5n3 (**b**) was incorporated into cellular lipids and some was elongated to 24:5n3

as 18:3n3 or 22:5n3 to 24:6n3 (Bazan et al., 1982; Delton-Vandenbroucke et al., 1997; Sprecher 2000; Voss et al., 1991). The 24:6n3 is then converted to 22:6n3 through peroxisomal β-oxidation (Sprecher 1999; Sprecher et al., 1999; Voss et al., 1991). The high content of 22:6n3 in all ELOVL4 expressing tissues except the skin

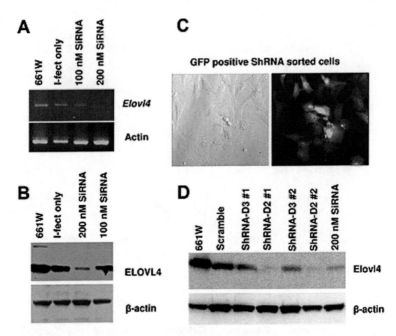

Fig. 27.3 siRNA and shRNA knock-down of mouse *Elovl4* in 661W cells; (**a**) *Elovl4* knock-down in 661W cells transfected with 100 or 200 nM anti-*Elovl4* siRNA smart-pools. *Elovl4* knock-down by the siRNA duplexes was assayed by RT-PCR. (**b**) Western blot analysis of ELOVL4 knock-down in 661W cells transfected with the pool of 4 siRNA duplexes 72 h after transfection. The *bottom panel* is β-actin loading control. (**c**) 661W cells transfected and sorted for GFP-positive cells expressing the pSilencer-anti-*Elovl4*-shRNA under the human U6 promoter and GFP under the CMV promoter. After sorting, the GFP positive cells were expanded and used for subsequent experiments. (**d**) Western blot analysis of GFP-positive 661W cells stably expressing anti-*Elovl4*-shRNA and controls post-sorting

suggested a probable role of ELOVL4 protein in the biosynthetic pathway of 22:6n3 from its short chain precursors (Zhang et al., 2001). However, mutations in the *ELOVL4* gene results in a truncated protein that misroutes both mutant and wild-type protein from the endoplasmic reticulum, the site of fatty acid biosynthesis (Grayson and Molday 2005; Karan et al., 2005; Vasireddy et al., 2005)

We tested whether ELOVL4 protein is involved in the pathway of 22:6n3 synthesis by silencing its expression in cells that have endogenous expression of this protein, and determining the effect on C-24 PUFA formation from shorter chain PUFA precursors. Using non-radioactive and [^{14}C]-18:3n3, we showed that cone photoreceptor-derived 661W cells express the ELOVL4 protein (Fig. 27.1) and have the metabolic machinery necessary for the elongation of either 18:3n3 or 22:5n3 to longer chain n3 fatty acids up to C24 (Fig. 27.2a, b). However, when we silenced the ELOVL4 expression in 661W cells, no detectable changes were observed in the elongation of either 18:3n3 or 22:5n3 to longer chain fatty acids. Elongation and desaturation of 18:3n3 and 22:5n3 fatty acids in these cells proceeded unabated in

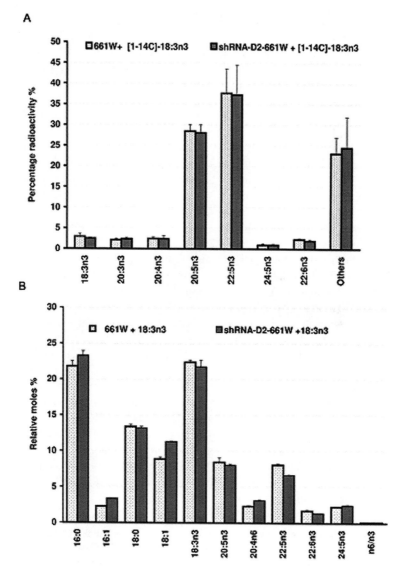

Fig. 27.4 Knock-down of ELOVL4 did not affect the elongation of [1-^{14}C]-18:3n3 to [^{14}C]-20:5n3, [^{14}C]-22:5n3 and [^{14}C]-24:5n3.; (**a**) Relative percentage radioactivity in ELOVL4 knock-down and wild type 661W cells supplemented with [1-^{14}C]-18:3n3. No differences in the formation of [^{14}C]-20:5n3, [^{14}C]-22:5n3, and [^{14}C]-24:5n3 were found between control (non-shRNA expressing cells) and the ELOVL4-knock-down cells. This suggests that ELOVL4 is not involved in the elongation of 18:3n3 to 20:5n3, of 20:5n3 to 22:5n3, and of 22:5n3 to 24:5n3 in these cells. (**b**) GC-FID results of elongation of 18:3n3 in wild type 661W cells and shRNA-D2-GFP positive cells. There were no differences in the elongation products

the same way as in the wild-type cells. These elongation steps could be mediated by the Δ5–7 elongase activity of the mouse ELOVL2 protein (Meyer et al., 2004). Elongation of 20:5n3 to 22:5n3 was also probably catalyzed by Δ5 elongase activity of the same enzyme (Meyer et al., 2004). This suggests ELOVL4 may not be involved in elongation of these steps in the pathway of 22:6n3 biosynthesis. We then evaluated Δ7 elongase activity in the pathway of 22:6n3 biosynthesis by incubating the cells with 22:5n3 while knocking down the expression of *Elovl4*. ELOVL4 knock-down did not have any effect on the elongation of 22:5n3 to 24:5n3 (data not shown). We, therefore, concluded that the ELOVL4 protein could either be playing a redundant role in biosynthesis of 22:6n3 or it may not be involved in the biosynthesis of 22:6n3 in the retina or in any tissues where it is expressed. These conclusions are also supported by recent studies on ELOVL4 using different mouse models (Cameron et al., 2007; Li et al., 2007; McMahon et al., 2007a, b; Vasireddy et al., 2007). Further, we designed experiments to test the hypothesis that the ELOVL4 protein is involved in synthesizing C26–C38 Very Long Chain Polyunsaturated Fatty Acids (VLC-PUFA), which are also found in ELOVL4 expressing tissues in minor quantities (Aveldano 1987). We presented an unequivocal evidence that indeed the ELOVL4 protein is involved in the biosynthesis of VLC-PUFA (Agbaga et al., 2008). The findings that ELOVL4 is involved in the biosynthesis of VLC-PUFA are in agreement with previous studies that showed that the skin of mice homozygous for *Elovl4* 5-bp deletion knock-in and *Elovl4* knock-out animals have greater total saturated FA (esp. 24:0 and 26:0) than that of their wild-type kin (Cameron et al., 2007; Li et al., 2007; McMahon et al., 2007a; Vasireddy et al., 2007). It also supported the studies by McMahon et al. (2007b) which showed that the retinas of *Stgd3*-knockin mice that carry one copy of the human pathogenic 5-bp deletion in the mouse *Elovl4* gene and one normal copy of the mouse *Elovl4* gene have deficiency in C32-C36 acyl phosphatidylcholine. Moreover, the 22:6n3 composition of those retinas was not different from the composition of the retinas from wild-type mice (McMahon et al., 2007b). The conclusion drawn from the current study is that ELOVL4 is not involved in the biosynthesis of 22:6n3 from shorter chain PUFA precursors.

Acknowledgments We thank Kimberly Henry for her technical support. This work was supported by National Eye Institute Grants EY04149, EY00871, and EY12190; National Center for Research Resources Grant RR17703; Research to Prevent Blindness, Inc., R01EY14052, Hope For Vision, Reynolds Oklahoma Center on Aging; and the Foundation Fighting Blindness.

References

Agbaga MP, Brush RS, Mandal MN et al (2008) Role of Stargardt-3 macular dystrophy protein (ELOVL4) in the biosynthesis of very long chain fatty acids. Proc Natl Acad Sci USA 105:12843–12848

Al-Ubaidi MR, Font RL, Quiambao AB et al (1992) Bilateral retinal and brain tumors in transgenic mice expressing simian virus 40 large T antigen under control of the human interphotoreceptor retinoid-binding protein promoter. J Cell Biol 119:1681–1687

Aveldano MI (1987) A novel group of very long chain polyenoic fatty acids in dipolyunsaturated phosphatidylcholines from vertebrate retina. J Biol Chem 262:1172–1179

Bazan HE, Careaga MM, Sprecher H et al (1982) Chain elongation and desaturation of eicos-apentaenoate to docosahexaenoate and phospholipid labeling in the rat retina in vivo. Biochim Biophys Acta 712:123–128

Benolken RM, Anderson RE, Wheeler TG (1973) Membrane fatty acids associated with the electrical response in visual excitation. Science 182:1253–1254

Bernstein PS, Tammur J, Singh N et al (2001) Diverse macular dystrophy phenotype caused by a novel complex mutation in the ELOVL4 gene. Invest Ophthalmol Vis Sci 42:3331–3336

Bligh EG, Dyer WJ (1959) A rapid method of total lipid extraction and purification. Can J Biochem Physiol 37:911–917

Cameron DJ, Tong Z, Yang Z et al (2007) Essential role of Elovl4 in very long chain fatty acid synthesis, skin permeability barrier function, and neonatal survival. Int J Biol Sci 3:111–119

DeMar JC Jr, Anderson RE (1997) Identification and quantitation of the fatty acids composing the CoA ester pool of bovine retina, heart, and liver. J Biol Chem 272:31362–31368

DeMar JC Jr, Wensel TG, Anderson RE (1996) Biosynthesis of the unsaturated 14-carbon fatty acids found on the N termini of photoreceptor-specific proteins. J Biol Chem 271:5007–5016

Delton-Vandenbroucke I, Grammas P, Anderson RE (1997) Polyunsaturated fatty acid metabolism in retinal and cerebral microvascular endothelial cells. J Lipid Res 38:147–159

Edwards AO, Donoso LA, Ritter R 3rd (2001) A novel gene for autosomal dominant Stargardt-like macular dystrophy with homology to the SUR4 protein family. Invest Ophthalmol Vis Sci 42:2652–2663

Grayson C, Molday RS (2005) Dominant negative mechanism underlies autosomal dominant Stargardt-like macular dystrophy linked to mutations in ELOVL4. J Biol Chem 280:32521–32530

Karan G, Yang Z, Howes K et al (2005) Loss of ER retention and sequestration of the wild-type ELOVL4 by Stargardt disease dominant negative mutants. Mol Vis 11:657–664

Leonard AE, Pereira SL, Sprecher H et al (2004) Elongation of long-chain fatty acids. Prog Lipid Res 43:36–54

Li W, Sandhoff R, Kono M et al (2007) Depletion of ceramides with very long chain fatty acids causes defective skin permeability barrier function, and neonatal lethality in ELOVL4 deficient mice. Int J Biol Sci 3:120–128

McMahon A, Butovich IA, Mata NL et al (2007a) Retinal pathology and skin barrier defect in mice carrying a Stargardt disease-3 mutation in elongase of very long chain fatty acids-4. Mol Vis 13:258–272

McMahon A, Jackson SN, Woods AS et al (2007b) A Stargardt disease-3 mutation in the mouse Elovl4 gene causes retinal deficiency of C32-C36 acyl phosphatidylcholines. FEBS Lett 581:5459–5463

Meyer A, Kirsch H, Domergue F et al (2004) Novel fatty acid elongases and their use for the reconstitution of docosahexaenoic acid biosynthesis. J Lipid Res 45:1899–1909

Morrison WR, Smith LM (1964) Preparation of Fatty Acid Methyl Esters and Dimethylacetals from Lipids with Boron Fluoride–Methanol. J Lipid Res 5:600–608

Salem N Jr, Litman B, Kim HY et al (2001) Mechanisms of action of docosahexaenoic acid in the nervous system. Lipids 36:945–959

Sprecher H (1999) An update on the pathways of polyunsaturated fatty acid metabolism. Curr Opin Clin Nutr Metab Care 2:135–138

Sprecher H (2000) Metabolism of highly unsaturated n-3 and n-6 fatty acids. Biochim Biophys Acta 1486:219–231

Sprecher H, Chen Q, Yin FQ (1999) Regulation of the biosynthesis of 22:5n-6 and 22:6n-3: a complex intracellular process. Lipids 34(Suppl):S153–S156

Tanito M, Brush RS, Elliott MH et al (2008) High levels of retinal membrane docosahexaenoic acid increase susceptibility to stress-induced degeneration. J Lipid Res 50(5):807–819

Tvrdik P, Westerberg R, Silve S et al (2000) Role of a new mammalian gene family in the biosynthesis of very long chain fatty acids and sphingolipids. J Cell Biol 149:707–718

Vasireddy V, Uchida Y, Salem N Jr et al (2007) Loss of functional ELOVL4 depletes very long-chain fatty acids (> or =C28) and the unique omega-O-acylceramides in skin leading to neonatal death. Hum Mol Genet 16:471–482

Vasireddy V, Vijayasarathy C, Huang J et al (2005) Stargardt-like macular dystrophy protein ELOVL4 exerts a dominant negative effect by recruiting wild-type protein into aggresomes. Mol Vis 11:665–676

Voss A, Reinhart M, Sankarappa S et al (1991) The metabolism of 7,10,13,16,19-docosapentaenoic acid to 4,7,10,13,16,19-docosahexaenoic acid in rat liver is independent of a 4-desaturase. J Biol Chem 266:19995–20000

Westerberg R, Tvrdik P, Unden AB et al (2004) Role for ELOVL3 and fatty acid chain length in development of hair and skin function. J Biol Chem 279:5621–5629

Zhang K, Kniazeva M, Han M et al (2001) A 5-bp deletion in ELOVL4 is associated with two related forms of autosomal dominant macular dystrophy. Nat Genet 27:89–93

Part II
Molecular Genetics and Candidate Genes

Chapter 28
Molecular Pathogenesis of Achromatopsia Associated with Mutations in the Cone Cyclic Nucleotide-Gated Channel CNGA3 Subunit

Xi-Qin Ding, J. Browning Fitzgerald, Alexander B. Quiambao, Cynthia S. Harry, and Anna P. Malykhina

Abstract Cone photoreceptor cyclic nucleotide-gated (CNG) channel is essential for central and color vision and visual acuity. Mutations in the cone channel subunits CNGA3 and CNGB3 are linked to achromatopsia and progressive cone dystrophy in humans. Over 50 mutations have been identified in the CNGA3 subunit. The R277C and R283W substitutions are among the most frequently occurring mutations. This study investigated the defects of these two mutations using a heterologous expression system. The wild type and mutant CNGA3 were expressed in HEK293 cells, the channel's expression and cellular localization were examined by immunoblotting and immunofluorecences labeling, and activity of the channel was evaluated by ratiometric $[Ca^{2+}]_i$ measurements and by electrophysiological recordings. By using this model system we observed dysfunction of the mutant channels. Co-expression of the mutant channel with the wild type subunit did not affect the wild type channel's activity. Immunofluorescence labeling showed apparent cytosol aggregation of the immunoreactivity in cells expressing the mutants. Thus these disease-causing mutations appear to induce loss of function by impairing the channel cellular trafficking and plasma membrane targeting. Therapeutic supplementation of the wild type transgene may help correct the visual disorders caused by these two mutations.

28.1 Introduction

Photoreceptor cyclic nucleotide-gated (CNG) channels play a central role in phototransduction. Rod and cone CNG channels comprise two structurally related subunit types; CNGA1 and CNGB1 for the rod channel, and CNGA3 and CNGB3

X.-Q. Ding (✉)
Department of Cell Biology, University of Oklahoma Health Sciences Center, 940 Stanton L. Young Blvd., Oklahoma City, OK 73104, USA
e-mail: xi-qin-ding@ouhsc.edu

R.E. Anderson et al. (eds.), *Retinal Degenerative Diseases*, Advances in Experimental Medicine and Biology 664, DOI 10.1007/978-1-4419-1399-9_28, © Springer Science+Business Media, LLC 2010

for the cone channel. Rod CNG channel complex has a stoichiometry of three CNGA1 subunits and one CNGB1 subunit (Weitz et al. 2002) while cone CNG channel is thought to contain two CNGA3 and two CNGB3 subunits (Peng et al. 2004). Like other members of this ion channel family, CNG channel A and B subunits contain six putative membrane-spanning segments, cytoplasmic amino- and carboxyl-termini, a cyclic nucleotide-binding domain, and a conserved pore region. Figure 28.1 shows membrane topology of the mouse CNGA3 subunit.

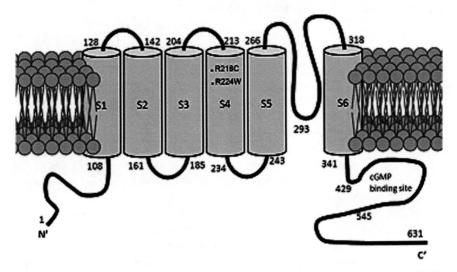

Fig. 28.1 Membrane topology of the mouse CNGA3 with locations of the R218C and R224W mutations indicated. cGMP binding site is between the residue 429 and 545

Cone vision mediated by CNG channel activation is essential for central and color vision and visual acuity. Naturally occurring mutations in *CNGA3* and *CNGB3* are associated with achromatopsia and progressive cone dystrophy (Kohl et al. 1998). Mutations in *CNGA3* and *CNGB3* account for 70% of all mutations found in achromatopsia patients. Nearly 50 mutations have been identified in the CNGA3 subunit. Among these mutations, the R277C and R283W substitutions are identified as the two most frequently occurring mutations (Wissinger et al. 2001). This work investigated the effects of the R277C and R283W mutations on the channel activity and cellular localization using a heterologous expression system. We found that both mutations abolish the channel activity and interfere with the channel plasma membrane localization. Thus the R277C and R283W mutations appear to cause loss of channel function by impairing the channel cellular trafficking and plasma membrane targeting. This work provides experimental evidence for understanding the pathogenesis of R277C and R283W mutations in the CNGA3 subunit.

28.2 Materials and Methods

28.2.1 Constructs, Cell Culture and Transfection

Construct encoding the full-length mouse CNGA3 was generated as we described previously (Ding et al. 2008). The R218C and R224W mutations in the mouse CNGA3 (Fig. 28.1), equivalent to the R277C and R283W mutations in the human CNGA3, respectively, were obtained by site-directed mutagenesis using the Quickchange Site-directed Mutagenesis Kit (Stratagene, La Jolla, CA). Cell culture and transfection was performed as described previously (Ding et al. 2008).

28.2.2 Ratiometric Measurement of Intracellular Ca^{2+} Concentration

The fluorescent indicator indo-1/AM was used to monitor Ca^{2+} influx through CNGA3 channels in cell suspensions. The assays were performed as described previously (Ding et al. 2008) using a PTI QuantaMaster spectrofluorometer (Photon Technology International). Briefly, cells ($\sim$48 h post-transfection) were harvested, washed, and loaded with 2 μM Indo-1/AM (Sigma-Aldrich) for 40 min at room temperature. After loading, cells were washed and resuspended in ECS buffer (140 mM NaCl, 5 mM KCl, 1 mM $MgCl_2$, 1.8 mM $CaCl_2$, 10 mM glucose, and 15 mM HEPES, pH 7.4) (2×10^6) for the assay. Ca^{2+} entry in response to 8-pCPT-cGMP (100 μM) was determined by ratiometric measurement which represents changes of free intracellular Ca^{2+} concentrations (expressed as a $\Delta340/380$ ratio). Data were analyzed and graphed using GraphPad Prism software (GraphPad software, San Diego, CA).

28.2.3 Electrophysiological Recordings

Standard whole-cell patch clamp recordings on cells grown on 35 mm culture dishes were performed as described previously (Malykhina et al. 2006; Fitzgerald et al. 2008). The pipette solution consisted of (in mM): K$^+$ aspartate 100, KCl 30, NaCl 5, $MgCl_2$ 2, Na-ATP 2, EGTA 1, HEPES 5 with pH 7.2 adjusted with KOH. Patch electrodes had resistances of 3–5 MΩ when filled with internal solution. Whole cell currents were recorded by using gap-free protocol with a holding potential at −50 mV. All experiments were performed at room temperature (23°C) and recorded using an Axopatch 200B amplifier (Axon Instrument, Foster City, CA). pCLAMP software (Axon Instruments) was used for data acquisition and analysis.

28.2.4 SDS-PAGE and Western Blot Analysis

SDS-PAGE and Western blot analysis was performed to detect expression of the wild type and mutant CNGA3 subunits using the rabbit polyclonal anti-CNGA3 as described previously (Ding et al. 2008; Matveev et al. 2008).

28.2.5 Immunofluorescence Labeling and Confocal Microscopy

Immunofluorescence labeling was performed as described previously (Ding et al. 2008; Matveev et al. 2008). Briefly cells were grown in DMEM medium on coverslips pre-coated with fibronectin (Sigma-Aldrich). Cells were washed, fixed with 4% (w/v) paraformaldehyde for 10 min at room temperature, and blocked for 1 h at room temperature in 5% BSA. Cells were then incubated with the rat monoclonal anti-CNGA3 (kindly provided by Dr. Benjamin Kaupp at the Institute of Neurosciences and Biophysics, Forschungszentrum, Jülich, Germany) (1:50) overnight at 4°C, followed by incubation with Alexa-conjugated goat anti-rat secondary antibody (1:1,000) for 1 h at room temperature. Vectashield^{TM} containing DAPI stain (Vector Laboratories) was used to mount the coverslips onto the slides.

The fluorescent signals were visualized using a 40X water immersion objective lens on an Olympus IX81-FV500 confocal laser scanning microscope (Olympus, Melville, NY) and analyzed with FluoView imaging software (Olympus) as described previously (Ding et al. 2008). Quantification of fluorescent labeling intensity was performed using FluoView to evaluate cellular distribution of the channel subunits. The plasma membrane localization of the wild type and mutant subunits was determined and expressed in terms of percent of total cellular fluorescence intensity. Data were analyzed and graphed using GraphPad Prism software (GraphPad software, San Diego, CA).

28.3 Results

28.3.1 The R218C and R224W Mutations Cause Loss of Channel Function

The concentration-dependent response of the wild type CNGA3 to cGMP stimulation has been characterized in our previous studies (Ding et al. 2008; Fitzgerald et al. 2008). The channel subunits were expressed in HEK293 cells and the mutation effects on the channel activity were investigated. With the functional assays we found that the two mutations had profound negative effects on the channel activity. As shown in Fig. 28.2a, the intracellular calcium response to cGMP (100 μM) stimulation was completely abolished in cells expressing the R218C mutant. The response in R224W mutant was lowered to less than 10% (as analyzed at 300 sec after cGMP stimulation) of the wild type response (Fig. 28.2a). The deficiency

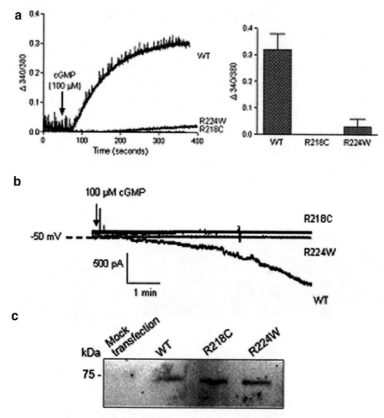

Fig. 28.2 The R218C and R224W mutations cause loss of channel function. **a.** Intracellular calcium response to 8-pCPT-cGMP (100 μM) stimulation in HEK293 cells expressing the wild type (WT), R218C and R224W mutants. The *left panel* shows the representative response curves and the *right panel* is the bar graph showing the quantitative analysis of the calcium measurement (at 300 s after cGMP stimulation) from 3 to 5 independently performed experiments. **b.** Representative patch-clamp recording profiles from HEK293 cells expressing the wild type, R218C and R224W mutants in response to 8-pCPT-cGMP (100 μM) stimulation. **c.** Western blot detection of the wild type, R218C and R224W mutant expression in HEK293 cells that had been transfected with the respective cDNAs

of the mutant channels was also confirmed by electrophysiological recordings. Figure 28.2b shows representative patch clamp recording profiles of the wild type, R218C and R224W mutants in response to 100 μM cGMP stimulation. No current was recorded in cells expressing the mutants, leading to the conclusion that the R218C and R224W mutations abolished the channel activity. While the physiological assays indicated abolished or severely reduced responses, Western blot analysis revealed similar levels of mutant expression when compared to wild type expression (Fig. 28.2c). These data together indicate channel deficiency, not expression levels, as that which contributes to loss of cone function in achromatopsia patients.

28.3.2 The R218C and R224W Mutations Cause Channel Mis-Localization

Immunofluorescence labeling was performed to determine cellular localization of the wild type and mutant channel subunits in cells. From these assays we observed that cells expressing the R218C and R224W mutants showed apparent cytosol aggregation of the immunofluorescent signal (Fig. 28.3a). Quantification analysis of immunofluorescence intensity showed that cells expressing the mutants displayed the decreased plasma membrane labeling compared to cells expressing the wild type subunit (Fig. 28.3b). This data indicates the mislocalization of mutants is a contributing factor to decreased cone function.

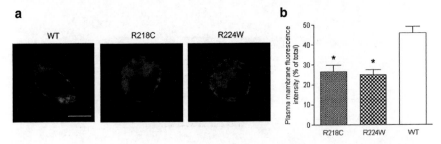

Fig. 28.3 The R218C and R224W mutations cause channel mis-localization. **a.** Representative confocal images showing cellular localization of the wild type, R218C and R224W mutants in HEK293 cells. Scale bar: 10 μm. **b.** The bar graph shows the quantitative analysis results of the plasma membrane fluorescence labeling intensities. *Bars* represent the means ± SEM of the number of cells (12 for the wild type, 15 for the R218C transfected, and 15 for the R224W transfected) from 3 independently performed experiments. Unpaired Student's t test was used for determination of the significance.*, $p < 0.05$

28.3.3 Co-Expression of The R218C and R224W Mutants with the Wild Type Channel Does Not Affect the Channel Activity

We examined the effects of co-expression of the mutant channel subunits with the wild type channel on the channel activity. Cells were co-transfected with equal amounts of the wild type cDNA and the mutant cDNA or pcDNA3.1 (the channel harboring plasmid) (10 μg of each per 100 mm dish) and assayed for intracellular calcium response to cGMP stimulation ~48 h post-transfection. From these assays we found that co-expression of the mutant channel with the wild type channel did not affect the wild type channel's activity. As shown in Fig. 28.4 the calcium responses to cGMP stimulation in cells co-expressing the wild type with R218C (Fig. 28.4a) or R224W (Fig. 28.4b) mutants were almost indistinguishable from those in cells expressing the wild type channel alone. This data indicates that the wild type channels do not form heterodimers with mutant channels. Or it indicates that the wild type/mutant heterodimers do form but the wild type channels are dominant in the complex.

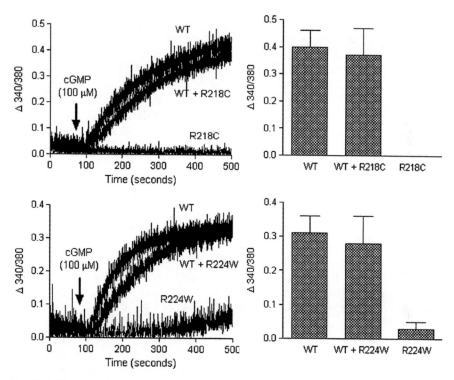

Fig. 28.4 Co-expression of the R218C or R224W mutants with the wild type subunit does not affect the channel activity. HEK293 cells were co-transfected with equal amounts of the wild type and R218C (**a**) or R224W (**b**) mutants and assayed for calcium response to 8-pCPT-cGMP (100 μM) stimulation ~48 h post-transfection. Shown in the *left panels* are the representative response curves and the *right panels* are the bar graphs showing the quantitative analysis of the calcium measurement at 400 s after 8-pCPT-cGMP stimulation from 3 to 6 independently performed experiments

28.4 Discussion

Achromatopsia is an inherited disorder that affects approximately 1 in every 33,000 Americans. The condition is associated with color blindness, visual acuity loss, extreme light sensitivity and nystagmus. To date, mutations in three genes, *CNGA3*, *CNGB3* and *Gnat2,* have been identified in achromatopsia patients. Indeed mutations in cone CNG channel are highly linked to various forms of achromatopsia and other types of cone degenerative diseases including early onset macular degeneration and progressive cone dystrophy. There are nearly 70 disease-causing mutations in *CNGA3* and *CNGB3* and these mutations account for 70% of the achromatopsia patients (Kohl et al. 1998; Wissinger et al. 2001; Nishiguchi et al. 2005).

Efforts are being made to explore the mechanism underlying the disease-causing mutations in cone CNG channel. Patel et al. (Patel et al. 2005) studied 4 mutations (Y181C, N182Y, L186F, and C191Y) in the S1 segment of human CNGA3.

They showed that the mutations resulted in loss of channel function and that the full-length mutant channel subunits were synthesized but were retained in the endoplasmic reticulum. They proposed a role of the S1 segment in both maturation and function of CNG channels. Faillace et al. (Faillace et al. 2004) studied 4 mutations (F294L, R296Q, N295Q, R302W; sequences in bovine CNGA3) in the S4 segment and demonstrated that the mutant channel failed to become glycosylated and arrive at the plasma membrane. This work implicated a role of the S4 segment in the channel proper intracellular processing and trafficking. Liu et al. (Liu and Varnum 2005) described an alteration in the channel membrane localization and gating properties in the two C-terminal mutants (N471S and R563H). Thus these studies suggest that an impaired cellular processing and membrane targeting is a common mechanism for a variety of mutations located at distinct regions of the channel subunit. The present work investigated the effects of the R218C and R224W mutations on the channel activity and cellular localization and showed that both mutations abolished the channel activity and interfered with the channel plasma membrane localization. These results are consistent with the previous findings by Faillace et al. (Faillace et al. 2004), supporting the view that S4 segment is critical for the channel cellular processing. With co-expression experiments we observed that co-expression of the mutant channel with the wild type subunit did not affect the wild type channel's activity. This observation is consistent with the clinical findings in which individuals with the heterozygous mutations show normal cone function and only individuals with homozygous mutations or compound heterozygous mutations experience cone defect symptoms. The channel subunit encoded by one wild type allele appears sufficient to maintain the normal channel activity. This observation may also suggest that the mutant channel subunits lack the ability to be recruited into the channel complexes.

Acknowledgments This work was supported by grants from the National Center For Research Resources (P20RR017703), the National Eye Institute (P30EY12190), the American Health Assistance Foundation, and the Presbyterian Health Foundation. We thank Dr. Benjamin Kaupp for providing the monoclonal anti-CNGA3 antibody.

References

Ding XQ, Fitzgerald JB, Matveev AV et al (2008) Functional activity of photoreceptor cyclic nucleotide-gated channels is dependent on the integrity of cholesterol- and sphingolipid-enriched membrane domains. Biochemistry 47:3677–3687

Faillace MP, Bernabeu RO, Korenbrot JI (2004) Cellular processing of cone photoreceptor cyclic GMP-gated ion channels: a role for the S4 structural motif. J Biol Chem 279: 22643–22653

Fitzgerald JB, Malykhina AP, Al-Ubaidi MR et al (2008) Functional expression of cone cyclic nucleotide-gated channel in cone photoreceptor-derived 661 W cells. Adv Exp Med Biol 613:327–334

Kohl S, Marx T, Giddings I et al (1998) Total colourblindness is caused by mutations in the gene encoding the alpha-subunit of the cone photoreceptor cGMP-gated cation channel. Nat Genet 19:257–259

Liu C, Varnum MD (2005) Functional consequences of progressive cone dystrophy-associated mutations in the human cone photoreceptor cyclic nucleotide-gated channel CNGA3 subunit. Am J Physiol Cell Physiol 289:C187–C198

Malykhina AP, Qin C, Greenwood-van Meerveld B et al (2006) Hyperexcitability of convergent colon and bladder dorsal root ganglion neurons after colonic inflammation: mechanism for pelvic organ cross-talk. Neurogastroenterol Motil 18:936–948

Matveev AV, Quiambao AB, Fitzgerald JB et al (2008) Native cone photoreceptor cyclic nucleotide-gated channel is a heterotetrameric complex comprising both CNGA3 and CNGB3: a study using the cone-dominant retina of Nrl–/– mice. J Neurochem 106(5):2042–2055

Nishiguchi KM, Sandberg MA, Gorji N et al (2005) Cone cGMP-gated channel mutations and clinical findings in patients with achromatopsia, macular degeneration, and other hereditary cone diseases. Hum Mutat 25:248–258

Patel KA, Bartoli KM, Fandino RA et al (2005) Transmembrane S1 mutations in CNGA3 from achromatopsia 2 patients cause loss of function and impaired cellular trafficking of the cone CNG channel. Invest Ophthalmol Vis Sci 46:2282–2290

Peng C, Rich ED, Varnum MD (2004) Subunit configuration of heteromeric cone cyclic nucleotide-gated channels. Neuron 42:401–410

Weitz D, Ficek N, Kremmer E et al (2002) Subunit stoichiometry of the CNG channel of rod photoreceptors. Neuron 36:881–889

Wissinger B, Gamer D, Jagle H et al (2001) CNGA3 mutations in hereditary cone photoreceptor disorders. Am J Hum Genet 69:722–737

Chapter 29
Mutation Spectra in Autosomal Dominant and Recessive Retinitis Pigmentosa in Northern Sweden

Irina Golovleva, Linda Köhn, Marie Burstedt, Stephen Daiger, and Ola Sandgren

Abstract Retinal degenerations represent a heterogeneous group of disorders affecting the function of the retina. The frequency of retinitis pigmentosa (RP) is 1/3500 worldwide, however, in northern Sweden it is 1/2000 due to limited migration and a 'founder' effect. In this study we identified genetic mechanisms underlying autosomal dominant and recessive RP present in northern Sweden. Several novel mutations unique for this region were found. In an autosomal recessive form of RP, Bothnia dystrophy caused by mutations in the *RLBP1* gene, bi-allelic mutations R234W, M226K and compound heterozygosity, M226K+R234W was detected.

In dominant form of RP mapped to 19q13.42 a 59 kb genomic deletion including the *PRPF31* and three other genes was found.

These data provide additional information on the molecular mechanisms of RP evolvement and in the future might be useful in development of therapeutic strategies. Identification of the disease-causing mutations allowed introducing molecular genetic testing of the patients and their families into the clinical practice.

29.1 Introduction

Retinitis pigmentosa (RP) is a group of inherited retinal disorders with a considerable genetic variation. Typical signs of the disease are night blindness and progressive loss of the peripheral visual field, characteristic pigment deposition in the retina, attenuation of the retinal blood vessels, and optic disc pallor.

A form of autosomal dominant RP (adRP) in patients with night blindness in the first and second decade, progressive visual field loss in later life, along with asymptomatic individuals though having an affected parent and an affected child was mapped to 19q13.4 (Al-Maghtheh et al., 1994) (RP11, MIM 600138). A putative human ortholog of yeast pre m-RNA splicing factor, *PRPF31* was reported

---

I. Golovleva (✉)
Department of Medical and Clinical Genetics, Medical Biosciences, Umeå University, 901 85, Umeå, Sweden
e-mail: irina.golovleva@medbio.umu.se

R.E. Anderson et al. (eds.), *Retinal Degenerative Diseases*, Advances in Experimental Medicine and Biology 664, DOI 10.1007/978-1-4419-1399-9_29,
© Springer Science+Business Media, LLC 2010

as a disease causing gene (Vithana et al., 2001). To date 42 *PRPF31* mutations are listed in the Human Genome Mutation Database and among these only 9 are missense, while the rest are deletions, insertions, indels and splicing mutations (http://www.hgmd.cf.ac.uk/ac/all.php).The majority of the mutations would result in truncated proteins due to exon skipping and premature stop codons (Vithana et al., 2001; Martinez-Gimeno et al., 2003; Sato et al. 2005; Sullivan et al., 2006), therefore, haploinsuffiency was suggested as a mechanism of RP11 evolvement (Vithana et al., 2001).

A rather large group of patients with a variant of autosomal recessive RP (arRP), Bothnia dystrophy (BD) (MIM 180090) has been identified in northern Sweden (Burstedt et al. 1999; 2001). The phenotype is characterized by night blindness in early childhood, retinitis punctata albescens (RPA) in young adulthood and a progressive macular and peripheral retinal degeneration (Burstedt et al. 2001).

The disease was reported to be associated with a bi-allelic c.700C>T mutation in the *RLBP1* gene (p.R234W). The majority of the reported cases carried *RLBP1* mutations in homozygous state although compound heterozygotes have also been described (http://www.hgmd.cf.ac.uk/ac/all.php). Sequence changes involving single nucleotides are not the only type of mutation affecting the *RLBP1* gene. In a patient with RPA a large homozygous deletion was recently described (Humbert et al. 2006).

In our inventory work on retinal dystrophies in northern Sweden, we found among patients with a BD phenotype homozygotes and heterozygotes for the c.700C>T mutation. The patients heterozygous for the c.700C>T mutation appeared to be carriers of the second mutation in the *RLBP1* gene, c.677T>A.

Thus, in this study we report a novel genomic deletion including almost the entire *PRPF31* gene in two families with adRP linked to 19q13.42 and compound heterozygosity in the *RLBP1* gene in arRP of Bothnia type.

29.2 Materials and Methods

29.2.1 Patients and Ophthalmologic Examinations

Patients residing in the four counties of northern Sweden with a population of 880,000 were included in this study. All of them had a history of night blindness and a clinical diagnosis of either arRP or adRP. The study followed the tenets of the Declaration of Helsinki, and consent was obtained from all individuals. Standard ophthalmologic examination included fundus photography and visual field testing. Dark adaptation tests and full-field ERGs were performed in selected cases.

29.2.2 Molecular Genetic Analysis

DNA was extracted from peripheral blood and used for linkage analysis with the ABI PRISM Linkage Mapping set version 2.5 (Applied Biosystems) as described elsewhere (Köhn et al. 2007). Sequence analysis of coding exons and adjacent intronic sequences of candidate genes was performed as described by Köhn et al. (2007). The products of the sequencing reactions obtained with Big Dye® Terminator v3.1 Cycle Sequencing Kit (Applied Biosystems) were run on a 3730 xl DNA analyzer (Applied Biosystems).

DNA from two BD patients carrying the *RLBP1* c.700C>T mutation on one allele were subjected to microarray genotyping designed and manufactured according to the APEX technology (Pastinen et al. 1997). (http://www.asperbio.com). Genetic testing was performed using the arRP array for both patients and in addition patient 223:3 was analysed with the autosomal dominant retinitis pigmentosa (adRP) array taking into account that only one mutation was detected in the BD patients. The arRP array included testing for 501 known mutations in 16 genes. adRP panel comprised 347 mutations in 13 genes (information about testing is available on http://www.asperophthalmics.com).

MLPA was done according to Sullivan et al. (2006) with a set of probes designed by this group in combination with the Retinitis Pigmentosa Kit (MRC Holland, http://www.mrc-holland.com/pages/indexpag.html). Additionally, we used *VSTM1* probe with following sequences forward 5′ – GGGTTCCCTAA GGGTTGGAccttcacggacctgaagcctaaggatgctgggag; reverse 5′ – gtactttgtgcctacaa-gacaacagcctcccatgagtggTCTAGATTGGATCTTGCTGGCAC (DNA Technology, Denmark). The collected raw data were analysed with ABI Prism GeneMapper Software v3.0 (Applied Biosystems). The ratio of 1.0 indicates the presence of two alleles (normal diploid) and 0.5 or 1.5 suggests either deletion or duplication of the target sequence, respectively. The breakpoint region was defined using long range PCR across the deletion with forward primer *VSTM* F1 5′– GATAGAGGAGGTTTTGCTCTGAC and reverse primer *PRPF31* 13R 5′ – CGGACCCTGCAGAAGCAGAGCGTCGTAT. PCR product was cloned into pGEM-T Easy (Promega) vector and positive clones were sequenced. Allele specific PCR on genomic DNA was done as described elsewhere using specific primers for both mutant and wild type alleles (BP-F 5′ – TGAAAGAGAGAAGGGGCTCA, BP-R 5′ – GTGGCCTCGTTTACCTGTGT, cDNA *PRPF31* 12F 5′ – ATCGAGGAGGACGCCT).

29.3 Results and Discussion

29.3.1 *adRP*

In one of two families with adRP at least 2 individuals were obligate carri-ers of the mutation since they had both an affected parent and offspring (VII:8, VII:15) (Fig. 29.1). Significant LOD scores with a maximum of 7.58 at the marker D19S926 at 19q13.42 were revealed in the region spanning nearly 1.77 Mb. The reconstructed haplotypes in both families confirmed segregation of adRP with markers D19S924, D19S927, D19S926, D19S418 and D19S605. Since no disease causing mutations were detected by PCR-based methods in *RDH13, SYT5, PPP1R12C, PRKCG, CACNG6, 7, 8* and *PRPF31*genes we considered testing for large genomic deletions using MLPA examining *PRPF31, RHO, RP1,* and *IMPDH1* genes. A large genomic deletion including *TFPT, NDUFA3, OSCAR* genes and 11 exons of the *PRPF31* gene was detected (Fig. 29.2). Based on the MLPA results indicating a normal ratio for the *VSTM1* probe and probes for exons 12-14 of the *PRPF31*, we applied a long range PCR with *VSTM1* and exon 13 *PRPF31* primers (Fig. 29.2b) and obtained a ~7 kb PCR fragment. Sequencing of this product revealed a deletion of 58,733 nucleotides with breakpoints in intron 11 of the *PRPF31* gene and in LOC441864 (ref|NT_011109.15|Hs19_11266), similar to osteoclast-associated receptor isoform 5 (Fig. 29.2b–d). Allele specific PCR with primers set shown at Fig. 29.2c revealed presence of the mutation in affected individuals, obligatory carriers and also several asymptomatic members (Fig. 29.1b). None of 20 simplex adRP cases or 94 healthy controls (188 control chromosomes) from the matched population demonstrated the mutant allele (data not shown).

PRPF31 codes for a protein needed for splicing in all cell types although its pathologic effect is seen only in rod photoreceptors, causing adRP with incomplete penetrance. PRPF31 is a 61 kDa protein, part of the U4/U6-U5 tri-snRNP complex (Makarova et al. 2002). The proposed mechanism of adRP (RP11) evolvement is haploinsufficiency rather than a dominant negative effect (Vithana et al. 2001). Identification of the large genomic deletion with almost entire loss of *PRPF31* gene

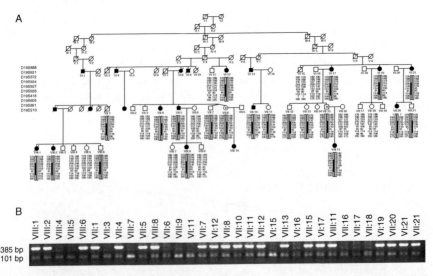

Fig. 29.1 Haplotype analysis (**a**) and segregation of the mutation (**b**) in the family 78. **a** – filled symbols indicate affected individuals, while empty symbols indicate unaffected. Symbols with represent an asymptomatic gene carrier. Only disease haplotypes shared by affected individuals in both families are boxed. **b** – allele-specific PCR where a band of 385 bp indicates the mutant allele and a band of 101 bp indicates presence of the internal PCR control, as a result of wild type and mutant allele's amplification

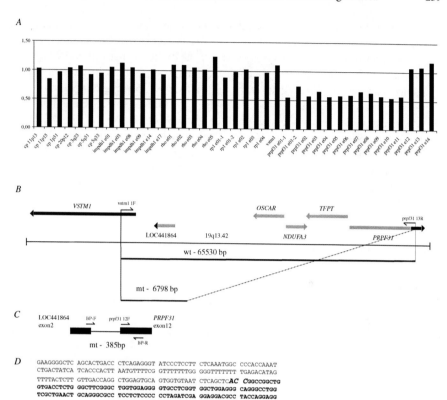

Fig. 29.2 Genomic deletion including *PRPF31* gene in adRP. **a** – a deletion detected by MLPA in VII:20 from family 078. **a** P235 Retinitis Pigmentosa kit (MRC Holland) along with the *VSTM1* probe was applied. The graph indicates presence of one gene copy with probes for exons 1–11 in the *PRPF31* gene (ratio is ~0.5). Two gene copies are present with the probes for *IMPDH1, RHO, RP1* and for exons 12–14 in the *PRPF31* (ratio is ~1.0). **b** – schematic representation of the genomic region 19q13.42 in proximity to *PRPF31*. PCR primers *VSTM1* 1F and *PRPF31* 13R were applied to amplify across the deleted region (the estimated size of a wild type allele is 65,530 bp and can not be amplified by PCR). PCR fragment of ~7 kb (mutant allele) was obtained by long range PCR, subcloned into pGEM-T Easy vector and sequenced. **c** – localisation of allele specific primers. Primers sequences and allele specific PCR are described in Materials and Methods and Results and Discussion. PCR with allele-specific primers BP-F and BP-R primers used for segregation analysis (Figs. 29.1B and 29.2B) resulted in 385 bp fragment representing a mutant allele. **d** – a partial sequence across the deletion. Nucleotide sequence belonging to the predicted gene 'similar to osteoclast-associated receptor isoform 5' and intron 11 in the *PRPF31* gene is shown. ACC at breakpoint shown in bold can be part of either LOC441864 or *PRPF31*

in this study provides additional evidence for haploinsuffciency as the mechanism in adRP pathogenesis.

Molecular methods used for mutation detection are mainly based on PCR and, therefore, large genomic rearrangements are easily missed. The deletion encompassing almost 59 kb of genomic sequence includes three genes additional to *PRPF31* and breakpoints occur in intron 11 of *PRPF31* and within the predicted gene, LOC441864, annotated as 'similar to osteoclast-associated receptor isoform 5'. A number of *Alu*-repeats in *PRPF31* introns can prone to internal unequal recombination resulting in a deletion; however the exact mechanism is not known.

Due to the size of the deletion we could expect a severe phenotype in our families as reported previously (Abu-Safieh et al. 2006). However, among our patients there were individuals with quite preserved visual fields and recordable ERGs at their 50 s. No additional symptoms associated with the genetic defects in *NDUFA3*, *TFPT* or *OSCAR* was observed. In conclusion, identification of such large deletion involving the *PRPF31* gene reveals additional evidence that haploinsufficiency is a molecular mechanism of evolvement of adRP with incomplete penetrance. Identification of deletion breakpoint provides an important tool for molecular testing and genetic counselling of these patients.

29.3.2 Bothnia Dystrophy

67 out of 121 individuals affected with arRP were homozygous and 10 were heterozygous for the c.700C>T mutation in the *RLBP1*. Simultaneous evaluation of 501 mutations known as a cause of arRP performed by arrayed APEX technology in two BD patients (027:4 and 223:3, Fig. 29.3a) revealed besides the one known to us

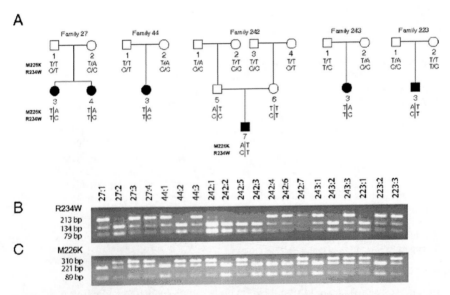

Fig. 29.3 Allelic c.677T>A and c.700C>T mutations in families to probands diagnosed with arRP of Bothnia dystrophy. Detection of both mutations was done by PCR-RFLP. **a.** Pedigree charts of 5 families where filled symbols indicate affected individuals, while empty symbols indicate unaffected. **b.** c.700C>T mutation abolishes a *Msp*I restriction site and results in one fragment of 213 bp. **c.** c.677T>A mutation abolishes a *Nsp*I restriction site and results in one fragment of 310 bp

RLBP1 c.700C>T (p.R234W) a second mutation, c.677T>A, resulting in p.M226K. Segregation analysis in five tested families showed that c.700C>T and c.677T>A were allelic and the patients were compound heterozygotes, [677T>A]+[700C>T] (Fig. 29.3). None of BD patients homozygous for c.700C>T carried c.677T>A mutation. Allele frequency of the c.677T>A mutation was 1 in 233. Two homozygotes for the *RLBP1* c.677T>A mutation were found in RP population from northern Sweden.

Testing of a BD patient (223:3) with the adRP panel which included 347 known mutations in 13 genes resulted in detection of only one sequence change, c.40C>T in exon 1 of carbonic anhydrase, *CAIV* (p.R14W). The p.R14W mutation was reported as a cause of adRP, RP17 (Rebello et al. 2004; Yang et al. 2005). Testing of all compound *RLBP1* heterozygotes for the presence of c.40C>T revealed absence of the *CAIV* c.40C>T in nine carriers of *RLBP1* c.[677T>A]+[700C>T] while its presence was detected in 223:3 and his unaffected mother (223:2). 6 carriers of *CAIV* c.40C>T were detected among 143 healthy blood donors (data not shown).

29.4 Conclusions

The prevalence of nonsyndromic RP is approximately 1/2000 in Västerbotten County in the northern part of Sweden. This can be explained by 'founder' effect, isolation of population in small villages and low migration rate. To date, at least 40 causative genes and loci have been identified in nonsyndromic RP but one can expect that only a limited number of mutated genes causes retinal degenerations in such populations like the northern Swedish.

We identified a large group of patients with similar clinical appearance and an identical underlying genetic defect. 67 patients have a biallelic mutation in the *RLBP1* gene, c.700C>T (p.R234W). Molecular testing in 10 patients with a phenotype similar to BD revealed two mutations, c.700C>T and c.677T>A. Based on allele frequency of c.700C>T (3/200) and c.677T>A (1/233) in a control population we expect that c.700C>T was the first mutation to appear in northern Sweden. Analysis of all ten c.[677T>A]+[700C>T] BD patients and 143 healthy control individuals for the p.R14W mutation in CAIV revealed the presence of this sequence variant in 4% of the population from northern Sweden. The phenotype of the *RLBP1* compound heterozygote carrying also CAIV p.R14W could not be distinguished from the other BD patients and no signs of retinal degenerative changes were detected in his 61 year-old mother carrying the same sequence variant.

In summary, the high frequency of arRP observed in northern Sweden is due to the presence of two mutations in the *RLBP1* gene, c.677T>A and c.700C>T. The patients are either homozygotes or compound heterozygotes. All 79 patients originating from Västerbotten County, with a population of 257,000 inhabitants presented the BD-like phenotype. Bothnia dystrophy is caused by loss of CRALBP function due to changed physical features and impaired activity of retinoid binding.

The CAIV p.R14W known as a cause of RP17 found in one of BD patients is not pathogenic in population of northern Sweden.

Furthermore, a novel mutation unique in patients of Swedish origin, a large genomic deletion resulting in almost entire loss of *PRPF31*and three additional genes was identified as the cause of adRP with reduced penetrance. Identification of the deletion breakpoints allowed development of a simple tool for molecular testing of this genetic subtype of adRP.

References

Abu-Safieh L, Vithana EN, Mantel I et al (2006) A large deletion in the adRP gene PRPF31: evidence that haploinsufficiency is the cause of disease. Mol Vis 12:384–388

Al-Maghtheh M, Inglehearn CF, Keen TJ et al (1994) Identification of a sixth locus for autosomal dominant retinitis pigmentosa on chromosome 19. Hum Mol Genet 3:351–354

Burstedt MSI, Forsman-Semb K, Golovleva I et al (2001) Ocular phenotype of Bothnia dystrophy, an autosomal recessive retinitis pigmentosa associated with an P.R234Wmutation in the *RLBP1* gene. Arch Ophthalmol 119:260–267

Burstedt MSI, Sandgren O, Holmgren G et al (1999) Bothnia dystrophy caused by mutation in the cellular retinaldehyde-binding protein gene (*RLBP1*) on chromosome 15q26. Invest Ophthalmol Visl Sci 40:995–1000

Humbert G, Delettre C, Senechal A et al (2006) Homozygous deletion related to Alu repeats in *RLBP1* causes retinitis punctata albescens. Invest Ophthalmol Vis Sci 47:4719–4724

Köhn L, Kadzhaev K, Burstedt MSI et al (2007) Mutation in PYK2-binding domain of the PITPNM3 causes autosomal dominant cone dystrophy (CORD5). Eur J Hum Genet 15: 664–671

Makarova OV, Makarov EM, Liu S et al (2002) Protein 61 K, encoded by a gene (PRPF31) linked to autosomal dominant retinitis pigmentosa, is required for U4/U6*U5 tri-snRNP formation and pre-mRNA splicing. EMBO J 21:1148–1157

Martinez-Gimeno M, Gamundi MJ, Hernan I et al (2003) Mutations in the pre-mRNA splicing-factor genes PRPF3, PRPF8, and PRPF31 in Spanish families with autosomal dominant retinitis pigmentosa. Invest Ophthalmol Vis Sci 44:2171–2177

Pastinen T, Kurg A, Metspalu A et al (1997) Minisequencing: a specific tool for DNA analysis and diagnostics on oligonucleotide arrays. Genome Res 7:606–614

Rebello G, Ramesar R, Vorster A et al (2004) Apoptosis-inducing signal sequence mutation in carbonic anhydrase IV identified in patients with the RP17 form of retinitis pigmentosa. Proc Natl Acad Sci USA 101:6617–6622

Sato H, Wada Y, Itabashi T, Nakamura M, Kawamura M, Tamai M (2005) Mutations in the pre-mRNA splicing gene, PRPF31, in Japanese families with autosomal dominant retinitis pigmentosa. Am J Ophthalmol 140:537–540

Sullivan LS, Bowne SJ, Seaman CR et al (2006) Genomic rearrangements of the PRPF31 gene account for 2.5% of autosomal dominant retinitis pigmentosa. Invest Ophthalmol Vis Sci 47:4579–4588

Vithana EN, Abu-Safieh L, Allen MJ et al (2001) A human homolog of yeast pre-mRNA splicing gene, PRPF31, underlies autosomal dominant retinitis pigmentosa on chromosome 19q13.4 (RP11). Mol Cell 8:375–381

Yang Z, Alvarez BV, Chakarova C et al (2005) Mutant carbonic anhydrase 4 impairs pH regulation and causes retinal photoreceptor degeneration. Hum Mol Genet 14:255–265

Chapter 30
1 Rhodopsin Mutations in Congenital Night Blindness

Suzanne D. McAlear, Timothy W. Kraft, and Alecia K. Gross

Abstract While there are over 100 distinct mutations in the rhodopsin gene that are found in patients with the degenerative disease autosomal dominant retinitis pigmentosa (ADRP), there are only four known mutations in the rhodopsin gene found in patients with the dysfunction congenital stationary night blindness (CSNB). CSNB patients have a much less severe phenotype than those with ADRP; the patients only lose rod function which affects their vision under dim light conditions, whereas their cone function remains relatively unchanged. The known rhodopsin CSNB mutations are found clustered around the site of retinal attachment. Two of the mutations encode replacements of neutral amino acids with negatively charged ones (A292E and G90D), and the remaining two are neutral amino acid replacements (T94I and A295V). All four of these mutations have been shown to constitutively activate the apoprotein in vitro. The mechanisms by which these mutations lead to night blindness are still not known with certainty, and remain the subject of some controversy. The dominant nature of these genetic defects, as well as the relative normalcy of vision in individuals with half the complement of wild type rhodopsin, suggest that it is an active property of the mutant opsin proteins that leads to defective rod vision rather than a loss of some needed function. Herein, we review the known biochemical and electrophysiological data for the four known rhodopsin mutations found in patients with CSNB.

30.1 Introduction

Rhodopsin is the dim-light visual pigment found in rod cells of the vertebrate retina. It is composed of an apoprotein opsin and its ligand, 11-*cis* retinal, which is covalently attached to the protein through a protonated Schiff base linkage to

A.K. Gross (✉)
University of Alabama at Birmingham, WORB 618, 924 18th Street South, Birmingham, AL 35295, USA
e-mail: agross@uab.edu

R.E. Anderson et al. (eds.), *Retinal Degenerative Diseases*, Advances in Experimental Medicine and Biology 664, DOI 10.1007/978-1-4419-1399-9_30,
© Springer Science+Business Media, LLC 2010

lysine 296 in the seventh transmembrane helix. While there are over 100 distinct mutations in the rhodopsin gene that are found in patients with the degenerative disease autosomal dominant retinitis pigmentosa (ADRP), there are only four known rhodopsin mutations found in patients with the dysfunction congenital stationary night blindness (CSNB). All four of these display a dominant pattern of inheritance (adCSNB). CSNB patients have a much less severe phenotype than those with ADRP; the patients only lose rod function which affects their vision under dim light conditions, whereas their cone function remains relatively unchanged. The known rhodopsin CSNB mutations are found clustered around the site of retinal attachment. Two of the mutations encode replacements of neutral amino acids with negatively charged ones (A292E and G90D), and the remaining two are neutral amino acid replacements (T94I and A295V). All four of these mutations have been shown to constitutively activate the apoprotein in vitro. The mechanisms by which these mutations lead to night blindness are still not known with certainty and remain the subject of some controversy. The dominant nature of these genetic defects, as well as the relative normalcy of photopic vision in individuals with half the complement of wild type (WT) rhodopsin (Dryja et al. 1993; Sieving et al. 1995; al-Jandal et al. 1999; Zeitz et al. 2008), suggest that it is an active property of the mutant opsin proteins that leads to defective rod vision rather than a loss of some needed function. Biochemical studies of the mutant rhodopsins have been carried out on recombinant proteins expressed in cultured mammalian cells, and electrophysiology has been carried out on transgenic animals expressing them. In addition, results from electroretinography studies (ERG) of rod-driven responses in patients add to our understanding of how these proteins function in the human rods. Herein, we review the known biochemical and electrophysiological data for the four known rhodopsin mutations found in patients with CSNB.

30.2 Properties of Rhodopsin CSNB Mutants

30.2.1 Spectral and Photochemical Properties

All vertebrate rod pigments share the same basic structure: a 40 kDa apoprotein arranged in seven transmembrane (TM) helices, with a chromophore attached *via* a protonated Schiff base bond on a conserved Lys residue on TM7. The positive charge on the Schiff base nitrogen is stabilized through an electrostatic interaction, or salt bridge, with the carboxylate on the counterion Glu113 (Sakmar et al. 1989; Nathans 1990; Zhukovsky et al. 1992). This negative charge perturbs the pKa of the Schiff base to ~16 (Steinberg et al. 1993), so that it is always protonated under physiological conditions. Upon absorption of a photon, 11-*cis* retinal isomerizes to all-*trans* retinal, causing a series of conformational and spectrophotometrically detectable changes to occur, ultimately leading to the active conformation of photoexcited rhodopsin, metarhodopsin II (MII). To reset rhodopsin back to its dark state, the Schiff base between Lys296 and all-*trans* retinal is hydrolyzed, and the chromophore dissociates, allowing a new molecule of 11-*cis* retinal to bind to the active site and covalently attach to Lys296.

While opsin alone does not absorb light in the visible region, 11-*cis* retinal free in solution has a λ_{max} of 380 nm, and an 11-*cis* retinal protonated Schiff base (PSB) molecule, such as an 'acid-trapped' acid-denatured rhodopsin, has a λ_{max} of 440 nm. In rods, dark rhodopsin absorbs maximally at 500 nm. The difference in the λ_{max} values of the pigment from that of the PSB free in solution has been termed the 'opsin-shift' (Nakanishi et al. 1980). The active conformation of the receptor, MII, absorbs maximally at 380 nm, characteristic of an unprotonated Schiff base.

The absorbance spectrum of A292E rhodopsin is similar to that of WT rhodopsin (Dryja et al. 1993). However, the absorption maxima of the other three CSNB mutants are shifted towards the blue: G90D absorbs maximally at 483 nm (Rao et al. 1994), T94I at 478 nm (Gross et al. 2003), and A295V at 482 nm (Zeitz et al. 2008). The slight blue-shift in the absorption spectrum indicates the retinal binding interaction has been perturbed slightly in these mutants. All four rhodopsin CSNB mutants are photobleachable with visible light to yield a MII species that absorbs maximally at 380 nm, indicative of an unprotonated Schiff base attachment.

Another indication that the structure of G90D rhodopsin is significantly different from that of WT rhodopsin is shown through hydroxylamine treatment. Dark WT rhodopsin is resistant to chemical bleach by hydroxylamine treatment, whereas G90D rhodopsin reacts with hydroxylamine, yielding a retinal oxime with a λ_{max} = 367 nm (Sieving et al. 2001). This result implies that the retinal binding pocket is more accessible to hydroxylamine in the G90D mutant, and therefore may be structurally more similar to MII.

30.2.2 Retinal Binding Kinetics of Rhodopsin CSNB Mutants

Another measurable property of rhodopsin that distinguishes the CSNB mutants from one another is the kinetics of regeneration. Using stopped-flow spectrophotometry on detergent solubilized and purified rhodopsin mutants in the context of a stabilizing mutation N2C, D282C which is known to significantly increase the stability of the apoprotein (Xie et al. 2003), the rate of the Schiff base formation upon addition of 11-*cis* retinal to opsin was found to be 80-fold slower for the G90D mutant than for WT opsin, but not for the A292E or T94I mutants (Gross et al. 2003). This effect is likely due to interference with the salt bridge between Lys296 and the counterion Glu113 that holds the protein in an inactive conformation. Even though the acidic amino acid glutamate is introduced at position 292, it does not seem to interfere with the salt bridge in the same manner.

Another property important for rhodopsin function that can be measured spectrophotometrically is the rate of MII decay, which must precede regeneration in functioning rods. For A292E and G90D that generate a protonated MII upon exposure to light, the rate of MII decay was determined after exposure to light passed through a 480 nm cut-on filter, followed by recording successive spectra until no further absorbance decrease was observed. For samples that bleach immediately to 380 nm maximum with an unprotonated MII after exposure to light (such as WT, T94I and A295V), the rate of MII decay is measured by taking into consideration that 11-*cis* retinal binds faster than MII decays. The rhodopsin in the sample was selectively activated in the presence of excess 11-*cis* retinal, and the rate of regeneration of the photopigment was monitored. The MII decay was 8-fold slower for T94I (Gross et al. 2003) and 1.7-fold slower for A295V (Zeitz et al. 2008). However, slower MII decay is unlikely to affect the in vivo night blindness phenotype because the signal termination by phosphorylation of the receptor and arrestin binding occurs faster than MII decays (Ng and Henikoff 2001).

30.2.3 Activity of CSNB Mutants

The ability of the rod visual system to detect single photons requires that rhodopsin remains dormant in the dark; indeed this is the case. The half-life for spontaneous activation of rhodopsin is ~49 years (Baylor et al. 1980). However, because each rod contains 10^8 rhodopsin molecules, thermal activation results in spontaneous fluctuations of activity that resemble single-photon events, on the order of every 100–200 s in dark-adapted rods (Baylor et al. 1984). Dark noise measurements indicate that rod noise limits behavioral sensitivity and sets the limit for absolute sensitivity of vision. If rhodopsin thermal activity were increased only a small amount (Barlow 1988) or if a genetic mutation resulted in constitutively active opsins (Rao et al. 1994), the aberrant signals generated within the rod would compete with dim external stimuli and desensitize night vision. The mechanism by which the four known rhodopsin mutations cause the underlying pathophysiology in CSNB patients remains the subject of some controversy, but one hypothesis is that their ability to activate the phototransduction cascade without bound all-*trans* retinal plays an important role. The highly amplified nature of this cascade means that low levels of activity may have significant physiological consequences.

30.2.3.1 In Vitro *Assays of CSNB Mutants*

One striking common phenotype of the four known CSNB rhodopsin mutations is that they constitutively activate transducin, the G-protein coupled to rhodopsin, in vitro. When 11-*cis* retinal is bound, all of the CSNB rhodopsin mutants activate transducin with kinetics similar to that of WT rhodopsin (Dryja et al. 1993; Rao et al. 1994; Gross et al. 2003; Zeitz et al. 2008); i.e., there is no detectable activity in the dark, but very high levels upon photoisomerization to all-*trans* retinal. However, a difference is observed in the absence of chromophore. While WT opsin does not activate transducin under the conditions of the assay, all of the known rhodopsin CSNB mutants activate transducin in the absence of chromophore and light, a property referred to as constitutive activation. There is a range of constitutive activation among the mutants: A292E > G90D ≈ A295V > T94I.

30.2.3.2 Electrophysiological Studies on Transgenic Animal Models

Mice heterozygous for G90D rhodopsin (expressing G90D as a transgene on a heterozygous knock-out background, $G^{+/-}$, $R^{+/-}$) exhibited considerable loss of rod sensitivity. The desensitization of the photoresponse increased with the number of G90D alleles expressed (Sieving et al. 2001). G90D formed a pigment that supported normal photoactivation of transduction leading to rod responses in vivo. Therefore the desensitization seen in these mice could not be explained simply by a decreased quantal catch or by an inability to generate a photoresponse.

In the dark the membrane current noise arises from fluctuations in the cGMP concentrations [cG] which themselves reflect the balance of the local activities of PDE and guanylyl cyclase. Thermal activation of rhodopsin, producing a true R*, results in a single photon event whereas spontaneous activation of transducin or PDE would result in a smaller, shorter local decrease in [cG] and contribute to the continuous noise component of the rod photoreceptor dark noise (Rieke and Baylor 1996). Single photon events themselves vary in amplitude in different species, large (0.6–1.0 pA) in frog, toad and monkey, moderate 0.3 pA in rodents and much smaller in the salamander. Mutations in rhodopsin that destabilize the ground state could increase the probability of a thermal isomerization or result in a meta-stable or partially activated rhodopsin enzyme that flips back and forth resulting in low levels of transducin activation. The discovery that bleached opsin itself activates transducin as well as PDE (Cornwall and Fain 1994; Melia et al. 1997) adds another possible explanation for rod desensitization: excess free opsin.

However, free opsin can be quenched by the addition of excess exogenous chromophore. In *Xenopus* just this case was elegantly demonstrated by Jin et al. (2003) where the dramatic changes in kinetics and sensitivity of rods from three CNSB mutants (G90D, T94I, and A292E) were completely restored by the addition of 11-*cis* retinal. WT or mutant bovine rhodopsin with EGFP followed by a repeat of the last eight C-terminal amino acids of rhodopsin (1D4) fused to the C terminus was introduced under the *Xenopus* opsin promoter. The authors performed suction micropipette recordings on individual WT rods or those expressing A292E, G90D or T94I before and after incubation with 11-*cis* retinal. The sensitivity curve of rods expressing G90D was shifted to the right compared with WT rods (Fig. 30.1a). After incubation with 11-*cis* retinal, the sensitivity of G90D rods was rescued to WT levels. If desensitization were due to thermal isomerization of the chromophore, then the addition of 11-*cis* retinal would have no effect. Similar results were seen for rods expressing T94I as well as those expressing A292E.

In the G90D mouse ($G^{+/-}$, $R^{+/+}$) single cell recordings showed a doubling of the stimulus strength required to evoke a 50% maximal response with a 0.1 log unit (20%) reduction of rhodopsin content compared to WT mice. And for dim light responses the time-to-peak was 25% faster in the G90D expressing rods (Sieving et al. 2001). In the same study, the $G^{+/-}$, $R^{+/-}$ genotype showed about a 25% higher rhodopsin content. The rod responses of this genotype were studied as a massed receptor potential by pharmacologically eliminating bipolar responses with 2-amino-4-phosphonobutyrate (APB) and blocking the slow PIII with barium.

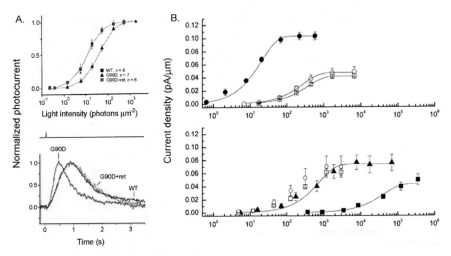

Fig. 30.1 Activity of G90D in transgenic rods. **a.** *Top*: Intensity-response curves of isolated trans-genic *Xenopus* rods expressing wild type (WT) rhodopsin (squares), G90D rhodopsin (triangles) or G90D rhodopsin after treatment with 11-*cis* retinal (*grey filled circles*). *Bottom*: Dim-flash kinetics of isolated rods expressing WT or G90D rhodopsin with and without addition of 11-*cis* retinal (adapted from Jin et al 2003). **b.** *Top*: Intensity-response curves from isolated trans-genic mouse rods. Data from isolated WT rods (*filled circles*), from $D^{+/+}$ rods before treatment with 11-*cis* retinal (*open squares*) and from $D^{+/+}$ rods after addition of 11-*cis* retinal (*open circles*). *Bottom*: Intensity-response curves from $D^{+/-}$; $R^{-/-}$ rods before (*filled squares*) and after (*filled triangles*) incubation with 11-*cis* retinal, and from $D^{+/-}$; $R^{-/-}$; $Rpe65^{-/-}$ rods before (*open squares*) and after (*open circles*) incubation with 11-*cis* retinal (adapted from Dizhoor et al. 2008)

Those results showed a rod response in the $G^{+/-}$, $R^{+/-}$ and the $R^{+/-}$ genotypes that appeared more similar to the light adapted $R^{+/+}$ than the massed receptor potential of the dark-adapted $R^{+/+}$ strain.

Earlier, Makino recorded from the rods of mice with only 50% of the normal rhodopsin content and found the expected reductions of sensitivity (about 70%). However, they also found a small acceleration in the time to peak of the response (14%) and a greater reduction of the integration time (almost 30%) indicating more profound effects on the inactivation phase of the phototransduction cascade (Lem et al. 1999). Thus the loss of 50% of the functioning rhodopsin can by itself alter the phototransduction cascade.

Sieving and colleagues further investigated their mouse model of CSNB, mea-suring single cell responses in their D$^+$ ($G^{+/-}$, $R^{-/-}$) and D$^{+/+}$ ($G^{+/+}$, $R^{-/-}$) lines. The ERG desensitization was confirmed and the integration time, dim flash sensitivity and dominant time constants were measured and found to be substantially reduced compared to WT rod responses. Moreover, these changes were not reversed by prior bathing in lipid vesicle containing 11-*cis* retinal (Fig. 30.1b), a treatment effective in the *Xenopus* model of the same disorder (Fig. 30.1a), and effective in reversing sensitivity losses in an RPE65$^{-/-}$ mouse model (Fig. 30.1b). Similar results were obtained in rods from $G90D^{+/-}$, $R^{+/-}$ that mimic more closely the heterozygous state of this autosomal dominant disease (Dizhoor et al. 2008).

There are at least three mechanisms that can alter the dominant time constant and saturation time of the light responses of rods to bright light flashes: (1) Continuous presence of background light; (2) Recent history of background light (novel form of adaptation) (Krispel et al. 2003); (3) molecular adaptations or manipulations that increase the content or effective concentration of RGS9 (Krispel et al. 2006). The presence of background light leads to reduced photocurrent and lower internal calcium along with the concomitant change in basal levels of PDE and guanylyl cyclase. The other two mechanisms need not necessarily change calcium levels to affect their influences on light response.

One cannot properly conclude equivalence to background light without specifically comparing the effects of background light to reproduce both the sensitivity and kinetic changes in the dim light response as well as the saturating light responses. Noise analysis of the membrane current or photoreceptor voltage can separate out the single photon vs. continuous noise provided the single photon response is large and may be able to address the issue of spontaneous PDE activation vs. partially activated rhodopsin as well.

30.3 Proposed Mechanisms of CSNB Mutations

Multiple studies have confirmed that rod cells of human CSNB patients and of animal models of CSNB are desensitized as if there was a consistent low basal stimulation that confounds vision under dim-light conditions. It is as though the rods are partially light adapted. The desensitization has been proposed to be due to constitutively active mutant opsins (Dryja et al. 1993; Jin et al. 2003), or thermal isomerization of the chromophore to cause activation of mutant rhodopsin without light (Sieving et al. 1995) or to activate rhodopsin.

30.3.1 Desensitization Due to Mutant Opsin Activity in Xenopus

One proposed model of CSNB is that constitutive activation of the A292E opsin causes rod cell desensitization (Dryja et al. 1993). At any given time there would be some opsin not bound to either 11-*cis* retinal or all-*trans* retinal that could theoretically activate the phototransduction cascade in the absence of light as observed in vitro. This model is further supported by the fact that constitutive activation of the phototransduction cascade is a common phenotype of all four known rhodopsin CSNB mutations in vitro. In addition, there are CSNB mutations of genes that encode other proteins of the phototransduction cascade including the β subunit of rod cGMP phosphodiesterase 6 (Gal et al. 1994) and the alpha subunit of transducin (Szabo et al. 2007), that both appear to be constitutively active.

The mechanism for constitutive activation is thought to be disruption of the salt bridge between Glu113 and Lys296 that holds the protein in an inactive conformation. For A292E and G90D the introduced negative residues compete with Glu113 for interaction with Lys296. For the other two, it is likely the position of the mutation that affects salt bridge formation. The location of the T94I mutation must be important because replacing threonine at position 94 with eight different amino acids all resulted in constitutively active proteins (Gross et al. 2003). For A295V, it was proposed that the introduction of the non-polar, β-branched amino acid valine may restrict movement of the polypeptide in the vicinity of the salt bridge (Zeitz et al. 2008). This model was tested in a study on transgenic *Xenopus laevis* tadpole models of CSNB mutations mentioned above (Jin et al. 2003). The addition of 11-*cis* retinal restored WT sensitivity of rods expressing G90D (Fig. 30.1a), A292E or T94I (Jin et al. 2003). Therefore, the results support the model that constitutively active free opsin is causing the reduced sensitivity of rod cells.

30.3.2 Proposed Dark-Active Rhodopsin in Mouse

In contrast to the findings discussed above, loss of rod cell sensitivity in G90D transgenic mouse rods is not rescued by the addition of 11-*cis* retinal (Fig. 30.1b) (Dizhoor et al. 2008). These data do not support the model of active free opsin causing desensitization of rod cells expressing G90D. Data from the same study does not support the proposed 'dark-light' model in which the CSNB mutations reduce rod sensitivity due to thermal isomerization of the chromophore in mutant rhodopsin; that is to say it does not appear to be photon-like noise (Sieving et al. 1995). Noise levels of WT and $G90D^{+/-}$, $R^{+/-}$ were very similar, and noise for WT cells exposed to the estimated equivalent light produced by G90D in the dark was higher (Dizhoor et al. 2008). Because the noise in the G90D expressing rods was not higher than that of WT rods, a highly active G90D rhodopsin is likely not the cause of the apparent 'light' causing the rod cells to desensitize. Ultimately, the authors propose that the rod cell desensitization is due to an active G90D rhodopsin with low gain (Dizhoor et al. 2008).

G90D opsin is more active in *Xenopus* rods than in mouse rods. Perhaps the differences in results are due to model system differences as the rhodopsin expressed in the *Xenopus* model was bovine and the rhodopsin expressed in the mouse model was human. A mammalian rhodopsin expressed in *Xenopus* tadpoles can yield a different phenotype than the endogenous rhodopsin. For example, dark rearing P23H transgenic *Xenopus* rescued retinal degeneration due to light sensitivity when bovine or human P23H rhodopsin was expressed, but not *Xenopus* P23H rhodopsin (Tam and Moritz 2007).

Human patients with the G90D mutation do not recover sensitivity even after long periods of dark adaptation (Sieving et al. 1995). If active G90D opsin is the cause of desensitization, the patients will never recover sensitivity similar to the *Xenopus* G90D rods after addition of exogenous chromophore because there is always (at best) a 1:1 molar ratio of rhodopsin to 11-*cis* retinal (Dowling 1960) so that in situ the RPE and retina together never recreate the experimental situation created with excess chromophore in the single-cell experiments.

30.4 Future Studies

Further work is needed to resolve the remaining uncertainties concerning the mechanisms by which rhodopsin mutations lead to night blindness. The degree to which constitutive activity is a causative factor in retinal degeneration is a matter to explore further. While some G90D rhodopsin mutation patients undergo slight degeneration with age (Sieving et al. 1995), the T94I, A295V and A292E rhodopsin mutant patients show quite minimal degeneration (Dryja et al. 1993; al-Jandal et al. 1999; Zeitz et al. 2008). K296M/E rhodopsin mutants display a high level of constitutive activity in vitro (Robinson et al. 1992), and those mutations are found in patients with ADRP (Keen et al. 1991; Sullivan et al. 1993).

Acknowledgments The authors thank T.G. Wensel and V.E. Wotring for critical comments on this manuscript. Our research is supported by grants from the EyeSight Foundation of Alabama, the Karl Kirchgessner Foundation, and by NIH grant EY019311.

References

al-Jandal N, Farrar GJ, Kiang A-S et al (1999) A novel mutation within the rhodopsin gene (Thr-94-Ile) causing autosomal dominant congenital stationary night blindness. Hum Mutat 13: 75–81

Barlow HB (1988) The thermal limit to seeing. Nature 334:296–297

Baylor DA, Matthews G, Yau KW (1980) Two components of electrical dark noise in road retinal rod outer segments. J Physiol 309:591–621

Baylor DA, Nunn BJ, Schnapf JL (1984) The photocurrent, noise and spectral sensitivity of rods of the monkey Macaca fascicularis. J Physiol (Lond) 357:575–607

Cornwall MC, Fain GL (1994) Bleaching pigment activates transducin in isolated rods of the salamander retina. J Physiol (Lond) 480:261–279

Dizhoor A, Woodruff M, Olshevskaya E et al (2008) Night blindness and the mechanism of constitutive signaling of mutant G90D rhodopsin. J Neurosci 28:11662–11672

Dowling JE (1960) Chemistry of visual adaptation in the rat. Nature 188:114–118

Dryja TP, Berson EL, Rao VR et al (1993) Heterozygous missense mutation in the rhodopsin gene as a cause of congenital stationary night blindness. Nat Genet 4:280–283

Gal A, Orth U, Baehr W et al (1994) Heterozygous missense mutation in the rod cGMP phosphodiesterase beta-subunit gene in autosomal dominant stationary night blindness. Nat Genet 7:551

Gross AK, Rao VR, Oprian DD (2003) Characterization of rhodopsin congenital night blindness mutant T94I. Biochemistry 42:2009–2015

Gross AK, Xie G, Oprian DD (2003) Slow binding of retinal to rhodopsin mutants G90D and T94D. Biochemistry 42:2002–2008

Jin S, Cornwall MC, Oprian DD (2003) Opsin activation as a cause of congenital night blindness. Nat Neurosci 6:731–735

Keen TJ, Inglehearn CF, Lester DH et al (1991) Autosomal dominant retinitis pigmentosa: four new mutations in rhodopsin, one of the in the retinal attachment site. Genomics 11:199–205

Krispel CM, Chen D, Melling N et al (2006) RGS expression rate-limits recovery of rod photoresponses. Neuron 51:409–416

Krispel CM, Chen CK, Simon MI et al (2003) Novel form of adaptation in mouse retinal rods speeds recovery of phototransduction. J Gen Physiol 122:703–712

Lem J, Krasnoperova NV, Calvert PD, et al (1999) Morphological, physiological and biochemical changes in rhodopsin knockout mice. Proc Natl Acad Sci USA 96:736–741

Melia TJ, Cowan CW, Angelson JK et al (1997) A comparison of the efficiency of G protein activation by ligand-free and light-activated forms of rhodopsin. Biophys J 73:3182–3191

Nakanishi K, Balogh-Nair V, Arnaboldi M et al (1980) An external point-charge model for bacteriorhodopsin to account for its purple color. J Am Chem Soc 102:7945–7947

Nathans J (1990) Determinants of visual pigment absorbance: identification of the retinylidene Schiff's base counterion in bovine rhodopsin. Biochemistry 29:9746–9752

Ng PC, Henikoff S (2001) Predicting deleterious amino acid substitutions. Genome Res 11: 863–874

Rao V, Cohen GB, Oprian DD (1994) Rhodopsin mutation G90D and a molecular mechanism for congenital night blindness. Nature 367:639–642

Rieke F, Baylor DA (1996) Molecular origin of continuous dark noise in rod photoreceptors. Biophys J 71:2553–2572

Robinson PR, Cohen GB, Zhukovsky EA et al (1992) Constitutively active mutants of rhodopsin. Neuron 9:719–725

Sakmar TP, Franke RR, Khorana HG (1989) Glutamic acid-113 serves as the retinylidene Schiff base counterion in bovine rhodopsin. Proc Natl Acad Sci USA 86:8309–8313

Sieving PA, Fowler ML, Bush RA et al (2001) Constitutive "light" adaptation in rods from G90D rhodopsin: a mechanism for human congenital nightblindness without rod cell loss. J Neurosci 21:5449–5460

Sieving PA, Richards JE, Naarendorp F et al (1995) Dark-light: model for nightblindness from the human rhodopsin Gly-90 –> Asp mutation. Proc Natl Acad Sci 92:880–884

Steinberg G, Ottolenghi M, Sheves M (1993) pKa of the protonated Schiff base of bovine rhodopsin: A study with artificial pigments. Biophys J 64:1499–1502

Sullivan JM, Scott KM, Falls HF et al (1993) A novel rhodopsin mutation at the retinal binding site (LYS 296 MET) in ADRP. Invest Ophthalmol Vis Sci 34:1149

Szabo V, Kreienkamp H-J, Rosenberg T et al (2007) p.Gln200Glu, a putative constitutively active mutant of rod á-transducin (*GNAT1*) in autosomal dominant congenital stationary night blindness. Hum Mutat 28:741–742

Tam B, Moritz O (2007) Dark rearing rescues P23H rhodopsin-induced retinal degeneration in a transgenic Xenopus laevis model of retinitis pigmentosa: a chromophore-dependent mechanism characterized by production of N-terminally truncated mutant rhodopsin. J Neurosci 27(34):9043–9053

Xie G, Gross AK, Oprian DD (2003) An opsin mutant with increased thermal stability. Biochemistry 42:1995–2001

Zeitz C, Gross AK, Leifert D et al (2008) Identification and functional characterization of a novel rhodopsin mutation associated with autosomal dominant CSNB. Invest Ophthalmol Visc Sci 49:4105–4114

Zhukovsky EA, Robinson PR, Oprian DD (1992) Changing the location of the Schiff base counterion in rhodopsin. Biochemistry 31:10400–10405

Chapter 31
GCAP1 Mutations Associated with Autosomal Dominant Cone Dystrophy

Li Jiang and Wolfgang Baehr

Abstract We discuss the heterogeneity of autosomal dominant cone and cone-rod dystrophies (adCD, and adCORD, respectively). As one of the best characterized adCD genes, we focus on the GUCA1A gene encoding guanylate cyclase activating protein 1 (GCAP1), a protein carrying three high affinity Ca^{2+} binding motifs (EF hands). GCAP1 senses changes in cytoplasmic free $[Ca^{2+}]$ and communicates these changes to GC1, by either inhibiting it (at high free $[Ca^{2+}]$), or stimulating it (at low free $[Ca^{2+}]$). A number of missense mutations altering the structure and Ca^{2+} affinity of EF hands have been discovered. These mutations are associated with a gain of function, producing dominant cone and cone rod dystrophy phenotypes. In this article we review these mutations and describe the consequences of specific mutations on GCAP1 structure and GC stimulation.

We discuss the heterogeneity of autosomal dominant cone and cone-rod dystrophies (adCD, and adCORD, respectively). As one of the best characterized adCD genes, we focus on the GUCA1A gene encoding guanylate cyclase activating protein 1 (GCAP1), a protein carrying three high affinity Ca^{2+} binding motifs (EF hands). GCAP1 senses changes in cytoplasmic free $[Ca^{2+}]$ and communicates these changes to GC1, by either inhibiting it (at high free $[Ca^{2+}]$), or stimulating it (at low free $[Ca^{2+}]$). A number of missense mutations altering the structure and Ca^{2+} affinity of EF hands have been discovered. These mutations are associated with a gain of function, producing dominant cone and cone rod dystrophy phenotypes. In this article we review these mutations and describe the consequences of specific mutations on GCAP1 structure and GC stimulation.

W. Baehr (✉)

Department of Biology; Department of Ophthalmology, Department of Neurobiology and Anatomy; John A. Moran Eye Center; University of Utah Health Science Center, Salt Lake City, UT 84112, USA

e-mail: wbaehr@hsc.utah.edu

R.E. Anderson et al. (eds.), *Retinal Degenerative Diseases*, Advances in Experimental   273
Medicine and Biology 664, DOI 10.1007/978-1-4419-1399-9_31,
© Springer Science+Business Media, LLC 2010

31.1 Heterogeneity of Autosomal Dominant Cone and Cone-Rod Dystrophies

Cone and cone-rod dystrophies (CD and CRD, respectively) are rare diseases and highly heterogeneous. Major hallmarks are photophobia, reduced central visual acuity, achromatopsia, but preserved peripheral vision mediated by rod photoreceptors at early stages (Hamel 2007). CD and CRD are diagnosed mainly on the basis of changes in the photopic and scotopic electroretinogram, but also by fundoscopy and optical coherence tomography (Wissinger et al. 2008; Wolfing et al. 2006). CD and CRD are most often caused by mutations in genes expressed in photoreceptors, such as *CRX*, *RIM1*, *PITPNM3*, *UNC119*, *GUCY2D* and *GUCA1A* associated with multiple functions, including gene regulation, regulation of cGMP synthesis, and regulation of Ca^{2+} entry at the photoreceptor synapse (Table 31.1).

The transcription factor CRX, a factor essential for the maintenance of mammalian photoreceptors, regulates the expression of several outer segment proteins such as visual pigments and arrestin (Furukawa et al. 1999). A number of missense mutations and truncations, presumably null alleles, have been discovered in families with CORD3, but is unclear whether the phenotype is caused by a dominant negative effect of a truncated protein or by haploinsufficiency (Freund et al. 1997; Swain et al. 1997). Human *RIM1*, a putative effector protein for the small GTPase rab3 involved in synaptic exocytosis was shown to be associated with CORD7 (Johnson et al. 2003; Wang et al. 1997). RIM1 is a large multidomain protein localizing to the synaptic ribbon and possibly involved in regulation of glutamate release (Schoch et al. 2002). The CORD7 missense mutation was identified in a region interacting with synaptic proteins like the a_{1D} subunit of L-type Ca^{2+} channels (Johnson et al. 2003). *UNC119* encodes a protein termed UNC119/RG4, related to PrBP/δ (*PDE6d*), a prenyl binding protein (Zhang et al. 2007). The mutation, UNC119/RG4(K57ter), was incorporated into a transgene producing a slowly progressing rod/cone dystrophy (Kobayashi et al. 2000). It was recently discovered that UNC119/RG4 interacts with CaBP4, a synaptic Ca^{2+}-binding protein in photoreceptors (Haeseleer, 2008) and with ribeye (Alpadi et al. 2008), suggesting a possible function in synaptic transmission (Kobayashi et al. 2000).The membrane-associated phosphatidylinositol transfer protein (*PITPNM3*), a human homolog of the D. melanogaster *rdgB* gene, is expressed ubiquitously, and also in retina, particularly the OPL and Müller cells (Tian and Lev 2002). The CORD5 mutation is located in the C-terminal region of *PITPNM3*, but the functional consequences of the mutation are unclear (Kohn et al. 2007).

31.2 Guanylate Cyclase 1 (GC1) and GCAP1

By far the best characterized genes associated with dominant CD/CRD are *GUCY2D* (CORD6), encoding photoreceptor guanylate cyclase 1 (retGC-1 or GC1), and *GUCA1A*, encoding the Ca^{2+}-binding protein GCAP1 (CORD3). Both of these

Table 31.1 Genetic loci associated with dominant cone dystrophies. Column 1, chromosomal localization. Column 2, disease nomenclature according to RetNet. Column 3, Online Mendelian Inheritance in Man (OMIM) nomenclature. Column 4, gene symbol. Column 5, function of the gene product. Column 6, references

Gene	Chromosome	OMIM	Function	Defect	References
CRX (CORD3)	19q13.3	120970	Transcription factor	Multiple missense mutations	(Swain et al. 1997; Freund et al. 1997)
GUCA1A(CORD3)	6p21.1	602093	Guanylate cyclase activator	Y99C;N104K; I143NT;	Review: (Baehr and Palczewski 2007)
GUCY2D (CORD6)	17p13.1	601777	Photoreceptor guanylate cyclase	E837D, R838A, R838H, R838C, T839M	(Perrault et al. 1996); review: (Baehr and Palczewski 2007)
PITPNM3 (CORD5)	17p13.2	600977	Involved in photoreceptor membrane renewal; *Drosophila* homolog is retinal degeneration B (*rdgB*)	Q626H	(Kohn et al. 2007)
QRX (CORD11)	18q21.1-q21.3	600624	Transcription factor	R87Q R137G	(Wang et al. 2004)
RIMS1 (CORD7)	6q13	603649	Function unknown; ribbon synapse-associated	R844H	(Johnson et al. 2003)
UNC119	17q11.2	604011	Function unknown; localizes to rod and cone cytoplasm and ribbon synapses	K57ter	(Kobayashi et al. 2000)

genes are expressed at high levels in photoreceptors and locate to the outer segments where phototransduction takes place. GC1 is a transmembrane protein with a large amino-terminal ECD of unknown function, a kinase-like homology domain possibly involved in autophosphorylation, a dimerization domain, and a catalytic domain. GC1 is Ca^{2+}-insensitive in its purified form. Its Ca^{2+} sensitivity on the outer segment disk membrane is mediated by guanylate cyclase-activating proteins (GCAPs) (Fig. 31.1). GCAPs are Ca^{2+}-binding proteins belonging to the calmodulin superfamily equipped with four EF hand motifs. GC1 and GCAP1 interact intracellularly since GCAP1 is present in the cytoplasm (deletion of the extracellular domain does not affect GC stimulation by GCAP1). The side of contact at GC1 involves the kinase-like domain because its deletion diminished the stimulation by GCAP1. GCAP1 in turn interacts with GC1 through the N-terminal region around the EF1

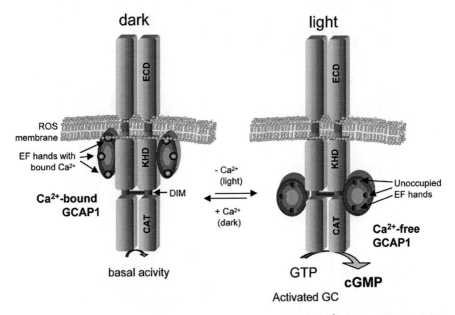

Fig. 31.1 Cartoon of the activation of GC1 by GCAP1. At high free Ca^{2+} (*dark*), GCAP and GC form a complex, but enzymatic activity is very low (basal activity is needed to maintain micromolar cGMP in the cytoplasm). At low free Ca^{2+} (*light*), GCAP1 converts into an activator of GC and GC activity accelerates. GCAPs are Ca^{2+}-binding proteins belonging to the calmodulin superfamily equipped with four EF hand motifs. GC1 and GCAP1 interact intracellularly since GCAP1 is present in the cytoplasm (deletion of the extracellular domain does not affect GC stimulation by GCAP1). The side of contact at GC1 involves the kinase-like domain because its deletion diminished the stimulation by GCAP1. GCAP1 in turn interacts with GC1 through the N-terminal region around the EF1 motif. A number of mutations causing dominant cone-rod dystrophy in GUCY2D are restricted to the dimerization domain. Some of the important missense mutations of the dimerization domain are E837D, R838A, R838H, R838C, T839M (Payne et al. 2001; Downes et al. 2001; Wilkie et al. 2000). Interestingly, the three disease mutations at residue 838 are nonequivalent. They exhibit GC activity equal or superior to WT GC at low free $[Ca]_{free}$ in the order R838C< R838H< R838A and showed a higher affinity for GCAP1 than WT GC (Wilkie et al. 2000)

motif. A number of mutations causing dominant cone-rod dystrophy in GUCY2D are restricted to the dimerization domain. Some of the important missense mutations of the dimerization domain are E837D, R838A, R838H, R838C, T839M (Payne et al., 2001; Downes et al., 2001; Wilkie et al., 2000). Interestingly, the three disease mutations at residue 838 are non-equivalent. They exhibit GC activity equal or superior to WT GC at low free $[Ca]_{free}$ in the order R838C<R838H<R838A and showed a higher affinity for GCAP1 than WT GC (Wilkie et al., 2000).

31.3 The EF Hand Motifs of GCAP1

GCAPs are N-myristoylated neuronal Ca^{2+} sensors with three functional high affinity Ca^{2+}-binding sites termed EF hands. The structure of GCAP1 in its Ca^{2+}-bound form has been determined recently in high resolution (Stephen et al. 2007). The structure shows that in the Ca^{2+}-bound state, the N-terminal acyl side chain is buried deeply between an N-terminal and a C-terminal helix, in contrast to the closely related recoverin, where the myristoyl group is exposed to the solvent (Fig. 31.2).

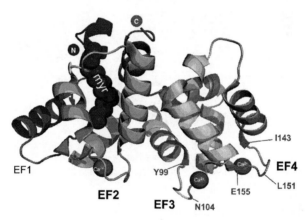

Fig. 31.2 Structure of GCAP1 (adapted from Baehr and Palczewski 2009). N-terminal (*blue*) and C-terminal (*red*) helices bury the myristoyl group attached to Gly-2. The EF hands are solvent exposed and shown with bound Ca^{2+}. The EF1 motif is incompetent for Ca^{2+} binding. Approximate locations of residues associated with cone dystrophy are depicted in *red*

The EF hands consist of a helix-loop-helix secondary structure that chelates Ca^{2+} ions. EF hands also have affinity for Mg^{2+} ions but the interaction is several orders of magnitude weaker (Gifford et al. 2007). The loop consists of 12 amino acids rich in acidic residues providing oxygen ligands for Ca^{2+} coordination. The N-terminal region contains a EF hand motif (EF1) in which Ca^{2+} coordination is prevented by lack of acidic side chains (Palczewski et al. 2004). EF hands 2–4 are fully functional, canonical EF-hand Ca^{2+}-binding sites. Their individual roles have been explored mostly by site-directed mutagenesis, and recording of conformational changes in the absence and presence of Ca^{2+} and/or Mg^{2+} (Rudnicka-Nawrot et al. 1998; Otto-Bruc et al. 1997; Peshenko and Dizhoor 2007; Sokal et al. 1999).

31.4 GUCA1A Mutations Associated with adCD and adCRD

Pathogenic mutations of residues flanking EF3 and EF4, as well as within the EF3 and EF4 loop of GCAP1 are associated with autosomal dominant cone or cone-rod dystrophy (Baehr and Palczewski 2007). These mutations are Y99, N104, I143, L151, E155 (Sokal et al. 1998; Dizhoor et al. 1998; Nishiguchi et al. 2004; Wilkie et al. 2001; Jiang et al. 2005; Sokal et al. 2005). The residue Y99 is located adjacent to the EF3 hand and I143 adjacent to the EF4 hand. N104 is located in EF3, and E155G, L151F are located in EF4 (Figs. 31.2, 31.3).

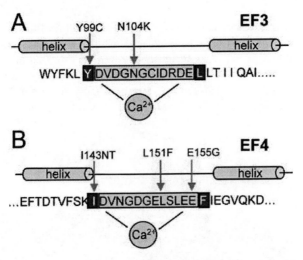

Fig. 31.3 Cartoon of the EF3 and EF4 hand motifs in GCAP1. The 12 amino acids comprising the Ca^{2+}-binding loop are boxed and shaded *blue*, flanking hydrophobic amino acids are highlighted on *dark blue* background. Mutations linked to adCD are identified by *red arrows*

When replaced by amino acids with different chemical properties, the mutant residues can disrupt coordination of Ca^{2+} to the mutant loop and change the Ca^{2+} sensitivity of GCAP1. As a result, mutant GCAPs are not fully inactivated at dark Ca^{2+} levels, leading to the persistent stimulation of GC1 in the dark, elevated cGMP and Ca^{2+} levels, and cell death.

31.5 EF3: The GCAP1(Y99C) and GCAP1(N104K) Mutations

Y99 is a hydrophobic amino acid that does not distort the helix N-terminal to EF3. However, replacement of Y99 by a Cys residue (Y99C), the first mutation in GCAP1 linked to dominant cone dystrophy, had adverse effects on the structure of EF3 and Ca^{2+}-binding (Sokal et al. 1998; Dizhoor et al. 1998). When Y99 was replaced by Trp, a hydrophobic residue, biological activity of mutant GCAP1 was unchanged (Sokal et al. 1999). Analysis of the EF3-hand motif Ca^{2+} binding kinetics with the Y99W mutant (W3Cys-), exploiting the intrinsic Trp fluorescence of Trp99, showed a significant increase in the Trp fluorescence intensity of W3-GCAP1(w⁻) in the presence of high Ca^{2+}, reflecting a conformational change (Sokal et al. 1999). Thus, the EF3-hand motif is a key region for conversion of GCAP1 from activator to inhibitor, consistent with mutations in this region being causative of cone dystrophy.

N104 occupies a position in the EF3 loop that is critical for Ca^{2+} coordination by providing oxygen of the amide side chain for coordination. N104K likely weakens Ca^{2+} coordination at EF3 under physiological conditions preventing formation of the Ca^{2+}-bound structure that is essential for inhibiting GC catalytic activity. The GCAP1 crystal structure implies that mutations in EF3 may distort contacts of the kinked C-terminal helix with the N-terminal helix of GCAP1. In contrast to wild-type GCAP1, GCAP1(N104K) is more susceptible to proteolysis at 1 mM Ca^{2+}. The reason for this distinction is the inability of the mutant GCAP1 to assume the tight Ca^{2+}-bound form of GCAP1 which is less accessible to trypsin. We conclude that the N104K mutation introduces a structural change that is irreversible even at 1 mM Ca^{2+}.

31.6 EF4: The GCAP1(I143NT), GCAP1(L151F) and GCAP1(E155G) Mutations

Another pathogenic mutation of a flanking hydrophobic residue (I143NT) (Nishiguchi et al. 2004) was observed in EF4, emphasizing the importance of an intact N-terminal helix for Ca^{2+} binding. Substitution of Ile143, positioned at the N-terminal end of EF4, by two polar residues changes the orientation of the N-terminal -helix, distorting the loop conformation that is essential for Ca^{2+} binding, and decreasing the affinity for Ca^{2+}. Changes in these positions among other Ca^{2+}-binding proteins have also been shown to impair Ca^{2+} coordination (Falke et al. 1994). Biochemical analysis showed that the GCAP1(I143NT) mutant adopted a conformation susceptible to proteolysis, and its properties suggest that it is incompletely inactivated by high Ca^{2+} concentrations as should occur with dark adaptation.

An A464G transition in the *GUCA1A* gene (Wilkie et al. 2001) changed amino acid Glu155 in the EF4-hand motif to Gly. Ca^{2+} binding at the EF4-hand motif does not affect structural changes of GCAP1 to the same extent as at the EF3-hand motif, as shown measuring intrinsic fluorescence as a function of Ca^{2+} using a Trp at position 142 (Sokal et al. 1999). However, it exerts similar dominant effects on GC1 stimulation as does GCAP1(Y99C). The residue Glu155 of GCAP1 is invariant in all GCAPs (Palczewski et al. 2004); an invariant Glu at position 12 of the EF-hand loop, contributing both of its side-chain oxygen atoms to the metal-ion coordination, has been shown to be essential for Ca^{2+} coordination (Nakayama et al. 1992; Falke et al. 1994).

In the L151F mutation, one hydrophobic residue (L) replaces another (F) which is not much bulkier than L. The resulting phenotype of adCD is therefore surprising.

However, the pathogenic properties of the GCAP1(L151F) mutations described in this article are supported by several independent observations. First, the mutation decreases the Ca^{2+} sensitivity of GC stimulation, an effect also seen in other EF hand mutations. Second, the recombinant GCAP1-L151F is susceptible to proteolysis. Third, molecular dynamics of WT GCAP1 and GCAP1(L151F) confirmed that a significant change in the structure of mutant GCAP1 influences the binding of Ca^{2+} in EF4 and EF2. Fourth, the L151F mutations have been independently identified in a large Utah pedigree with dominant cone dystrophy. The reason for the discrepancy in phenotype (adCD versus adCORD) is unclear, but anomalies in the rod response may be slow in developing and may depend on the genetic background.

31.7 Conclusion

All EF hand mutations alter the Ca^{2+} sensitivity of GCAP1, leading to the constitutive stimulation of GC1 at high $[Ca^{2+}]$ limiting its ability to fully inactivate GC1 under physiological dark conditions. Persistent stimulation of GC by the mutant proteins is predicted to lead to elevated levels of cGMP in the dark-adapted retina, which in turn causes a higher percentage of cGMP-gated channels in the plasma membrane to be opened. The altered physiological cGMP levels may be subtle and thus cause relatively slow retinal degeneration. The reason for the mostly cone-specific degeneration in response to this physiological defect is not understood. GCAP1 may be more active in cones than rods, or, alternatively, it may reflect other differences in cGMP metabolism between rods and cones. Animal models with homologous dominant GCAP1 mutations will be helpful to address this uncertainty. A mouse line expressing GCAP1(Y99C) was generated and shown to shift the Ca^{2+} sensitivity of GCs in photoreceptors, keeping it partially active at 250 nM free Ca^{2+}, the normal resting Ca^{2+} concentration in darkness (Olshevskaya et al. 2004).

References

Alpadi K, MagupalliVG, Kappel S et al (2008) RIBEYE recruits Munc119, a mammalian ortholog of the Caenorhabditis elegans protein unc119, to synaptic ribbons of photoreceptor synapses. J Biol Chem 283:26461–26467

BaehrW, Palczewski K (2007) Guanylate cyclase-activating proteins and retina disease. Subcell Biochem 45:71–91

Baehr W, Palczewski K (2009) Focus on Molecules: Guanylate cyclase-activating proteins (GCAPs). Exp Eye Res 89:2–3

Dizhoor AM, Boikov SG, Olshevskaya E (1998) Constitutive activation of photoreceptor guanylate cyclase by Y99C mutant of GCAP-1. J Biol Chem 273:17311–17314

Downes SM, Payne AM, Kelsell RE et al (2001) Autosomal dominant cone-rod dystrophy with mutations in the guanylate cyclase 2D gene encoding retinal guanylate cyclase-1. Arch Ophthalmol 119:1667–1673

Falke JJ, Drake SK, Hazard AL et al (1994) Molecular tuning of ion binding to calcium signaling proteins. Quantative Rev Biophys 27:219–290

Freund CL, Gregory EC, Furukawa T et al (1997) Cone-rod dystrophy due to mutations in a novel photoreceptor-specific homeobox gene (CRX) essential for maintenance of the photoreceptor. Cell 91:543–553

Furukawa T, Morrow EM, Li T et al (1999) Retinopathy and attenuated circadian entrainment in Crx-deficient mice. Nat.Genet 23:466–470

Gifford JL, Walsh MP, Vogel HJ (2007) Structures and metal-ion-binding properties of the Ca^{2+} binding helix-loop-helix EF-hand motifs. Biochem J 405:199–221

Haeseleer F (2008) Interaction and Colocalization of CaBP4 and Unc119 (MRG4) in Photoreceptors. Invest Ophthalmol Vis Sci 49:2366–2375

Hamel CP (2007) Cone rod dystrophies. Orphanet J Rare Dis 2:7

Jiang L, Katz BJ, Yang Z et al (2005) Autosomal dominant cone dystrophy caused by a novel mutation in the GCAP1 gene (GUCA1A). Mol Vis 11:143–151

Johnson S, Halford S, Morris AG et al (2003) Genomic organisation and alternative splicing of human RIM1, a gene implicated in autosomal dominant cone-rod dystrophy (CORD7). Genomics 81:304–314

Kobayashi A, Higashide T, Hamasaki D (2000) HRG4 (UNC119) mutation found in cone-rod dystrophy causes retinal degeneration in a transgenic model. Invest Ophthalmol Vis Sci 41:3268–3277

Kohn L, Kadzhaev K, Burstedt MS et al (2007) Mutation in the PYK2-binding domain of PITPNM3 causes autosomal dominant cone dystrophy (CORD5) in two Swedish families. Eur J Hum Genet 15:664–671

Nakayama S, Moncrief ND, Kretsinger RH (1992) Evolution of EF-hand calcium-modulated proteins II. Domains of several subfamilies have diverse evolutionary histories. J Mol Evol 34:416–448

Nishiguchi KM, Sokal I, Yang L et al (2004) A Novel Mutation (I143NT) in Guanylate Cyclase-Activating Protein 1 (GCAP1) Associated with Autosomal Dominant Cone Degeneration. Invest Ophthalmol Vis Sci 45:3863–3870

Olshevskaya EV, Calvert PD, Woodruff ML et al (2004) The Y99C mutation in guanylyl cyclase-activating protein 1 increases intracellular Ca^{2+} and causes photoreceptor degeneration in transgenic mice. J Neurosci 24:6078–6085

Otto-Bruc A, Buczylko J, Surgucheva Icka-Nawrot M et al (1997) Functional reconstitution of photoreceptor guanylate cyclase with native and mutant forms of guanylate cyclase activating protein 1. Biochemistry 36:4295–4302

Palczewski K, Sokal I, Baehr W (2004) Guanylate cyclase-activating proteins: structure, function, and diversity. Biochem Biophys Res Commun 322:1123–1130

Payne AM, Morris AG, Downes SM et al (2001) Clustering and frequency of mutations in the retinal guanylate cyclase (GUCY2D) gene in patients with dominant cone-rod dystrophies. J Med Genet 38:611–614

Perrault I, Rozet J-M, Calvas P et al (1996) Retinal-specific guanylate cyclase gene mutations in Leber's congenital amaurosis. Nature Genet 14:461–464

Peshenko IV, Dizhoor AM (2007) Activation and inhibition of photoreceptor guanylyl cyclase by guanylyl cyclase activating protein 1 (GCAP-1): the functional role of Mg^{2+}/Ca^{2+} exchange in EF-hand domains. J Biol Chem 282:21645–21652

Rudnicka-Nawrot M, Surgucheva I, Hulmes JD et al (1998) Changes in biological activity and folding of guanylate cyclase-activating protein 1 as a function of calcium. Biochemistry 37:248–257

Schoch S, Castillo PE, Jo T et al (2002) RIM1alpha forms a protein scaffold for regulating neurotransmitter release at the active zone. Nature 415:321–326

Sokal I, Dupps WJ, Grassi MA et al (2005) A GCAP1 missense mutation (L151F) in a large family with autosomal dominant cone-rod dystrophy (adCORD). Invest Ophthalmol Vis Sci 46:1124–1132

Sokal I, Li N, Surgucheva I et al (1998) GCAP1(Y99C) mutant is constitutively active in autosomal dominant cone dystrophy. Mol Cell 2:129–133

Sokal I, Otto-Bruc AE, Surgucheva I et al (1999) Conformational changes in guanylyl cyclase-activating protein 1 (GCAP1) and its tryptophan mutants as a function of calcium concentration. J Biol Chem 274:19829–19837

Stephen R, Bereta G, Golczak M et al (2007) Stabilizing function for myristoyl group revealed by the crystal structure of a neuronal calcium sensor, guanylate cyclase-activating protein 1. Structure 15:1392–1402

Swain PK, Chen S, Wang QL et al (1997) Mutations in the cone-rod homeobox gene are associated with the cone-rod dystrophy photoreceptor degeneration. Neuron 19:1329–1336

Tian D, Lev S (2002) Cellular and developmental distribution of human homologues of the Drosophilia rdgB protein in the rat retina. Invest Ophthalmol Vis Sci 43:1946–1953

Wang QL, Chen S, Esumi N et al (2004) QRX, a novel homeobox gene, modulates photoreceptor gene expression. Hum Mol Genet 13:1025–1040

Wang Y, Okamoto M, Schmitz F et al (1997) Rim is a putative Rab3 effector in regulating synaptic-vesicle fusion. Nature 388:593–598

Wilkie SE, Li Y, Deery EC et al (2001) Identification and functional consequences of a new mutation (E155G) in the gene for GCAP1 that causes autosomal dominant cone dystrophy. Am J Hum Genet 69:471–480

Wilkie SE, Newbold RJ, Deery E et al (2000) Functional characterization of missense mutations at codon 838 in retinal guanylate cyclase correlates with disease severity in patients with autosomal dominant cone-rod dystrophy. Hum Mol Genet 9:3065–3073

Wissinger B, Dangel S, Jagle H et al (2008) Cone dystrophy with supernormal rod response is strictly associated with mutations in KCNV2. Invest Ophthalmol Vis Sci 49:751–757

Wolfing JI, Chung M, Carroll J et al (2006) High-resolution retinal imaging of cone-rod dystrophy. Ophthalmology 113:1019

Zhang H, Li S, Doan T et al (2007) Deletion of PrBP/{delta} impedes transport of GRK1 and PDE6 catalytic subunits to photoreceptor outer segments. Proc Natl Acad Sci USA 104:8857–8862

Chapter 32
Genotypic Analysis of X-linked Retinoschisis in Western Australia

Tina Lamey, Sarina Laurin, Enid Chelva, and John De Roach

Abstract X-linked Retinoschisis is a leading cause of juvenile macular degeneration. Four Western Australian families affected by X-Linked Retinoschisis were analysed using DNA and clinical information from the Australian Inherited Retinal Disease (IRD) Register and DNA Bank. By direct sequencing of the RS1 gene, three genetic variants were identified; 52+1G > T, 289T > G and 416delA. 289T > G has not been previously reported and is likely to cause a substitution of a membrane binding residue (W92G) in the functional discoidin domain. All clinically diagnosed individuals showed typical electronegative ERGs. The 52+1G > T obligate carrier also recorded a bilaterally abnormal rod ERG and mildly abnormal photopic responses. mfERG trace arrays showed reduced response densities in the paramacular region extending futher temporally for each eye.

Further analyses are currently underway for Stargardt's disease, autosomal dominant and autosomal recessive retinitis pigmentosa, and Leber's congenital amaurosis.

32.1 Introduction

Juvenile X-linked Retinoschisis (XLRS) is a common form of inherited juvenile macular degeneration caused by mutations in the Retinoschisin (RS1) gene (Forsius et al. 1973; George et al. 1995). Symptoms caused by splitting of inner and sometimes peripheral retinal layers typically present between 5 and 10 years of age and progress mildly until the 4th decade of life followed by more progressive deterioration (Deutman 1971; Kellner et al. 1990). Disease severity and progression exhibit significant variability even between affected siblings, hence they are likely

T. Lamey (✉)
Department of Medical Technology and Physics, Sir Charles Gairdner Hospital, Hospital Avenue, Nedlands, WA, 6009, Australia
e-mail: john.deroach@health.wa.gov.au

R.E. Anderson et al. (eds.), *Retinal Degenerative Diseases*, Advances in Experimental Medicine and Biology 664, DOI 10.1007/978-1-4419-1399-9_32,
© Springer Science+Business Media, LLC 2010

to depend on factors other than mutation alone (Forsius et al. 1973; Eksandh et al. 2005; Pimenides et al. 2005). Since RS1 exhibits complete penetrance (Forsius et al. 1973), the most likely theory is that modifier genes may play a role.

The small, six exon RS1 gene (Xp 22.2) is expressed only in retinal tissues and encodes the extracellular, 201-amino acid peripheral membrane protein, Retinoschisin (RS). Its function in photoreceptor membrane adhesion (Wu et al. 2005) is afforded by the highly conserved, 157 amino acid discoidin domain (DD; cys 63 to cys 219) present in many cell adhesion and cell signalling proteins (Wu and Molday 2003; Wu et al. 2005; Molday et al. 2007).

XLRS pathology predominantly arises from missense mutations in exons four to six (The Retinoschisis Consortium 1998; Hewitt et al. 2005) often causing protein misfolding and intracellular retention and degradation (Wang et al. 2002).

With the liklihood of successful human gene therapy in the forseeable future, it is our aim at the Australian Inherited Retinal Disease Register and DNA Bank to progressively expand the once Western Australian specific database (est. 1984) and DNA bank (est. 2001), to include all Australian families affected inherited retinal disease (IRD). This now rapidly growing database currently contains information on 2300 individuals dating back to 1976, and includes results of electrophysiological, psychophysical and ophthalmic tests, family and personal history details, best known diagnoses, and more recently, disease causing mutations. Information and DNA will be made available to approved researchers and we anticipate that in time, the resource may contribute to the improvement of diagnostic and prognostic accuracy and help guide Australian patients for future therapies as well as funding towards research most applicable to the Australian IRD community.

With our initial focus on Retinoschisis, Stargardt's disease, autosomal dominant retinitis pigmentosa, and Leber's congenital amaurosis we recently undertook to first analyse genomic DNA of Western Australian families for disease causing mutations. The small Retinoschisis study is presented here.

32.2 Methodology

Four of five Western Australian families on the IRD Register, containing individuals clinically diagnosed with XLRS who had not before participated in similar research were included in the study. Informed consent was obtained from all research participants in accordance with Sir Charles Gairdner Hospital Human Research Ethics Committee's approval guidelines.

32.2.1 Molecular Genetic Studies

Blood (30mL EDTA) and saliva samples (Oragene Saliva Kit) were collected from 10 individuals clinically diagnosed with XLRS and their family members. Genomic

DNA was extracted from blood leukocytes and saliva samples by the Western Australian DNA Bank (www.wadb.org.au) and analysed for disease causing mutations in RS1. The six exons and flanking intronic regions of RS1 were amplified by PCR using published, exon flanking intronic primers (Sauer et al. 1997). Amplified DNA was purified and directly sequenced (Macrogen, Seoul). Sequences were compared (Sequencher 4.8) to human RS1 reference sequence (NM_000330.2).

Likely pathogenicity of novel variants was confirmed by DNA sequencing of family members and 135 X chromosomes from unrelated individuals with no known family history of retinal disease and deemed normal following electrophysiological, ophthalmological and psychophysical tests.

32.2.2 Electrophysiological Studies

The electrophysiological tests reported in this paper were perfomed to International Society for Clinical Electrophysiology of Vision (ISCEV) standards. Full-field and multifocal (mf) electroretinograms (ERGs) were recorded using HK-loop and Burian-Allen contact lens electrodes respectively on LKC UTAS 3000 and EDI VERIS™ Science data acquisition systems. Results were analysed by comparison to aged-matched normal ranges.

32.3 Results

32.3.1 RS1 Mutations in Western Australian Families

An RS1 mutation was confirmed for each clinically diagnosed individual. In total, three distinct genetic variants from four families were identified, one being novel (Table 32.1). These include; (1) an exon one splice donor mutation (52+1G>T) found in two families, (2) an exon four missense genetic variant (289T>G), and (3) an exon five, frameshift mutation (416delA). Comparison of clinical data (ophthalmological, electrophysiological and psychophysical) did not indicate a correlation between patient genotype and the manifestation of clinical symptoms.

Table 32.1 XLRS mutations identified in the RS1 gene within the Western Australian population. To the best of our knowledge, the 289T>G genetic variant observed is novel

No. Families	Exon/IVS	Nucleotide Δ	Predicted effect	Novel/Reported
2	IVS 1	52+1 G>T	Splicing defect	Reported
1	4	289T>G	W92G	Novel
1	5	416delA	Early termination	Reported

32.3.2 Compromised Full-Field and mfERG in an Obligate Carrier with 52+1G > T Mutation

Full-field and mfERG tracings from the affected male with a 52+1G > T mutation were typical for XLRS with reduced b-wave amplitudes and response densities respectively (Fig. 32.1a, b). A related obligate carrier, heterozygous for this mutation, similarly recorded a bilaterally abnormal rod ERG with delayed b-waves as well as mildly abnormal photopic responses; cone and flicker ERG tracings showed slightly reduced and delayed b-wave amplitdues respectively. mfERG trace arrays showed reduced response density in the paramacular region extending futher temporally for each eye (Fig. 32.1a, b).

32.3.3 Likely Pathogenicity of the Novel 289T > G Genetic Variant

32.3.3.1 Family Information

In this family, the proband was the only individual clinically diagnosed with XLRS (Fig. 32.2a; III:1). The proband reported however, that his younger male sibling had very recently began to suffer similar visual symptoms (age 17) but had not yet consulted an ophthalmologist. He also reported that maternal uncles (Thailand) suffered similar visual symptoms. None have seen a medical practitioner for diagnosis.

32.3.3.2 Patient Information

Upon presentation at age 18, fundus examination revealed the proband's perifoveal retina was spokewheel in appearance accompanied by a peripheral retinal sheen, but no schisis. Electroretinographic findings were typical for an XLRS diagnosis; scotopic, photopic and flicker tracings revealed severely reduced b-wave amplitudes and slightly delayed a-waves. Pattern ERG was normal. Eight years later a mfERG trace array showed responses with normal mophology but delayed latencies as well as reduced densities throughout the central retina, being more severe in the macula.

32.3.3.3 Genetic Information

This 289T > G single base substitution found in exon four is likely to cause a W92G amino acid change in the discoidin domain of the translated product and to the best of our knowledge has not before been reported in the literature (Fig. 32.2b).

Fig. 32.1 (continued) (*right*). (**a**) mfERG first order kernel results; full-field trace arrays, response densities and latencies in rows 1–3 respectively. (**b**) Full-field ERG results; rod, maximal rod-cone, cone and flicker waveforms in *rows* 1–4 respectively. Amplitude (uV) is plotted on the Y axis and time (ms) on the X axis

(A)

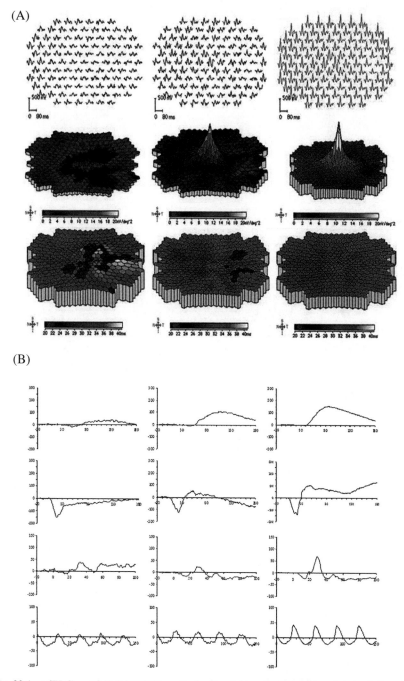

(B)

Fig. 32.1 mfERG and full-field ERG results for the right eyes of an affected male (*left*) and his carrier sister (*middle*) each with a 52+G > T mutation, as well as an aged matched, normal control

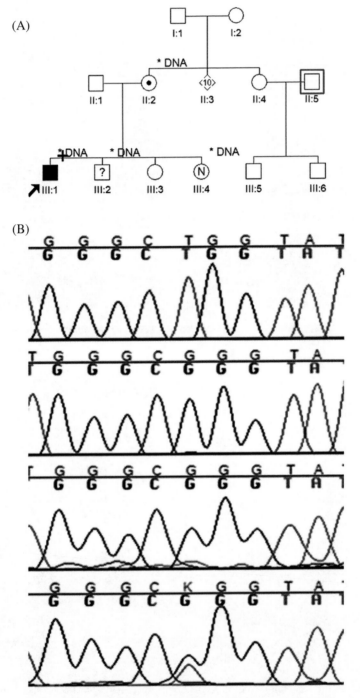

Fig. 32.2 (a) A three generation pedigree of a family with a 289T > G single base substitution in the RS1 gene. Four individuals were analysed for RS1 mutations (*DNA above right of symbol).

```
                                    62                                                     114
H.sapiens      NP_035432.1    HKPLGFESGEVTPDQITCSNPEQYVGWYSSWTANKARLNSQGFGCAW-LSKFQD

C.lupus        XP_548882.2    HKPLGFESGEVTPDQITCSNLDQYVGWYSSWTANKARLNSQGFGCAW-LSKYQD

O.cunniculus   NP_001103293.1 HKPLGFESGEVTADQITCSNPEQYVGWYSSWTANKARLNSQGFGCAW-LSKFQD

M.musculus     NP_035432.3    HKPLGFESGEVTPDQITCSNPEQYVGWYSSWTANKARLNSQGFGCAW-LSKYQD

G.gallus       NP_001128447.1 HKPLGFESGAVTPDQISCSNPEQYTGWYSSWTANKARLNGQGFGCALALSKYQD

D.rerio        NP_001003438.1 HKPLGFEAGSVASDQISCSNEDQYTGWFSSWTPNRARLNSQGFGCAW-LSKFQD
```

Fig. 32.3 ClustalW alignment of RS proteins shows the tryptophan residue at position 92 (W92; boxed) has been highly conserved throughout evolution

ClustalW RS protein sequence alignment shows W92 is highly conserved, even in *Danio rerio* (Fig. 32.3).

Sequencing of 135 control X chromosomes confirmed this variant was not present in the normal population (data not shown). DNA sequencing of family members revealed the proband's mother was heterozygous for this variant, the symptomatic younger brother did in fact posess the same novel 289T > G single base substitution, while the younger sister did not harbour any change (Fig. 32.2a, b).

32.4 Discussion

In this study we revealed the genetic diagnosis of individuals affected by XLRS in four Western Australian families. The exon five, frameshift 416delA mutation has previously been reported resulting in premature termination in the discoidin domain hence abrogating normal RS structure (The Retinoschisis Consortium 1998) making intra-cellular retention and degradation very likely. Clincal data was not presented for this family as the ophthalmic report indicated that in addition to Retinoschisis, an RP type syndrome was likley.

Also previously reported, the 52+1G > T missense mutation was found in two Western Australian families and is likely to result in a splicing defect predicted to cause a deleterious insertion or deletion towards the end of the leader sequence, a motif important in secretion of RS from the endoplasmic reticulum (Mashima et al. 1999). We showed that the full-field and mfERG results for an affected

◄──

Fig. 32.2 (continued) *Solid square* indicates affected male, in this case the proband (III:1; *arrow*). *Central dot* within a *circle* indicates carrier female (II:2). *Question mark* within a *box* indicates a possibly affected male (III:2). A circle containing the letter 'N' indicates a non-carrier female (III:4). (**b**) Electropherograms for part of the RS1 nucleotide sequence from exon four is shown in order from top to bottom for (1) an unrelated, normal control, (2) the proband (III:1) in which the 289T > G substitution was observed, (3) the proband's symptomatic brother (III:2) in which this change was also observed, (4) the proband's mother II:2, heterozygous for this change and marked by the letter *K*. The position of nucleotide 289T is marked by an arrow (*top*)

male with this mutation were typical for XLRS (Piao et al. 2003; Tantri et al. 2004; Tsang et al. 2007). The carrier, heterozygous for 52+1G>T recorded an abnormal mfERG trace array, sometimes observed in XLRS obligate carriers (Kim et al. 2006). Interestingly, the abnormal full-field ERG observed, is not usually seen in XLRS carriers. The likely explanation for this is unfavourably biased X-inactivation (Lyon 1962) or alternatively, the presence of another underlying condition.

To the best of our knowledge the 289T>G genetic variant has not before been reported. This single base substitution causes a W92G amino acid change. Importantly, the highly conserved W92 is one of three aromatic amino acids proposed to form the membrane lipid anchorage site (Fraternali et al. 2003) confirmed by site directed mutatengesis; the W92C mutant reduced the ability of RS to anchor to the preferred lipid moiety, phosphatidylserine, by 30–50% in vitro (Vijayasarathy et al. 2007). While the effect of a W92G transition in RS has not been confirmed experimentally, replacement of the large, hydrophobic, aromatic membrane binding tryptophan with the ambivalent and smallest of all amino acids, glycine, is likely to negatively affect anchorage as demonstrated for other membrane binding proteins (Ortega-Gutierrez and Lopez-Rodriguez 2005). Hence even if extracellular RS is present in this case, is is unlikely to be properly functional.

Given that (1) the 289T>G genetic variant was the the only change detected in RS1 DNA of the proband, (2) the proband's mother is heterozygous for this single base substitution, (3) this change was absent from 135 control X chromosomes, and (4) it causes a change in a crucial membrane binding residue in a protein that functions to bind photoreceptor and bi-polar cell membranes, there is strong evidence to suggest that 289T>G is pathogenic.

That RS1 is a small gene with retinal specific expression patterns makes this gene a suitable candidate for gene delivery gene therapies. Characterisation of disease causing mutations in patients affected by inherited retinal diease is an important preceeding step for such therapies, but also contributes towards a better understanding of the clinical manifestation of these diseases.

Acknowledgments The authors gratefully acknowledge the Western Australian Retinitis Pigmentosa Foundation for their generous funding, and the assistance of the Western Australian DNA Bank (NHMRC Enabling Facility) with DNA samples for this study.

References

Deutman AF (1971) Sex-linked retinoschisis. In: Deutman AF (ed) The hereditary dystrpohies of the posterior pole of the eye. Van Gorcum, Assen, Netherlands

Eksandh L, Andreasson S, Abrahamson M (2005) Juvenile x-linked retinoschisis with normal scotopic b-wave in the electroretinogram at an early stage of the disease. Ophthalmic Genet 26(3):111–117

Forsius H, Krause U, Helve J et al (1973) Visual acuity in 183 cases of x-chromosomal retinoschisis. Can J Ophthalmol 8(3):385–393

Fraternali F, Cavallo L, Musco G (2003) Effects of pathological mutations on the stability of a conserved amino acid triad in retinoschisin. FEBS Lett 544(1–3):21–26

George ND, Yates JR, Moore AT (1995) X linked retinoschisis. Br J Ophthalmol 79(7):697–702

Hewitt AW, FitzGerald LM, Scotter LW et al (2005) Genotypic and phenotypic spectrum of x-linked retinoschisis in australia. Clin Exp Ophthalmol 33(3):233–239

Kellner U, Brummer S, Foerster MH et al (1990) X-linked congenital retinoschisis. Graefes Arch Clin Exp Ophthalmol 228(5):432–437

Kim DY, Neely KA, Sassani JW et al (2006) X-linked retinoschisis: novel mutation in the initiation codon of the xlrs1 gene in a large family. Retina 26(8):940–946

Lyon MF (1962) Sex chromatin and gene action in the mammalian x-chromosome. Am J Hum Genet 14:135–148

Mashima Y, Shinoda K, Ishida S et al (1999) Identification of four novel mutations of the xlrs1 gene in japanese patients with x-linked juvenile retinoschisis. Mutation in brief no. 234. Online. Hum Mutat 13(4):338

Molday LL, Wu WW, Molday RS (2007) Retinoschisin (rs1), the protein encoded by the x-linked retinoschisis gene, is anchored to the surface of retinal photoreceptor and bipolar cells through its interactions with a na/k atpase-sarm1 complex. J Biol Chem 282(45):32792–32801

Ortega-Gutierrez S, Lopez-Rodriguez ML (2005) Cb1 and cb2 cannabinoid receptor binding studies based on modeling and mutagenesis approaches. Mini Rev Med Chem 5(7): 651–658

Piao CH, Kondo M, Nakamura M et al (2003) Multifocal electroretinograms in x-linked retinoschisis. Invest Ophthalmol Vis Sci 44(11):4920–4930

Pimenides D, George ND, Yates JR et al (2005) X-linked retinoschisis: clinical phenotype and rs1 genotype in 86 uk patients. JMedGenet 42(6):e35

Sauer CG, Gehrig A, Warneke-Wittstock R et al (1997) Positional cloning of the gene associated with x-linked juvenile retinoschisis. Nat Genet 17(2):164–170

Tantri A, Vrabec TR, Cu-Unjieng A et al (2004) X-linked retinoschisis: a clinical and molecular genetic review. Surv Ophthalmol 49(2):214–230

The Retinoschisis Consortium (1998) Functional implications of the spectrum of mutations found in 234 cases with x-linked juvenile retinoschisis. Hum Mol Genet 7(7):1185–1192

Tsang SH, Vaclavik V, Bird AC et al (2007) Novel phenotypic and genotypic findings in x-linked retinoschisis. Arch Ophthalmol 125(2):259–267

Vijayasarathy C, Takada Y, Zeng Y et al (2007) Retinoschisin is a peripheral membrane protein with affinity for anionic phospholipids and affected by divalent cations. Invest Ophthalmol Vis Sci 48(3):991–1000

Wang T, Waters CT, Rothman AM et al (2002) Intracellular retention of mutant retinoschisin is the pathological mechanism underlying x-linked retinoschisis. Hum Mol Genet 11(24):3097–3105

Wu WW, Molday RS (2003) Defective discoidin domain structure, subunit assembly, and endoplasmic reticulum processing of retinoschisin are primary mechanisms responsible for x-linked retinoschisis. J Biol Chem 278(30):28139–28146

Wu WW, Wong JP, Kast J et al (2005) Rs1, a discoidin domain-containing retinal cell adhesion protein associated with x-linked retinoschisis, exists as a novel disulfide-linked octamer. J Biol Chem 280(11):10721–10730

Chapter 33
Mutation Frequency of IMPDH1 Gene of Han Population in Ganzhou City

Li Shumei, Luo Xiaoting, Zeng Xiangyun, Hu Liqun, Xiong Liang, and Li Sisi

Abstract

Objective: Mutations in the inosine monophosphate dehydrogenase 1 gene (IMPDH1) have recently been discovered that IMPDH1 gene plays a critical role in pathogenesis of autosomal dominant retinitis pigmentosa (adRP). Aiming towards an understanding of the molecular background of retinitis pigmentosa (RP), this paper investigates the mutation frequency of IMPDH1 genes in the Han patients with adRP in Ganzhou City.

Methods: The whole blood samples were collected randomly from 56 adRP patients and 62 unrelated normal controls who were residents of Han population in Ganzhou City, and then their genomic DNA samples were extracted respectively. Genic polymorphism was examined by the polymerase chain reaction and restriction-fragment-length polymorphisms (PCR-RFLP). The statistical significance of the data was further analyzed by SPSS 14.0 software.

Results: Mutation rate of IMPDH1 gene had no significance between in adRP patients and in the normal control by exact probabilities in 2×2 table ($p = 0.232$). The mutation frequency of IMPDH1gene in the Han samples was 3.6%.

Conclusion: The mutation frequency of IMPDH1 gene of the Han population in Ganzhou city was similar as approximately 2–5% of the adRP cases among Americans of European origin and Europeans.

33.1 Introduction

Retinitis pigmentosa (RP) is a group of inherited retinal degenerative disorders characterized by progressive degeneration of the midperipheral retina, leading to night blindness, visual field constriction, and eventual loss of visual acuity (Gandra et al.

L. Shumei (✉)
Department of Preventive Medicine, Gannan Medical College, Ganzhou, China
e-mail: gnyxylsm@163.com

R.E. Anderson et al. (eds.), *Retinal Degenerative Diseases*, Advances in Experimental Medicine and Biology 664, DOI 10.1007/978-1-4419-1399-9_33, © Springer Science+Business Media, LLC 2010

2008). It is one of the leading causes of blindness in adults with an incidence of around 1 in 3,500 worldwide (Hims et al. 2003). RP has a strong genetic component with multiple modes of inheritance including autosomal dominant (adRP), autosomal recessive (arRP), X-linked (xLRP) and apparent digenic forms (Wang et al. 2001). The autosomal dominant forms have been associated with 16 different loci, and for 15 of these, the causative genes have been identified including: PRPF3 (1q21.2), SEMA4A (1q22), RHO (3q22), GUCA1B (6p21.1), RDS(6p21.2), RP9 (7q14), IMPDH1 (7q32), RP1 (8q12), ROM1 (11q12), NRL (14q11), PRPF8 (17p13), CA4 (17q23), FSCN2 (17q25), CRX (19q13.3), and PRPF31 (19q13.4) (Zhao et al. 2006).

Inosine monophosphate dehydrogenase (IMPDH) proteins form homotetramers and catalyze the rate limiting step of de novo guanine synthesis by oxidizing IMP to xanthosine-5′-monophosphate (XMP) with reduction of nicotinamide adenine dinucleotide (NAD). Two closely related human IMPDH isoforms, types 1 and 2, have been identified, each consisting of 514 amino acids with 84% sequence identity. IMPDH genes are found in virtually every organism, and the gene and amino acid sequences are highly conserved across species. The isoforms are encoded by 2 distinct genes, IMPDH1 and IMPDH2 (inosine monophosphate dehydrogenase 1 and 2), located at 7q31.3–q32 and 3p21.2–p24.2, respectively. Gene expression of the 2 isoforms is differently regulated in various tissues and cell populations, and they are not mutually redundant (Bremer et al. 2007). Mutations in IMPDH1 cause the RP10 form of autosomal dominant RP (adRP) (Kennan et al. 2002). IMPDH1 is located on chromosome 7q32.1 and encodes the enzyme IMPDH1.

In this study, we surveyed a population of patients with adRP to determine the range and the frequency of IMPDH1 mutations. The clinical heterogeneity of mutations in genes associated with retinal degeneration has been demonstrated many times (Bowne et al. 2006). Therefore, we analyzed patients with specifically autosomal recessive RP (arRP) to investigate the possibility that mutations in IMPDH1 cause alternate phenotypes.

33.2 Materials and Methods

33.2.1 Subjects

This study was performed in accordance with the Declaration of Helsinki, with informed consent obtained in all cases. Most subjects examined in this study were diagnosed at one of the following sites: (1) Department of Ophthalmology of the 1st Affiliated Hospital, Gannan Medical College; (2) Department of Ophthalmology of the People Hospital of Ganzhou City. The research at each academic institution was approved by the respective human subjects' review board.

33.2.2 DNA Extraction

The whole blood samples were collected randomly from 56 adRP patients and 62 unrelated normal controls who were residents of Han population in Ganzhou City, and then their genomic DNA samples were extracted respectively by the DNA extraction kit (Shenggong, PRC).

33.2.3 Amplification of IMPDH1 Genes

Exon 7 of the IMPDH 1 gene was amplified by PCR. According to the reference (Yu et al. 2007), the peculiar primes were 5'-CAGTGGAATCTCTGGAGTGGTC-3' and 5'-CCT2GGGTCCTCATAAACCTC-3' which were synthesized by Shanghai Shenggong biology engineering company. The total volume of polymerase chain reaction (PCR) was 10 ul which included 6 ul of DNA sample, 2 pmol of positive prime and negative prime respectively, 2.5 mmol/L dNTP, 1 ul of 10 × PCR Buffer and 0.5 U Taq DNA polymerase enzyme. All PCRs were carried out in a SX-240B thermal cycler (Shunda, PRC). The reactions were incubated for 10 min at 96°C which was followed by 34 cycles of denaturation (96°C, 1 min), annealing (50°C, 30 s), extension (68°C, 3 min), final extension (68°C, 10 min) and were then held at 4°C.

33.2.4 RFLP Analysis

Msp restriction endonuclease (Shenggong, PRC) was selected for DNA digestion. The volume of enzymatical digestion was 20 ul. IMPDH 1 gene amplicons (10 ul/reaction) of each sample were enzymatically digested by Msp I(0.2 ul/reaction) at 37°C for 9 h. PCR-product restriction fragments (20 ul) were separated by electrophoresis (TAE buffered agarose gels) at 5 V/cm for 2 h and stained with ethidium bromide. Each gel included 50 bp DNA ladder markers. RFLPs were visualized using UV light, and images were recorded using a Gel Documentation Digital Imaging system.

33.2.5 Statistical Analysis

The statistical significance of the data was further analyzed by SPSS 14.0 software. The rates were compared by χ^2 test, and $\alpha = 0.05$ was size of test.

33.3 Results

Mutation rate of IMPDH1 gene had no significance between in adRP patients and in the normal control by exact probabilities in 2×2 table ($p = 0.232$). The mutation frequency of IMPDH1gene in the Han samples was 3.6%. Group distribution $\chi^2 = 1.635$, $p > 0.5$. The allelic distribution of the gene was in accordance with Hardy-Weinberg equilirium.

33.4 Discussion

The identification of IMPDH1 as the causitive gene in the RP10 form of adRP had implicated a nucleotide biosynthesis pathway in a degeneration of the retina (Kennan et al. 2003). The IMPDH1 gene encodes a protein subunit of 514 amino acid residues, with the active IMPDH1 enzyme consisting of a homotetramer of these subunits. Each monomer of the protein possesses two domains; the larger forms a barrel which contains the active site loop and the smaller is comprised of two tandem cystathionine-beta-synthase dimer domains (Nimmesgern et al. 1999). It was difficult to speculate how precisely mutations within the IMPDH1 gene may bring about the pathology. One possibility was that, while not in the active site of the enzyme, the mutation might cause a reduction in the levels of guanine nucleotides available to photoreceptors which it appeared, might be relying almost solely on IMPDH1 for maintaining their guanine nucleotide reserves.

The mutation frequency of IMPDH1 gene was approximately 2–5% of the adRP cases among Americans of European origin and Europeans (Bowne et al. 2006; Bowne et al. 2002; Wada et al. 2005). The mutation frequency of IMPDH1 gene of the Han population in Ganzhou city was similar as this. The evidence implicating the *IMPDH1* gene as a cause of dominant RP includes the identification of different missense mutations in different families, the observation that none of these mutations is found among normal controls, and the observation that the mutations perfectly cosegregate with RP. There is no reported comparison of the clinical features of patients with mutations in this gene versus those with mutations in other identified RP genes. The most frequent mutation, Asp226Asn, appeared to cause at least as much loss of rod function as cone function. Patients with this form of RP retain, on average, two to five times more ERG amplitude per unit of remaining visual area than patients with three other forms of dominant RP (Wada et al. 2005). Bowne et al. (2006) reported that IMPDH1 mutations did not alter enzyme activity and demonstrated that these mutants altered the recently identified single-stranded nucleic acid binding property of IMPDH. Subsequent studies are needed to further elucidate the nucleic acid binding property of IMPDH1 and its relevance to photoreceptor biology and retinal disease.

References

Bowne SJ, Sullivan LS, Blanton SH et al (2002) Mutations in the inosine monophosphate dehydrogenase 1 gene (IMPDH1) cause the RP10 form of autosomal dominant retinitis pigmentosa. Hum Mol Genet 11(5):559–568

Bowne SJ, Sullivan LS, Mortimer SE et al (2006) Spectrum and frequency of mutations in IMPDH1 associated with autosomal dominant retinitis pigmentosa and leber congenital amaurosis. Invest Ophthalmol Vis Sci 47(1):34–42

Bremer S, Rootwelt H, Bergan S (2007) Real-time PCR determination of IMPDH1 and IMPDH2 expression in blood cells. Clin Chem. 53(6):1023–1029

Gandra M, Anandula V, Authiappan V et al (2008) Retinitis pigmentosa: mutation analysis of RHO, PRPF31, RP1, and IMPDH1 genes in patients from India. Mol Vis 14:1105–1113

Hims MM, Diager SP, Inglehearn CF (2003) Retinitis pigmentosa: genes, proteins and prospects. Dev Ophthalmol 37:109–125

Kennan A, Aherne A, Bowne SJ et al (2003) On the role of IMPDH1 in retinal degeneration. Adv Exp Med Biol 533:13–18

Kennan A, Aherne A, Palfi A et al (2002) Identification of an IMPDH1 mutation in autosomal dominant retinitis pigmentosa (RP10) revealed following comparative microarray analysis of transcripts derived from retinas of wild-type and Rho(–/–) mice. Hum Mol Genet 11(5): 547–557

Nimmesgern E, Black J, Futer O et al (1999) Biochemical analysis of the modular enzyme inosine 5'-monophosphate dehydrogenase. Protein Expr Purif 17(2):282–289

Wada Y, Sandberg MA, McGee TL et al (2005) Screen of the IMPDH1 gene among patients with dominant retinitis pigmentosa and clinical features associated with the most common mutation, Asp226Asn. Invest Ophthalmol Vis Sci. 46(5):1735–1741

Wang Q, Chen Q, Zhao K et al (2001) Update on the molecular genetics of retinitis pigmentosa. Ophthalmic Genet. 22(3):133–154

Yu Y, Yang H, Yu Y et al (2007) Mutations of the IMPDH 1 gene in patients correlated with autosomal dominant retinitis pigmentosa family. Rec Adv Ophthalmol 27(9):649–652

Zhao C, Lu S, Zhou X et al (2006) A novel locus (RP33) for autosomal dominant retinitis pigmentosa mapping to chromosomal region 2cen-q12.1. Hum Genet 119(6):617–623

Part III
Diagnostic, Clinical, Cytopathological and Physiologic Aspects of Retinal Degeneration

Chapter 34
Reversible and Size-Selective Opening of the Inner Blood-Retina Barrier: A Novel Therapeutic Strategy

Matthew Campbell, Anh Thi Hong Nguyen, Anna-Sophia Kiang, Lawrence Tam, Paul F. Kenna, Sorcha Ni Dhubhghaill, Marian Humphries, G. Jane Farrar, and Peter Humphries

Abstract The inner Blood-Retina-barrier (iBRB) remains a key element in retarding the development of novel therapeutics for the treatment of many ocular disorders. The iBRB contains tight-junctions (TJ's) which reduce the space between adjacent endothelial cells lining the fine capillaries of the retinal microvasculature to form a selective and regulatable barrier. We have recently shown that in mice, the iBRB can be transiently and size-selectively opened to molecules with molecular weights of up to approximately 1 kDa using an siRNA-mediated approach involving suppression of the tight junction protein, claudin-5. We have systemically delivered siRNA targeting claudin-5 to retinal capillary endothelial cells in mice and through a series of tracer experiments and magnetic-resonance-imaging (MRI), we have shown a transient and size-selective increase in permeability at the iBRB to molecules below 1 kDa. The potential to exploit this specific compromise in iBRB integrity may have far reaching implications for the development of experimental animal models of retinal degenerative disorders, and for enhanced delivery of therapeutic molecules which would normally not traverse the iBRB. Using RNAi-mediated opening of the iBRB, the systemic delivery of low molecular weight therapeutics could in principle, hold real promise as an alternative to repeated intraocular inoculation of compounds. Results demonstrated here in mouse models, should lead to a 'humanized' form of systemic delivery as opposed to the hydrodynamic approach used in our work to date.

34.1 Introduction

The human retina has the highest oxygen consumption per weight of any tissue in the body. The high metabolic rate of the neural retina underlines the need for a distinct and regulated blood supply, and this is mediated via the Blood Retinal Barrier

M. Campbell (✉)
Ocular Genetics Unit, Department of Genetics, Trinity College Dublin, Dublin 2, Ireland
e-mail: matthew.campbell@tcd.ie

R.E. Anderson et al. (eds.), *Retinal Degenerative Diseases*, Advances in Experimental Medicine and Biology 664, DOI 10.1007/978-1-4419-1399-9_34,
© Springer Science+Business Media, LLC 2010

(BRB). At the inner retina, retinal capillaries arising from the central artery permeate the retina only as far as the inner nuclear layer (INL), with the outer segments of the retina remaining avascular. Very similar in structure and function to the blood brain barrier (BBB), the BRB in the retina allows for the maintenance of neural tissue environments through the regulation of ion concentrations, water permeability, delivery of amino acids and sugars, and by preventing the exposure of the neural tissue to circulatory factors such as antibodies and immune cells (Antonetti et al. 1999). In contrast to the BBB, however, the BRB consists of both an inner blood retinal barrier (iBRB) and an outer blood retinal barrier (oBRB). The iBRB comprises retinal endothelial cells, which line the micro-vessels allowing for the maintenance of blood vessel integrity and preserving the vessel's homeostasis while the oBRB is made up of retinal pigment epithelial (RPE) cells and Bruch's membrane, and it acts as a filter to restrict the passage of macromolecules.

Both the iBRB and oBRB contain tight junctions that confer highly selective properties on barrier function. Tight junctions are formed at the apical periphery of endothelial cells of the iBRB (Fig. 34.1). They perform the dual role of creating a primary barrier to the diffusion of solutes through the paracellular pathway, while also maintaining cell polarity as a boundary between the apical and basolateral plasma membrane domains Sakakibara et al. (1997).

Tight junctions are complex structures, which are composed of a series of integral and peripheral membrane proteins. The transmembrane proteins of the tight junction include occludin, junctional adhesion molecule (JAM) and claudins 1–20. These proteins extend into the paracellular space, creating the seal characteristic of the tight junction (Fanning and Anderson 1998; Riesen et al. 2002).

Occludin and the claudins are transmembrane proteins associated with the tight junction and have previously been shown to interact homotypically with proteins on adjacent endothelial cells. In 2003, claudin-5 knockout mice were reported, and were shown to have a compromised BBB. The authors concluded that while removal of claudin-5 compromises the function of the BBB by allowing it to become permeable to molecules of up to approximately 800 Da, the barrier could still form, remaining intact and impervious to larger molecules (Nitta et al. 2003).

Claudin-5 is highly expressed in the plasma membrane of retinal microvascular endothelial cells under normal conditions in vivo while hypoxia significantly reduces the level of claudin-5 in the membrane of these cells. In addition, inhibition of claudin-5 expression using RNAi leads to a reduction of transendothelial electrical resistance in bEND.3 cells even under normoxic conditions (Koto et al. 2007).

It has been proposed that claudin-5 may play a role in the formation of paracellular pores or channels that function in mediating selective ion permeability (Anderson et al. 2001). It is clear however that removal of claudin-5 from the tight junction will cause a size-selective increase in the permeability of the tight junction.

Here, we describe the first report of reversible and controlled RNAi mediated size-selective opening of the paracellular pathway of the iBRB, representing a novel approach for delivery of a wide range of small molecules to the inner retina. This method of reversible iBRB modulation may pave the way for controlled delivery

The Tight Junction

Apical (Blood Side)

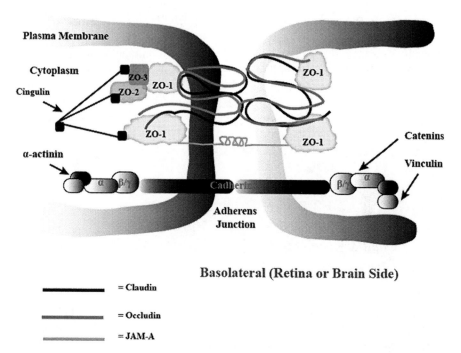

Basolateral (Retina or Brain Side)

_____ = Claudin

_____ = Occludin

_____ = JAM-A

Fig. 34.1 The tight junction is expressed at the apical periphery of both endothelial and epithelial cells of the blood retinal barrier (BRB). Occludin and claudins are the transmembrane proteins represented as a network of fibrils encircling the apical end of the lateral membrane in freeze-fracture images of the tight junction. The integral membrane proteins zonula occludens-1, -2, -3 (ZO-1, -2, and -3) allow for the scaffolding of the transmembrane proteins (Fanning and Anderson 1998) and have also been implicated in intracellular signaling pathways

of therapeutic agents to the retina in a range of degenerative retinal conditions that currently offer little or no prospect of effective treatment.

34.2 Materials and Methods

34.2.1 Animal Experiments and Experimental Groups

All experiments involving the use of C57/BL6 mice were assessed and approved by an internal ethics committee in Trinity College Dublin (TCD) prior to all experimentation. All studies carried out in the Ocular Genetics Unit in TCD adhere to the ARVO statement for the use of Animals in Ophthalmic and Vision Research. C57/BL6 mice were sourced from Jackson Laboratories and bred on-site at the Ocular Genetics Unit in TCD.

34.2.2 Web-Based siRNA Design Protocols Targeting Claudin-5

Initially, four siRNAs targeting Claudin-5 were tested and the most efficient used in further studies. Sequences of the claudin-5 siRNA used in this study were as follows. Sense sequence: CGUUGGAAAUUCUGGGUCUUU. Antisense sequence: AGACCCAGAAUUUCCAACGUU. Non-targeting control siRNA targeting human rhodopsin was used as a non-targeting control since rhodopsin is only expressed in photoreceptor cells in the retina and at low levels in the pineal gland of the brain. Sense sequence: CGCUCAAGCCGGAGGUCAAUU. Antisense sequence: UUGACCUCCGGCUUGAGCGUU.

34.2.3 In Vivo Delivery of siRNA to Murine Retinal Capillary Endothelial Cells by Large Volume Hydrodynamic Injection

Rapid high pressure, high volume tail vein injections were carried out essentially as previously successfully used at this laboratory (Kiang et al. 2005; Campbell et al. 2008). Wild type C57/Bl6 mice of weight 20–30 g were individually restrained inside a 60-ml volume plastic tube. The protruding tail was warmed for 5 min prior to injection under a 60-W lamp and the tail vein clearly visualized by illumination from below. 20 micrograms of targeting siRNA, or non-targeting siRNA made up with PBS to a volume in mls of 10% of the body weight in grams was injected into the tail vein at a rate of 1 ml/s using a 26-guage (26G 3/8) needle.

34.2.4 Indirect Immunostaining of Retinal Flatmounts

Retinas were permeabilised and blocked with 5% Normal Goat Serum (NGS) in PBS with 0.5% Triton X-100 for 2 h at room temperature. Rabbit anti-Claudin-5 (Zymed, California) was incubated on sections overnight at 4°C. Following incubation, retinas were washed 6 times in PBS and subsequently blocked again with 5% NGS for 2 h at room temperature. Secondary rabbit IgG-Cy3, (Jackson-Immunoresearch, Europe) was incubated with the sections at 37°C for 4 h followed by 10 washes with PBS.

34.2.5 Assessment of BRB Integrity by Perfusion of Hoechst (H33342)

Following RNAi-mediated ablation of transcripts encoding claudin-5 mice were per-fused through the left ventricle of the beating heart and @ 37°C with 500 μl/g body weight of PBS containing 100 μg/ml Hoechst stain H33342 (Sigma Aldrich, Ireland) 24, 48, 72 h and 1 week post-hydrodynamic delivery of claudin-5 siRNA. Following perfusion, the whole eye was dissected and placed in 4% PFA pH 7.4 for 4 h and subsequently washed 4 × 15 mins with PBS. Eyes were cryoprotected using a sucrose gradient, 12 μm cryosections were cut using a cryostat.

34.2.6 Magnetic Resonance Imaging (MRI)

Following injection of siRNA and using appropriate controls, BRB integrity to a molecule of 742 Daltons was assessed via MRI, using a dedicated small rodent Bruker BioSpec 70/30 (i.e. 7T, 30 cm bore) with an actively shielded USR Magnet. BBB integrity was then visualised in high resolution T_1 weighted MR images before and after injection of a 0.1 mM /L/kg bolus of Gd-DTPA (Gadolinium diethylene-triamine pentaacetic acid), administered via the tail vein. Following injection of Gd-DTPA, repeated 3 min T_1-weighted scans were performed over a period of 30 min, and images shown are representative of the final scans of this 30 min period.

34.3 Results

34.3.1 Claudin-5 Levels in Retinal Flatmounts

Following hydrodynamic tail vein delivery of siRNA targeting claudin-5, levels of expression of this tight junction protein were shown to dramatically decrease at 24 and 48 h post-injection. The pattern of expression of claudin-5 72 h post-injection of siRNA appeared similar to that of mice receiving a non-targeting siRNA (Fig. 34.2).

34.3.2 Perfusion of Hoechst 33342 (562 Da) in Mice Post-Delivery of Claudin-5 Sirna

Following suppression of claudin-5 at the iBRB in mice, Hoechst 33342 was per-fused through the left ventricle of the heart. After preparation of 12 μm retinal cryosections, it was observed that iBRB permeability was manifested by INL stain-ing at 24 h post injection of claudin-5 siRNA and both INL and ONL staining 48 h post-injection of siRNA targeting claudin-5. This increase in iBRB permeability

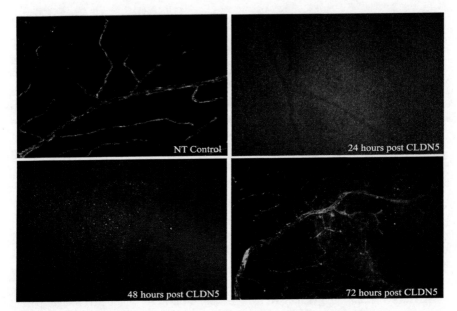

Fig. 34.2 Retinal flatmount analysis of claudin-5 expression in the retinas of mice receiving a non-targeting (NT) siRNA showed distinct peripheral staining of claudin-5 in the retinal vasculature. This peripheral staining appeared diffuse and discontinuous in the retinas of mice 24 and 48 h post-injection of siRNA targeting claudin-5, with levels returning to normal 72 h post-injection of siRNA

was shown to be a transient event as 72 h post injection of siRNA, there was no extra-vascular staining of the nuclear layers of the retina (Fig. 34.3).

34.3.3 MRI Analysis of Ibrb Integrity Following Rnai of Claudin-5

Forty-eight hours post injection of siRNA targeting claudin-5, mice were injected with the MRI tracer molecule Gd-DTPA (742 Da). As evidenced by Gd-DTPA deposition within the eye, the iBRB was shown to be compromised in that dark contrasting was observed both in the retina and in the vitreous region of the mouse eye (Fig. 34.4).

34.4 Discussion

The retinal microvasculature plays an essential role in supplying the high-energy demanding retina with oxygen-enriched blood. The endothelial cells that line these fine capillaries have evolved 'tight junctions', which form a selective and regulatable barrier. However, oxygen can still diffuse from these cells, and other essential materials can be delivered to the retina by special transporters located in the membranes

Hoechst 33342 (562 Da) perfusion 24, 48, 72 hours and 1 week post HTV
delivery of siRNA targeting CLDN5

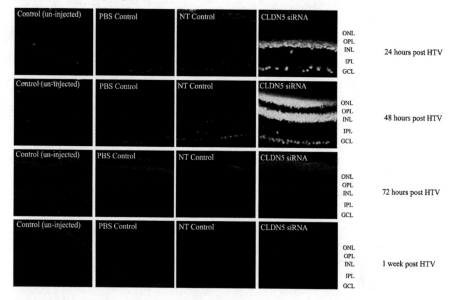

Fig. 34.3 Extravasation of Hoechst 33342 was evident in 12 μm retinal cryosections, with the Inner Nuclear Layer (INL) appearing stained at 24 h and distinct Outer Nuclear Layer (ONL) staining at 48 h post delivery of CLDN5 siRNA. In all control groups, Hoechst staining was manifested solely in the nuclei of retinal blood vessels which diffuse within the retina as far as the Outer Plexiform Layer (OPL). Scale bar approx. 20 μm. (IPL) Inner Plexiform Layer; (GCL) Ganglion Cell Layer

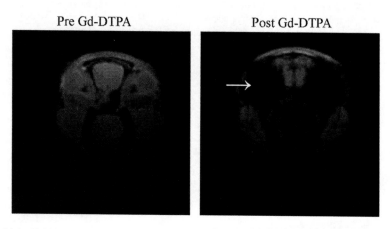

Fig. 34.4 48 h post injection of siRNA targeting claudin-5, Gd-DTPA permeation was evident within the eyes of mice. The image to the *left* represents a T1-weighted MRI image of a mouse 48 h post-injection of claudin-5 siRNA pre-Gd-DTPA injection. The image to the *right* shows the same mouse post-Gd-DTPA injection, showing enhanced contrasting due to Gd-DTPA extravasation within the eye

of the endothelial cells. Complete breakdown of the iBRB would have disastrous consequences for overall retina function. However, if transient, reversible opening of the barrier could be achieved, an avenue would be available for experimental delivery to the retina, in animals such as mice, of agents which may modulate neuronal function.

We have herein described a method whereby the iBRB can be induced to become transiently and size-selectively permeable to molecules below approximately 1 kDa. Although this is an experimental approach using a hydrodynamic technique of inoculation, a viral mediated delivery system could in principle 'humanize' this approach to allow for the delivery of a wide range of therapeutics to the inner retina.

The potential to exploit transient compromises in iBRB integrity also has far reaching implications for the development of experimental animal models of neurodegenerative diseases of the retina, for therapeutic applications involving drug delivery/drug screening in mice and for advancing our understanding of iBRB function in general.

Acknowledgments This work was supported by the Wellcome Trust, Fighting Blindness Ireland, and Science Foundation Ireland.

References

Anderson JM (2001) Molecular structure of tight junctions and their role in epithelial transport. News Physiol Sci 16:126–130

Antonetti DA, Barber AJ, Hollinger LA et al (1999) Vascular endothelial growth factor induces rapid phosphorylation of tight junction proteins occludin and zonula occluden 1. A potential mechanism for vascular permeability in diabetic retinopathy and tumors. J Biol Chem Aug 13 274(33):23463–23467

Campbell M, Kiang AS, Kenna PF et al (2008) RNAi-mediated reversible opening of the blood-brain barrier. J Gene Med 10(8):930–947

Fanning AS, Anderson JM (1998) PDZ domains and the formation of protein networks at the plasma membrane. Curr Top Microbiol Immunol 228:209–233

Kiang AS, Palfi A, Ader M et al (2005) Toward a gene therapy for dominant disease: validation of an RNA interference-based mutation-independent approach. Mol Ther 12(3):555–561

Koto T, Takubo K, Ishida S et al (2007) Hypoxia disrupts the barrier function of neural blood vessels through changes in the expression of claudin-5 in endothelial cells. Am J Pathol 170(4):1389–1397

Nitta T, Hata M, Gotoh S et al (2003) Size-selective loosening of the blood-brain barrier in claudin-5-deficient mice. J Cell Biol 161(3):653–660

Riesen FK, Rothen-Rutishauser B, Wunderli-Allenspach H (2002) A ZO1-GFP fusion protein to study the dynamics of tight junctions in living cells. Histochem Cell Biol 117(4):307–315 AprEpub 2002 Mar 29

Sakakibara A, Furuse M, Saitou M et al (1997) Possible involvement of phosphorylation of occludin in tight junction formation. J Cell Biol Jun 16 137(6):1393–1401

Chapter 35
Spectral Domain Optical Coherence Tomography and Adaptive Optics: Imaging Photoreceptor Layer Morphology to Interpret Preclinical Phenotypes

Jungtae Rha, Adam M. Dubis, Melissa Wagner-Schuman, Diane M. Tait, Pooja Godara, Brett Schroeder, Kimberly Stepien, and Joseph Carroll

Abstract Recent years have seen the emergence of advances in imaging technology that enable in vivo evaluation of the living retina. Two of the more promising techniques, spectral domain optical coherence tomography (SD-OCT) and adaptive optics (AO) fundus imaging provide complementary views of the retinal tissue. SD-OCT devices have high axial resolution, allowing assessment of retinal lamination, while the high lateral resolution of AO allows visualization of individual cells. The potential exists to use one modality to interpret results from the other. As a proof of concept, we examined the retina of a 32 year-old male, previously diagnosed with a red-green color vision defect. Previous AO imaging revealed numerous gaps throughout his cone mosaic, indicating that the structure of a subset of cones had been compromised. Whether the affected cells had completely degenerated or were simply morphologically deviant was not clear. Here an AO fundus camera was used to re-examine the retina (~6 years after initial exam) and SD-OCT to examine retinal lamination. The static nature of the cone mosaic disruption combined with the normal lamination on SD-OCT suggests that the affected cones are likely still present.

35.1 Introduction

Human trichromacy relies on three different cone types in the retina; long- (L), middle- (M), and short- (S) wavelength-sensitive. Dichromatic color vision results from the functional loss of one cone class. One central question has been whether individuals with this form of red-green color-blindness have lost one population of cones or whether they have normal numbers of cones filled with either of two instead

J. Carroll (✉)
Department of Ophthalmology; Department of Cell Biology; Neurobiology, and Anatomy; Department of Biophysics, Medical College of Wisconsin, The Eye Institute, Milwaukee, WI, USA
e-mail: jcarroll@mcw.edu

R.E. Anderson et al. (eds.), *Retinal Degenerative Diseases*, Advances in Experimental Medicine and Biology 664, DOI 10.1007/978-1-4419-1399-9_35,
© Springer Science+Business Media, LLC 2010

of three pigments. It has become clear that the answer to this question depends upon the genotype. Two main causes of inherited red-green color vision deficiency have been identified. The most common cause is rearrangement of the L/M opsin genes (Xq 28) resulting either in the deletion of all but one visual pigment gene, or in the production of a gene array in which the first two genes both encode a pigment of the same spectral class (Deeb et al. 1992; Jagla et al. 2002; Nathans et al. 1986; Neitz et al. 2004; Ueyama et al. 2003). The second general cause is the introduction of an inactivating mutation in either the first or second gene in the array.

These two different causes of inherited color vision defects might be expected to lead to different retinal phenotypes. It is thought that all photoreceptors destined to become L or M cones will express either the first or second gene in the X-chromosome array (Hayashi et al. 1999). In the case of gene rearrangements, all cone photoreceptors are expected to express a gene that encodes a functional pigment. However in the case of the inactivating mutation, a fraction of the photoreceptors will express a pigment that is not functional and, in fact, may be deleterious to the viability of the cell. Recently it was discovered that there are different retinal phenotypes among red-green color blind individuals. Carroll et al. (2005) found that in individuals having either a single-gene array, or an array in which the first two genes both encode a pigment of the same spectral class, the cone mosaic is normal in appearance. In contrast, in an individual with a deuteranopic phenotype in whom the M-opsin gene (OPN1MW; MIM:303800) in the array encoded a pigment with an inactivating mutation, a dramatic loss of healthy cones was observed. This is consistent with the authors' hypothesis that cells expressing the mutant pigment degenerated (Carroll et al. 2004).

Here we re-examined this individual with a disrupted cone mosaic using adaptive optics (AO) to determine whether there has been any change in the appearance of the cone mosaic over time. In addition, we evaluated the photoreceptor layer using spectral domain optical coherence tomography (SD-OCT) in an effort to deduce whether the cones expressing the mutant pigment degenerated completely or whether they have simply been functionally compromised. AO and SD-OCT provide complementary views of the living retina, and efforts to advance our understanding on how the images from these two modalities relate to one another will improve the clinical utility of each.

35.2 Materials and Methods

35.2.1 Subjects

A 32 year old male (NC) was previously reported as having a novel M-opsin sequence in transmembrane IV (leucine 153, isoleucine 171, alanine 174, valine 178, alanine 180; '*LIAVA*') (Carroll et al. 2004; Neitz et al. 2004). Initial examination took place in January of 2003, with first follow-up in December of 2004, and the most recent exam in November of 2008. Complete ophthalmic exam revealed no abnormalities at any of the three visits. Best-corrected visual acuity was 20/16.

Retinal imaging was done using adaptive optics and SD-OCT (see below). Sixty individuals with clinically normal vision were imaged using Bioptigen™ SD-OCT as controls for outer nuclear layer analysis. Written informed consent was obtained from all subjects. The study conforms to the Declaration of Helsinki and was approved by the Children's Hospital of Wisconsin Institutional Review Board.

35.2.2 Adaptive Optics Retinal Imaging

Images of NC's cone mosaic were obtained using a newly developed AO ophthalmoscope housed at the Medical College of Wisconsin. The head was stabilized using a dental impression on a bite bar. The subject's eye was dilated and accommodation suspended through use of a combination of Phenylephrine Hydrochloride (2.5%) and Tropicamide (1%). In a continuous closed-loop fashion, the eye's monochromatic aberrations were measured over a 6.8-mm pupil with a Shack-Hartmann wavefront sensor and corrected for them with a 52-channel deformable mirror (Imagine Eyes, Orsay, France). Details on the Mirao52 deformable mirror have been previously published (Fernández et al. 2006).

Once a wavefront correction was obtained, a retinal image was acquired by illuminating the retina with a 1.8° diameter, 500 ms flash. A fiber-coupled near infrared source was used for imaging, which consists of a 200 mW SLD (center wavelength of 837.8 nm, 14.1-nm spectral bandwidth FWHM) and 110 m of multimode step index fiber (Fiberguide Industries, Stirling, NJ USA). The optical role of the fiber was to reduce the spatial coherence of the laser and prevent speckle noise that confounds interpretation of the retinal image. The fiber has a 0.22 numerical aperture, core diameter of 365 μ and core refractive index of 1.457 at 0.633 nm wavelength. The function of the step index multimode fiber has been described in detail (Rha et al. 2006). The exposure at the cornea was 2 mW, well below the maximum permissible exposure for continuous intrabeam viewing recommended by ANSI (Z136 2007). A back-illuminated scientific-grade 12-bit charge-coupled device (CCD) (Cam1M100-SFT, Sarnoff Imaging) captured aerial images of the retina whose acquisition was triggered with a mechanical shutter. This CCD is a frame transfer camera with a light sensitive area of 1,024 × 512 pixels. During each 500 ms exposure, continuous images of the retina are collected at a frame rate of 167 fps with 6 ms exposure.

Because of non-uniformity in gain across the CCD array and circuitry artifacts with the Sarnoff camera, background correction is necessary. Figure 35.1a shows a raw retinal image containing cone structure (object) and the Gaussian beam profile, CCD circuit and dust (noise). A background correction procedure was developed to correct these artifacts. Figure 35.1b shows a 'defocused image', which includes only noise. Correction of the raw retinal image for noise, and subsequent registration of multiple frames, results in the image in Figure 35.1c.

The position of cone photoreceptors in the adaptive optics images were identified using previously described automated Matlab software (Li and Roorda 2007) and manual identification by two of the authors. Cone density was measured using previously described methods (Carroll et al. 2004).

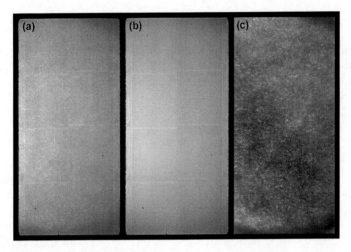

Fig. 35.1 Processing retinal images from the Medical College of Wisconsin Adaptive Optics Ophthalmoscope. (**a**) Raw image from the CCD camera (~1.8° × ~0.9°). (**b**) Noise image comprised of dust, beam profile, and CCD circuit. (**c**) Processed retinal image (noise removed, registered average of 20 individual frames)

35.2.3 Spectral Domain Optical Coherence Tomography

In addition to the patient with the *LIAVA* M opsin, SD-OCT imaging was performed in 60 normal subjects (30 male, 30 female), ranging in age from 20 to 49 years-old, with a mean of 34.5 years. A Zeiss IOL Master (Dublin, CA) was used to measure axial length of each eye, and SD-OCT scan lengths were corrected for inter-individual differences in axial length based on Leung et al. (2007). Axial length in our subjects ranged from 21.96 to 29.93 mm, as such actual macular scan lengths ranged from 3.68 to 5.01 mm. The SD-OCT imaging protocol included a fast volume scan (512 A scans/B scan; 50 B scans in a nominal 4 × 4 mm volume). Additional high-resolution line scans were obtained (1,000 A-scans/B scan; 100 repeated line scans) through the center of fixation, which was cross-referenced with the volumetric scan to ensure coincidence with the foveal pit. Scans from each eye were directly exported and read into ImageJ (http://www.rsb.info.nih.gov/ij/) for processing. Frames from scans that were distorted due to large saccades or eye blinks were removed. A rigid body registration using the ImageJ plugin 'StackReg' was applied to generate a stabilized frame sequence for subsequent averaging (Thévenaz et al. 1998). The internal limiting membrane (*ILM*), outer plexiform layer (*OPL*), external limiting membrane (*ELM*) and retinal pigmented epithelium (*RPE*) were manually segmented. The distance between the ILM and RPE provided total retinal thickness while the distance between the OPL and ELM provided the outer nuclear layer (ONL) thickness.

35.3 Results

35.3.1 Cone Photoreceptor Mosaic Topography

To determine whether there were any structural changes since the initial imaging, three patches of retina between 1 and 1.5° temporal eccentricity were subject to detailed analysis. In order to make a direct comparison of cone locations, we first precisely co-registered the image from the initial imaging session to that from the most recent session (as the images were acquired on different adaptive optics cameras, the retinal magnification was different). Shown in Fig. 35.2a is an image from 1.25° temporal retina taken in November 2008. Figure 35.2b shows an overlay of identified cone coordinates, the cone density at this location is 21,367 cones/mm^2.

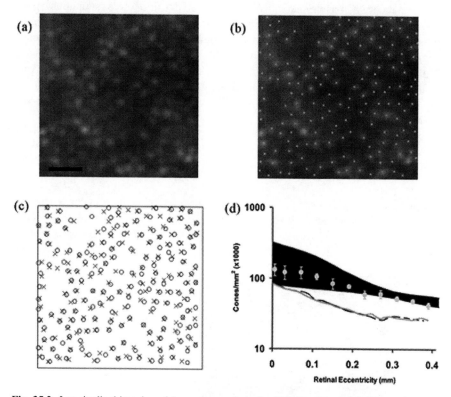

Fig. 35.2 Longitudinal imaging of the cone mosaic in the LIAVA retina. (**a**) Cone mosaic image from 1.25° temporal retina, taken November 2008 on the Medical College of Wisconsin Adaptive Optics Ophthalmoscope. Scale bar = 20 microns (**b**) Same image as in (**a**), with cone locations identified as *dots*. (**c**) Comparison of cone locations in (**b**) (*crosses*) to that from the exact same retinal location taken about 6 years prior (*open circles*). (**d**) Plot of cone density as a function of eccentricity. *Shaded region* represents normal bounds from histology data (Curcio et al. 1990) and *filled circles* represent average ± 1 SD values from adaptive optics data (Carroll et al. 2005). Density data for patient NC is plotted as a *black dashed line* (November 2008) and a *gray line* (January 2003)

Figure 35.2c shows a comparison of cone coordinates from this patch of retina from the initial and most recent imaging sessions. Over this period spanning nearly 6 years, there has been virtually no change in the microstructure of the mosaic, as indicated by the close agreement of cone positions. This analysis was repeated on two other retinal locations and the average discrepancy between images was only 832 cones/mm^2 (the equivalent of five cone misidentifications). Owing to the high contrast and low spatial frequency of the gaps in the cone mosaic, it was qualitatively determined that the same gaps present in the initial images still remain (*data not shown*).

To quantitatively evaluate the gross topography of the cone mosaic, we compared cone density between the two imaging sessions. Figure 35.2d shows cone density as a function of retinal eccentricity for patient NC compared to normals. Compared to imaging (Carroll et al. 2005) and histology (Curcio et al. 1990) data from normal retina, patient NC has dramatically reduced cone density. There is an approximate 35% reduction in cone numerosity across the central retina. However, the precipitous decline in density from the fovea remains, with the curve shifted vertically, suggesting that normal cone migration and foveal packing took place. Also shown in Fig. 35.2d is the density curve from the initial evaluation (January 2003). Compared to the most recent examination, cone density appears unchanged, suggesting that the morphological disruption we observed is static in nature over at least a 6-year period.

35.3.2 Outer Nuclear Layer Thickness

Previous work has shown significant variation in 'normal' ONL thickness (Jacobson et al. 2007; Jacobson et al. 2005). We also observed significant variability in ONL thickness among the 60 normal subjects (Fig. 35.3a). The ONL thickness is greatest

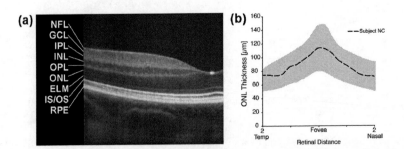

Fig. 35.3 SD-OCT imaging in the *LIAVA* retina. (**a**) Line scan through the central fovea of patient NC, main retinal layers are labeled: NFL = nerve fiber layer, GCL = ganglion cell layer, IPL = inner plexiform layer, INL = inner nuclear layer, OPL = outer plexiform layer, ONL = outer nuclear layer, ELM = external limiting membrane, IS/OS = inner/outer segment junction, RPE = retinal pigment epithelium. (**b**) ONL thickness across horizontal meridian in normal subjects (*shaded gray*, ±2 SD) and patient NC with *LIAVA* M-opsin (*dashed black line*). Thickness data is presented as right eye equivalents

under the foveal pit, and falls off by nearly half by 2 mm eccentricity, reflecting the significant non-uniformity in cone density across the macular region (Curcio et al. 1990). Interestingly in the patient with the *LIAVA* M opsin there was no abnormality observed on the SD-OCT (Fig. 35.3b), despite the reduction in cone numerosity observed with adaptive optics.

35.4 Discussion

Based on the packing density of the cone photoreceptors, one would predict that the ONL thickness should be dependent on the number of photoreceptors present. Therefore it is curious that despite an apparent reduction in cone number in the *en face* AO images, no disruption in the SD-OCT was observed. One possible explanation is that the ONL thickness is maintained by glial cells, much like how RNFL thickness remains normal in RP patients despite significant axonal loss (Hood et al. 2009). Alternatively, it is possible that affected cone cells have not completely degenerated and their cell bodies remain in the ONL layer. However, we do know that even if structurally present, these cones are not contributing to function as seen by both the dichromatic phenotype (Carroll et al. 2004) and AO microperimetric findings (Makous et al. 2006). More generally, the disconnect between the AO and SD-OCT results suggests that a 'normal' OCT image does not necessarily imply that there is normal function of the retina. As shown here, cellular damage of the photoreceptors can still exist, and this warrants further investigation for determining the absolute sensitivity of both imaging modalities. This study highlights the potential utility of using SD-OCT to aid in the interpretation of AO. There is also clinical value in using AO to decipher SD-OCT abnormalities, however the full diagnostic potential of this relationship has yet to be realized, though integration with functional measures will aid in this effort (Choi et al. 2006; Duncan et al. 2007).

Acknowledgments The authors thank Dr. Alf Dubra for technical assistance with the adaptive optics control software & Dr. Tom Connor for helpful discussion. This study was supported by NIH Grants EY017607, EY001931, & EY014537, Fight for Sight, The E. Matilda Ziegler Foundation for the Blind, The Karl Kirchgessner Foundation, the RD & Linda Peters Foundation, the Gene & Ruth Posner Foundation, and an unrestricted departmental grant from Research to Prevent Blindness. JC is the recipient of a Career Development Award from Research to Prevent Blindness.

References

Carroll J, Neitz M, Hofer H et al (2004) Functional photoreceptor loss revealed with adaptive optics: an alternate cause for color blindness. Proc Natl Acad Sci USA 101(22):8461–8466

Carroll J, Porter J, Neitz J et al (2005) Adaptive optics imaging reveals effects of human cone opsin gene disruption. Invest Ophthalmol Vis Sci 46 ARVO E-Abstract:4564

Choi SS, Doble N, Hardy JL et al (2006) In vivo imaging of the photoreceptor mosaic in retinal dystrophies and correlations with visual function. Invest Ophthalmol Vis Sci 47(5):2080–2092

Curcio CA, Sloan KR, Kalina RE et al (1990) Human photoreceptor topography. J Comp Neurol 292:497–523

Deeb SS, Lindsey DT, Hibiya Y et al (1992) Genotype-phenotype relationships in human red/green color-vision defects: molecular and psychophysical studies. Am J Hum Genet 51:687–700

Duncan JL, Zhang Y, Gandhi J et al (2007) High-resolution imaging with adaptive optics in patients with inherited retinal degeneration. Invest Ophthalmol Vis Sci 48:3283–3291

Fernández EJ, Vabre L, Hermann B et al (2006) Adaptive optics with a magnetic deformable mirror: Applications in the human eye. Opt Express 14(20):8900–8917

Hayashi T, Motulsky AG, Deeb SS (1999) Position of a 'green-red' hybrid gene in the visual pigment array determines colour-vision phenotype. Nat Genet 22:90–93

Hood DC, Lin CE, Lazow MA et al (2009) Thickness of receptor and post-receptor retinal layers in patients with retinitis pigmentosa measured with frequency-domain optical coherence tomography (fdOCT). Invest Ophthalmol Vis Sci 50(5):2328–2336

Jacobson SG, Aleman TS, Cideciyan AV et al (2007) Human cone photoreceptor dependence on RPE65 isomerase. Proc Natl Acad Sci USA 104(38):15123–15128

Jacobson SG, Aleman TS, Cideciyan AV et al (2005) Identifying photoreceptors in blind eyes caused by RPE65 mutations: Prerequisite for human gene therapy success. Proc Natl Acad Sci USA 102(17):6177–6182

Jagla WM, Jägle H, Hayashi T et al (2002) The molecular basis of dichromatic color vision in males with multiple red and green visual pigment genes. Hum Mol Genet 11:23–32

Leung CK, Cheng ACK, Chong KKL et al (2007) Optic disc measurements in myopia with optical coherence tomography and confocal scanning laser ophthalmoscopy. Invest Ophthalmol Vis Sci 48(7):3178–3183

Li KY, Roorda A (2007) Automated identification of cone photoreceptors in adaptive optics retinal images. J Opt Soc Am A Opt Image Sci Vis 24(5):1358–1363

Makous W, Carroll J, Wolfing JI et al (2006) Retinal microscotomas revealed with adaptive-optics microflashes. Invest Ophthalmol Vis Sci 47(9):4160–4167

Nathans J, Piantanida TP, Eddy RL et al (1986) Molecular genetics of inherited variation in human color vision. Science 232:203–210

Neitz M, Carroll J, Renner A et al (2004) Variety of genotypes in males diagnosed as dichromatic on a conventional clinical anomaloscope. Vis Neurosci 21:205–216

Rha J, Jonnal RS, Thorn KE et al (2006) Adaptive optics flood-illumination camera for high speed retinal imaging. Opt Express 14(10):4552–4569

Thévenaz P, Ruttimann UE, Unser M (1998) A pyramid approach to subpixel registration based on intensity. IEEE Trans Image Process 7(1):27–41

Ueyama H, Li Y-H, Fu G-L et al (2003) An A-71C substitution in a green gene at the second position in the red/green visual-pigment gene array is associated with deutan color-vision deficiency. Proc Natl Acad Sci USA 100(6):3357–3362

Z136 ASC (2007) American national standard for safe use of lasers. Orlando.

Chapter 36
Pharmacological Manipulation of Rhodopsin Retinitis Pigmentosa

Hugo F. Mendes, Raffaella Zaccarini, and Michael E. Cheetham

Abstract Mutations in rhodopsin cause autosomal dominant retinitis pigmentosa. The majority of these mutations (class II) lead to protein misfolding. The misfolded protein is retained in the ER then retrotranslocated into the cytoplasm for degradation by the proteasome. If degradation fails, the protein can aggregate to form intracellular inclusions. In addition, the mutant rod opsin exerts a dominant negative effect on the wild-type protein. Here, we review these pathways and how different drug treatments can affect mutant rod opsin. Interestingly, drugs targeted at general protein stability (kosmotropes) or improving the cellular folding and degradation machinery (molecular chaperone inducers and autophagy induction) reduced P23H rod opsin aggregation and inclusion formation together with associated caspase activation and cell death, but did not enhance mutant protein processing or reduce the dominant negative effects. In contrast, pharmacological chaperones (retinoids) enhanced P23H folding and reduced the dominant negative effects, as well as reducing the other gains of function. Therefore, targeting the toxic gain of function did not require improved folding, whereas reducing the dominant negative effects required improved folding. These studies suggest that some forms of rhodopsin retinitis pigmentosa could be treated by targeting protein folding and/or reducing protein aggregation.

36.1 Introduction

Mutations in rhodopsin are the most common cause of autosomal dominant retinitis pigmentosa (ADRP) OMIM 180380. Disease-causing rhodopsin mutations can be categorised by their effects on rhodopsin structure, function and localisation when expressed in cultured cells or photoreceptors. We recently classified rhodopsin

M.E. Cheetham (✉)
UCL Institute of Ophthalmology, London, EC1V 9EL, UK
e-mail: michael.cheetham@ucl.ac.uk

R.E. Anderson et al. (eds.), *Retinal Degenerative Diseases*, Advances in Experimental Medicine and Biology 664, DOI 10.1007/978-1-4419-1399-9_36,
© Springer Science+Business Media, LLC 2010

mutations into 6 types based on their biochemical and cellular consequences (Mendes et al., 2005). The most common, type II (e.g. P23H), cause the misfolding of the protein.

Protein folding is a complex process. The folding energy landscape for a polypeptide often includes several off-pathway non-native states, in addition to the state occupied by the native conformation. Changes in the primary amino acid sequence and cellular stress can compromise folding efficiency, shifting the equilibrium away from the native state and towards intermediates that can result in increased production of off-pathway products that can aggregate. Protein misfolding can lead to a variety of diseases, including loss of function diseases like cystic fibrosis, antitrypsin deficiency and gain of function diseases related to protein aggregation; such as Huntington's, Parkinson's, Alzheimer's and prion diseases. The misfolding mutations in rhodopsin show similarities with these forms of neurodegeneration.

In transfected cells, rhodopsin bearing class II mutations in the transmembrane, intradiscal or cytoplasmic domains fail to translocate to the plasma membrane and accumulate within the endoplasmic reticulum (ER) (Sung et al., 1991; Illing et al., 2002; Saliba et al., 2002). These mutant proteins trapped within the cell cannot form a functional visual pigment with 11-*cis*-retinal (Sung et al., 1991), and are found in a complex with the ER-resident chaperones GRP78 (BiP) and GRP94, supporting the notion that they are incorrectly folded (Chapple et al., 2001; Kosmaoglou et al., 2008). Interestingly, the failure of one copy of rhodopsin to translocate to the outer segment per se does not appear to be sufficient to cause retinitis pigmentosa, rather it appears that misfolded rhodopsin acquires a 'gain of function' that leads to cell death.

The precise mechanisms by which rhodopsin misfolding leads to photoreceptor cell death still remain to be clarified, but most likely involves one, if not several, of the following initiators and/or accelerators (reviewed in Mendes et al., 2005): induction of the unfolded protein response (Lin et al., 2007); UPS inhibition (Illing et al., 2002); cytotoxic protein aggregates; interference with normal protein traffic; protein sequestration or dominant negative effects (Saliba et al., 2002; Rajan and Kopito 2005). This understanding of potential disease mechanisms can be used to develop potential treatments. For example, we have recently shown that a variety of drug treatments can be used to counteract the toxic effects associated with rod opsin misfolding and aggregation (Mendes and Cheetham 2008).

36.2 Pharmacological Strategies for Misfolding Mutant Rod Opsin

36.2.1 Pharmacological Chaperones

As disease-causing misfolding proteins, including mutant rod opsin, may not be inherently non-functional several therapeutic strategies can target the manipulation of folding and consequent trafficking through the secretory pathway. One of these strategies involved the use of pharmacological chaperones, such as the rod opsin chromophore (11-*cis*-retinal) and its retinoid analogues (e.g. 9-*cis*-retinal).

Several studies have suggested that these compounds have the potential to correct misfolding of mutant rod opsin by binding specifically to near-native forms and stabilising the protein structure. Li and colleagues (1998) showed that a vitamin A supplemented diet reduced the rate of decline of the ERG a-wave and b-wave in class II T17M transgenic mice. In vitro studies suggested that 9-*cis*-retinal increased the amount of P23H rod opsin reaching the plasma membrane (Saliba et al., 2002). Furthermore, the introduction of 11-*cis*-7-ring-retinal, a 7 membered ring analogue of 11-*cis*-retinal, to stable cell lines expressing P23H rod opsin also resulted in the folding of mutant protein (Noorwez et al., 2003). A similar effect was observed when 9-*cis*-retinal and 11-*cis*-retinal were added during rod opsin synthesis in cell culture (Noorwez et al., 2004).

Importantly, the improvement in folding promoted by these pharmacological chaperones also decreased the toxic gain of function and dominant-negative effects associated with P23H rod opsin expression in SK-N-SH neuroblastoma cells (Mendes and Cheetham 2008). Treatment with 9-*cis*-retinal and 11-*cis*-retinal resulted in a reduction in inclusion incidence and protein aggregation, increased the presence of mature glycosylated P23H rod opsin species, and protected against cell death and caspase activation suggesting a reduction of the gain of function effects of mutant rod opsin. Significantly, the dominant-negative effects of P23H rod opsin were also alleviated by these pharmacological chaperones, as the retention of wild-type rod opsin in the ER associated with the expression of the mutant protein was reduced. These data suggest that if 11-*cis*-retinal were present in the inner segment during rhodopsin biogenesis and could bind rod opsin, it would potentially stabilise class II mutant rod opsin folding, and decrease the gain of function and dominant negative effects. Furthermore, bright light exposure would isomerise the 11-*cis*-retinal and exacerbate the gain of function and dominant negative effects of the class II mutants and this may contribute to the acceleration in retinal degeneration caused by light in class II rhodospin animal models (Wenzel et al., 2005).

36.2.2 Kosmotropes

A group of low molecular weight compounds named kosmotropes, or chemical chaperones, have been reported to improve the folding and reduce aggregation of proteins involved in a variety of human diseases associated with protein misfolding, such as CFTR (Zeitlin et al., 2002). Kosmotropes include polyols such as glycerol; solvents such as dimethyl sulfoxide (DMSO); methylamines such as trimethylamine-N-oxide (TMAO); fatty acids such as 4-phenylbutyric acid (4-PBA); and sugars such as trehalose among others. Unlike pharmacological chaperones, the effects of kosmotropes are non-specific and might involve the hydration of proteins (Back et al. 1979) or the reduction of the free movement of proteins to prevent the aggregation of partially folded proteins (Singer and Lindquist 1998).

DMSO, TMAO, 4-PBA and trehalose were effective at reducing protein aggregation and inclusion incidence in SK-N-SH cells expressing P23H rod opsin (Mendes and Cheetham 2008). Furthermore, this correlated with protection against cell death and caspase activation induced by mutant rod opsin expression. However, unlike retinoids, kosmotropes did not appear to promote the trafficking of the mutant protein or alleviate the dominant-negative effects associated with P23H rod opsin. Therefore, it appeared that the gain of function effects could be alleviated by increasing the degradation of the aggregation prone species and reducing inclusion incidence rather than by assisting protein folding per se.

36.2.3 Molecular Chaperone Inducers

All secreted proteins are subject to ER quality control, the primary mediators of which are molecular chaperones that not only sample and help polypeptides to fold but also evaluate the conformations of their substrates. If folding is delayed or an illegitimate conformation arises, the substrate is either subjected to additional folding cycles or is selected for a process termed ER-associated degradation (ERAD) (Vembar and Brodsky 2008). Molecular chaperones recognise hydrophobic residues or unstructured backbone regions in misfolded proteins and promote the folding process through cycles of substrate binding and release regulated by their nucleotide binding, hydrolysis and facilitated by cofactor proteins (Kosmaoglou et al., 2008: Kosmaoglou and Cheetham 2008). There is now ample evidence in a variety of in vivo and in vitro models that the manipulation of the chaperone machinery can be used to alleviate toxicity associated with misfolded protein disorders. For example, Cummings and colleagues (1998) first showed that the overexpression of a chaperone decreased ataxin-1 aggregation in a model of spinocerebellar ataxia type 1 and several chaperones have now been shown to protect against polyglutamine-induced neurodegeneration (e.g. Westhoff et al., 2005; Howarth et al., 2007).

A pharmacological approach has been attempted in several models of neurodegenerative diseases using the Hsp90 inhibitors geldanamycin, radicicol, 17-allylamino-17-demethoxygeldanamycin (17-AAG). The rationale for using these Hsp90 inhibitors at low doses to induce molecular chaperones is based on the autoregulation of heat shock factor 1 (HSF1) by chaperones. HSF1 is usually bound to a molecular chaperone complex containing Hsp90 and other chaperones and is kept in an inactive state unless a stress signal is detected. Hsp90 inhibitors disrupt the chaperone: HSF1 complex and release the HSF1, which is then activated and increases the expression of chaperone proteins. This approach has been used in a cell model of Huntington's disease where treatment of COS-1 cells with geldanamycin induced the expression of Hsp40, Hsp70 and Hsp90 and inhibited polyglutamine expanded Huntingtin exon 1 protein aggregation in a dose-dependent manner (Sittler et al., 2001).

In the rhodopsin RP cell model, geldanamycin, radicicol and 17-AAG alleviated the gain of function effects induced by P23H rod opsin. Treatment with these compounds reduced protein aggregation and inclusion incidence which correlated with protection against cell death and caspase activation (Mendes and Cheetham 2008). However, these Hsp90 inhibitors did not promote the processing of P23H rod opsin beyond the ER or affect the dominant-negative effect of the mutant opsin (Mendes and Cheetham 2008). As with kosmotropes, the reduction of inclusion incidence and increased degradation of aggregate prone species, without the promotion of protein folding appeared to be sufficient to reduce the gain of function mechanisms induced by the mutant protein.

Another chaperone inducer celastrol, a quinone methide triterpene, which is an active component from Chinese herbal medicine with potent anti-inflammatory and anti-oxidative effects, in addition to activating HSF1, was less successful in the RP cell model, as it was toxic at concentrations that were starting to be effective at reducing protein aggregation and inclusion formation (Mendes and Cheetham 2008).

36.2.4 Autophagy Inducers

In addition to the proteasome, autophagy plays a major role in protein degradation in eukaryotic cells. Autophagy is upregulated when the proteasome is inhibited and P23H rod opsin aggregation inhibits the proteasome (Illing et al., 2002). Furthermore, autophagy may play a role in the degradation of mutant rhododpsin, as the autophagic marker proteins, Atg7, Atg8 (LC3), and LAMP-1 co-localised with P23H rod opsin in cells (Kaushal 2006).

Autophagy can be induced by inhibiting the mammalian target of rapamycin (mTOR) with rapamycin and related drugs, as mTOR negatively regulates autophagy. Induction of autophagy with rapamycin and analogues protected against neurodegeneration and decreased the levels of inclusions in a mouse model of Huntington's disease (Ravikumar et al., 2004). Furthermore, Sarkar and colleagues (2007) demonstrated that the effects of rapamycin on autophagy substrates such as mutant huntingtin and α-synuclein were enhanced by the presence of trehalose.

Rapamycin protected against the toxic gain of function effects (reducing aggregation, inclusion formation and cell death) associated with P23H rod opsin expression and, importantly, this effect was enhanced by the presence of trehalose (Mendes and Cheetham 2008). Similar to kosmotropes and chaperone inducers, however, rapamycin did not promote mutant rod opsin processing or inhibit the dominant-negative effects.

36.3 Conclusion

These in vitro studies suggest that a pharmacological approach could be used to alleviate the gain of function and dominant-negative effects of misfolded mutant rod opsin (Fig. 36.1). This could be achieved by promoting the folding of the mutant rod opsin (retinoids; Fig. 36.1a), reducing protein aggregation (Fig. 36.1b)

Fig. 36.1 Schematic representation of a rod photoreceptor inner segment and potential pharmacological intervention in rhodopsin retinitis pigmentosa. Gain of function and dominant-negative effects of misfolded mutant rod opsin could be alleviated by pharmacological chaperones, such as 9-*cis*-retinal and 11-*cis*-retinal, which assist the folding of mutant protein (**a**). Kosmotropes, molecular chaperone inducers could alleviate the gain of function effects by reducing aggregation (**b**) and/or promoting proteasomal degradation (**c**). Rapamycin could reduce the toxic gain of function effects of mutant rod opsin by increasing autophagy (**d**)

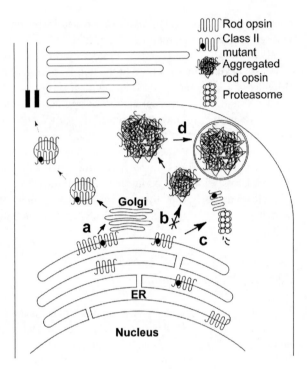

and promoting degradation of aggregate prone species (Fig. 36.1c), or stimulating autophagy (Fig. 36.1d). It is now necessary to establish the effects of these compounds, or potential combination therapies based on targeting multiple pathways, in photoreceptors in vivo prior to the translation to the clinic.

Acknowledgments This work is supported by the British Retinitis Pigmentosa Society (BRPS), Fight for Sight, the Daphne Jackson Trust and National Institute for Health Research (NIHR).

References

Back JF, Oakenfull D, Smith MB (1979) Increased thermal stability of proteins in the presence of sugars and polyols. Biochemistry 18:5191–5196

Chapple JP, Grayson C, Hardcastle AJ et al (2001) Unfolding retinal dystrophies: a role for molecular chaperones?. Trends Mol Med 7:414–421

Cummings CJ, Mancini MA, Antalffy B et al (1998) Chaperone suppression of aggregation and altered subcellular proteasome localization imply protein misfolding in SCA1. Nat Genet 19:148–154

Howarth JL, Kelly S, Keasey MP et al (2007) Hsp40 molecules that target to the ubiquitin-proteasome system decrease inclusion formation in models of polyglutamine disease. Mol Ther 15:1100–1105

Illing ME, Rajan RS, Bence NF et al (2002) A rhodopsin mutant linked to autosomal dominant retinitis pigmentosa is prone to aggregate and interacts with the ubiquitin proteasome system. J Biol Chem 277:34150–34160

Kaushal S (2006) Effect of rapamycin on the fate of P23H opsin associated with retinitis pigmentosa (an American Ophthalmological Society thesis). Trans Am Ophthalmol Soc 104:517–529

Kosmaoglou M, Cheetham ME (2008) Calnexin is not essential for mammalian rod opsin biogenesis. Mol Vis 14:2466–2474

Kosmaoglou M, Schwarz N, Bett JS et al (2008) Molecular chaperones and photoreceptor function. Prog Ret Eye Res 27:434–449

Li T, Sandberg MA, Pawlyk BS et al (1998) Effect of vitamin A supplementation on rhodopsin mutants threonine17methionine and proline347serine in transgenic mice and in cell cultures. Proc Natl Acad Sci USA 95:11933–11938

Lin JH, Li H, Yasumura D et al (2007) IRE1 signaling affects cell fate during the unfolded protein response. Science 318:944–949

Mendes HF, Cheetham ME (2008) Pharmacological manipulation of gain-of-function and dominant-negative mechanisms in rhodopsin retinitis pigmentosa. Hum Mol Genet 17:3043–3054

Mendes HF, van der Spuy J, Chapple JP et al (2005) Mechanisms of cell death in rhodopsin retinitis pigmentosa: implications for therapy. Trends Mol Med 11:177–185

Noorwez SM, Kuksa V, Imanishi Y et al (2003) Pharmacological chaperone-mediated in vivo folding and stabilization of the P23H-opsin mutant associated with autosomal dominant retinitis pigmentosa. J Biol Chem 278:14442–14450

Noorwez SM, Malhotra R, McDowell JH et al (2004) Retinoids assist the cellular folding of the autosomal dominant retinitis pigmentosa opsin mutant P23H. J Biol Chem 279:16278–16284

Rajan RS, Kopito RR (2005) Suppression of wild-type rhodopsin maturation by mutants linked to autosomal dominant retinitis pigmentosa. J Biol Chem 280:1284–1291

Ravikumar B, Vacher C, Berger Z et al (2004) Inhibition of mTOR induces autophagy and reduces toxicity of polyglutamine expansions in fly and mouse models of Huntington disease. Nat Genet 36:585–595

Saliba RS, Munro PM, Luthert PJ et al (2002) The cellular fate of mutant rhodopsin: quality control, degradation and aggresome formation. J Cell Sci 115:2907–2918

Sarkar S, Davies JE, Huang Z et al (2007) Trehalose, a novel mTOR-independent autophagy enhancer, accelerates the clearance of mutant huntingtin and alpha-synuclein. J Biol Chem 282:5641–5652

Singer MA, Lindquist S (1998) Multiple effects of trehalose on protein folding in vitro and in vivo. Mol Cell 1:639–648

Sittler A, Lurz R, Lueder G et al (2001) Geldanamycin activates a heat shock response and inhibits huntingtin aggregation in a cell culture model of Huntington's disease. Hum Mol Genet 10:1307–1315

Sung CH, Schneider BG, Agarwal N et al (1991) Functional heterogeneity of mutant rhodopsins responsible for autosomal dominant retinitis pigmentosa. Proc Natl Acad Sci USA 88:8840–8844

Vembar SS, Brodsky JL (2008) One step at a time: endoplasmic reticulum-associated degradation. Nature 9:944

Wenzel A, Grimm C, Samardzija M et al (2005) Molecular mechanisms of light-induced photoreceptor apoptosis and neuroprotection for retinal degeneration. Prog Retin Eye Res 24:275–306

Westhoff B, Chapple JP, van der Spuy J et al (2005) HSJ1 is a neuronal shuttling factor for the sorting of chaperone clients to the proteasome. Curr Biol. 15:1058–1064

Zeitlin PL, Diener-West M, Rubenstein RC et al (2002) Evidence of CFTR function in cystic fibrosis after systemic administration of 4-phenylbutyrate. Mol Ther 6:119–126

Chapter 37
Targeted High-Throughput DNA Sequencing for Gene Discovery in Retinitis Pigmentosa

Stephen P. Daiger, Lori S. Sullivan, Sara J. Bowne, David G. Birch, John R. Heckenlively, Eric A. Pierce, and George M. Weinstock

Abstract The causes of retinitis pigmentosa (RP) are highly heterogeneous, with mutations in more than 60 genes known to cause syndromic and non-syndromic forms of disease. The prevalence of detectable mutations in known genes ranges from 25 to 85%, depending on mode of inheritance. For example, the likelihood of detecting a disease-causing mutation in known genes in patients with autosomal dominant RP (adRP) is 60% in Americans and less in other populations. Thus many RP genes are still unknown or mutations lie outside of commonly tested regions. Furthermore, current screening strategies can be costly and time-consuming.

We are developing targeted high-throughput DNA sequencing to address these problems. In this approach, a microarray with oligonucleotides targeted to hundreds of genes is used to capture sheared human DNA, and the sequence of the eluted DNA is determined by ultra-high-throughput sequencing using next-generation DNA sequencing technology. The first capture array we have designed contains 62 full-length retinal disease genes, including introns and promoter regions, and an additional 531 genes limited to exons and flanking sequences. The full-length genes include all genes known to cause at least 1% of RP or other inherited retinal diseases. All of the genes listed in the RetNet database are included on the capture array as well as many additional retinal-expressed genes. After validation studies, the first DNA's tested will be from 89 unrelated adRP families in which the prevalent RP genes have been excluded. This approach should identify new RP genes and will substantially reduce the cost per patient.

37.1 Introduction

The genetic causes of inherited retinal diseases, even a "simple' category such as autosomal dominant retinitis pigmentosa (adRP), are extremely heterogeneous.

S.P. Daiger (✉)
School of Public Health, Human Genetics Center; Department of Ophthalmology and Visual Science, University of Texas Health Science Center, Houston, TX, USA
e-mail: stephen.p.daiger@uth.tmc.edu

R.E. Anderson et al. (eds.), *Retinal Degenerative Diseases*, Advances in Experimental Medicine and Biology 664, DOI 10.1007/978-1-4419-1399-9_37,
© Springer Science+Business Media, LLC 2010

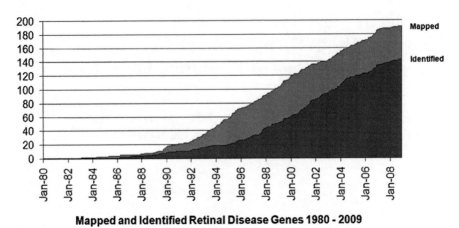

Mapped and Identified Retinal Disease Genes 1980 - 2009

Fig. 37.1 Graph of mapped and identified retinal disease genes from 1980, the beginning of the modern era of gene discovery, through December 2008 (RetNet 2009)

More than 190 genes causing inherited retinal diseases have been identified (Fig. 37.1), including at least 40 causing non-syndromic retinitis pigmentosa and 20 causing syndromic forms of RP (Daiger et al. 2007; RetNet 2009). In addition to many disease-causing genes, there are often many different mutations at each locus, and different mutations within the same gene may cause strikingly different diseases. Further, in spite of the large number of genes identified to date, the fraction of patients in which a mutation can be found by screening the known genes is often low. For example, screening known genes in adRP families leads to identification of a disease-causing mutation in 60% of cases among Americans of European origin and less frequently among other populations (Fig. 37.2). Thus there are many retinal disease genes that have not been identified yet.

Next generation sequencing techniques, that is, novel gene selection and targeting methods followed by massively-parallel, ultra-high-throughput sequencing, offer a rapid, efficient way to find disease-causing mutations in affected individuals and to discover new disease genes (Albert et al. 2007). We are applying these

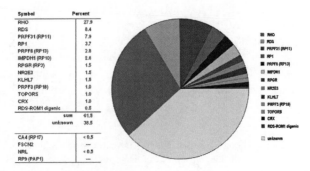

Fig. 37.2 Fraction of mutations detected in known adRP genes in a cohort of 228 adRP families (Sullivan et al. 2006; Sullivan et al. 2006a; Gire et al. 2007; Bowne et al. 2008; and unpublished)

methods to finding genes and mutations causing adRP, focusing on a cohort of 89 families in which conventional testing failed to detect mutations in known genes (Sullivan et al. 2006; Sullivan et al. 2006a; Gire et al. 2007; Bowne et al. 2008). That is, these families have mutations in novel adRP genes or mutations in known genes that are not readily detectable, for example, mutations outside of coding regions.

Our approach is to address these possibilities by targeting a large number of known and candidate retinal disease genes using oligonucleotide capture arrays followed by ultra-high-throughput sequencing. In addition to the many candidates for gene discovery, the capture arrays include non-coding sequences of known retinal disease genes to detect subtle mutations. We refer to this approach as the VisionCHIP. 'VisionCHIP' stands for Comprehensive High-Throughput Interrogation of Patient DNAs for Vision Research.

The first disease targeted for study is adRP – because of the availability of families enriched in novel genes and mutations, and because many of the families are large enough to test segregation of potentially pathogenic mutations, a major problem in assessing rare variants. However, the VisionCHIP approach, once optimized and validated, will be equally applicable to other forms of inherited retinal disease.

37.2 Methods

37.2.1 Selection of Families

In earlier and continuing research, we have ascertained and acquired DNA samples from over 500 families with a diagnosis of adRP (Sullivan et al. 2006). Among these, we have selected families with at least (i) three generations of inheritance and multiple affected females or (ii) two affected generations, three or more affected individuals and male-to-male transmission. That is, these families are more likely to have dominant RP and less likely to have an X-linked mode of inheritance. This is our adRP cohort; at present, there are 228 families in the cohort, approximately 85% white, 5% Hispanic, 5% African American, and 5% Asian and other.

The 228 families in the adRP cohort have been screened for mutations by a number of methods: sequencing of known genes (Sullivan et al. 2006), deletion testing using multiplex ligation-dependent probe amplification (MLPA) (Sullivan et al. 2006a), linkage mapping (Sullivan et al. 2005) and candidate gene screening (Gire et al. 2007; Bowne 2008). To date we have found mutations in 61% of these families (Fig. 37.2 and unpublished), leaving 89 for gene discovery. The additional adRP patients who are not part of the cohort are available for further screening of likely candidate genes.

37.2.2 VisionCHIP Gene Selection

Version 1 of the VisionCHIP contains 593 genes divided into three categories in terms of sequence overage:

1. genes less than 100 kb in length, known to cause some form of retinal degeneration, which will be sequenced completely (51 genes);
2. genes larger than 100 kb in length, known to cause some form of retinal degeneration, which will have all exons and some non-coding regions sequenced (11 genes); and
3. genes that are potential candidates for retinal degeneration which will have exons and exon-flanking regions sequenced (531 genes).

Genes in categories 1 and 2 were derived from the RetNet database of retinal disease genes (RetNet 2009). Genes that are known to cause 1% or more of cases of retinitis pigmentosa, juvenile macular degeneration, or cognate diseases were selected for full-length sequencing because these genes are most likely to have disease-causing mutations, and some mutations may fall outside of coding regions (Daiger et al. 2007).

Genes in category 3 came from multiple sources, including the EyeSAGE database (Bowes Rickman et al. 2006), and the human homologs of genes coding for proteins found in mouse photoreceptor outer segments and axonemes (Liu et al. 2007). Additional candidates were chosen from the retinal literature, while others were found in public databases such as NEIBank (2008), UniGene (2008), Entrez (2008), the Human Protein Reference Database (2008), and BioGRID (2008). Characteristics of chosen genes include high levels of retina/photoreceptor/eye/cilia expression; interaction with known disease genes; sequence similarity to known retinal disease genes; identification in screens of retinal gene expression; similarity in expression patterns to known retinal disease genes; candidate genes proposed by other investigators; and genes previously tested in our laboratory as potential candidates.

Figure 37.3 shows the chromosomal distribution of the first set of genes chosen for the VisionCHIP.

37.2.3 VisionCHIP Validation

To optimize and validate the VisionCHIP, we are focusing on controls with known adRP mutations, including deletions, and on 21 families from the adRP cohort without known mutations. The 21 families each have multiple affected members immediately available for segregation testing. In addition, three of the largest families are being tested for genome-wide linkage using Affymetrix 6.0 SNP Arrays. The linkage testing will provide genotypes for independent validation of SNPs within VisionCHIP genes, and may implicate linkage regions containing targeted retinal genes.

The current iteration of the VisionCHIP is being fabricated by NimbleGen Inc. (Roch). An alternative capture method is under development at the Genome Sequencing Center, Washington University (WU-GSC), St. Louis. Patient DNAs are subjected to whole-genome amplification, and then sheared, ligated with universal

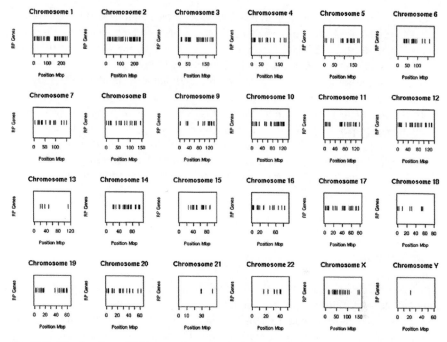

Fig. 37.3 Map location of 593 genes chosen for inclusion on the first iteration of the VisionCHIP

primers and individual 'bar codes', pooled and captured. The eluted, targeted DNA is then amplified and sequenced using 454 FLX (Roche), 454 Titanium (Roche) and/or Solexa (Illumina) ultra-high-throughput, massively parallel sequencers. Sequencing and sequence assembly are underway at WU-GSC. We anticipate 5–10 Mb of diploid sequence, 30–50-fold depth, for nearly 600 retinal genes, from each of the 21 families. In practice, we are actually testing pairs of affected individuals from each family (as far apart in the pedigree as possible) to generate preliminary segregation information for each variant observed.

37.2.4 Evaluating Potentially Pathogenic Variants

Because of the extensive sequencing of retinal genes, including introns and promoter regions, we anticipate that a significant fraction of patients will be found to have novel, rare variants in known RP genes and rare variants in many candidate genes. We are focusing on the RP genes first. Bioinformatics analysis of amino acid substitutions involves application of PolyPhen and related programs (Grantham 1974; Ng and Henikoff 2003; Stone 2007). Intronic sequences will be examined for possible splice-altering mutations using a combination of NNSPLICE and ASSP (alternative splice site predictor) (Wang and Marin 2006). Promoter regions will be determined and analyzed using programs such as PromoterInspector and Dragon Promoter Finder (Bajic et al. 2002; Scherf et al. 2001). Additional computational methods for ranking possible pathogenicity are in Sullivan et al. (2006). Investigators at the WU-GSC have successfully applied a suite of computational tools to identify pathogenic somatic mutations in adenocarcinoma (Ding et al. 2008).

In order to detect copy number variants (CNVs), especially deletions, we will examine genotypes of SNPs within each gene, looking for extended regions of homozygosity. We also plan to work with WU-GSC to look for gene regions that appear to be over or under represented and to determine if this correlates with CNVs. Our existing panel of adRP patients with large PRPF31 deletions will be used as controls (Sullivan et al. 2006a).

37.3 Conclusion

The VisionCHIP approach to finding retinal disease genes, based on targeted capture and ultra-high-throughput sequencing, is only one step towards whole-genome sequencing to identify mutations causing single-gene Mendelian disorders. Whole-genome sequencing will become widely available in as little as 5 years, possibly based on single-molecule techniques. The problem lies not with the sequencing technology but with analyzing and understanding the resulting genotypes. Humans are heterozygous for a nucleotide substitution roughly every 1,000 bp; of these, roughly 1 in 20 are rare, non-polymorphic variants. With the conservative estimate that 1 in 10 of *these* are potentially pathogenic based on computational analysis, each individual will be heterozygous for a potential disease-causing variant every 200 kb. Therefore, we anticipate detecting dozens of possible mutations per person with the first iteration of the VisionCHIP, and thousands when whole-genome sequences become routinely available. This estimate does not include indels, copy number variants, variable repeats or other DNA variants.

Determining pathogenicity of rare variants will be a major challenge to medical genetics for the foreseeable future. We believe that autosomal dominant retinitis pigmentosa offers a model system for addressing this problem. First, even though many adRP genes are not yet known, many disease-causing genes and mutations, and disease pathways, have been identified already. Also, retinal biology is a highly developed science. Thus there is a strong scientific background against which to judge novel genes and variants. Second, many multi-generation adRP families are available for segregation analysis – perhaps the most powerful means to assess pathogenicity. Finally, there are many functional assays for retinal gene mutations including in vitro systems, single-cell models, animal models and powerful imaging techniques for localizing and characterizing retinal proteins. Taken together, these approaches are likely to reveal several or many new adRP genes and many novel mutations.

Support Supported by grants from the Foundation Fighting Blindness, The Gustavus and Louise Pfeiffer Research Foundation, the Herman Eye Fund, and NIH grants EY007142 and EY005235.

References

Albert TJ, Molla MN, Muzny DM et al (2007) Direct selection of human genomic loci by microarray hybridization. Nat Methods 4:903–905

Bajic VB, Seah SH, Chong A et al (2002) Dragon promoter finder: recognition of vertebrate RNA polymerase II promoters. Bioinformatics 18:198–199

BioGRI D (2008) A general repository for interaction datastes, http://www.thebiogrid.org/. Accessed December 1

Bowes Rickman C, Ebright JN, Zavodni ZJ et al (2006) Defining the human macula transcriptome and candidate retinal disease genes using EyeSAGE. Invest Ophthalmol Vis Sci 47:2305–2316

Bowne SJ, Sullivan LS, Gire AI et al (2008) Mutations in the TOPORS gene cause 1% of autosomal dominant retinitis pigmentosa (adRP. Mol Vis 14:922–927

Daiger SP, Bowne SJ, Sullivan LS (2007) Perspective on genes and mutations causing retinitis pigmentosa. Arch Ophthalmol 125:151–158

Ding L, Getz G, Wheeler DA et al (2008) Somatic mutations affect key pathways in lung adenocarcinoma. Nature 455:1069–1075

Entrez G (2008) NCBI Entrez Gene database, http://www.ncbi.nlm.nih.gov/sites/entrez?db=gene. Accessed December 1

Gire AI, Sullivan LS, Bowne SJ et al (2007) The Gly56Arg mutation in NR2E3 accounts for 1–2% of autosomal dominant retinitis pigmentosa. Mol Vis 13:1970–1975

Grantham R (1974) Amino acid difference formula to help explain protein evolution. Science 185:862–864

Human Protein Reference Database (2008) HPRD, http://www.hprd.org/. Accessed December 1

Liu Q, Tan G, Levenkova N et al (2007) The proteome of the mouse photoreceptor sensory cilium complex. Mol Cell Proteomics 6:1299–1317

NEIBank (2008) NEI database of eye tissue ESTs, http://neibank.nei.nih.gov/. Accessed December 1

Ng PC, Henikoff S (2003) SIFT: Predicting amino acid changes that affect protein function. Nucleic Acids Res 31:3812–3814

RetNet (2009) The Retinal Information Network, http://www.sph.uth.tmc.edu/RetNet/. Stephen P. Daiger, PhD, Administrator, The Univ. of Texas Health Science Center at Houston. Accessed December 1

Scherf M, Klingenhoff A, Frech K et al (2001) First pass annotation of promoters on human chromosome 22. Genome Res 11:333–340

Stone EM (2007) Leber congenital amaurosis – a model for efficient genetic testing of heterogeneous disorders: LXIV Edward Jackson Memorial Lecture. Am J Ophthalmol 144:791–811

Sullivan LS, Bowne SJ, Birch DG et al (2006) Prevalence of disease-causing mutations in families with autosomal dominant retinitis pigmentosa (adRP): a screen of known genes in 200 families. Invest Ophthalmol Vis Sci 47:3052–3064

Sullivan LS, Bowne SJ, Seaman CR et al (2006a) Genomic rearrangements of the PRPF31 gene account for 2.5% of autosomal dominant retinitis pigmentosa. Invest Ophthalmol Vis Sci 47:4579–4588

Sullivan LS, Bowne SJ, Shankar SP et al (2005) Linkage mapping in families with autosomal dominant retinitis pigmentosa (adRP). Invest Ophthalmol Vis Sci 46 E-Abstract 2293

UniGene (2008) NCBI UniGene database, http://www.ncbi.nlm.nih.gov/sites/entrez?db=unigene. Accessed December 1

Wang M, Marin A (2006) Characterization and prediction of alternative splice sites. Gene 366: 219–227

Chapter 38
Advances in Imaging of Stargardt Disease

Y. Chen, A. Roorda, and J. L. Duncan

Abstract Stargardt disease (STGD1) is an autosomal-recessively inherited condition often associated with mutations in ABCA4 and characterized by accumulation of autofluorescent lipofuscin deposits in the retinal pigment epithelium (RPE). Non-invasive imaging techniques including fundus autofluorescence (FAF), spectral domain optical coherence tomography (SD-OCT) and adaptive optics scanning laser ophthalmoscopy (AOSLO) have the potential to improve understanding of vision loss in patients with STGD. We describe a comprehensive approach to the study of patients with STGD. Measures of retinal structure and FAF were correlated with visual function including best-corrected visual acuity (BCVA), color vision, kinetic and static perimetry, fundus-guided microperimetry and full-field and multifocal electroretinography. Mutation analysis of the ABCA4 gene was carried out by sequencing the complete coding region. Preliminary data suggest that a combination of imaging modalities may provide a sensitive measure of disease progression and response to experimental therapies in patients with STGD.

38.1 Introduction

Stargardt disease/ fundus flavimaculatus (STGD/FF) is the most common form of hereditary macular dystrophy in childhood, affecting 1 in 10,000 individuals (Bither and Berns 1988). The progression of vision loss in autosomal recessive STGD is usually rapid in childhood and young adulthood, but may be unpredictable and often does not correlate with the severity of fundus lesions (Klevering et al. 2002; Klevering et al. 2002; Rotenstreich et al. 2003). Fundus photographs of early disease range from a beaten-bronze appearance to atrophy, often presenting with characteristic yellow-white flecks at the level of the retinal pigment epithelium (RPE) (Armstrong et al. 1998). Histology shows the accumulation of lipofuscin,

J.L. Duncan (✉)
Department of Ophthalmology, University of California, San Francisco, CA, USA
e-mail: duncanj@vision.ucsf.edu

R.E. Anderson et al. (eds.), *Retinal Degenerative Diseases*, Advances in Experimental Medicine and Biology 664, DOI 10.1007/978-1-4419-1399-9_38,
© Springer Science+Business Media, LLC 2010

a lipid-containing fluorophoric by-product of photoreceptor digestion, inside the RPE (Sparrow and Boulton 2005). In advanced STGD, lipofuscin is associated with atrophy of photoreceptors, RPE, and choroidal vasculature concurrent with central vision loss (Rotenstreich et al. 2003). Fluorescein angiograms of STGD/FF often show a characteristic 'dark choroid,' superimposed by non-homogenous hyperfluorescent regions in the posterior pole (Fishman et al. 1987).

Eighty percent of patients with clinical STGD/FF have mutations in the ABCA4 gene, a phospholipid flippase found in the outer disc segments of photoreceptors involved in retinoid recycling (Allikmets 1997; Kitiratschky et al. 2008). ABCA4 defects lead to the intracellular accumulation of A2E in RPE cells (Radu et al. 2004). A2E is cytotoxic to the RPE in high concentrations (Sparrow et al. 2003) and can be visualized in living eyes using fundus autofluorescence (FAF).

This manuscript will review three non-invasive imaging techniques used in diagnosing and characterizing STGD/FF, fundus autofluorescence (FAF), optical coherence tomography (OCT), and adaptive-optics scanning laser ophthalmoscopy (AOSLO), and describe methods to evaluate cone and RPE cell structure in patients with STGD/FF.

38.2 Fundus Autofluorescence

FAF, a non-invasive imaging technique used to visualize lipofuscin, originates from the RPE layer; its distribution pattern in the normal retina is elevated in the parafoveal area, reduced in the fovea and towards the periphery, and absent over the optic disc and large blood vessels (Delori et al. 1995a; Delori et al. 2001; von Ruckmann et al. 1995; von Ruckmann et al. 1997). Abnormally increased FAF suggests RPE dysfunction, while decreased FAF indicates RPE atrophy and photoreceptor death (Lois et al. 2000; von Ruckmann et al. 1995). Most FAF images are acquired with a confocal scanning laser ophthalmoscopy system, which gathers light from a single optical plane, effectively reducing AF from sources anterior to the retina (Sharp et al. 2004).

Abnormalities in AF intensity, texture, and/or topographic distribution can be found in a spectrum of macular degenerative diseases (Cideciyan et al. 2004; Delori et al. 1995; Delori et al. 2000; Lois et al. 2004; von Ruckmann et al. 1997; Wabbels et al. 2006). The abnormal increase of RPE lipofuscin is likely the first detectable change in STGD/FF, with its continuous accumulation used as a likely marker for early disease progression (Cideciyan et al. 2004). Studies of early STGD/FF have consistently demonstrated abnormal AF, although with wide variation in pattern and degree. In some patients, AF images reveal areas of atrophy or flecks not seen on fundus photographs, suggesting its potential in detecting early disease (Boon et al. 2008; Lois et al. 1999). Recent studies have correlated FAF to visual function. Lois et al. (2004) demonstrated that STGD eyes without photoreceptor dysfunction as measured by pattern ERG had either normal AF throughout the macula or normal AF at the fovea surrounded by focally increased AF. In contrast, those with photoreceptor dysfunction had variably decreased AF at the fovea, presumably reflecting advanced disease with RPE and photoreceptor atrophy. Cideciyan et al. (2004) proposed a disease sequence model for ABCA4-associated retinopathies based on FAF findings. Early detectable disease is characterized by diffusely increased FAF in the posterior pole, and is followed by the appearance of focally increased FAF flecks in the perifoveal region. In late disease, FAF decreases due to dysfunction and eventual loss of RPE cells, leading to photoreceptor degeneration and death (Cideciyan et al. 2004).

Most FAF studies have relied on qualitative descriptions, characterizing the intensity as decreased, normal, or increased, with significant inter-observer variability (Lois et al. 2000; Sunness et al. 2006). Images captured by different systems show variability in absolute signal intensity and contrast, due to discrepancies in detector gain, argon laser amplification value, and normalization value (Bellmann et al. 2003). Furthermore, FAF intensity cannot be directly correlated with lipofuscin accumulation, due to absorption of fluorescence by a number of ocular structures, including melanin pigments, nerve fibers, capillaries, and lens opacities (Delori et al. 2001).

38.3 OCT

OCT is a non-invasive technique that provides high-resolution axial images of the retina, with depth resolution better than 3 μm (Drexler and Fujimoto 2008; Podoleanu and Rosen 2008). A low coherence infrared source is used to image the retina and a portion of coherent backscattered light is detected using an optical interferometer (Podoleanu and Rosen 2008). Depth and intensity information from captured signal light are converted digitally to visualize structural morphology of intraretinal layers (Drexler and Fujimoto 2008). Spectral domain OCT (SD-OCT) is the most advanced OCT method available and provides high resolution, fast scanning speeds, high repeatability, and the capacity for transverse C-scans and the 3D mapping of single retinal layers (Forte et al. 2008; Gupta et al. 2008; Leung et al. 2008).

Macular thickness and other retinal architectural OCT features provide useful information on the transverse and axial location of retinal lesions, atrophy, and other microstructural changes seen in STGD. OCT has revealed disruption or absence of inner and outer photoreceptor segment layers with or without thinning of other intraretinal layers, and visual acuity loss correlated with central foveal thickness in atrophic areas in patients with STGD (Ergun et al. 2005).

38.4 Adaptive Optics Scanning Laser Ophthalmoscope

AOSLO uses a wavefront sensor to measure ocular aberrations and compensates for them using a deformable mirror, providing non-invasive, high-resolution images of the retina (Roorda et al. 2002; Zhang et al. 2006). Achieving higher contrast and a transverse resolution of 2 μm, it is capable of imaging individual cones and single leukocytes moving through retinal capillaries (Martin and Roorda 2005; Roorda et al. 2002). Multiple frames from the same video can be added together and averaged to improve the signal-to-noise ratio, producing clearer images where most, if not all, photoreceptors are resolved (Zhang et al. 2006). Cones in healthy eyes are clearly visualized as bright spots arranged in organized hexagonal arrays with regular spacing, while cones in eyes with retinopathies show abnormal morphology, spacing, and packing patterns (Choi et al. 2006; Duncan et al. 2007; Roorda et al. 2007; Wolfing et al. 2006; Yoon et al. 2008).

Images of patients with inherited retinal degenerations, using both flood-illuminated AO ophthalmoscopes (Choi et al. 2006) and AOSLO systems (Duncan et al. 2007; Wolfing et al. 2006), have observed increased cone spacing/reduced cone density compared to normals, as well as hyper-reflective lesions in regions where cones and RPE were absent clinically. AO images of a patient with juvenile macular dystrophy showed an irregular cone mosaic where retinal sensitivity was reduced (Choi et al. 2006). A regular array of RPE cells in an annular region surrounding the cone-preserved fovea was visualized in 2 eyes with cone-rod dystrophy (Roorda et al. 2007). AOSLO imaging of members of a family with a mitochondrial mutation causing NARP syndrome (neurogenic muscle weakness, ataxia, and retinitis pigmentosa) showed three predominant cone spacing patterns: normal, increased within a contiguous mosaic, and patchy cone loss with increased spacing, the latter of which correlated with the most severe impairment in visual function (Yoon et al. 2008).

The use of AOSLO to study patients with inherited retinal degenerations both during disease progression and in response to experimental therapies requires accurate and reliable identification of not only normal cones but of also irregularly shaped and packed cones. Although software-based automated algorithms have achieved over 90% agreement between automated and manual methods (Li and Roorda 2007), unambiguous identification of cones is not always reliable using either method. Lack of visible cones may not always indicate photoreceptor loss, but could instead be due to poor image resolution or scattering from media anterior to the photoreceptors. Conversely, small, bright features in an AOSLO image are not always photoreceptors. For this reason, cone spacing is reliably quantified only in regions where cone mosaics can be identified unambiguously. The criteria for an unambiguous cone array is the appearance of multiple, similar-sized features arranged in a close-packed array, in addition to the presence of the expected laminar appearance of the photoreceptor inner and outer segment layers in a corresponding SD-OCT cross-section. An example of four imaging modalities used to image the nasal aspect of a normal fovea is illustrated in Fig. 38.1.

Although each of the reviewed imaging modalities has been established as a reliable diagnostic tool, a combination of imaging modalities including evaluation of structure on a cellular level may yield the most comprehensive

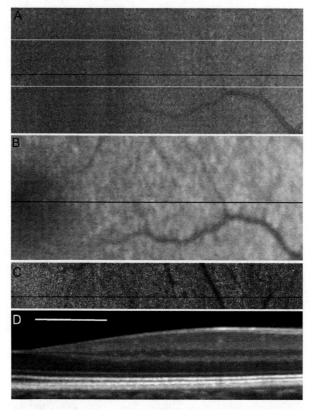

Fig. 38.1 Images of the right eye of a normal subject. The fovea is on the *left edge* of the image. Scale bar is 1° (∼ 300 μ) (**a**) fundus photograph, (**b**) FAF, (**c**) AOSLO and (**d**) SD-OCT. The *black lines* on **a**, **b** and **c** indicate the exact location of the SD-OCT scan. The thin *white lines* on (**a**) indicate the exact bounds for the AOSLO image overlay. Image (**b**) shows the expected decrease in AF toward the fovea. The AOSLO image shows resolved photoreceptors with increasing spacing with distance from the fovea (*left to right*). The OCT image shows the typical layered structure, including well-defined *inner* and *outer segments* expected for a healthy photoreceptor layer

characterization of the disease phenotype in STGD/FF patients. High-resolution images of the macula were obtained using AOSLO and SD-OCT in 5 patients with STGD and 10 age-similar normal subjects. A STGD patient with vision reduced to 20/200 and eccentric fixation nasal to the anatomic fovea shows regions of irregular and reduced FAF that correlate with increased cone spacing and loss of the photoreceptor inner and outer segment layers closer to the anatomic fovea on SD-OCT, while cone spacing is preserved adjacent to the optic nerve where FAF is more uniform (Fig. 38.2).

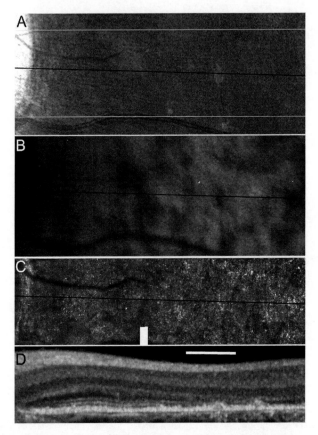

Fig. 38.2 Images of the left eye of a STGD patient. The edge of the optic disc is on the *left edge* of the image. The scale bar is 1° (∼ 300 μ) (**a**) fundus photograph (**b**) FAF, (**c**) AOSLO and (**d**) SD-OCT. The *dark lines* indicate the location of the OCT cross section. The thin *white lines* on (**a**) indicate the bounds of the AOSLO frame. FAF is mottled throughout the image with the exception a band around the optic disc. Uniform FAF corresponds with a regular array of cone photoreceptors in the AOSLO image and is further confirmed in the SD-OCT image by the presence of a laminar structure corresponding to photoreceptor *inner* and *outer segments*

38.5 Conclusion

STGD/FF is a complex retinal degenerative disease with variable disease presentation and progression. Better understanding of disease pathogenesis will require longitudinal data integration and analyses using multiple parameters, many of which can be acquired through the three imaging modalities reviewed above. Each technology has value in identifying disease severity and progression, but each also has intrinsic limitations that the other methods can complement. FAF can track lipofuscin accumulation, OCT can visualize cross-sectional retinal structure and AOSLO can directly visualize photoreceptor morphology to yield valuable insights into the temporal and topographic patterns of cone death. Understanding disease progression on a high-resolution scale will be essential in developing and monitoring response to therapies as they become available.

Acknowledgments Supported by a Career Development Award, Physician Scientist Award and Unrestricted Grant from Research to Prevent Blindness (JLD); a Career Development Award and Clinical Center Grant from the Foundation Fighting Blindness (JLD, AR); NIH-NEI grants EY00415, EY002162 (JLD), EY014375 (AR); That Man May See, Inc. (JLD); The Bernard A. Newcomb Macular Degeneration Fund (JLD); Hope for Vision (JLD); and the Karl Kirchgessner Foundation (JLD).

References

Allikmets R (1997) A photoreceptor cell-specific ATP-binding transporter gene (ABCR) is mutated in recessive Stargardt macular dystrophy. Nat Genet 17:122

Armstrong JD, Meyer D, Xu S et al (1998) Long-term follow-up of Stargardt's disease and fundus flavimaculatus. Ophthalmology 105:448–457

Bellmann C, Rubin GS, Kabanarou SA et al (2003) Fundus autofluorescence imaging compared with different confocal scanning laser ophthalmoscopes. Br J Ophthalmol 87:1381–1386

Bither PP, Berns LA (1988) Stargardt's disease: a review of the literature. J Am Optom Assoc 59:106–111

Boon CJ, Jeroen Klevering B, Keunen JE et al (2008) Fundus autofluorescence imaging of retinal dystrophies. Vision Res 48:2569–2577

Choi SS, Doble N, Hardy JL et al (2006) In vivo imaging of the photoreceptor mosaic in retinal dystrophies and correlations with visual function. Invest Ophthal Vis Sci 47:2080–2092

Cideciyan AV, Aleman TS, Swider M et al (2004) Mutations in ABCA4 result in accumulation of lipofuscin before slowing of the retinoid cycle: a reappraisal of the human disease sequence. Hum Mol Genet 13:525–534

Delori FC, Dorey CK, Staurenghi G et al (1995a) In vivo fluorescence of the ocular fundus exhibits retinal pigment epithelium lipofuscin characteristics. Invest Ophthal Vis Sci 36:718–729

Delori FC, Fleckner MR, Goger DG et al (2000) Autofluorescence distribution associated with drusen in age-related macular degeneration. Invest Ophthal Vis Sci 41:496–504

Delori FC, Goger DG, Dorey CK (2001) Age-related accumulation and spatial distribution of lipofuscin in RPE of normal subjects. Invest Ophthal Vis Sci 42:1855–1866

Delori FC, Staurenghi G, Arend O et al (1995b) In vivo measurement of lipofuscin in Stargardt's disease–fundus flavimaculatus. Invest Ophthal Vis Sci 36:2327–2331

Drexler W, Fujimoto JG (2008) State-of-the-art retinal optical coherence tomography. Prog Retin Eye Res 27:45–88

Duncan JL, Zhang Y, Gandhi J et al (2007) High-resolution imaging with adaptive optics in patients with inherited retinal degeneration. Invest Ophthal Vis Sci 48:3283–3291

Ergun E, Hermann B, Wirtitsch M et al (2005) Assessment of central visual function in Stargardt's disease/fundus flavimaculatus with ultrahigh-resolution optical coherence tomography. Invest Ophthal Vis Sci 46:310–316

Fishman GA, Farber M, Patel BS et al (1987) Visual acuity loss in patients with Stargardt's macular dystrophy. Ophthalmology 94:809–814

Forte R, Cennamo GL, Finelli ML et al (2009) Comparison of time domain stratus OCT and spectral domain SLO/OCT for assessment of macular thickness and volume. Eye (London) 23:2071–2078

Gupta V, Gupta P, Singh R et al (2008) Spectral-domain cirrus high-definition optical coherence tomography is better than time-domain stratus optical coherence tomography for evaluation of macular pathologic features in uveitis. Am J Ophthalmol 145:1018–1022

Kitiratschky VB, Grau T, Bernd A et al (2008) ABCA4 gene analysis in patients with autosomal recessive cone and cone rod dystrophies. Eur J Hum Genet 16:812–819

Klevering BJ, Blankenagel A, Maugeri A et al (2002) Phenotypic spectrum of autosomal recessive cone-rod dystrophies caused by mutations in the ABCA4 (ABCR) gene. Invest Ophthal Vis Sci 43:1980–1985

Leung CK, Cheung CY, Weinreb RN et al (2008) Comparison of macular thickness measurements between time domain and spectral domain optical coherence tomography. Invest Ophthal Vis Sci 49:4893–4897

Li KY, Roorda A (2007) Automated identification of cone photoreceptors in adaptive optics retinal images. J Opt Soc Am A Opt Image Sci Vis 24:1358–1363

Lois N, Halfyard AS, Bird AC et al (2000) Quantitative evaluation of fundus autofluorescence imaged "in vivo" in eyes with retinal disease. Br J Ophthalmol 84:741–745

Lois N, Halfyard AS, Bird AC et al (2004) Fundus autofluorescence in Stargardt macular dystrophy-fundus flavimaculatus. Am J Ophthalmol 138:55–63

Lois N, Holder GE, Fitzke FW et al (1999) Intrafamilial variation of phenotype in stargardt macular dystrophy-fundus flavimaculatus. Invest Ophthal Vis Sci 40:2668–2675

Martin JA, Roorda A (2005) Direct and noninvasive assessment of parafoveal capillary leukocyte velocity. Ophthalmology 112:2219–2224

Podoleanu AG, Rosen RB (2008) Combinations of techniques in imaging the retina with high resolution. Prog Retin Eye Res 27:464–499

Radu RA, Mata NL, Bagla A et al (2004) Light exposure stimulates formation of A2E oxiranes in a mouse model of Stargardt's macular degeneration. Proc Natl Acad Sci USA 101:5928–5933

Roorda A, Romero-Borja F, Donnelly W, III et al (2002) Adaptive optics scanning laser ophthalmoscopy. Opt Express 10:405–412

Roorda A, Zhang Y, Duncan JL (2007) High-resolution in vivo imaging of the RPE mosaic in eyes with retinal disease. Invest Ophthal Vis Sci 48:2297–2303

Rotenstreich Y, Fishman GA, Anderson RJ (2003) Visual acuity loss and clinical observations in a large series of patients with stargardt disease. Ophthalmology 110:1151–1158

Sharp PF, Manivannan A, Xu H et al (2004) The scanning laser ophthalmoscope–a review of its role in bioscience and medicine. Phys Med Biol 49:1085–1096

Sparrow JR, Boulton M (2005) RPE lipofuscin and its role in retinal pathobiology. Exp Eye Res 80:595–606

Sparrow JR, Fishkin N, Zhou J et al (2003) A2E, a byproduct of the visual cycle. Vision Res 43:2983–2990

Sunness JS, Ziegler MD, Applegate CA (2006) Issues in quantifying atrophic macular disease using retinal autofluorescence. Retina 26:666–672

von Ruckmann A, Fitzke FW, Bird AC (1995) Distribution of fundus autofluorescence with a scanning laser ophthalmoscope. Br J Ophthalmol 79:407–412

von Ruckmann A, Fitzke FW, Bird AC (1997) Fundus autofluorescence in age-related macular disease imaged with a laser scanning ophthalmoscope. Invest Ophthal Vis Sci 38:478–486

Wabbels B, Demmler A, Paunescu K et al (2006) Fundus autofluorescence in children and teenagers with hereditary retinal diseases. Graefes Arch Clin Exp Ophthalmol 244:36–45

Wolfing JI, Chung M, Carroll J et al (2006) High-resolution retinal imaging of cone-rod dystrophy. Ophthalmology 113:1019.e1

Yoon MK, Roorda A, Zhang Y et al (2009) Adaptive optics scanning laser ophthalmoscopy images demonstrate abnormal cone structure in a family with the mitochondrial DNA T8993C mutation. Invest Ophthal Vis Sci 50:1838–1847

Zhang Y, Poonja S, Roorda A (2006) MEMS-based adaptive optics scanning laser ophthalmoscopy. Opt Lett 31:1268–1270

Chapter 39
Protamine Sulfate Downregulates Vascular Endothelial Growth Factor (VEGF) Expression and Inhibits VEGF and Its Receptor Binding in Vitro

Jianbin Hu, Chao Qu, Yufeng Yu, Ma Ping, Dong Wei, and Dong Dandan

Abstract

Objective: To investigate protamine sulfate inhibition of expression of the vascular endothelial growth factor (VEGF) and VEGF-VEGFR binding in vitro and to find a new drug that inhibits neovascularization, which can potentially be used to treat angiogenic eye diseases such as diabetic retinopathy and age-related macular degeneration (AMD).

Methods: Monkey retinal vascular endothelial cells (RF/6A) were cultured in vitro and different concentrations of protamine sulfate were added to the vascular endothelial cells after three passages. VEGF expression level was examined by ELISA and immunohistochemistry after the cells were treated with protamine sulfate.

Results: VEGF expression decreased in a dose-dependent pattern in 10–80 μg/ml of protamine sulfate. We also found that protamine sulfate could inhibit VEGF to bind to its receptor, VEGFR.

Conclusion: Protamine sulfate could inhibit VEGF expression and VEGF-VEGFR binding in vitro. Protamine sulfate may be used for inhibiting neovascularization in angiogenic eye diseases.

Angiogenic eye diseases such as diabetic retinopathy (DR), age-related macular degeneration (AMD) and retinal vein occlusion are the main blindness-causing diseases. Previous studies indicated that VEGF and its receptor were involved in the pathogenesis, development and prognosis of these diseases. VEGF inhibition drugs have been used successfully in clinical treatment, but the cost is prohibitive.

J. Hu (✉)
Department of Ophthalmology, Sichuan Academy of Medical Sciences and Sichuan Provincial People's Hospital, Sichuan 610072, China
e-mail: jbinhy@hotmail.com

R.E. Anderson et al. (eds.), *Retinal Degenerative Diseases*, Advances in Experimental Medicine and Biology 664, DOI 10.1007/978-1-4419-1399-9_39,
© Springer Science+Business Media, LLC 2010

Protamine sulfate is a common, inexpensive anti-coagulation drug widely used for anti-coagulation in cases when heparin has been overused in the clinic. Recent studies suggest that protamine sulfate can inhibit tumor growth, probably through inhibiting vascular growth of the tumor. In this study we showed that protamine sulfate could inhibit VEGF and the binding of VEGF and its receptor, implying that protamine sulfate may inhibit blood vessel growth through inhibition of the VEGF pathway. This study further suggested that protamine sulfate may be potentially used to treat angiogenic eye diseases.

39.1 Materials and Methods

39.1.1 Cell Culture

Monkey retinal vascular endothelial cells (RF/6A) cells were cultured under normal oxygen or hypoxic condition. The hypoxic condition was modified based on the description of Eichler et al. (2004). In brief, the cell culture plate was put into a plastic bag, and the plastic bag was sealed completely. The mixture gas of 950 ml/L N_2, 35 ml/L CO_2 and 15 ml/L O_2 was supplied through oxygen pipe. A plastic bag with cell culture plate was then put into a 37°C cell incubator, and the mixture gas was supplied every 24 h. Different concentrations of protamine sulfate (0, 20, 40, 80, 160 ug/ml) were added to the medium of the cultured cells after passage of 24 h. The concentration of VEGF in the medium was measured by ELISA method at different times after the protamine sulfate was added (0, 24, 48, 96 h). Four days after the passage, the cells fully covered the plates; immunocytochemical (ICC) analysis was then performed on the cells to determine the binding efficiency of VEGF and its receptor.

39.1.2 Semi-Quantitative Assay of VEGF Expression in the Culture Cells by ICC

Two methods of scoring were used for the semi-quantitative of VEGF expression in the culture cells by ICC. In the first method, the cells were scored according to the density of the ICC staining, in which 0 represents no staining, 1 represents light staining, 2 represents staining with brown-yellow color, and 3 represents dark brown color. The total scores were obtained by multiplying the score of each group times the percentage of cells in the group. The second method of score was based on the condition of the staining particle, 1 for small-particle staining cells, 2 for clear particle-staining cells and 3 for big, dark-staining cells. The total scores were obtained by multiplying the score of each group times the percentage of cells in the group. The final scores were determined by adding the scores from the first method with the scores from the second method. Five fields were randomly selected for analysis. The data were further analyzed through MetaMorph/DP10/BX41 microimaging analyzer system for semi-quantity of VEGF expression.

39.1.3 VEGF Expression was Determined by ELISA

The sandwich ELISA method was used for the measurement of the VEGF expression. The VEGF monoclonal antibody was used for coating and the VEGF polyclonal antibody (Santa Cruz, CA USA) was used for detection. By this method, the detection sensitivity of VEGF was 9 pg/ul and reception rate was 102%. The assay was performed according to the instructions of the kit (Quantikineo, CA USA). The OD was analyzed to calculate the VEGF concentration using regression analysis according to the standard curve.

39.1.4 Statistical Analysis

The data was further analyzed using SPSS software (Windows 13.0). Then Dunnett comparison was used for comparisons of different groups.

39.2 Results

39.2.1 The Maximum Inhibition of VEGF Expression by Protamine Sulfate

We found that the VEGF expression was inhibited by protamine sulfate with a dose-dependent pattern from 10 to 80 ug/ml of protamine. The maximum inhibition was observed when 80 ug/ml of protamine sulfate was used. We observed that VEGF expression was reduced 47% from 810 to 383 pg/ml when 80 ug/ml of protamine sulfate was used for inhibition of VEGF expression. However, we also found that the VEGF expression could not be inhibited when 160 ug/ml of protamine sulfate was used; the reason remains unclear. Most cells died when 640 ug/ml of protamine sulfate was used for VEGF inhibition. Taken together, 80 ug/ml of protamine sulfate causes the inhibition of maximum VEGF expression (Fig. 39.1).

39.2.2 Protamine Sulfate Inhibits the RF/6A Cell VEGF Expression at the Hypoxic Condition

The cells were divided into four groups including normal control group, hypoxia group, and normal with protamine sulfate treatment group and hypoxia with protamine sulfate treatment group. The final concentration of protamine sulfate is 80 ug/ml. The cells were cultured for 5 days, then 50 ul of culture medium from each group was used for VEGF measurement and 50 ul of fresh medium was added to the culture plate to keep the total volume constant. In order to have enough nutrition for the cells, we kept 20 ml medium in the plates. VEGF was detected at 0, 24, 48, 72 and 96 h after the addition of protamine sulfate. We found that (1) the

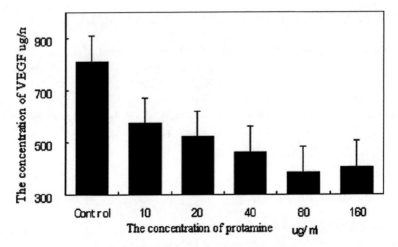

Fig. 39.1 The inhibition of VEGF expression by protamine sulfate of different concentrations. VEGF expression was inhibited by protamine sulfate with a dose-dependent pattern. The maximum inhibition of VEGF expression was observed with 80 ug/ml of protamine sulfate

VEGF expression in hypoxic condition was always higher than that of normal condition, and the VEGF expression increased significantly at 72 h, 96 h and 120 days (p <0.05). (2) The VEGF expression in hypoxia with protamine sulfate treatment group was significantly higher than that of the hypoxia group at 72 and 96 h (p <0.05, p <0.01, respectively). Accordingly, protamine sulfate could inhibit VEGF expression at hypoxic condition (Fig. 39.2).

39.2.3 Protamine Sulfate Inhibits the Binding of VEGF to Its Receptor

The four groups of cells were smeared on slides for immunocytochemistry studies after 96 h of culture (Fig. 39.3b). The semi-quantity results were as follows: A = 2.70 ± 0.06, B = 5.02 ± 0.20, C = 1.03 ± 0.16, D = 3.75 ± 0.63, X2 analysis with single factor showed significant difference between different groups(F = 43.43, P = 1.02E-06; between group A and group C and between group B and group D(t = 7.10, P = 0.00086; t = 2.79; P = 0.038) (Fig. 39.3a). The staining color in protamine sulfate groups was obviously slighter than those in their control groups in normal or hypoxic condition. These results can be explained by two possibilities: (1) protamine sulfate inhibited the binding of VEGF to its receptors; (2)protamine sulfate inhibited VEGF expression, so the VEGF-VEGFR complex was reduced. In any event, protamine sulfate can inhibit the binding of VEGF and its receptor in hypoxic condition.

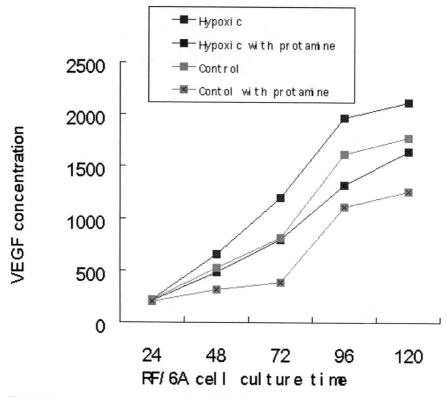

Fig. 39.2 Time course of VEGF expression inhibited by protamine sulfate (80 ug/ml) in vascular endothelial cells. VEGF expression level was measured by the semi-quantity method of ICC under normal and hypoxic condition with or without treatment of protamine sulfate

39.3 Discussions

Protamine sulfate is a weak anti-coagulation drug, and it is an antagonist of heparin. Recent studies have suggested that protamine sulfate has a function to inhibit tumor growth through inhibition of new blood vessels of the tumor cells. Since the angiogenic eye diseases such as AMD, diabetic retinopathy and retinal vein occlusion have a similar pathway of new blood vessel development as in tumor cells, so the drugs used for inhibition of new blood vessels of tumors can be tested for potential use for treatment of the angiogenic eye diseases, as well (Barfod and Larsen 1974). It is well known that VEGF is a critical factor of angiogenesis, so we studied the inhibition effect of protamine sulfate on VEGF and investigated the potential use in treatment of angiogenic eye diseases.

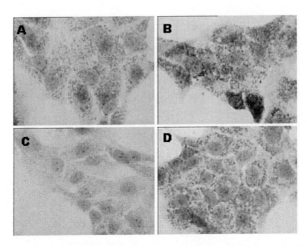

Fig. 39.3 Protamine sulfate inhibits the binding of VEGF and its receptor. RF/6A vascular cells were cultured in different conditions for 96 h with and without protamine sulfate treatment and VEGF was examined by immunocytochemistry assay. **a.** Normal control group: small, homogenous brown particles in cytoplasm; **b.** Hypoxia control group:1big, dark particles unevenly distributed in cytoplasm; **c.** Normal group with protamine sulfate treatment: smaller, homogenous lighter staining particles in cytoplasm compared to those in **a**. **d.** Hypoxia with protamine sulfate treatment group; the particles were bigger but lighter compared to those in group **b**

39.3.1 The Inhibition Effect of Protamine Sulfate on VEGF

In 1998, Gilbert et al. found that VEGF and its receptor were expressed in retinas of normal and diabetic mice using the in situ hybridization method (Heiduschka et al. 2008). They also found that the VEGF and VEGFR2 expression level increased in the retinas of diabetic mice. It was evident that the neovascularization of diabetic retinopathy is because of hypoxia (Eichler et al. 2004). Forooghian et al. (2007) found that the VEGF expression level increased dramatically in ARPE-19 cells after 24 h of hypoxic condition culture, because VEGF expression is regulated by hypoxia-inducible factor (HIF). Our study also confirmed that VEGF expression increased significantly in RF/6A cells after 72 and 96 h of hypoxic condition compared to that of normal condition ($p < 0.01$ and $p < 0.05$, respectively). Protamine sulfate can inhibit VEGF expression of RF/6A cells in both normal and hypoxic condition.

39.3.2 Inhibition of the Binding Between VEGF and Its Receptor

VEGF receptor 2 (VEGFR2) binding with VEGF secreted by the cell itself or other cells activate the downstream signal and cause angiogenesis. VEGF receptor 1 (VEGFR1) has neuron protection function (Wu et al. 2007). We found that protamine sulfate reduced the VEGF amount at the cell surface in the immunocyto-chemistry studies, maybe because protamine sulfate can directly inhibit the binding of VEGF to its receptor or protamine sulfate may inhibit VEGF receptor expression. Though VEGF can be secreted by other surrounding cells besides endothelial cells, protamine sulfate inhibits downstream signaling by inhibiting binding of VEGF to its receptor binding, even if the concentration of VEGF coming from cells other than endothelial cells is very hogh. So, protamine sulfate can potentially inhibit the neovascularization.

39.3.3 The Potential Use of Protamine Sulfate Inhibition of Angiogenic Eye Diseases

It was ascertained that the neovascularization because of hypoxia and increase of VEGF expression is one of the mechanisms of age-related macular degeneration (AMD), diabetic retinopathy (DR) and retinal vein occlusion pathogenesis. The increase of VEGF plays a critical role in the development of neovascularization. In this study, we showed that protamine sulfate can inhibit VEGF expression and binding between VEGF and its receptor. On this basis, we conclude that protamine sulfate can potentially be used to treat angiogenic eye disease in clinic. The in vivo study will be investigated to further evaluate this potential value of protamine sulfate in angiogenic eye diseases.

Acknowledgments The Study was supported by the National Natural Foundation of China; Sichuan Provincial Foundation for People Coming Back from Studying Abroad; Sichuan Academy of Medical Sciences & Sichuan Provincial People's Hospital.

References

Barfod NM, Larsen B (1974) Increased growth-inhibiting effect on tumour cells of protamine sulfate after Polymerization. Eur J Cancer 10(11):765–769

Eichler W, Yafai Y, Wiedemann P et al (2004) Angiogenesis-related factors derived from retinal glial (Müller) cells inhypoxia. Neuroreport 15(10):1633–1637

Forooghian F, Razavi R, Timms L (2007) Hypoxia-inducible factor expression in human RPE cells. Br J Ophthalmol 91(10):1406–1410

Gilbert RE, Vranes D, Berka JL et al (1998) Vascular endothelial growth factor and its receptors in control and diabetic rat eyes. Lab Invest 78(8):1017–1027

Heiduschka P, Julien S, Hofmeister S et al (2008) Bevacizumab (Avasin) does not harm retinal function after intravireal injection as shown by electrorenitography in abult mice. Retina 28(1):46–55

Wu WC, Kao YH, Hu PS et al (2007) Geldanamycin, a HSP90 inhibitor, attenuates the hypoxia-induced vascular endothelial growth factor expression in retinal pigment epithelium cells in vitro. Exp Eye Res 85(5):721–773

Chapter 40
Computer-Assisted Semi-Quantitative Analysis of Mouse Choroidal Density

Yun-Zheng Le

Abstract Geographic atrophy is a dry form of age-related macular degeneration (AMD) and a leading cause of blindness in the United States. The mechanism of the disease is unknown and there is no treatment for the disease at present. During aging and the development of geographic atrophy, there is a significant decrease in choroidal density. Since mouse is the only mammal that allows precise genomic manipulation, in vivo studies with genetically altered mice are likely to provide more mechanistic insights about the pathogenic mechanisms of the disease. To establish an efficient and quantitative procedure measuring choroidal density in mice for studies related to choroidal biology and geographic atrophy, we developed a computer-assisted semi-quantitative procedure for mouse choroidal density. In this study, mouse choroidal vessels were immunostained with anti-CD31 antibody and were detected by fluorescently labeled secondary antibody. Confocal or fluorescent microscopic images were analyzed with Adobe Photoshop software to determine the relative density of choroidal vessels. This procedure is relatively simple to perform and can be utilized to measure choroidal density efficiently in mouse models, which may be useful for preclinical studies relevant to the pathogenic mechanisms and therapeutics of geographic atrophy.

40.1 Introduction

Geographic atrophy is a dry form of age-related macular degeneration (AMD) that causes a severe central vision loss in 3.5% of people over 75 years of age in the United States and constitutes approximately 25% of AMD patients with severe central vision loss (Sunness 1999; Zarbin 2004). During aging and AMD, there is a

Y.-Z. Le (✉)
Departments of Medicine and Cell Biology, Dean A. McGee Eye Institute, Harold Hamm Oklahoma Diabetes Center, University of Oklahoma Health Sciences Center, Oklahoma, OK 73104, USA
e-mail: yun-le@ouhsc.edu

R.E. Anderson et al. (eds.), *Retinal Degenerative Diseases*, Advances in Experimental Medicine and Biology 664, DOI 10.1007/978-1-4419-1399-9_40,

significant decrease in choroidal density (Ramrattan et al. 1994). Patients with geographic atrophy demonstrate a lower choroidal blood flow (Grunwald et al. 1998). Experimental and clinical evidence suggests that abnormal interaction between the RPE and choroid is associated with the loss of choroidal density (Klein et al. 1997; McLeod et al. 2002; Sarks et al. 1988; Sarks 1976; Sunness 1999; Zarbin 2004). Abnormal choroidal development is also associated with the loss of retinal integrity in experimental mice (Marneros et al. 2005). Mouse is the only mammal that allows precise genomic manipulation. Therefore, in vivo studies with genetically altered mice are likely to provide more mechanistic insights about the pathogenic mechanisms of the disease. To establish an efficient and quantitative procedure measuring choroidal density in mice for studies related to choroidal development and degeneration, we developed a computer-assisted semi-quantitative method for choroidal density using immunostained mouse choroid. We herein describe the experimental procedure.

40.2 Methods

40.2.1 Immunohistochemial Staining of Choroidal Endothelia

Eyes from albino mice were enucleated and immersed in 4% paraformaldehyde in PBS for 2 h. The choroid/RPE layer was carefully dissected. The RPE cells were then carefully brushed off with a hair loop. The remaining choroidal vessels were washed three times with PBS, blocked with 5% serum containing 1% Triton X-100 in PBS for 1 h, and incubated with a polyclonal anti-CD31 antibody (BD Pharmingen, San Diego, CA) at 37°C for 2 h. The anti-CD-31 antibody stained choroidal vessels were incubated with FITC-conjugated secondary antibody (Chemicon, Temecula, CA), flat-mounted, and imaged with either a fluorescent microscope or confocal microscope.

40.2.2 Analysis of Choriodal Density with Photoshop 8.0

To quantify choroidal density, fluorescent images of the immunostained choroidal layer were obtained with confocal microscope or fluorescent microscope. Adobe Photoshop 8.0 software was used to calculate choroidal density. The threshold tool (under the adjustment in image) of the software was selected to convert a fluorescent image (Fig. 40.1a) to a black-white image (Fig. 40.1b), in which white area represented choroidal vessels. The threshold was then adjusted to make white area appeared as painted choroidal vessels (Fig. 40.1b), similarly to that in color or grayscale images. The percentage of white area in the adjusted image was calculated with the histogram tool of the software and was used to represent relative choroidal density (Fig. 40.1b). Comparison of a particular region among animals was achieved based on relative choroidal density obtained from identical image window.

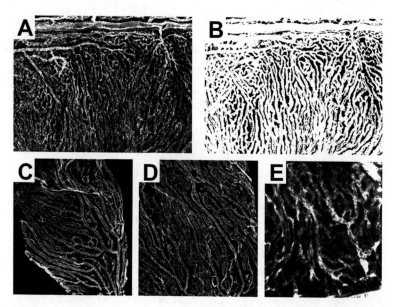

Fig. 40.1 Semi-quantitative analysis of choroidal density. (**a**) a grayscale image showing anti-CD31 antibody stained choroidal vessels of a wild-type mouse. (**b**) a *black-white* image converted from **a**. The *white area* is a representation of choroidal density and its value was 67.3%, calculated by Adobe Photoshop 8.0 software. (**c–d**) choroidal vessel images from identical region of an RPE-specific VEGF knockout (KO) mouse (**c**) and wild-type control (**d**). The calculated choroidal densities in the conditional VEGF KO mouse and wild-type control were 48.6 and 64.5%, respectively. The conditional VEGF KO mouse demonstrated a 24.7% loss of choroidal density, compared with that of the wild-type control (defined as 100%). The size of choroidal vessels was also reduced in the conditional VEGF KO mouse. (**e**) choroidal vessel image from a pigmented mouse

40.3 Results and Discussion

40.3.1 Analysis Of Choroidal Density

In this study, we utilized Photoshop 8.0 imaging software and converted fluorescent choroidal vessel images to black-white images. As demonstrated, a fluorescent image of immunostained choroidal vessels (Fig. 40.1a) can be converted to a black-white image (Fig. 40.1b). Since the white area in this black-white image was a representation of choroidal density, the value of the white area in Fig. 40.1b could be calculated by Adobe Photoshop and many other computer programs. The conversion of fluorescent images into black-white images is critical to the methodology and makes it possible to calculate the area of choroidal vessels, rather than fluorescent intensity, which was difficult to control in experiments. Since the result is not affected by the intensity of fluorescent images, we could use this method to compare images generated from different experiments. In our effort to investigate the function of the RPE-produced vascular endothelial growth factor (VEGF), we used this method to confirm its role in choroidal development. Figure 40.1c–d demonstrated a 24.7% reduction of choroidal density in an RPE-specific VEGF knockout mouse, as reported previously (Marneros et al. 2005). Since the procedure simplifies a three-dimensional structure to two-dimensional, the method may only be considered as semi-quantitative.

40.3.2 Usefulness of the Methodology

Choroidal vasculature provides approximately 70–80% of retinal blood circulation and thus is vital to the function and maintenance of the retina. To study the biology of choroid and outer blood retina barrier, attempts have been made to imaging choroidal vessels. Immunohistostaining of alkaline phosphatase for choroidal vessels is effective with human and primates (McLeod et al. 2002; Otsuji et al. 2002). However, the method does not work well with mice (Dr. G. Lutty, personnel communication). The reproducibility of corrosion cast (Majji et al. 2000) for mouse choroidal vessel is not easy to control, at least not in our hands. The leakage of fluorescin-conjugated large molecular weight dextran is an issue in visualization choroidal vessels with angiography. Taken together, there has not been a uniform and reliable methodology for imaging mouse choroidal vessels. The experimental procedure described in this study allows us to visualize choroidal density within one day, which is relatively efficient. Although images obtained in this study is two dimensional, they gave a similar readout (Fig. 40.1) as that derived from corrosion cast (Majji et al. 2000). There are also technical challenges associated with this method. For pigmented mice, it is more difficult to obtain reproducible results and images are usually less clear (Fig. 40.1e). The choroid is organized as dense vessels in wild-type mice, the method developed in this study may not be suitable for detecting subtle changes in the choroidal vasculature, which is a weakness of all other methods described above. However, a moderate change in choroidal density, as well as the size of choroidal vessels, can be detected and quantified (Fig. 40.1c–d).

40.3.3 Summary

At present, a major challenge in preclinical studies in dry-AMD field is the difficulties to image pathological changes in choroidal vasculature. The procedure developed in this study may be a supplement to existing methods. However, given the difficulties in imaging choroid, a dense vascular network with vessels overlaying closely, a combination of methods including those discussed above and ultrastructural analysis may be required to detect the changes in choroidal vasculature. Since mouse is the only mammal that allows precise genomic manipulation, semi-quantitative analyses of choroidal density in genetically altered mice is likely to provide more insights about the pathogenic mechanisms and therapeutic strategies for geographic atrophy.

Acknowledgments I thank W. Zheng, Dr. L. Zheng, and M. Zhu for technical assistance and Dr. M. Tanito for the tutorial of Adobe Photoshop program. This study was supported by NIH grants RR17703, and EY12190, ADA grant 1-06-RA-76, AHAF grant M2008-059, FFB grant BR-CMM-0808-0453-UOK and unrestricted grants from Hope for Vision and Research to Prevent Blindness.

References

Grunwald JE, Hariprasad SM, DuPont J et al (1998) Foveolar choroidal blood flow in age-related macular degeneration. Invest Ophthalmol Vis Sci 39:385–390

Klein R, Klein BE, Jensen SC et al (1997) The five-year incidence and progression of age-related maculopathy: the Beaver Dam Eye Study. Ophthalmology 104:7–21

Majji AB, Cao J, Chang KY et al (2000) Age-related retinal pigment epithelium and Bruch's membrane degeneration in senescence-accelerated mouse. Invest Ophthalmol Vis Sci 41: 3936–3942

Marneros AG, Fan J, Yokoyama Y et al (2005) Vascular endothelial growth factor expression in the retinal pigment epithelium is essential for choriocapillaris development and visual function. Am J Pathol 167:1451–1459

McLeod DS, Taomoto M, Otsuji T et al (2002) Quantifying changes in RPE and choroidal vasculature in eyes with age-related macular degeneration. Invest Ophthalmol Vis Sci 43:1986–1993

Otsuji T, McLeod DS, Hansen B et al (2002) Immunohistochemical staining and morphometric analysis of the monkey choroidal vasculature. Exp Eye Res 75:201–208

Ramrattan RS, van der Schaft TL, Mooy CM et al (1994) Morphometric analysis of Bruch's membrane, the choriocapillaris, and the choroid in aging. Invest Ophthalmol Vis Sci 35:2857–2864

Sarks SH (1976) Ageing and degeneration in the macular region: a clinico-pathological study. Br J Ophthalmol 60:324–341

Sarks JP, Sarks SH, Killingsworth MC (1988) Evolution of geographic atrophy of the retinal pigment epithelium. Eye 2(Pt 5):552–577

Sunness JS (1999) The natural history of geographic atrophy, the advanced atrophic form of age-related macular degeneration. Mol Vis 5:25

Zarbin MA (2004) Current concepts in the pathogenesis of age-related macular degeneration. Arch Ophthalmol 122:598–614

Chapter 41
Thioredoxins 1 and 2 Protect Retinal Ganglion Cells from Pharmacologically Induced Oxidative Stress, Optic Nerve Transection and Ocular Hypertension

Yasunari Munemasa, Jacky M.K. Kwong, Seok H. Kim, Jae H. Ahn, Joseph Caprioli, and Natik Piri

Abstract Oxidative damage has been implicated in retinal ganglion cell (RGC) death after optic nerve transection (ONT) and during glaucomatous neuropathy. Here, we analyzed the expression and cell protective role of thioredoxins (TRX), key regulators of the cellular redox state, in RGCs damaged by pharmacologically induced oxidative stress, ONT and elevated intraocular pressure (IOP). The endogenous level of thioredoxin-1 (TRX1) and thioredoxin-2 (TRX2) in RGCs after axotomy and in RGC-5 cells after glutamate/buthionine sulfoximine (BSO) treatment showed upregulation of TRX2, whereas no significant change was observed in TRX1 expression. The increased level TRX-interacting protein (TXNIP) in the retinas was observed 2 and 5 weeks after IOP elevation. TRX1 level was decreased at 2 weeks and more prominently at 5 weeks after IOP increase. No change in TRX2 levels in response to IOP change was observed. Overexpression of TRX1 and TRX2 in RGC-5 treated with glutamate/BSO increased the cell survival by 2- and 3-fold 24 and 48 h after treatment, respectively. Overexpression of these proteins in the retina increased the survival of RGCs by 35 and 135% 7 and 14 days after ONT, respectively. In hypertensive eyes, RGC loss was approximately 27% 5 weeks after IOP elevation compared to control. TRX1 and TRX2 overexpression preserved approximately 45 and 37% of RGCs, respectively, that were destined to die due to IOP increase.

41.1 Introduction

Oxidative stress implicated in neurodegenerative diseases such as Alzheimer's, Parkinson, Huntington's, and amyotrophic lateral sclerosis, has also been proposed to be an important factor in retinal ganglion cell (RGC) death after optic nerve

N. Piri (✉)
Jules Stein Eye Institute, UCLA, Los Angeles, CA 90095, USA
e-mail: piri@jsei.ucla.edu

R.E. Anderson et al. (eds.), *Retinal Degenerative Diseases*, Advances in Experimental Medicine and Biology 664, DOI 10.1007/978-1-4419-1399-9_41, © Springer Science+Business Media, LLC 2010

transection (ONT), tissue hypoxia, ischemia, axonal transport disruption and during glaucomatous neurodegeneration (Tezel 2006; Kumar and Agarwal 2007). Cell defensive mechanisms against oxidative damage involve superoxide dismutase, the glutathione (GSH,) and thioredoxin (TRX) systems.

The TRX system is a ubiquitous thiol-reducing system that includes TRX proteins, TRX-interacting protein (TXNIP), TRX reductase (TRXR), and NADPH. TRX proteins, cytoplasmic TRX1 and mitochondrial TRX2, protect against oxidative damage by scavenging intracellular reactive oxygen species (ROS), which leads to their oxidation. The oxidized TRX can be converted back to its reduced form by TRXR in the presence of NADPH. In addition to protection from oxidative stress, TRX proteins perform a variety of biological functions including regulation of apoptotic cell death (Masutani et al. 2005). TRX1 negatively regulates the ASK1-JNK/P38 apoptotic pathway by binding and inhibiting the kinase activity of ASK1, which plays an important role in ROS-induced cellular responses (Saitoh et al. 1998). Oxidative stress leads to dissociation of TRX1 from the ASK1, allowing ASK1 to form a fully activated complex by recruitment of TRAF2 and TRAF6. TRX2 is an essential regulator of ROS level in mitochondria. TRX2 anti-apoptotic characteristics are associated with the regulation of pro-apoptotic BCL-XL level and mitochondrial outer membrane permeability (Wang et al. 2006). The role of TRX2 in cell survival was demonstrated in TRX2-deficient mice, which is characterized by massive apoptosis and early embryonic death (Nonn et al. 2003).

TRX activity and expression is negatively regulated by TXNIP. TXNIP directly interacts with catalytic active center of TRX and inhibits the interaction of the TRX with other proteins including with the proliferation associated gene or ASK-1, causing cells to be more sensitive to oxidative stress (Nishiyama et al. 1999).

The aim of this study was to analyze the involvement of the proteins of the TRX system in RGC degeneration and evaluate the neuroprotective effect of TRX1 and TRX2 overexpression after pharmacological induction of oxidative stress, as well as in ONT and ocular hypertension rat models (Munemasa et al. 2008, 2009).

41.2 Methods

41.2.1 Animals

The use of animals for this study was approved by the Animal Research Committee of the University of California, Los Angeles, and was performed in compliance with the ARVO Statement for the Use of Animals in Ophthalmic and Vision Research.

To generate the ONT model, the optic nerve of the anesthetized adult male Wistar rat was exposed through a lateral conjunctival incision, the optic nerve sheath was incised 2 mm longitudinally, starting 3 mm behind the globe and a cross-section of the optic nerve was made without damaging the adjacent blood supply.

A rat ocular hypertension model was generated as described previously (Ishii et al. 2003). Briefly, anesthetized rats were injected intracamerally with 10 µl of

35% India ink in 0.01 M PBS. Five days later, approximately 200 laser burns were delivered ab externo to the pigmented trabecular band at dye laser setting of 532 λm, 200 μm diameter, 150–200 mW, and 0.2 s duration. IOP measurements were monitored once a week in the awake state 1 h after initiation of the dark phase.

41.2.2 RGC Counting

For ONT model: retrograde labeling to identify RGCs was performed by placing a small piece of Gelfoam soaked with dextran tetramethylrhodamine (DTMR) to the proximal cut surface of the optic nerve after ONT. For elevated IOP model: the number of RGCs was determined 5 weeks after IOP elevation by retrograde labeling of these cells with DTMR applied to the proximal cut surface of the axotomized optic nerve 48 h before animals were sacrificed. RGCs were counted at 1, 2, and 3 mm from the center of the optic nerve in retinal quadrant under fluorescent microscopy at 200× magnification.

41.2.3 RGC Isolation

RGC isolation from adult rat retinas was performed with magnetic beads coated with Thy-1 monoclonal antibody (Kwong et al. 2006).

41.2.4 Western Blot Analysis

Immunoblot analysis was carried out as described previously (Piri et al. 2007). Briefly, 2–5 μg of protein was separated on a 12.5% SDS-polyacrylamide gel and transferred to the polyvinylidene membrane. After blocking with 5% non-fat milk, the membranes were incubated with primary polyclonal antibodies against TXNIP, TRX1, TRX2, or β-actin overnight at 4°C and followed by incubation with peroxidase-conjugated secondary antibodies. The signals were visualized with an ECL plus Detection Kit and quantified with NIH Images software.

41.2.5 RGC-5 Culture and Transfection

RGC-5 cells were maintained in Dulbecco's modified Eagle's medium containing 10% fetal bovine serum, 100 U/ml penicillin, and 100 μg/ml streptomysin. EGFP-tagged TRX1 and TRX2 expression plasmid DNAs were introduced into the RGC-5 cells with the calcium phosphate-mediated transfection.

41.2.6 Cell Viability Assay

Cells were seeded on the 96-well plate (5×10^3 cells/well) and treated with 5 mM or 10 mM glutamate and 0.5 mM buthionine sulfoximine (BSO). Twenty-four or 48 hours after treatment, cells were incubated with 10 µl of water-soluble tetrazolium salt-1 solution and the absorbance was measured at 450 nm.

41.2.7 In Vivo Electroporation (ELP)

ELP-mediated gene delivery was performed as described previously (Dezawa et al. 2002; Ishikawa et al. 2005). DNA (4 µl; 10 µg) was injected into the vitreous cavity 0.5 mm posterior to the limbus. ELP parameters were as follows: electric field strength of 6 V/cm, pulse durations of 100 ms, stimulation pattern of five pulses at a frequency of one pulse/second. After a 10 min pause, five more pulses with the same parameters were delivered.

41.2.8 Statistical Analysis

Data are presented as the mean ± standard deviation. Differences among groups were analyzed by one-way ANOVA, followed by the Scheffé or Mann-Whitney test. $P<0.05$ was considered statistically significant.

41.3 Results

41.3.1 Expression of TRX1, TRX2 and TXNIP in the Retina After ONT and IOP Elevation and in RGC-5 Cells with Induced Oxidative Stress

Immunohistochemical analysis of TXNIP, TRX1 and TRX2 spatial expression showed similar distribution of these proteins in untreated rat retina with most abundant expression in the RGC layer, nerve fiber layer and inner nuclear layer. The majority of TXNIP-, TRX1- and TRX2-positive cells in the GCL was co-localized with RGCs.

41.3.1.1 TRX Expression in RGC-5 Cells in Response to Oxidative Stress

Oxidative stress in RGC-5 cells was induced by glutamate/BSO treatment. BSO is known to reduce the level of GSH with consequent increase in ROS and activation of apoptotic pathways, while glutamate regulates cellular redox status. The effect of the oxidative stress on the level of TRX expression in RGC-5 cells was determined by immunoblot. An increase in TRX2 (1.7-fold) and TRX1 (1.4-fold) expression was observed 12 and 18 h after treatment, respectively.

41.3.1.2 The Levels of TRX Proteins After ONT

Significant loss of RGCs was observed starting day 5 after ONT. By day 7 and by day 14 after ONT, approximately 50% and more than 90% of RGCs were lost, respectively. The levels of TRX1 and TRX2 proteins in whole retinal extracts were not changed significantly after ONT compared to the controls. Since western blot analysis of the whole retinal extract may be not sensitive to detect modulation in TRX expression in RGCs (RGCs constitute a small percent of retinal cells), TRX1 and TRX2 levels were analyzed in purified RGCs. TRX1 level was elevated approximately 1.4-fold 7 days after ONT, whereas TRX2 expression was increased approximately 1.3- and 2-fold 1 and 3 days after ONT, respectively.

41.3.1.3 The Levels of TRX Proteins After IOP Elevation

Increased IOP was sustained for 5 weeks, with a maximum of 32.1 ± 7.7 mmHg at 1 week. The changes in TRX1, TRX2 and TXNIP expression levels induced by IOP elevation were analyzed in whole retinal extracts with immunoblotting. Approximately 1.5-fold increase in TXNIP expression was observed in retinas 2 and 5 weeks after IOP elevation compared to the controls, whereas TRX1 level was decreased somewhat at 2 weeks and more prominently at 5 weeks. TRX2 level was not significantly affected by IOP elevation.

41.3.2 The Effect of TRX1 and TRX2 Overexpression on RGC Survival

EGFP tagged TRX1 and TRX2 expressing plasmids, pEGFP-C1-TRX1 and pCMV-hTRX2-EGFP (Tanito et al. 2005; Wang et al. 2006), were used to evaluate the cell protective effect of these proteins in response to glutamate/BSO-induced oxidative stress, after ONT and IOP elevation.

41.3.2.1 TRX1 and TRX2 Overexpression Protects RGC-5 cells Against Oxidative Stress

Similar to endogenous TRX proteins, EGFP-tagged TRX1 expression was localized in the cytoplasm, while EGFP-tagged TRX2 was co-localized with Mitotracker, indicating its mitochondrial localization. The transfection efficiencies were 67 and 63% for TRX1 and TRX2 expressing plasmids, respectively. To induce dose-dependent oxidative cell death, RGC-5 cells were treated with glutamate/BSO. A significant increase in cell survival was achieved by TRX1 overexpression: approximately 2-fold 24 h after exposure to 5 mM or 10 mM glutamate with BSO,

2.5- and 3-fold 48 h after treatment with 5 mM and 10 mM glutamate/BSO, respectively (Fig. 41.1a and b). TRX2 overexpression had significant cell protective effect against 5 mM glutamate with BSO treatment compared to glutamate/BSO treated non-transfected cells. This effect was not significant when cells were treated with 10 mM glutamate with BSO.

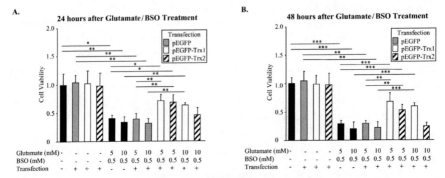

Fig. 41.1 The effect of TRX1 and TRX2 overexpression on RGC-5 survival. Cell protective effect of TRX1 overexpression was observed 24 (**a**) and 48 (**b**) hours after treatment with 5.0 or 10.0 mM glutamate and BSO ($n = 5$–11; $*P<0.05$, $**P<0.005$, $***P<0.0005$). TRX2 overexpression had cell protective effect 24 (**a**) and 48 (**b**) hours after treatment with 5.0 mM glutamate and BSO ($n = 5$–11; $*P<0.05$, $**P<0.005$, $***P<0.0005$)

41.3.2.2 TRX1 and TRX2 Overexpression Increases RGC Survival After ONT

ELP-mediated transfection was used to deliver EGFP-tagged TRX1 and TRX2 expressing plasmids to retinal cells. The RGC transfection efficiency was evaluated by counting EGFP-positive cells co-localized with DTMR-labeled RGCs and the total number of DTMR-labeled RGCs. Approximately 35% of RGCs were transfected with TRX1-EGFP or TRX2-EGFP. The cell protective effect of TRX1 and TRX2 overexpression was evaluated 7 and 14 days after ONT. In 7 days ONT retinas, $1,232 \pm 43$ and $1,205 \pm 93$ RGCs/mm^2 were present after TRX1 or TRX2 transfection, respectively, compared to 921 ± 75 cells/mm^2 of control (Fig. 41.2a). In 14 days ONT retinas, 419 ± 125 and 398 ± 58 cells/mm^2 were remained after TRX1 and TRX2 transfection, respectively, versus 176 ± 27 cells/mm^2 of control (Fig. 41.2b).

41.3.2.3 TRX1 and TRX2 Overexpression Increases RGC Survival After IOP Elevation

The efficiency of RGC transfection with EGFP-tagged TRX1 and TRX2 expressing plasmids was evaluated as described above by colocalization of EGFP-positive cells with DTMR-labeled RGCs. We have noticed that RGCs in the nasal retina were consistently more efficiently transfected than in other areas. Therefore, RGCs were counted in the two nasal retinal quadrants. Approximately 44 and 42% of RGCs

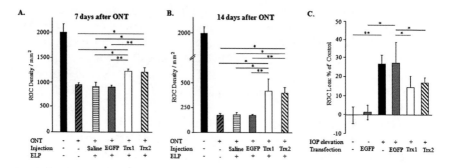

Fig. 41.2 The effect of TRX1 and TRX2 overexpression on RGC survival after ONT (**a** and **b**) and IOP elevation (**c**). (**a** and **b**). TRX1 and TRX2 overexpression increased RGC survival by approximately 35 and 135% 1 and 2 weeks after ONT, respectively ($n = 4$–7; *$P < 0.05$, **$P < 0.001$). (**c**). Approximately 45 and 37% of RGC that were destined to die due to elevated IOP were preserved by TRX1 and TRX2 overexpression, respectively ($n = 5$–14; *$P < 0.05$, **$P < 0.005$)

were expressing TRX1-EGFP or TRX2-EGFP, respectively. RGCs constituted approximately 70% of all transfected cells in the GCL. The RGC protective effect of TRX1 and TRX2 overexpression was evaluated 5 weeks after IOP elevation. At this time point the loss of RGCs in non-transfected retinas was approximately 27% compared to the control. RGC loss in EGFP-TRX1 or EGFP-TRX2 transfected retinas was approximately 15 and 17%, respectively, compared to the non-transfected or pEGFP-transfected control eyes (Fig. 41.2c).

41.4 Discussion

RGC degeneration after ONT and during glaucomatous neurodegeneration was associated with oxidative damage due to increased ROS levels. ROS have direct neurotoxic effects on RGCs and also contribute to secondary degeneration by affecting glial function (Thanos et al. 1993). The current study was initiated with the aim to determine the role of TRX proteins, important regulators of the cellular redox state, in RGC protection against ONT- and elevated IOP-induced oxidative injury.

TRX cytoprotective effect was first analyzed in RGC-5 cells treated with glutamate and BSO. Although overexpression of both TRX1 and TRX2 had a cytoprotective effect against oxidative stress induced by these agents, the effect of TRX1 was more potent than by TRX2. Based on data observed in RGC-5 cells, we analyzed the effect of these proteins on RGC survival after ONT and IOP elevation. ONT shifts the cellular redox status toward oxidation, which may lead to cell death by affecting mitochondrial functions or caspase activation (Nguyen et al. 2003). The survival of RGCs was shown to depend on redox state and stimulated by ROS scavengers (Geiger et al. 2002). In our study, TRX1 and TRX2 overexpression increased RGC survival by approximately 35 and 135% 1 and 2 weeks after axotomy, respectively. More pronounced effect of TRX proteins at two compared to

1 week after ONT could be explained by attenuation of secondary events associated with increased oxidative damage: RGCs dying early after axotomy may damage neighboring RGCs or lead to activation of microglial cells, which in turn could contribute to secondary RGC degeneration. Induced expression of nitric oxide (NO) synthase by injured RGCs and glial cells and subsequent NO toxicity associated with cellular oxidation has been implicated in RGC death after ONT (Koeberle and Ball 1999).

TRX overexpression also supported RGC survival after IOP elevation. TRX1 and TRX2 preserved approximately 45 and 37% of cells, respectively, that were destined to die due to high IOP. We believe that the observed neuroprotective effect of TRX1 and TRX2 could be even higher considering relatively low efficiency of ELP-mediated RGC transfection with TRX-expression constructs. Approximately 30% of transfected cells were non-RGCs, including glial cells and since oxidative stress-induced dysfunction of glial cells has been proposed to play a role in secondary neuronal damage in glaucoma (Tezel and Wax 2003), TRX overexpression may decrease the impact of oxidative stress in these cells and thus contribute to RGC survival.

References

Dezawa M, Takano M, Negishi H et al (2002) Gene transfer into retinal ganglion cells by in vivo electroporation: a new approach. Micron 33:1–6

Geiger LK, Kortuem KR, Alexejun C, Levin LA (2002) Reduced redox state allows prolonged survival of axotomized neonatal retinal ganglion cells. Neuroscience 109:635–642

Ishii Y, Kwong JM, Caprioli J (2003) Retinal ganglion cell protection with geranylgeranylacetone, a heat shock protein inducer, in a rat glaucoma model. Invest Ophthalmol Vis Sci 44:1982–1992

Ishikawa H, Takano M, Matsumoto N et al (2005) Effect of GDNF gene transfer into axotomized retinal ganglion cells using in vivo electroporation with a contact lens-type electrode. Gene Ther 12:289–298

Koeberle PD, Ball AK (1999) Nitric oxide synthase inhibition delays axonal degeneration and promotes the survival of axotomized retinal ganglion cells. Exp Neurol 158:366–381

Kumar DM, Agarwal N (2007) Oxidative stress in glaucoma: a burden of evidence. J Glaucoma 16:334–343

Kwong JM, Lalezary M, Nguyen JK et al (2006) Co-expression of heat shock transcription factors 1 and 2 in rat retinal ganglion cells. Neurosci Lett 405:191–195

Masutani H, Ueda S, Yodoi J (2005) The thioredoxin system in retroviral infection and apoptosis. Cell Death Differ 12:991–998

Munemasa Y, Ahn JH, Kwong JM et al (2009) Redox proteins thioredoxin 1 and thioredoxin 2 support retinal ganglion cell survival in experimental glaucoma. Gene Ther 16:17–25

Munemasa Y, Kim SH, Ahn JH et al (2008) Protective effect of thioredoxins 1 and 2 in retinal ganglion cells after optic nerve transection and oxidative stress. Invest Ophthalmol Vis Sci 49:3535–3543

Nguyen SM, Alexejun CN, Levin LA (2003) Amplification of a reactive oxygen species signal in axotomized retinal ganglion cells. Antioxid Redox Signal 5:629–634

Nishiyama A, Matsui M, Iwata S et al (1999) Identification of thioredoxin-binding protein-2/vitamin D(3) up-regulated protein 1 as a negative regulator of thioredoxin function and expression. J Biol Chem 274:21645–21650

Nonn L, Williams RR, Erickson RP et al (2003) The absence of mitochondrial thioredoxin 2 causes massive apoptosis, exencephaly, and early embryonic lethality in homozygous mice. Mol Cell Biol 23:916–922

Piri N, Song M, Kwong JM et al (2007) Modulation of alpha and beta crystallin expression in rat retinas with ocular hypertension-induced ganglion cell degeneration. Brain Res 1141:1–9

Saitoh M, Nishitoh H, Fujii M et al (1998) Mammalian thioredoxin is a direct inhibitor of apoptosis signal-regulating kinase (ASK) 1. EMBO J 17:2596–2606

Tanito M, Kwon YW, Kondo N (2005) Cytoprotective effects of geranylgeranylacetone against retinal photooxidative damage. J Neurosci 25:2396–2404

Tezel G (2006) Oxidative stress in glaucomatous neurodegeneration: mechanisms and consequences. Prog Retin Eye Res 25:490–513

Tezel G, Wax MB (2003) Glial modulation of retinal ganglion cell death in glaucoma. J Glaucoma 12:63–68

Thanos S, Mey J, Wild M (1993) Treatment of the adult retina with microglia-suppressing factors retards axotomy-induced neuronal degradation and enhances axonal regeneration in vivo and in vitro. J Neurosci 13:455–466

Wang D, Masutani H, Oka S et al (2006) Control of mitochondrial outer membrane permeabilization and Bcl-xL levels by thioredoxin 2 in DT40 cells. J Biol Chem 281:7384–7391

Chapter 42
Near-Infrared Light Protect the Photoreceptor from Light-Induced Damage in Rats

Chao Qu, Wei Cao, Yingchuan Fan, and Ying Lin

Abstract

Background: A project originally developed for NASA plant growth experiments in space demonstrating the Light-Emitting Diode (LED) could promote the wound healing. Further study showed that the LED's could protect cells by stimulating the basic energy processes in the mitochondria of each cell.

Objective: The purpose of this study was to assess the effects of 670 nm LED to protect the photoreceptor from the light-induced damage in a rodent model.

Methods: SD rats were randomly assigned to one of eight groups: untreated control group, the LED-treated control group, three light-induced damage groups, and three LED-protected groups. The rats were exposed to constant light for 3 h of different illuminations of 900, 1,800 and 2,700 lux, respectively. The LED treatment (50 mW) were done for 30 min, 3 h before the light damage and 0, 24 and 48 h after the light damage. Using the electroretinogram as a sensitive indicator of retinal function, and the histopathologic change was showed as a proof of the protective effect of LED treatment.

Results: The 900 lux illumination for 3 h did not cause damage to the retina of rats, however, the 1,800 lux illumination for 3 h caused significant damage to ONL of an approximate half retina, which caused the swing of ERG b wave to be 431 μV. With the LED protection: the damage of ONL was near 1/6 of retina, which was significantly reduced than the ones without LED protection ($P < 0.01$); and the swing of ERG b wave was recorded to be 1,011 μV, which was

Y. Fan (✉)

Department of Ophthalmology, Sichuan Academy of Medical Sciences & Sichuan Provincial People's Hospital, Sichuan 610072, China

e-mail: lucyjeffersonqu@hotmail.com

This work was supported by National Natural Science Funds No: 30771220; by Provincial Funds No: 303005002082 & 303005002127037

R.E. Anderson et al. (eds.), *Retinal Degenerative Diseases*, Advances in Experimental Medicine and Biology 664, DOI 10.1007/978-1-4419-1399-9_42, © Springer Science+Business Media, LLC 2010

increased significantly than the ones without LED protection ($P < 0.01$). The illumination of 2,700 lux for 3 h caused severe damage to the rats' retinas and the LED could not protect them significantly in both of morphology and function ($P > 0.05$, $P > 0.05$).

Conclusions: 670 nm LED treatment has an evident protective effect on retinal cells against light-induced damage, which may be an innovative and non-invasive therapeutic approach to prevent or to delay age-related macular degeneration.

42.1 Introduction

Light-emitting diodes (LED) arrays, which consist of light in the far-red to near-infrared region (NIR) of the spectrum (630–1,000 nm), were developed for National Aeronautics and Space Administration manned space flight experiments (Whelan et al. 2001). Thenceforth Whelan and others designed a serial of animal experiments and clinical trails, the results of which indicted the LED could prevent the development of oral mucositis in pediatric bone marrow transplant patients (Whelan et al. 2002), accelerate wound healing in genetically diabetic mice (Whelan et al. 2003), reduce TCDD-induced mortality in the developing chick embryo (Yeager et al. 2006, 2005), improve recovery from ischemic injury in the heart (Sommer et al. 2003), and attenuate degeneration in the injured optic nerve (Eells et al. 2004, 2003). The mechanism of LED therapy, commonly referred to as 'Photobiomodulation', has been shown to stimulate signaling pathways resulting in improved mitochondrial energy metabolism, antioxidant production, and cell survival (Desmet et al. 2006). Whelan proposed that NIR-LED photobiomodulation represents an innovative and non-invasive therapeutic approach for the treatment of tissue injury and disease processes in which mitochondrial dysfunction is postulated to play a role including age-related macular degeneration (Eells et al. 2004).

The light-induced retinal damage (LIRD) profile in the SD rat manifests similarities to advanced human atrophic AMD, so which was chosen as the optimal animal model to research the mechanism of AMD (Marc et al. 2008). Recent observations demonstrating the importance of mitochondrial function and the high metabolic demands of rods make it likely that loss of calcium homeostasis, free radical damage, and any other processes leading to mitochondrial failure may also be of significance in light induced damage (Barron et al. 2001; Missiaen et al. 2000; Carmody et al. 1999).

The present studies extended the LED investigations to an in vivo system to determine whether 670-nm LED treatment would attenuate the retinal degeneration in an animal model of light-damage, implications for age related macular degeneration.

42.2 Material and Methods

42.2.1 Animal

Animals were cared for and handled according to the Association for Research in Vision and Ophthalmology (ARVO) statement for the use of animals in vision and ophthalmic research, with the University of Oklahoma Faculty of Medicine guidelines for use of animals in research. Thirty two SD rats, which weighed 250–350 g, were randomly assigned to one of eight groups: untreated control group, LED control group, six light-induced damage groups and in them three with LED-protection. All animals were born and raised in a 12-h-on and 12-h-off bright cyclic light environment.

42.2.2 Light Damage

Four cages were placed in a light box and each rat was housed separately in individual chambers to prevent them from shielding each other from the light. The rats, which were neither dilated nor anesthetized, were exposed to constant light for 3 h of different illuminations of 900, 1,800 and 2,700 lux, respectively. Then the rats were put back into the animal room with the cyclic light for 5 days, ant then into a dark room overnight for the Electroretinograms examination.

42.2.3 670 nm LED Treatment

GaAlAs LED arrays of 670-nm wavelength (LED) bandwidth 25–30 nm at 50% power were obtained from Quan-tum Devices. Rats were anesthetized with a ketamine-xylazine mixture. The LED array was positioned directly over the animal heads at a distance of 1 in. Treatment was consisted of irradiation at 670 nm for 30 min resulting in a power intensity of 50 mW/cm^2 and an energy density of 90 J/cm. The LED treatment was done 3 h before the light damage and 0, 24 and 48 h after the light damage.

42.2.4 Evaluation of Photoreceptor Cell Function by Electroretinography

The SD rats were kept in total darkness overnight before ERG recording. Animals were anesthetized with a ketamine-xylazine mixture. Pupils were dilated with 1.0% tropicamide and 2.5% phenylephrine HCl. A circular silver wire, recording electrode, was positioned on the cornea, a reference electrode was positioned on the mouth, and a ground electrode was placed on one foot (Cao et al. 2001). The duration of white-light stimulation was 10 ms with a 60-s delay between flashes at seven light intensities presented in ascending order, beginning below threshold, to record the b-wave sensitivity curves and allow calculation of the saturated b-wave amplitude (Bmax). B-wave amplitude was measured between a- and b-wave peaks for quantitative analysis.

42.2.5 Morphological Evaluation of Photoreceptor Rescue by Quantitative Histology

Animals were killed by an overdose of carbon dioxide after electroretinographic testing. The eyes were enucleated, fixed, embedded in paraffin, and 5 μm think sections were cut along the vertical meridian. In each of the superior and inferior hemispheres, outer nuclear layer (ONL) thickness was measured at nine defined points as described (Li et al. 2006; Kong et al. 2006). In each of the experiments where ONL thickness was quantified, a single section from each of 8 eyes was measured.

42.2.6 Statistical Analysis

Results are expressed as mean±SD. Differences were assessed by one-way ANOVA and by t test. A P value less than 0.05 was considered significant.

42.3 Results

42.3.1 LED Attenuated the Light Damage Area in Retinas

The retinas, especially the outer nuclear layer, did not alter in the control, LED control, and light damage groups of 900 lux with or without LED protection (Fig. 42.1a–d). The extent of the degeneration retinas, explored to constant light (1,800 lux) for 3 h, decreased from approximately 1/2 to 1/6 after LED protections (Fig. 42.1e, f). Performing, a continue section cutting along the vertical meridian, we found that the damage extension were within a small circle, the center of which seems at the vertical meridian through the optic nerve head shown in Fig. 42.2. In most cases in group F, the damage region is located in the superior retina.

42.3.2 LED Protected the Morphology of Light Damage Retina

The extent of photoreceptor degeneration in rats was evaluated by measuring the thickness of outer nuclear layers (ONL) (Fig. 42.3). The area under every line stood for the amount of survival cells in ONL of each retina. Thus, the area between every line and the control one stood for the amount of lost cells in ONL induced by light

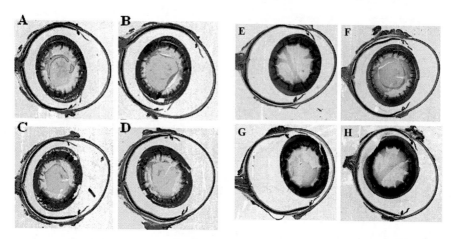

Fig. 42.1 The extent of light-induced retina damage. (**a**) Untreated control (**b**) LED control (**c,e,g**) 3 h constant light damage of different illuminations of 900, 1,800 and 2,700 lux, respectively. (**d,f,h**) 3 h constant light damage of different illuminations of 900, 1,800 and 2,700 lux, respectively+LED treatment for 30 min, 3 h before the light damage and 0, 24 and 48 h after the light damage. (**a~d**) Without significant morphologic alteration in retinae. (**e~h**) the *black double arrow* indicates the light-induced damage area, in which the outer nuclear layer (ONL) becomes thinner

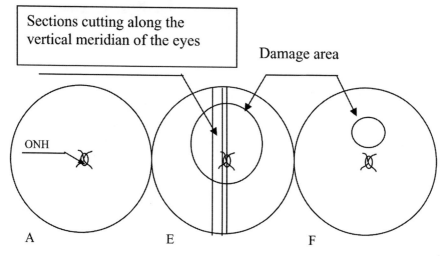

Fig. 42.2 Two-dimensional schematic diagram of light-induced retina damage area. (**a**), Untreated control. (**e**), 3 h constant light damage of illuminations of 1,800 lux, (**f**) 3 h constant light damage of illuminations of 1,800 lux, +LED treatment for 30 min, 3 h before the light damage and 0, 24 and 48 h after the light damage

damage. There was a significant difference of lost cell between group E and LED-protected F ($p < 0.01$), both of which were exposed to illumination of 1,800 lux for 3 h. However, there was no significant difference between group G and LED-protected H ($p > 0.05$), which were both of 2,700 lux. Then, an interesting event

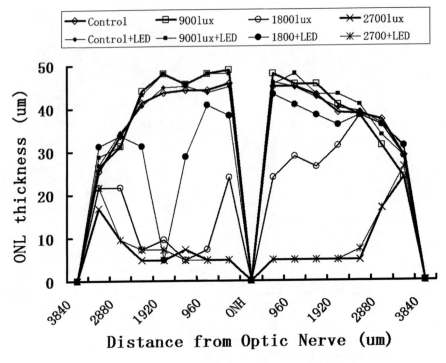

Fig. 42.3 A measurements of ONL thickness of the light-induced damage retina

emerged: the amount of lost cells in superior and inferior retina was significantly different in group E ($p < 0.01$) and F ($p < 0.01$), however, not in other groups.

The high magnification pictures were provided for group E and F. Three hours of exposure to constant light (1,800 lux) reduced the thickness of the ONL of photorecepor cell nuclei from the normal 10–13 rows in control animal (Fig. 42.4a) to 2–3 rows (Fig. 42.4e, f) in the most severe degenerated region of the retinas, while the IS and OS layer disappear simultaneously. However, with the LED protection (Fig. 42.4f), there was significant rescue of photoreceptors with the ONL having 2–5 rows of nuclei.

42.3.3 LED Protected the Function of Light Damage Retina

The effect of LED-treatment on retinal function was determined by electroretinography 5 days after exposure to constant light for 3 h. Histograms of B_{max} values are presented in Fig. 42.5. The B_{max} did not alter in the LED control and light damage groups of 900 lux (with or without LED protection) compared with the untreated control. Exposure to illumination of 1,800 lux obviously reduced the b-wave amplitudes to 40% in group E. There was a significant difference between group E and F,

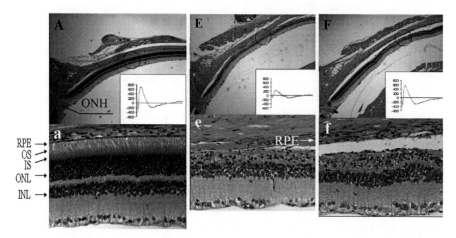

Fig. 42.4 The morphological and functional alteration of the retina explored to 1,800 lux for 3 h. (**a**) Control: the *black arrow* indicates the optic nerve head, and the *small circle* indicates where the high magnification was taken (HE, ×200). The *inset* shows a typical normal ERG waveform. (**e**) 3 h constant light damage of illuminations of 1,800 lux. (**f**) 3 h constant light damage of illuminations of 1,800 lux, +LED treatment for 30 min, 3 h before the light damage and 0, 24 and 48 h after the light damage. RPE, retinal pigment epithelium; OS, outer segment; IS, inner segment; ONL, outer nuclear layer; INL, inner nuclear layer; ONH, optic nerve head; LED, light-emitting diode

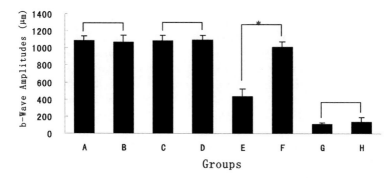

Fig. 42.5 Functional evaluation by electroretinogram (ERG). Electroretinography (ERG) was performed at the 6 day after light damage. Data show a dramatic reduction in (*E, G* and *H*) b-wave amplitudes in rats compared to the untreated control. There is a difference between group *E* and *F*, which was preserved by LED irradiation. Data from eight independent experiments were averaged (mean±SD, $n=8$)

which were preserved by LED irradiation. As expected, exposure to constant light of 2,700 lux for 3 h almost completely abolished the ERG response (Fig. 42.5 g), which did not increase after the LED treatment (Fig. 42.5 h) ($P > 0.05$).

42.4 Discussions

Results of this study demonstrate the therapeutic benefit of LED irradiation in the survival and functional recovery of the retina in vivo after light-induced damage. We provide in vivo evidence that 670 nm LED photo-irradiation reduces the retinal lesion by light microscope and quantitative histology, and attenuates the damage of retinal function in rod and cone pathways by measuring the ERG b wave. The mechanism of LED irradiation emphasizes to the organism absorption of near-infrared light and subsequent cellular biochemical alteration, obviously, it is different from the 'light precondition' reported by Liu et al. (1998). Liu et al. (1998) found that the preconditioning with bright light, that could help the animal resistant to subsequent light damage, by evoking two opposing processes: a fast degenerative process and a relatively slower protective process, which needs 2 days to develop fully. We gave the LED treatment 3 h before the light damage, however it is too short to develop the protective process. Besides, the power intensity of led in present study is 50 mW/cm^2, which is not as bright as described in Liu C group's article, 115–130 cd.

Despite the cellular mechanisms underlying LED treatment for light damage remain uncertain, the junction of both current theory about the LED and light damage may give us a reasonable explanation. The continued research efforts have provided a wealth of information on LED treatment and light damage. Gene discovery studies conducted using microarray technology documented a significant up-regulation of gene expression in pathways involved in mitochondrial energy production and antioxidant cellular protection (Wong-Riley et al. 2005). Britton Chance's group reported about 50% of near-infrared light (NIL) is absorbed by mitochondrial chromophores such as cytochrome c oxidase (Beauvoit et al. 1994).Cytochrome oxidase is an integral membrane protein and contains four redox active metal centers: the dinuxlear Cu$_A$, Cu$_B$, heme a and heme a3, all of which have absorbance in the red to near-infrared range detectable in vivo near-infrared spectroscope (Cooper and Springett 1997). Cytochrome c oxidase is the terminal enzyme of the electron transport system of all eukaryotes (Krab and Wikström 1987), oxidizing its substrate cytochrome c and reducing molecular oxygen including free radical oxygen to water. Meanwhile, it is an important energy-generating enzyme critical for the proper functioning of almost all cells, especially those of highly oxidative organs and tissue such as the brain and retina.

Recent observations demonstrate the loss of calcium homeostasis, free radical damage, and any other processes lead to mitochondrial failure in light damage process (Barron et al. 2001; Missiaen et al. 2000; Carmody et al. 1999). Penn et al. (1987) have reported an increased antioxidant levels in the animal retinas, which were raised in a bright rearing environment. He implied the antioxidants could ameliorate light-induced retinal degeneration, suggesting a role for oxidative stress in photoreceptor cell death. Carmody RJ group's study (Carmody et al. 1999) demonstrates an early and sustained increase in intracellular reactive oxygen species accompanied by a rapid depletion of intracellular glutathione in an in vitro model of photoreceptor apoptosis. Those early changes in the cellular redox state lead to a disruption of mitochondrial transmembrane potential, ultimately result in cell apoptosis. Chen (1993) has proved that the blue light with a fatal dose could inhibit the cytochrome oxidase irreversibly, and then lead to redistribution of chlorine and potassium in the inner and outer segments, damage to the mitochondria in the inner segments, edema in the inner and outer segments, and progressive degeneration of photoreceptor cells. So the dysfunction of cytochrome oxidase is the fuse to the cell apoptosis.

Based on above factors, the mechanism of LED treatment for light damage was speculated like that: Absorbing the NIL, the cytochrome c oxidase oxidizes its substrate cytochrome c and reduces the free radical oxygen to water and produces substantial deoxidize substance and ATP for the activity of the Na/K-ATPase to retain the physiological ions' distribution, balance the intracellular osmotic pressure and prevent the cellular edema and apoptosis.

In the past decade, mitochondrial genomic instability was investigated as an important factor in mitochondrial impairment resulting in age-related changes and age-related pathology. Focused on the relationship between mitochondria and AMD, those researches found that the acquired mitochondrial (mt) DNA deletion (Barron et al. 2001) or damage (Wang et al. 2008) and mtDNA control region SNPs (Udar et al. 2009) increased with aging in the retina, particularly in the foveal region, which was consistent with the decline in mitochondrial function with age. Genomic alterations and the consequent events including altered mitochondrial translation, import of nuclear-encoded proteins, and ATP synthase activity would be the susceptibility factors underlying the development of AMD (Nordgaard et al. 2008). Since the LED treatment could enhance the mitochondrial function by stimulating the cytochrome oxidase to resist light damage, it probably could prevent or delay the age-related macular degeneration as a mitochondria-related disease.

References

Barron MJ, Johnson MA, Andrews RM et al (2001) Mitochondrial abnormalities in ageing macular photoreceptors. Invest Ophthalmol Vis Sci 42(12):3016–3022
Beauvoit B, Kitai T, Chance B (1994) Contribution of the mitochondrial compartment to the optical properties of the rat liver: a theoretical and practical approach. Biophys J 67(6):2501–2510
Cao W, Tombran-Tink J, Elias R et al (2001) In vivo protection of photoreceptors from light damage by pigment epithelium-derived factor. Invest Ophthalmol Vis Sci 42:1646–1652
Carmody RJ, McGowan AJ, Cotter TG (1999) Reactive oxygen species as mediators of photoreceptor apoptosis in vitro. Exp Cell Res 248:520–530
Chen E (1993) Inhibition of enzymes by short-wave optical radiation and its effect on the retina. Acta Ophthalmol Suppl 208:1–50
Cooper CE, Springett R (1997) Measurement of cytochrome oxidase and mitochondrial energetics by near-infrared spectroscopy. Philos Trans R Soc Lond B Biol Sci 352(1354):669–676
Desmet KD, Paz DA, Corry JJ et al (2006) Clinical and experimental applications of NIR-LED photobiomodulation. Photomed Laser Surg 24(2):121–128
Eells JT, Henry MM, Summerfelt P et al (2003) Therapeutic photobiomodulation for methanol-induced retinal toxicity. Proc Natl Acad Sci USA 100:3439–3444
Eells JT, Wong-Riley MT, VerHoeve J et al (2004) Mitochondrial signal transduction in accelerated wound and retinal healing by near-infrared light therapy. Mitochondrion 4:559–567

Kong L, Li F, Soleman CE et al (2006) Bright cyclic light accelerates photoreceptor cell degeneration in tubby mice. Neurobiol Dis 21:468–477

Krab K, Wikström M (1987) Principles of coupling between electron transfer and proton translocation with special reference to proton-translocation mechanisms in cytochrome oxidase. Biochim Biophys Acta 895(1):25–39

Li C, Tang Y, Li F, et al (2006) 17beta-estradiol (betaE2) protects human retinal Müller cell against oxidative stress in vitro: evaluation of its effects on gene expression by cDNA microarray. Glia 53(4):392–400

Liu C, Peng M, Laties AM et al (1998) Preconditioning with bright light evokes a protective response against light damage in the rat retina. J Neurosci 18(4):1337–1344

Marc RE, Jones BW, Watt CB et al (2008) Extreme retinal remodeling triggered by light damage: implications for age related macular degeneration. Mol Vis 14:782–806

Missiaen L, Robberecht W, van den Bosch L et al (2000) Abnormal intracellular Ca2_homeostasis and disease. Cell Calcium 28:1–21

Nordgaard CL, Karunadharma PP, Feng X et al (2008) Mitochondrial proteomics of the retinal pigment epithelium at progressive stages of age-related macular degeneration. Invest Ophthalmol Vis Sci 49(7):2848–2855

Penn JS, Naash MI, Anderson RE (1987) Effect of light history on retinal antioxidants and light damage susceptibility in the rat. Exp Eye Res 44(6):779–788

Sommer AP, Oron U, Pretorius AM et al (2003) A preliminary investigation into light-modulated replication of nanobacteria and heart disease. J Clin Laser Med Surg 21(4):231–235

Udar N, Atilano SR, Memarzadeh M et al (2009) Mitochondrial DNA haplogroups associated with age-related macular degeneration. Invest Ophthalmol Vis Sci 50(6):2966–2974

Wang AL, Lukas TJ, Yuan M et al (2008) Increased mitochondrial DNA damage and down-regulation of DNA repair enzymes in aged rodent retinal pigment epithelium and choroid. Mol Vis 14:644–651

Whelan HT, Buchmann EV, Dhokalia A et al (2003) Effect of NASA light-emitting diode irradiation on molecular changes for wound healing in diabetic mice. J Clin Laser Med Surg 21(2):67–74

Whelan HT, Connelly JF, Hodgson BD et al (2002) NASA light-emitting diodes for the prevention of oral mucositis in pediatric bone marrow transplant patients. J Clin Laser Med Surg 20:319–324

Whelan HT, Smits RL Jr, Buchman EV et al (2001) Effect of NASA light-emitting diode irradiation on wound healing. J Clin Laser Med Surg 19:305–314

Wong-Riley MT, Liang HL, Eells JT et al (2005) Photobiomodulation directly benefits primary neurons functionally inactivated by toxins: role of cytochrome c oxidase. J Biol Chem 280:4761–4771

Yeager RL, Franzosa JA, Millsap DS et al (2005) Effects of 670-nm phototherapy on development. Photomed Laser Surg 23:268–272

Yeager RL, Lim J, Millsap DS et al (2006) 670 nanometer light treatment attenuates dioxin toxicity in the developing chick embryo. J Biochem Mol Toxicol 20:271–278

Chapter 43
BDNF Improves the Efficacy ERG Amplitude Maintenance by Transplantation of Retinal Stem Cells in RCS Rats

Chunyu Tian, Chuan Chuang Weng, and Zheng Qin Yin

Abstract The aim of this study was to evaluate the efficacy of subretinal transplantation of rat retinal stem cell when combined with Brain-derived neurotrophic factor (BDNF) in a rat model of retinal degeneration – Royal College of Surgeons (RCS) rats. Retinal stem cells were derived from embryonic day 17 Long-Evans rats and pre-labeled with fluorescence pigment-DiI prior to transplant procedures. RCS rats received injections of retinal stem cells, stem cells+BDNF, phosphate buffered saline or BNDF alone ($n = 3$ eyes for each procedure). At 1, 2 and 3 months after transplantation, the electroretinogram (ERG) was assessed and the outer nuclear layer thickness measured. The eyes receiving retinal stem cell and stem cell+BDNF transplants showed better photoreceptor maintenance than the other groups ($P < 0.01$) at all time points. One month after retina transplantation, the amplitudes of rod-ERG and Max-ERG b waves were significantly higher the eyes with stem cells+BDNF ($P < 0.01$), however, this difference was not seen at two and three months post transplantation. BDNF treatment alone group (without transplanted cells) had no effect when compared to buffer injections. The present results indicate that BDNF can enhance the short-term efficacy of the retinal stem cell transplantation in treating retinal degenerative disease.

43.1 Introduction

Brain-derived neurotrophic factor (BDNF) has been shown to regulate many aspects of neuronal development in the central neural system, including survival, axonal and dendritic growth and synapse formation. In the retina, BDNF can support the survival and maintenance of the dendritic morphology of retinal ganglion cells

Z.Q. Yin (✉)
Southwest Hospital, Southwest Eye Hospital, Third Military Medical University, Chongqing 400038, People's Republic of China
e-mail: qinzyin@yahoo.com.cn

The authors Chunyu Tian and Zheng Qin Yin contributed equally to this work.

R.E. Anderson et al. (eds.), *Retinal Degenerative Diseases*, Advances in Experimental Medicine and Biology 664, DOI 10.1007/978-1-4419-1399-9_43,
© Springer Science+Business Media, LLC 2010

(Weber and Harman 2008) and protects photoreceptors from the damaging effects of constant light (Gauthier et al. 2005). Recently, it has been reported that BDNF also plays an important role in dendritic growth in response to enriched visual environments that control the development of retinal circuitry (Landi et al. 2007a, b). In addition, researchers found that, in the rat, BDNF can effectively minimize the retinal toxicity resulting from photodynamic therapy (Paskowitz et al. 2007).

Retinal degenerative conditions, such as age-related macular degeneration and retinitis pigmentosa, leads to irreversible loss of vision, and is a major problem around the world that lacks suitable clinic treatment. A more general approach for the treatment of photoreceptor loss may be cell-based therapy dependent on the strategy of photoreceptor replacement by cell transplantation (MacLaren et al. 2006; Bartsch et al. 2008; Djojosubroto and Arsenijevic 2008; Wang et al. 2008; West et al. 2008). However, cell-based therapeutic approaches for the replacement of photoreceptors in disease such as retinitis pigmentosa have been limited to date due to the minimal integration of donor cells into the outer nuclear layer (ONL) and their ability to participate in host retinal circuitry. One of the most important goals for retina transplantation is to protect visual function during the process of retinal degeneration. We investigated whether BDNF combined with retinal stem cell (RSC) transplantation could provide a better restoration of visual function in degenerating retinas compared to previous approaches to the problem.

43.2 Methods

43.2.1 Animals

Animals were treated in accordance with the NIH guidelines for the care and use of laboratory animals and ARVO Statement for the Use of Animals in Ophthalmic and Vision Research, under a protocol approved by the Institutional Animal Care and Use Committee of Third Military Medical University. All efforts were made to minimize animal suffering and to use only the minimum number of animals necessary to provide an adequate sample size for statistically meaningful scientific conclusions. Eighteen pigmented dystrophic RCS rats were used in this study, and received a unilateral subretinal injection of rat retinal stem cells (rSCs) ($n = 9$) or rSCs+BDNF (1 mg/ml, 5 ìg/animal, Sigma, US, $n = 9$). The other eye received a subretinal injection of phosphate buffered saline (PBS) ($n = 9$) or the BDNF solution alone (5 ìg/animal, $n=9$).

43.2.2 Cell Preparation and Subretinal Transplantation

Embryonic day 17 rats were obtained from pregnant Long Evans dams (Taconic, Hudson, NY), and rSCs harvested from the retinas under sterile conditions. Culture and purifying of rSCs has been described previously (Chen et al. 2008). One hour before surgery, rSCs neurospheres were gently dissociated into a cell suspension and then labeled with fluorescence marker, CM-DiI (2 ìg/ml, Millipore, US). rSCs were washed twice with medium and then diluted to a final concentration of 2×10^4/ìl in PBS or a solution containing 1 mg/ml BDNF and kept on ice until transplantation. Trypan blue dye exclusion was performed on the cell suspensions before and immediately after transplantation, which showed greater than 90 and 80% cell survival, respectively. All recipient RCS rats (at the age of P30) were anaesthetized with medelomidine hydrochloride (0.01 mg/10 g body wt, i.p., Dormitor, Pfizer) and placed in a head holder. The pupils were dilated with 1% tropicamide and the surfaces of the eye anesthetized with drops of 0.4% oxybuprocaine hydrochloride. A 5 ìl Hamilton syringe (26-gauge needle; Hamilton, Switzerland) containing the suspension of labeled rSCs was tangentially inserted through the conjunctiva and sclera into the subretinal space, causing a self-sealing wound tunnel. Cell suspensions were slowly injected (5 ìl/eye, 1×10^5 cells/eye in total) to produce a retinal detachment in the superior retina. The other eye received an injection with 5 ìl PBS or 5 ìl BDNF solutions (1 mg/ml). All surgical procedures were performed using an operating ophthalmic microscope. The cornea was punctured to reduce intraocular pressure and limit the efflux of cells. After subretinal transplantation, the fundus was examined using direct ophthalmoscopic observation.

43.2.3 Flash-Electroretinogram (F-ERG) Recordings

Animals were tested at 1, 2 and 3 months ($n = 3$ for each treatment at each time) after surgery. The rats were dark-adapted overnight then anesthetized i. m. with a combination of xylazine (5 mg/Kg, Sigma, US) and ketamine (50 mg/kg, Sigma, US). Body temperature was controlled at 37°C with a heating pad. A ground electrode needle was placed in the tail, and a reference electrode needle placed in the forehead. An F-ERG recording electrode consisting of a small silver ring positioned on the surface of the cornea by a drop of methyl cellulose was used to record responses at a gain of 1 k using a 30 HZ (EPIC-2000; Roland, Germany). ERG b waves were generated with flashes of white light at intensities ranging from -6.3 log cd-s. m^{-2} to 0.6 log cd-s. m^{-2}. Each ERG response represents the average of five flashes. For all F-ERG recordings, b-wave amplitude was measured from the a-wave trough baseline to the peak of b-wave, and b-wave latency was measured from the onset of the stimulus to the b-wave peak.

43.2.4 Histology and Quantification

Rats killed by anesthetic overdoes after recordings, the eyes enucleated and the eyecups fixed in 4% paraformaldehyde in PBS (0.01 M, pH 7.4). Eye cups were immersed in a graded series of sucrose solutions (10, 20 and 30% in 0.01 M PBS) at room temperature for 2 days, embedded in OCT and sectioned on a cryostat (15 ìm thickness, Leica CM1900). Sections were fixed to poly-L-lysine coated slides and the thickness of the ONL visualized by differential interference contrast (DIC) florescence microscope (Leica, Germany) and measured (Image Pro-plus 6.0 system) in 6 fields per sample ($n = 3$ each time point/group). We began to pick up the sections, once we found the DiI labeled cells in the retina and through the disappearance of donor cells. To find the survival donor cells transplanted in the subretinal spaces, we picked 20 sections each eye, which is totally 300 μm distance. And we counted the survival donor cells every 4 sections of these 20 sections of each eye to get the number of survival donor cells used to compare with each group. Sections we chose to measure the ONL thickness were picked from the sections which across the optic nerve ($n = 4$, each eye).

43.2.5 Data Analysis

Statistical analyses were performed using SPSS 15.0 for Windows. Data were presented as mean ± standard error of the mean (SEM). Statistical analyses were made using either Student's two-tailed t test or analysis of variance (ANOVA). Newman-Keuls procedure was used for multiple comparison analysis. Differences were considered to be significant at $P \leq 0.05$.

43.3 Results

43.3.1 ERG Amplitudes and Latencies

ERG wave amplitudes: Comparison of the rSCs and rSCs+BDNF groups at 1 mon revealed that the rSCs+BDNF group had significantly greater rod-ERG b wave (151 ± 31.5 ìv vs. 137 ± 35.3 ìv, $P < 0.01$, $n = 3$) and Max-ERG b wave (203.5 ± 27.4 ìv vs. 174 ± 33.4 ìv, $P < 0.01$) amplitudes; both groups had significantly higher amplitudes than PBS or BDNF injected eyes. However, recordings at 2 and 3 months showed no difference between rSCs+BDNF and rSCs groups for the amplitudes of the rod-ERG b and max-ERG b waves (2 mon; 47.5 ± 24.8 ìv vs. 49 ± 21.3 ìv; 96 ± 25.1 ìv vs. 95 ± 21.3 ìv, and 3 mon; 20.8 ± 5.4 ìv vs. 17.9 ± 6.2 ìv; 32 ± 12.5 ìv vs. 29.7 ± 12.4 ìv, respectively). Both amplitudes were still significantly higher than values recorded for PBS or BNDF eyes in the first and second month ($P < 0.05$).

ERG wave latencies: One month after surgery the latencies of the rod-ERG b and max-ERG b waves in rSCs+BDNF eyes were shorter ($P<0.05$) than in rSCs eyes (92 ± 7.9 ms vs. 95 ± 12.6 ms, and 71 ± 12.5 ms vs. 75 ± 21.7 ms, respectively). Similar to wave amplitudes, at 2 and 3 months after transplantation, there is no significant difference between the latencies of the rod-ERG b and max-ERG b waves ($P > 0.05$) between rSCs+BDNF and rSCs (2 mon; 100.3 ± 18.4 ms vs. 99 ± 17.9 ms; 84.5 ± 33.7 ms vs. 83.2 ± 31.6 ms, and 3 mon; 114.7 ± 32.7 ms vs.

115.9 ± 34.5 ms; 97.5 ± 35.4 ms vs. 97 ± 36.2 ms). Both latencies were still significantly shorter than times recorded for PBS or BNDF eyes in the first and second month ($P < 0.05$). Significant differences were not seen between any of the comparisons for the PBS vs. BDNF groups with respect to latency or amplitude (Fig. 43.1).

43.3.2 ONL Thickness

There were no significant differences between the thicknesses of the ONL in the rSCs and rSCs+BDNF eyes at any time (Fig. 43.2), however, ONL thickness in rSCs eyes at 1, 2 and 3 months after transplantation (34.8 ± 4.3 ìm, 19.1 ± 3.7 ìm and 13.2 ± 2 ìm; $n = 3$), were significantly greater than that seen in PBS injection eyes over the same time period (22.8 ± 2.1 ìm, 13 ± 2.7 ìm and 9.1 ± 1.5 respectively; $P < 0.01$). Similarly, the rSCs+BDNF eyes also showed significantly thicker ONLs (32.1 ± 7.9 ìm, 18 ± 0.4 ìm and 12.8 ± 2.4 ìm) than the BDNF injections alone ($P < 0.01$), which were 23.4 ± 4.1 ìm, 14 ± 1.8 ìm and 9.2 ± 1.8 ìm at 1, 2 and 3 months, respectively. There were no significant differences in ONL thickness between the PBS and BDNF injected.

43.3.3 Graft Cells Survival After Subretinal Transplantation

Graft cells can survival through 3 months after transplantation in both rSCs + BDNF eyes and rSCs eyes. The graft cells not only located in ONL but also migrated into INL after transplantation in both groups (Fig. 43.3). One month after transplantation, rSCs + BDNF eyes showed more grafts cells survival (139 ± 5 per eye, $n = 3$) than rSCs eyes (101.7 ± 9.9 per eye, $n = 3$) ($P < 0.05$). In 2 and 3 months after transplantation, there are no more difference between rSCs + BDNF eyes and rSCs eyes (106 ± 3.8 per eye vs. 94.7 ± 8.4 per eye and 70.7 ± 8.7 vs. 65.3 ± 6.4 per eye, $n = 3$, respectively, $P > 0.05$).

43.4 Discussion

Our results showed that BDNF can enhance the efficacy of rSCs subretinal transplantation, when assessed by ERG analysis. These results support previous studies by Marler et al. (2008) in which they used the animal model of light induced photoreceptor degeneration rat and transplanted adenovirus mediated gene delivery of BDNF of Müller cells in vitreous. They found that BDNF gene delivery to Müller glia can markedly increased the survival and structural integrity of light damaged photoreceptors (Gauthier et al. 2005). Also Ikeda in 2003 showed that BDNF shows protective effect and improves recovery of ERG b-wave in light induced photoreceptor damage (Ikeda et al. 2003). In 2008, Seiler et al. transplanted BDNF-treated retinal sheets into S 334ter lin3 rhodopsin retinal degenerate rats and found that

Latency (ms)   Amplitude (µV)

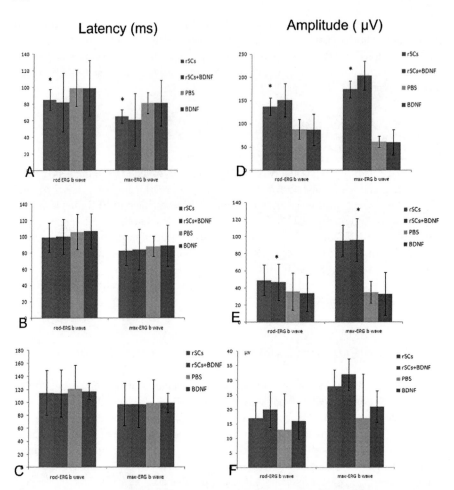

Fig. 43.1 ERG latency and amplitude measurements. (**a**) One month after transplantation, eyes receiving either rSCs or rSCs+BDNF transplants retained better ERG responses compared to eyes receiving PBS or BDNF injections ($P < 0.01$; *bars* represent the SEM). rSCs+BDNF eyes had significantly higher amplitude rod-ERG b (151 ± 31.5 iv vs. 137 ± 35.3 iv, $P < 0.01$, $n = 3$) and Max-ERG b waves (203.5 ± 27.4 iv vs. 174 ± 33.4 iv, $P < 0.01$) compared to rSCs eyes. The latencies of rod-ERG b and max-ERG b waves in rSCs+BDNF eyes are shorter than those seen in rSCs eyes (92 ± 7.9 ms vs. 95 ± 12.6 ms, $P < 0.05$, $n = 3$ and 71 ± 12.5 ms vs. 75 ± 21.7 ms, $P < 0.05$, $n = 3$). (**b**) At 2 months after transplantation, eyes receiving either rSCs or rSCs+BDNF transplants retained better ERG responses than PBS or BDNF, injected eyes ($P < 0.01$). However, there is no difference between rSCs or rSCs+BDNF eyes with respect to wave latencies and amplitude. (**c**) No differences were seen between groups

BDNF coating improved the head-tracking behavior and the electrophysiological responses of the host retina. However, transplanted whole retinal sheets have their limitations, for example it difficult for the sheets to integrate and make functional connections within the host neural retina (Zhang et al. 2003).

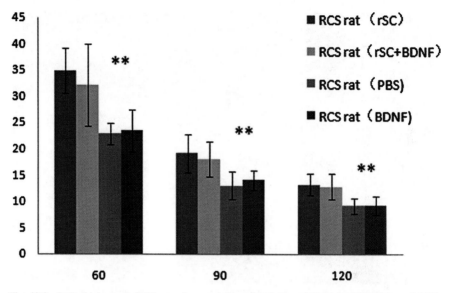

Fig. 43.2 ONL thickness in RCS rats after receiving transplants or injections. The mean and ONL thicknesses and SEMs are shown at 1, 2 and 3 months after rSCs or rSCs+ BDNF (5 ìl with 5 µg) /transplantation or PBS (5 ìl) or BDNF (5 ìl with 5 µg) injections into the subretinal space (**$P<0.01$). Y-axis is ONL thickness (µm)

Photoreceptor cell bodies are located in ONL of retina, therefore, measuring ONL thickness can indicate enhance cell survival and may represent the protection of the host retina (Fujieda and Sasaki 2008). In this study, we found both rSCs eyes and rSCs + BDNF eyes had thicker ONL layers compared to PBS and BDNF injected eyes ($P<0.01$) at each time point and thus suggesting that the rate of photoreceptor degeneration and cell death is slowed down to some degree. However, ONL thickness in rSCs+BDNF transplanted eyes was not significantly different from rSC transplants alone suggesting no added benefit from BDNF in terms of cell survival. Although several researchers have found that BDNF can maintain the morphology and support the survival of retinal ganglion cells (Weber and Harman 2008) and could protect photoreceptors from the damaging effects of constant light (Gauthier et al. 2005). Recent research has shown that exogenously applied BDNF can activate neuroprotective signaling pathways such as ERK1/2 and Akt and can upregulate endogenous production of BDNF by Müller cells in the mouse retina (Azadi et al. 2007). Others have demonstrated that BDNF and its receptor TrkB play a significant role in the regulation of neuronal growth, survival and synapse formation in the central nervous system and in the retina (Loeliger et al. 2008; Pinnock and Herbert 2008; Vissio et al. 2008; Xuan et al. 2008). Furthermore, BDNF-TrkB signaling regulated the maturational formation of new branches in ON-ganglion cells and controls cell-specific, experience-dependent remodeling of neuronal structures in the visual system (Liu et al. 2007; Grishanin et al. 2008; Marler et al. 2008).

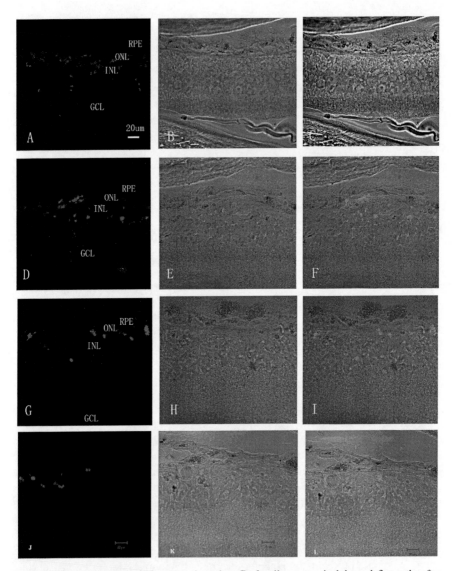

Fig. 43.3 Graft cells survival after transplantation. Graft cells can survival through 3 months after transplantation in both rSCs + BDNF eyes (**a–i**) and rSCs (**j, k, l**) eyes. One month after transplantation, rSCs + BDNF eyes (**a, b, c**) showed more grafts cells survival (139 ± 5 per eye, $n = 3$) than rSCs eyes (**j, k, l**, 101.7 ± 9.9 per eye, $n=3$) ($P<0.05$). In 2 and 3 months after transplantation, there are no more difference between rSCs + BDNF eyes (**d–f** and **g–i**) and rSCs eyes, $P>0.05$. Graft cells labeled with DiI. RPE: retina pigment epithelia; ONL: out nuclear layer; INL: inner nuclear layer; GCL: ganglion cell layer. Scale bar is 20 μm

However, BDNF when injected alone had no appreciable effect when compared to PBS injections, and enhanced the effect of rSCs transplantation. We figure that BDNF combined cell transplantation could get a better vision function restoration at first month after transplantation because of BDNF can help graft cells get a better survival rate. Or may be BDNF related signal pathway participate into synapse formation and host retina circuitry. In future, more work has to be done on this hypothesis.

Although rSCs+BDNF and rSCs transplants show a better maintenance of the ERG and ONL thickness than PBS and BDNF injections over the first two months albeit diminished, the enhancement due to rSCs+BDNF transplants was only apparent in the first month after the operation. We suggest that effects of the BDNF are limited due to diminished concentration of BDNF following transplantation. In the future, we will give the recipients multiple injections of exogenous BDNF to determine if a maintained concentration of BDNF is required to prolong the beneficial effects of rSCs transplantation.

Acknowledgments Supported by National Basic Research Program of China Grants 2007CB512203 and 2005CB724302 and by Nature Science Foundation of China Grant 30772371. The authors thank Dr. T. FitzGibbon for comments on earlier drafts of the manuscript and Ms. Yu Xiao Zeng for excellent technical support.

References

Azadi S, Johnson LE et al (2007) CNTF+BDNF treatment and neuroprotective pathways in the rd1 mouse retina. Brain Res 1129(1):116–129

Bartsch U, Oriyakhel W et al (2008) Retinal cells integrate into the outer nuclear layer and differentiate into mature photoreceptors after subretinal transplantation into adult mice. Exp Eye Res 86(4):691–700

Chen LF, Yin ZQ et al (2008) Differentiation and production of action potentials by embryonic rat retina stem cells in vitro. Invest Ophthalmol Vis Sci 49(11):5144–5150

Djojosubroto MW, Arsenijevic Y (2008) Retinal stem cells: promising candidates for retina transplantation. Cell Tissue Res 331(1):347–357

Fujieda H, Sasaki H (2008) Expression of brain-derived neurotrophic factor in cholinergic and dopaminergic amacrine cells in the rat retina and the effects of constant light rearing. Exp Eye Res 86(2):335–343

Gauthier R, Joly S et al (2005) Brain-derived neurotrophic factor gene delivery to muller glia preserves structure and function of light-damaged photoreceptors. Invest Ophthalmol Vis Sci 46(9):3383–3392

Grishanin RN, Yang H et al (2008) Retinal TrkB receptors regulate neural development in the inner, but not outer, retina. Mol Cell Neurosci 38(3):431–443

Ikeda K, Tanihara H et al (2003) Brain-dervied neurotrophic factor shows a protective effect and improves recovery of the ERG b-wave response in light-damage. J Neurochem 87(2):290–296

Landi S, Cenni MC et al (2007a) Environmental enrichment effects on development of retinal ganglion cell dendritic stratification require retinal BDNF. PLoS ONE 2(4):e346

Landi S, Sale A et al (2007b) Retinal functional development is sensitive to environmental enrichment: a role for BDNF. FASEB J 21(1):130–139

Liu X, Grishanin RN et al (2007) Brain-derived neurotrophic factor and TrkB modulate visual experience-dependent refinement of neuronal pathways in retina. J Neurosci 27(27):7256–7267

Loeliger MM, Briscoe T et al (2008) BDNF increases survival of retinal dopaminergic neurons after prenatal compromise. Invest Ophthalmol Vis Sci 49(3):1282–1289

MacLaren RE, Pearson RA et al (2006) Retinal repair by transplantation of photoreceptor precursors. Nature 444(7116):203–207

Marler KJ, Becker-Barroso E et al (2008) A TrkB/EphrinA interaction controls retinal axon branching and synaptogenesis. J Neurosci 28(48):12700–12712

Paskowitz DM, Donohue-Rolfe KM et al (2007) Neurotrophic factors minimize the retinal toxicity of verteporfin photodynamic therapy. Invest Ophthalmol Vis Sci 48(1):430–437

Pinnock SB, Herbert J (2008) Brain-derived neurotropic factor and neurogenesis in the adult rat dentate gyrus: interactions with corticosterone. Eur J Neurosci 27(10):2493–2500

Seiler MJ, Thomas BB et al (2008) BDNF-treated retinal progenitor sheets transplanted to degenerate rats: improved restoration of visual function. Exp Eye Res 86(1):92–104

Vissio PG, Canepa MM et al (2008) Brain-derived neurotrophic factor (BDNF)-like immunoreactivity localization in the retina and brain of Cichlasoma dimerus (Teleostei, Perciformes). Tissue Cell 40(4):261–270

Wang S, Girman S et al (2008) Long-term vision rescue by human neural progenitors in a rat model of photoreceptor degeneration. Invest Ophthalmol Vis Sci 49(7):3201–3206

Weber AJ, Harman CD (2008) BDNF preserves the dendritic morphology of alpha and beta ganglion cells in the cat retina after optic nerve injury. Invest Ophthalmol Vis Sci 49(6):2456–2463

West EL, Pearson RA et al (2008) Pharmacological disruption of the outer limiting membrane leads to increased retinal integration of transplanted photoreceptor precursors. Exp Eye Res 86(4):601–611

Xuan AG, Long DH et al (2008) BDNF improves the effects of neural stem cells on the rat model of Alzheimer's disease with unilateral lesion of fimbria-fornix. Neurosci Lett 440(3):331–335

Zhang Y, Arner K et al (2003) Limitation of anatomical integration between subretinal transplants and the host retina. Invest Ophthalmol Vis Sci 44(1):324–331

Chapter 44
The Role of Purinergic Receptors in Retinal Function and Disease

Michelle M. Ward, Theresa Puthussery, Kirstan A. Vessey, and Erica L. Fletcher

Abstract Extracellular ATP acts as a neurotransmitter in the central and peripheral nervous systems. In this review, the role of purinergic receptors in neuronal signaling and bi-directional glial-neuronal communication in the retina will be considered. There is growing evidence that a range of P2X and P2Y receptors are expressed on most classes of retinal neurons and that activation of P2 receptors modulates retinal function. Furthermore, neuronal control of glial function is achieved through neuronal release of ATP and activation of P2Y receptors expressed by Müller cells. Altered purinergic signaling in Müller cells has been implicated in gliotic changes in the diseased retina and furthermore, elevations in extracellular ATP may lead to apoptosis of retinal neurons.

44.1 Introduction

Extracellular ATP and other nucleotides are now recognized neurotransmitters that act in the peripheral and central nervous systems to facilitate neurotransmission and neuromodulation, and are also involved in developmental and disease processes (Abbracchio et al. 2008). In the following review, the role of purinergic receptors in retinal function and disease will be explored.

Two families of receptors respond to ATP and its degradation products; P1 receptors are solely activated by adenosine and P2 receptors (P2R) respond to extracellular nucleotides including ATP. The P2 receptor family can be further subdivided by the intracellular signaling pathway of the receptor. P2X receptors belong to the ionotropic class of receptors whilst P2Y receptors are members of the metabotropic receptor family. There are currently seven known subtypes of P2X receptor ($P2X_{1-7}$) and eight subtypes of P2Y receptors ($P2Y_{1, 2, 4, 6, 11, 12, 13, and 14}$;

M.M. Ward (✉)
Department of Anatomy and Cell Biology, The University of Melbourne, Grattan St, Parkville 3010, Victoria, Australia
e-mail: m.ward@unimelb.edu.au

R.E. Anderson et al. (eds.), *Retinal Degenerative Diseases*, Advances in Experimental Medicine and Biology 664, DOI 10.1007/978-1-4419-1399-9_44,
© Springer Science+Business Media, LLC 2010

Abbracchio et al. 2009). Both P2X and P2Y receptors are believed to play a role in neuronal and glial cell transmission and neurodegenerative diseases.

44.2 Mechanisms of ATP Release and Degradation

44.2.1 ATP Release

Under physiological conditions, ATP is released through a variety of mechanisms where it acts as a glio- and neurotransmitter. Like other conventional neurotransmitters, ATP is stored and released from secretory vesicles in the presynaptic terminal of neurons. It is thought to act as a co-transmitter in many cells, where it is released with both inhibitory (GABA) and excitatory (glutamate) neurotransmitters and neuropeptides (Sperlágh et al. 1998; Jo and Schlichter 1999; Jo and Role 2002). Until recently, the mechanism of ATP transport into secretory vesicles was unknown. However, a newly identified vesicular transporter, from the same family as the vesicular glutamate transporters (VGluTs), was shown to accumulate ATP, ADP and GTP (Sawada et al. 2008). Immunohistochemical analysis showed that the vesicular nucleotide transporter (VNUT) was expressed in a population of astrocytes however the localization of VNUT in other systems is yet to be thoroughly explored. In addition to exocytosis, ATP may also be released by ATP-binding cassette transporters, gap junction hemichannels and through P2X$_7$Rs (Fields and Burnstock 2006; Suadicani et al. 2006).

There is evidence for the storage and release of nucleotides from retinal cells. Cholinergic amacrine cells from the rabbit retina release ATP in conjunction with acetylcholine in response to light (Neal and Cunningham 1994) and cultured cholinergic-like amacrine cells from chick retina release ATP, likely via an exocytotic mechanism (Santos et al. 1999). In an eye-cup preparation of rat retina, light stimulation lead to an increase in extracellular ATP levels, purported to be released from amacrine and/or ganglion cells (Newman 2005). Non-neuronal cells are also a source of ATP in the retina. Extracellular ATP-mediated calcium waves are a feature of retinal astrocytes and Müller cells (Newman and Zahs 1997; Newman 2001) and ATP is also released from the retinal pigment epithelium (Mitchell 2001).

44.2.2 Degradation of ATP

Common to all neurotransmitters is the requirement for a mechanism for cessation of neurotransmission. In the following section we will discuss the methods of extracellular ATP degradation.

In the retina, deactivation of neurotransmission typically occurs through the re-uptake and recycling of neurotransmitter. Other mechanisms to terminate neurotransmission include receptor desensitization or enzymatic degradation of the signaling molecule in the extracellular space. In the case of extracellular nucleotide signaling, a family of surface bound ecto-enzymes, known as ectonucleotidases, hydrolyse and thereby inactivate, synaptically released ATP (Zimmermann 1996,

2000). Conversion of ATP to nucleotide diphosphates, and ultimately adenosine occurs in a step-wise manner involving a number of ecto-enzymes (ATP → ADP → AMP → adenosine).

Using an enzyme histochemical method, Puthussery et al. (2006) and Puthussery and Fletcher (2007) demonstrated ecto-ATPase activity (required for the first step of hydrolysis of ATP-ADP) was present in synaptic layers in the retina, providing a mechanism for the degradation of extracellular ATP. The presence of ecto-enzymes in the retina is further supported by functional studies that have shown endogenous production of adenosine following ATP release from glial cells, which can be prevented with the application of an ecto-enzyme inhibitor (Newman, 2003).

44.3 Purinergic Signaling in the Retina

44.3.1 Purinergic Modulation of Neuronal Signaling

There is an increasing body of work studying purinergic receptor expression in the retina. Many P2X and P2Y receptor subtypes have been localized to a diverse number of retinal cell classes including neurons and glia (Table 44.1), supporting a role for purinergic modulation of visual processing. Activation of $P2X_7Rs$ in the outer retina increases the photoreceptorally derived a-wave of the electroretinogram (Puthussery et al. 2006), whilst application of UTP, a P2YR agonist decreases the post-receptoral rod and cone b-waves of the electroretinogram (Ward et al. 2008); suggesting that purines modulate 'through' pathway transmission in the retina. OFF-cholinergic cells are also responsive to ATP through activation of $P2X_2Rs$, whilst blockade of P2 receptors with the antagonist PPADS altered firing rates of ON and OFF ganglion cells (Kaneda et al. 2008). Taken together, this data supports a role for ATP in neural modulation in ON and OFF pathways in the retina.

Table 44.1 Localization of purinergic receptors in the retina

P2 receptor	Cellular localization	References
$P2Y_1$	AC, GC, MC (rat, human, porcine), RPE	Fries et al. (2004, 2005)
$P2Y_2$	RPE, MC	Fries et al. (2004, 2005)
$P2Y_4$	RBC, MC, AC	Fries et al. (2004, 2005) and Ward et al. (2008)
$P2Y_6$	MC, RPE	Fries et al. (2004, 2005)
$P2X_2$	AC, GC	Taschenberger et al. (1999), Kaneda et al. (2004), Puthussery and Fletcher (2006) and Kaneda et al. (2008)
$P2X_3$	AC, GC	Wheeler-Schilling et al. (2001) and Puthussery and Fletcher (2007)
$P2X_7$	PR, HC, AC, GC, MC (human), MG	Pannicke et al. (2000), Innocenti et al. (2004), Puthussery and Fletcher (2004) and Puthussery et al. (2006)

44.3.2 ATP and Glial Transmission

The long held belief that glial cells in the central nervous system were solely responsible for neuronal support has recently changed. It is now thought that these cells may also play a role in the regulation of neuronal transmission (Fields and Stevens 2000). In the retina, there is evidence that the bi-directional communication between neurons and glial cells is in part controlled by purinergic transmission (Newman and Zahs 1998; Newman 2003, 2004, 2005).

Intercellular calcium waves have been observed to propagate between astrocytes in culture and in intact retinal tissue and are therefore thought to be involved in glial cell communication. Although originally believed to be mediated by gap junctional coupling between cells, physically isolated astrocytes in culture also display Ca^{2+} waves (Hassinger et al. 1996), suggesting that signal propagation relies on the release of an extracellular signaling molecule. In the retina, studies by Newman and Zahs (1997) and Newman (2001) have suggested that ATP acting as an extracellular messenger facilitates communication between retinal astrocytes and Müller cells. More recently, this work has extended to suggest that glial cells may also modulate neuronal transmission in the inner retina, however this is likely to be due to the action of adenosine on P1 receptors following ATP release from Müller cells and its subsequent hydrolysis in the extracellular milieu (Newman and Zahs 1998; Newman 2003, 2004; Newman and Volterra 2004).

Propagation of calcium waves by ATP is supported by anatomical evidence for purinergic receptors on Müller cells, although this remains contentious. Early studies suggested that P2XRs were present on Müller cells in human (Pannicke et al. 2000) and rat retina (Neal et al. 1998; Jabs et al. 2000), however, it is now apparent that P2YRs mediate Müller cell responses to ATP (Li et al. 2001). Li et al. (2001) suggested that intercellular calcium signalling in Müller cells was likely to arise via $P2Y_1R$ stimulation based on purinergic agonist sensitivity profiles of isolated cells. In agreement with the functional profiling, immunocytochemical studies from our laboratory found that $P2Y_1$ receptors are strongly expressed on Müller cell processes in the inner retina (Ward and Fletcher 2009).

44.4 The Role of Purinergic Receptors in Retinal Disease

The ubiquitous presence of ATP in all cells means that under pathological conditions such as ischemia, large amounts of ATP can be liberated from dead or dying cells (Franke et al. 2006). There is a growing body of evidence which suggests that extracellular ATP may be an important factor in retinal pathologies (Franke and Illes 2006). Whilst the excitotoxic properties of $P2X_7Rs$ have been considered in the retina (Innocenti et al. 2004; Zhang et al. 2005; Puthussery and Fletcher 2009), P2Y receptors appear more likely to be involved in gliotic events during disease (Uckermann et al. 2003; Iandiev et al. 2006).

The high permeability of $P2X_7Rs$ to Ca^{2+} ions and the potential for pore formation make them a potential contributor to neurodegenerative processes. Intravitreal injection of ATP into adult rat eyes leads to selective apoptosis of photoreceptors (Puthussery and Fletcher 2009), and there is an increase in P2X$_7$R mRNA in the retina of the BALBC*rds* mouse during the peak period of photoreceptor degeneration (Franke et al. 2005). Stimulation of P2X$_7$Rs on neonatal ganglion cells in culture causes an influx of extracellular calcium leading to cell death (Zhang et al. 2005) and increases in ocular pressure also lead to ganglion cell damage, likely to be mediated by P2X$_7$R activation (Resta et al. 2007; Reigada et al. 2008). Therefore, altered extracellular ATP signalling may be involved in ganglion cell death during glaucoma.

Reactive gliosis is a common feature of many retinal diseases including diabetic retinopathy (Mizutani et al. 1998), retinal detachment (Francke et al. 2005) and retinal degeneration (Eisenfeld et al. 1984). However, the underlying cause of glial cell change during disease is not well understood. Some recent studies have suggested that activation of P2Y receptors on Müller cells may regulate some of these changes. Following induced retinal detachment in rabbit retinae, it was shown that Müller cells in vivo were more responsive to ATP (Uckermann et al. 2003). Similarly, in a porcine model of retinal detachment, increases in Müller cell Ca^{2+} responses following application of ATP was found, as was a concomitant increase in the expression of P2Y$_{1 \, and \, 2}$ receptors in Müller cells (Iandiev et al. 2006). This is supported by studies on cultured guinea pig Müller cells, which were shown to respond to application of ATP with an increase in DNA synthesis, which suggests cellular proliferation (Moll et al. 2002; Milenkovic et al. 2003). In light of the important role of that purinergic receptors play in glial-glial and glial-neuronal signalling in the retina, it is possible that altered purinergic transmission contributes to glial cell dysfunction during disease.

44.5 Concluding Remarks

Our understanding of the role of extracellular ATP in modulation of retinal signalling is rapidly expanding. Furthermore, exciting findings suggest that changes in purinergic signalling may contribute to retinal pathologies, in particular glial cell function and photoreceptor death, and therefore may provide novel therapeutic interventions in the future.

References

Abbracchio MP, Burnstock G, Verkhratsky A et al (2009) Purinergic signalling in the nervous system: an overview. Trends Neurosci 32:19–29

Eisenfeld AJ, Bunt-Milam AH, Sarthy PV (1984) Müller cell expression of glial fibrillary acidic protein after genetic and experimental photoreceptor degeneration in the rat retina. Invest Ophthalmol Vis Sci 25:1321–1328

Fields RD, Burnstock G (2006) Purinergic signalling in neuron-glia interactions. Nat Rev Neurosci 7:423–436

Fields RD, Stevens B (2000) ATP: an extracellular signaling molecule between neurons and glia. Trends Neurosci 23:625–633

Francke M, Faude F, Pannicke T et al (2005) Glial cell-mediated spread of retinal degeneration during detachment: a hypothesis based upon studies in rabbits. Vision Res 45:2256–2267

Franke H, Illes P (2006) Involvement of P2 receptors in the growth and survival of neurons in the CNS. Pharmacol Ther 109:297–324

Franke H, Klimke K, Brinckmann U et al (2005) P2X(7) receptor-mRNA and -protein in the mouse retina; changes during retinal degeneration in BALBCrds mice. Neurochem Int 47: 235–242

Franke H, Krugel U, Illes P (2006) P2 receptors and neuronal injury. Pflugers Arch 452:622–644

Fries JE, Goczalik IM, Wheeler-Schilling TH et al (2005) Identification of P2Y receptor subtypes in human müller glial cells by physiology, single cell RT-PCR, and immunohistochemistry. Invest Ophthalmol Vis Sci 46:3000–3007

Fries JE, Wheeler-Schilling TH, Guenther E et al (2004) Expression of P2Y1, P2Y2, P2Y4, and P2Y6 receptor subtypes in the rat retina. Invest Ophthalmol Vis Sci 45:3410–3417

Hassinger TD, Guthrie PB, Atkinson PB et al (1996) An extracellular signaling component in propagation of astrocytic calcium waves. Proc Natl Acad Sci U S A 93:13268–13273

Iandiev I, Uckermann O, Pannicke T et al (2006) Glial cell reactivity in a porcine model of retinal detachment. Invest Ophthalmol Vis Sci 47:2161–2171

Innocenti B, Pfeiffer S, Zrenner E et al (2004) ATP-induced non-neuronal cell permeabilization in the rat inner retina. J Neurosci 24:8577–8583

Jabs R, Guenther E, Marquordt K et al (2000) Evidence for P2X(3), P2X(4), P2X(5) but not for P2X(7) containing purinergic receptors in Müller cells of the rat retina. Brain Res Mol Brain Res 76:205–210

Jo YH, Role LW (2002) Coordinate release of ATP and GABA at in vitro synapses of lateral hypothalamic neurons. J Neurosci 22:4794–4804

Jo YH, Schlichter R (1999) Synaptic corelease of ATP and GABA in cultured spinal neurons. Nat Neurosci 2:241–245

Kaneda M, Ishii T, Hosoya T (2008) Pathway-dependent modulation by P2-purinoceptors in the mouse retina. Eur J Neurosci 28:128–136

Kaneda M, Ishii K, Morishima Y et al (2004) OFF-cholinergic-pathway-selective localization of P2X2 purinoceptors in the mouse retina. J Comp Neurol 476:103–111

Li Y, Holtzclaw LA, Russell JT (2001) Müller cell Ca^{2+} waves evoked by purinergic receptor agonists in slices of rat retina. J Neurophysiol 85:986–994

Milenkovic I, Weick M, Wiedemann P et al (2003) P2Y receptor-mediated stimulation of Müller glial cell DNA synthesis: dependence on EGF and PDGF receptor transactivation. Invest Ophthalmol Vis Sci 44:1211–1220

Mitchell CH (2001) Release of ATP by a human retinal pigment epithelial cell line: potential for autocrine stimulation through subretinal space. J Physiol 534:193–202

Mizutani M, Gerhardinger C, Lorenzi M (1998) Muller cell changes in human diabetic retinopathy. Diabetes 47:445–449

Moll V, Weick M, Milenkovic I et al (2002) P2Y receptor-mediated stimulation of Müller glial DNA synthesis. Invest Ophthalmol Vis Sci 43:766–773

Neal M, Cunningham J (1994) Modulation by endogenous ATP of the light-evoked release of ACh from retinal cholinergic neurones. Br J Pharmacol 113:1085–1087

Neal MJ, Cunningham JR, Dent Z (1998) Modulation of extracellular GABA levels in the retina by activation of glial P2X-purinoceptors. Br J Pharmacol 124:317–322

Newman EA (2001) Propagation of intercellular calcium waves in retinal astrocytes and Müller cells. J Neurosci 21:2215–2223

Newman EA (2003) Glial cell inhibition of neurons by release of ATP. J Neurosci 23:1659–1666

Newman EA (2004) Glial modulation of synaptic transmission in the retina. Glia 47:268–274

Newman EA (2005) Calcium increases in retinal glial cells evoked by light-induced neuronal activity. J Neurosci 25:5502–5510

Newman EA, Volterra A (2004) Glial control of synaptic function. Glia 47:207–208

Newman EA, Zahs KR (1997) Calcium waves in retinal glial cells. Science 275:844–847

Newman EA, Zahs KR (1998) Modulation of neuronal activity by glial cells in the retina. J Neurosci 18:4022–4028

Pannicke T, Fischer W, Biedermann B et al (2000) P2X7 receptors in Müller glial cells from the human retina. J Neurosci 20:5965–5972

Puthussery T, Fletcher EL (2004) Synaptic localization of P2X7 receptors in the rat retina. J Comp Neurol 472:13–23

Puthussery T, Fletcher EL (2006) P2X2 receptors on ganglion and amacrine cells in cone pathways of the rat retina. J Comp Neurol 496:595–609

Puthussery T, Fletcher EL (2007) Neuronal expression of P2X3 purinoceptors in the rat retina. Neuroscience 146:403–414

Puthussery T, Fletcher EL (2009) Extracellular ATP induces retinal photoreceptor apoptosis through activation of purinoceptors in rodents. J Comp Neurol 513:430–440

Puthussery T, Yee P, Vingrys AJ et al (2006) Evidence for the involvement of purinergic P2X receptors in outer retinal processing. Eur J Neurosci 24:7–19

Reigada D, Lu W, Zhang M et al (2008) Elevated pressure triggers a physiological release of ATP from the retina: possible role for pannexin hemichannels. Neuroscience 157:396–404

Resta V, Novelli E, Vozzi G et al (2007) Acute retinal ganglion cell injury caused by intraocular pressure spikes is mediated by endogenous extracellular ATP. Eur J Neurosci 25:2741–2754

Santos PF, Caramelo OL, Carvalho AP (1999) Characterization of ATP release from cultures enriched in cholinergic amacrine-like neurons. J Neurobiol 41:340–348

Sawada K, Echigo N, Juge N et al (2008) Identification of a vesicular nucleotide transporter. Proc Natl Acad Sci U S A 105:5683–5686

Sperlágh B, Magloczky Z, Vizi ES et al (1998) The triangular septal nucleus as the major source of ATP release in the rat habenula: a combined neurochemical and morphological study. Neuroscience 86:1195–1207

Suadicani SO, Brosnan CF, Scemes E (2006) P2X7 receptors mediate ATP release and amplification of astrocytic intercellular Ca^{2+} signaling. J Neurosci 26:1378–1385

Taschenberger H, Juttner R, Grantyn R (1999) Ca^{2+}-permeable P2X receptor channels in cultured rat retinal ganglion cells. J Neurosci 19:3353–3366

Uckermann O, Uhlmann S, Weick M et al (2003) Upregulation of purinergic P2Y receptor-mediated calcium responses in glial cells during experimental detachment of the rabbit retina. Neurosci Lett 338:131–134

Ward MM, Fletcher EL (2009) Subsets of retinal neurons and glia express P2Y1 receptors. Neuroscience 160:555–566

Ward MM, Puthussery T, Fletcher EL (2008) Localization and possible function of P2Y(4) receptors in the rodent retina. Neuroscience 155:1262–1274

Wheeler-Schilling TH, Marquordt K, Kohler K et al (2001) Identification of purinergic receptors in retinal ganglion cells. Brain Res Mol Brain Res 92:177–180

Zhang X, Zhang M, Laties AM et al (2005) Stimulation of P2X7 receptors elevates Ca^{2+} and kills retinal ganglion cells. Invest Ophthalmol Vis Sci 46:2183–2191

Zimmermann H (1996) Biochemistry, localization and functional roles of ecto-nucleotidases in the nervous system. Prog Neurobiol 49:589–618

Zimmermann H (2000) Extracellular metabolism of ATP and other nucleotides. Naunyn Schmiedebergs Arch Pharmacol 362:299–309

Part IV
Macular Degeneration

Chapter 45
Fundus Autofluorescence Imaging in Age-Related Macular Degeneration and Geographic Atrophy

Srilaxmi Bearelly and Scott W. Cousins

Abstract The traditional method for documenting and quantifying geographic atrophy (GA) is color photography. This method has been shown to be reproducible in several clinical trials, including the Age-related Eye Disease Study (AREDS) and the natural progression of GA studies by Sunness et al. (AREDS No. 6, Am J Ophthalmol 132(5):668–681, 2001; Sunness et al., Invest Ophthalmol Vis Sci 40(8):1761–1769, 1999). Nevertheless, it can be difficult to distinguish between dead/nonfunctioning retinal pigment epithelium (RPE), living but depigmented RPE (RPE often release melanin granules upon injury), and yellowish coloration caused by large drusen or calcified regressed drusen. Two imaging technologies that seem promising are fundus autofluorescence (FAF) and spectral domain (high resolution) optical coherence tomography (SDOCT). Here we provide an overview of FAF imaging in the setting of age-related macular degeneration (AMD) and GA.

45.1 Background

Approximately 10 million Americans and 60 million individuals worldwide exhibit some form of age-related macular degeneration (AMD). Most affected patients manifest early AMD, characterized by sub retinal pigment epithelium (RPE) deposits called drusen. However, almost 20% of AMD patients progress to one of two late forms of AMD: geographic atrophy (GA) and neovascular AMD, both of which are associated with severe vision loss. The prevalence of GA and neovascular AMD are similar. Approximately 1.2 million individuals manifest neovascular AMD in at least one eye, but approximately 973,000 individuals exhibit geographic atrophy in at least one eye (Friedman et al. 2004). These prevalence rates are likely to double

S. Bearelly (✉)
The Duke Center for Macular Diseases, Duke Eye Center, Durham, NC, USA
e-mail: beare002@mc.duke.edu

R.E. Anderson et al. (eds.), *Retinal Degenerative Diseases*, Advances in Experimental Medicine and Biology 664, DOI 10.1007/978-1-4419-1399-9_45,
© Springer Science+Business Media, LLC 2010

by the age 2030. Since poor vision may result from either form of late AMD, novel approaches to management and treatment of GA are important.

The traditional method for documenting and quantifying GA is with color fundus photographs (CFP). This method has been shown to be reproducible in several clinical trials, including the Age-related Eye Disease Study (AREDS) and the natural progression of GA studies by Sunness et al. (AREDS No. 6 2001; Sunness et al. 1999). Nevertheless, it can be difficult to distinguish between dead/nonfunctioning RPE, living but depigmented RPE (RPE often release melanin granules upon injury), and yellowish coloration caused by large drusen or calcified regressed drusen. In addition, the predictive sensitivity of color photos is poor, and is capable of identifying only 5–7% of eyes that progress to late stages of AMD in 5 years (Klein et al. 1997). An imaging technology that seems promising in measuring and predicting GA is fundus autofluorescence (FAF) imaging (Fig. 45.1).

If FAF imaging is more reproducible and accurate as compared with the current gold standard, color fundus photos, this could potentially have a major impact on how we measure and follow GA in future prospective trials. Imaging could help stratify slow and fast progressors, and thus enable smaller trials with shorter duration and enhanced power. Without the development of methods for stratification of risk, trials for treatment of early AMD and GA will remain prohibitively large and expensive, making it difficult to test efficacy of novel therapeutic approaches.

45.2 Fundus Autofluorescence Overview

FAF is a photographic technique that measures emitted fluorescent light from the retina after excitation with 488 nm light. Emission is detected above 500 nm with a barrier filter. Although standard fundus cameras equipped with appropriate barrier filters can detect autofluorescence, the Heidelberg Retinal Angiograph, which is a confocal scanning laser ophthalmoscope (cSLO) equipped with excitation 488 nm solid-state laser and Heidelberg image analysis software, can register and average multiple FAF images. Typically from 9 to 15 single images are averaged in order to amplify the FAF signal. The source of FAF is not completely understood. Delori et al. demonstrated with spectrophotometric investigations that lipofuscin granules in the RPE monolayer contain the dominant fluorophores responsible for FAF imaging (Delori et al. 2001, 1995). Other potential fluorescent structures include photoreceptors (rhodopsin), and autofluorescence of vitreous and lens. The confocal nature of the HRA, however, limits the autofluorescence from other planes of the eye, and maximizes the signal from the plane of interest.

Figure 45.1 demonstrates the appearance by FAF and grayscale CFP with (a) normal macula, (b) multiple, large coalesced drusen consistent with AMD, and (c) geographic atrophy. The normal macula has a decrease in the FAF signal concentrically in the macula, which corresponds with the increased lutein and zeaxanthin

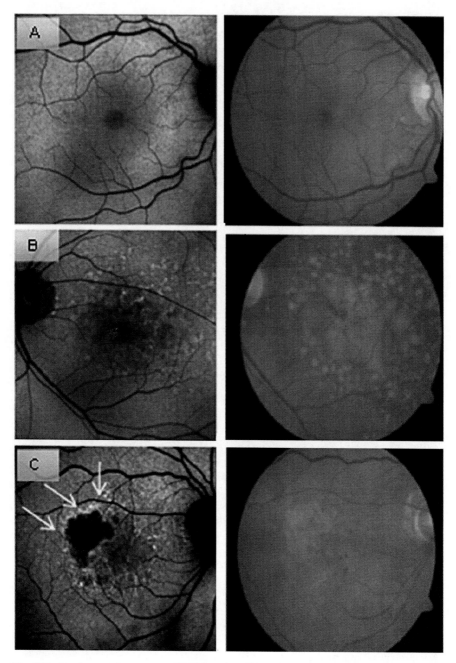

Fig. 45.1 Fundus autofluorescence (FAF) imaging (*first column*) and grayscale of color fundus photos (CFP) in patients with (**a**) normal, (**b**) multiple large coalesced drusen, and (**c**) late non-neovascular age-related macular degeneration (NNVAMD) with geographic atrophy (GA)

concentration. Drusen themselves do not typically correspond exactly to the autofluorescence in AMD. Different patterns of FAF have been described in early dry AMD, as described below.

A discrete area of GA is noted superotemporal to the fovea in image C of Fig. 45.1. This area of RPE death is easily demarcated on FAF as black (or absent autofluorescence). While CFP does show the demarcated area of GA with visibility of the underlying choroidal structures, the extent of GA especially inferiorly becomes obscured by depigmentation. This depigmentation of the RPE inferior to the fovea could be mistaken for dead RPE, and an overestimation of GA is possible. Such a patient may show no difference in progression by CFP, when in fact there is (ß error). The FAF image also shows an area of focal increase in autofluorescence around part of the perimeter of GA (arrows) or 'rim area focal hyperautofluorescence (RAFH)' indicative of increased lipfuscin load in these RPE cells.

45.3 FAF Findings in Early AMD with Drusen Only

Analysis of FAF patterns in the setting of non-neovascular AMD (NNVAMD) performed by Einbock et al. suggests that risk of progression may be stratified by pattern type. The International Fundus Autofluorescence Group has identified eight patterns: minimal change, focal increase, lace-like, reticular, speckled, patchy, linear and plaque-like patterns. While this is a qualitative approach to interpretation, patchy FAF may predict a higher risk of progression to neovascular changes, focal or plaque-like FAF in the macula may result in progression to geographic atrophy (Einbock et al. 2005). This heterogeneity of patterns may reflect underlying differences in cell kinetics and metabolism. Hyperpigmentation, seen clinically as clumping of pigment in the posterior pole, typically exhibits a higher level of FAF which is thought to be secondary to a higher level of RPE lipofuscin (Lois et al. 2002). The lack of correspondence between distribution of drusen and FAF supports the conclusion that drusen and autofluorescence represent independent measures of aging in the posterior pole. These FAF findings may exceed funduscopically visible alterations, suggesting that changes at the level of the RPE precede the occurrence of any visible lesions.

45.4 FAF Findings in Late AMD with Geographic Atrophy

It has been theorized that increased FAF may precede the enlargement of preexisting atrophy and the development of new atrophy over time (Holz et al. 2001). This supports the observation that excess lipofuscin in the RPE may be key in the progression of GA. In addition, the areas of increased FAF outside of GA may be associated with variable loss of retinal sensitivity as measured by fundus perimetry, thereby suggesting a functional correlate of excessive lipofuscin accumulation

(Schmitz-Valckenberg et al. 2004). Similar to identifiable patterns in early AMD, different patterns of FAF have been identified in the junctional zone outside GA separating atrophic and normal retina. These patterns are present with a high degree of symmetry in patients with bilateral geographic atrophy, pointing towards specific genetic contributions rather than non-specific aging processes. Different patterns may predict different rates of spread of pre-existing atrophy (Bindewald et al. 2005; Holz et al. 2007). Holz and colleagues recently stratified progression rates of GA according to FAF pattern type, and demonstrated in a subset analysis that there was significant difference between none/focally increased FAF and diffusely increased FAF (Holz et al. 2007). About 195 eyes from 129 patients were followed with repeated FAF imaging over a median follow-up of 1.8 years, and progression rates in eyes with the banded (1.81 mm^2/year) and diffusely increased (1.77 mm^2/year) pattern types demonstrated significantly faster rates of progression compared to eyes without FAF abnormalities (0.38 mm^2/year) and focally increased patterns (0.81 mm^2/year, $P < 0.0001$) (Holz et al. 2007). We propose a simpler categorical scheme, as well as a novel parameter called rim area focal hyperautofluorescence, or RAFH (Fig. 45.2).

45.5 Progression of Geographic Atrophy

Past studies of natural history progression of GA using color fundus photos reveals a mean progression rate of 2.6 mm^2/year, and median of 2.1 mm^2/year (Sunness et al. 2007). There is a high concordance rate between enlargement rates in 2 eyes of patients with bilateral GA (correlation coefficient, 0.76), and knowledge of prior rates of enlargement is the most significant factor in predicting subsequent enlargement rates (Sunness et al. 2007). Quantification of enlargement in this study was based on fundus photographs and involved several magnification steps (Sunness et al. 1999). Measurements of GA progression with FAF images reveals a mean progression of 1.74 mm^2/year (median, 1.52 mm^2/year) (Holz et al. 2007).

45.6 Mechanisms of Progression

Progression is best studied in the junctional zone at the margin of intact and dead RPE, where increased FAF may be noted in varying levels. Higher lipofuscin content as evidenced by increased FAF has demonstrated faster progression of RPE death (Holz et al. 2007). This increase in FAF is attributable to autophagy, phagocytosis of discarded photoreceptor cells and byproducts, and phagocytosis of dead RPE. In the area overlying increased FAF, there appears to be impaired photoreceptor function (Schmitz-Valckenberg et al. 2004; Scholl et al. 2004). A2E is the major fluorophore that has been identified as toxic by its detergent and phototoxic effects (Sparrow et al. 2003).

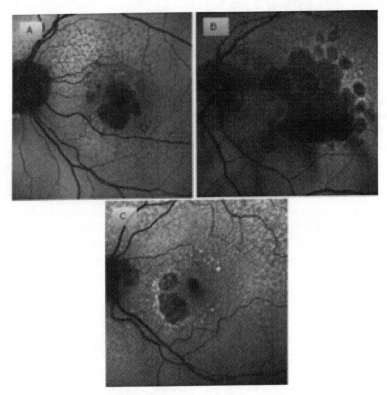

Fig. 45.2 Example of categorical scheme used to quantitate rim area focal hyperautofluorescence (RAFH). In category 1 (**a**), ≤ 1/3 of the 500 μm zone bordering the geographic atrophy (GA) had increased autofluorescence. For category 2 eyes (**b**), between 1/3 and 2/3, and in category 3 (**c**), ≥ 2/3 of this area had increased autofluorescence

45.7 Research to Prevent Progression

Several trials of new pharmacologic agents to slow progression of established GA have been proposed or initiated. One study investigates OT-551 (Othera Pharmaceuticals, Inc), a topical antioxidant eye drop which is now in phase II of clinical study. This agent, when metabolized to Tempol-H by corneal esterases, acts as a free-radical scavenger. In animal models of AMD, topical administration has demonstrated anti-inflammatory and anti-angiogenic effects (Wang et al. 1995). Ciliary neurotrophic factor (CNTF) is another agent in phase II of clinical study for atrophic AMD as well as advanced retinitis pigmentosa. In an animal model, CNTF slows the progression of photoreceptor degeneration (Sieving et al. 2006). Major advances in genetic knowledge implicate alterations in the inflammatory pathways in both wet and dry AMD, however this is not yet directly modifiable (Shaumberg et al. 2007).

Another new area of research to slow GA involves the reduction of serum retinol. Sirion Pharmaceuticals has initiated a randomized, double-masked and placebo controlled study of the safety and efficacy of 100 and 300 mg of fenretinide in the treatment of geographic atrophy. The active ingredient in fenretinide, N-(4-hydroxyphenyl) retinamide, promotes clearance of retinol and reduces the total retinol available for visual processing. This compound competes for binding sites on retinol binding protein (RBP), and may prevent binding of transthyretin. The altered moiety is then cleared through the urine by glomerular filtration. By reducing lipofuscin and A2E accumulation, this agent is theorized to reduce fundus autofluorescence and slow the progression of geographic atrophy (Radu et al. 2005). This 2 year trial has a targeted enrollment of 225 patients with three to five disc areas of geographic atrophy in at least one eye. The primary endpoint will be the deterioration of scotoma size or depth, defined as at least 5 points/loci losing light sensitivity from baseline by a clinically significant amount as measured by microperimetry. A secondary outcome is change from baseline in the area and intensity of fundus autofluorescence.

45.8 Discussion

Several ongoing clinical trials of GA are using FAF imaging as a clinical endpoint. Based on our studies, FAF imaging is likely to have a major impact in how we follow and predict geographic atrophy progression (studies submitted for publication). By potentially stratifying risk and enrolling patients at high risk of progression, the use of FAF imaging could further optimize clinical trial design for GA.

References

Age-Related Eye Disease Study (AREDS) Research Group (2001) The age-related eye disease study system for classifying age-related macular degeneration from stereoscopic color fundus photographs: AREDS report No. 6. Am J Ophthalmol 132(5):668–681

Bindewald A, Schmitz-Valkenberg S, Jorzik JJ et al (2005) Classification of abnormal fundus autofluorescence patterns in the junctional zone of geographic atrophy in patients with age related macular degeneration. Br J Ophthalmol 89(7):874–878

Delori FC, Dorey CK, Staurenghi G et al (1995) In vivo fluorescence of the ocular fundus exhibits retinal pigment epithelium lipofuscin characteristics. Invest Ophthalmol Vis Sci 36(3): 718–729

Delori FC, Goger DG, Dorey CK (2001) Age-related accumulation and spatial distribution of lipofuscin in the RPE of normal subjects. Invest Ophthalmol Vis Sci 42(8):1855–1866

Einbock W, Moessner A, Schnurrbusch UE et al (2005) Changes in fundus autofluorescence in patients with age-related maculopathy. Correlation to visual function: a prospective study. Graefes Arch Clin Exp Ophthalmol 243(4):300–305

Friedman DS, O'Colmain BJ, Munoz B et al (2004) Prevalence of age-related macular degeneration in the United States. Arch Ophthalmol 122(4):564–572

Holz FG, Bellman C, Staudt S et al (2001) Fundus autofluorescence and development of geographic atrophy in age-related macular degeneration. Invest Ophthalmol Vis Sci 42(5): 1051–1056

Holz FG, Bindewald-Wittich A, Fleckenstein M et al (2007) Progression of geographic atrophy and impact of fundus autofluorescence patterns in age-related macular degeneration. Am J Ophthalmol 143(3):463–472

Klein R, Klein BE, Jensen SC et al (1997) The five-year incidence and progression of age-related maculopathy: the Beaver Dam Eye Study. Ophthalmology 104(1):7–21

Lois N, Owens SL, Coco R et al (2002) Fundus autofluorescence in patients with age-related macular degeneration and high risk of visual loss. Am J Ophthalmol 133(3):341–349

Radu RA, Han Y, Bui TV et al (2005) Reductions in serum vitamin A arrest accumulation of toxic retinal fluorophores: a potential therapy for treatment of lipofuscin-based retinal diseases. Invest Ophthalmol Vis Sci 46(12):4393–4401

Schmitz-Valckenberg S, Bultmann S, Dreyhaupt J et al (2004) Fundus autofluorescence and fundus perimetry in the junctional zone of geographic atrophy in patients with age-related macular degeneration. Invest Ophthalmol Vis Sci 45(12):4470–4476

Scholl HP, Bellmann C, Dandekar SS et al (2004) Photopic and scotopic fine matrix mapping of retinal areas of increased fundus autofluorescence in patients with age-related maculopathy. Invest Ophthalmol Vis Sci 45(2):574–583

Shaumberg DA, Hankinson SE, Guo Q et al (2007) A prospective study of 2 major age-related macular degeneration susceptibility alleles and interaction with modifiable risk factors. Arch Ophthalmol 125(1):55–62

Sieving PA, Caruso RC, Tao W et al (2006) Ciliary neurotrophic factor (CNTF) for human retinal degeneration: phase I trial of CNTF delivered by encapsulated cell intraocular implants. Proc Natl Acad Sci USA 103(10):3896–3901

Sparrow JR, Fishkin N, Zhou J et al (2003) A2E, a byproduct of the visual cycle. Vision Res 43(28):2983–2990

Sunness JS, Bressler NM, Tian Y et al (1999) Measuring geographic atrophy in advanced age-related macular degeneration. Invest Ophthalmol Vis Sci 40(8):1761–1769

Sunness JS, Margalit E, Srikumaran D et al (2007) The long-term natural history of geographic atrophy from age-related macular degeneration: enlargement of atrophy and implications for interventional trials. Ophthalmology 114(2):271–277

Wang M, Lam TT, Fu J et al (1995) TEMPOL, a superoxide dismutase mimic, ameliorates light-induced retinal degeneration. Res Commun Mol Pathol Pharmacol 89(3):291–305

Chapter 46
Endoplasmic Reticulum Stress as a Primary Pathogenic Mechanism Leading to Age-Related Macular Degeneration

Richard T. Libby and Douglas B. Gould

Abstract Age-related macular degeneration (AMD) is a multi-factorial disease and a leading cause of blindness. Proteomic and genetic data suggest that activation or de-repression of the alternate complement cascade of innate immunity is involved in end-stage disease. Several lines of evidence suggest that production of reactive oxygen species and chronic oxidative stress lead to protein and lipid modifications that initiate the complement cascade. Understanding the triggers of these pathogenic pathways and the site of the primary insult will be important for development of targeted therapeutics. Endoplasmic reticulum (ER) stress from misfolded mutant proteins and other sources are an important potential tributary mechanism. We propose that misfolded-protein-induced ER stress in the retinal-pigmented epithelium and/or choroid could lead to chronic oxidative stress, complement deregulation and AMD. Small molecules targeted to ER stress and oxidative stress could allow for a shift from disease treatment to disease prevention.

46.1 Age Related Macular Degeneration Is a Leading Cause of Vision Loss

AMD is the leading cause of visual impairment in the elderly (Javitt 2003; Klaver et al. 2001; Klein et al. 1992) affecting an estimated 10 million Americans and 50 million people worldwide. AMD is clinically heterogeneous and is diagnosed irrespective of visual acuity. Late AMD is described as either dry or wet depending on the absence or presence of choroidal neo-vascularization (penetration of the choroidal vasculature into the subretinal space). Most patients have dry AMD where focal degeneration of photoreceptors, RPE and choriocapillaris in the macula (together called geographic atrophy) impairs visual acuity over time. In contrast,

D.B. Gould (✉)
Departments of Ophthalmology and Anatomy and Institute for Human Genetics, University of California at San Francisco, San Francisco, CA 94143, USA
e-mail: gouldd@vision.ucsf.edu

R.E. Anderson et al. (eds.), *Retinal Degenerative Diseases*, Advances in Experimental Medicine and Biology 664, DOI 10.1007/978-1-4419-1399-9_46,
© Springer Science+Business Media, LLC 2010

in wet AMD there is often sudden and acute vision loss because of choroidal neo-vessels. The presence of wet and dry lesions within the same eye, the observations of dry AMD progressing to wet AMD, and the lack of significant differences in the frequency of risk alleles of predisposing genes between the two sub-groups support the notion that common mechanisms underlie all disease classes.

46.2 Oxidative Stress and Complement Activation are Common Pathways in End-Stage Disease

Important studies of human eyes showed components of the alternate complement pathway of innate immunity, and acute phase response proteins of the systemic arm of innate immunity, accumulated at the RPE/Bruch's membrane interface in AMD patients. These observations led to the hypothesis that activation/de-repression of the alternate complement pathway, and a smoldering inflammatory response, might be central to AMD pathogenesis (Crabb et al. 2002; Hageman et al. 2001). Genetic data support this contention, and loci containing genes encoding components of the alternate complement pathway are reproducibly associated with disease risk (Edwards et al. 2005; Hageman et al. 2005; Haines et al. 2005; Klein et al. 2005). Complement activation/de-repression appears to be a common end-stage pathway where other tributary mechanisms have converged. However, the cellular mechanisms preceding complement activation/de-repression are largely unknown. Unfortunately, identifying primary mechanisms for age-related diseases is often confounded by complex genetic interactions (Klaver et al. 1998) and a lifetime of variable exposure to environmental factors. Several factors are implicated in AMD pathogenesis, including high fat diet (Cho et al. 2001; Seddon et al. 2003), pathogen load (Kalayoglu et al. 2005), increased light exposure (Taylor et al. 1990), choroidal hypoperfusion (Friedman et al. 1995), and cigarette smoking (Klein et al. 1993). Importantly, these associations, and several other lines of evidence (Beatty et al. 2000; Decanini et al. 2007; Shen et al. 2007; Suzuki et al. 2007), strongly support a role for oxidative stress as a primary trigger of AMD pathogenesis.

Oxidative stress refers to the cellular or molecular damage caused by reactive oxygen species. In addition to abnormally oxidized proteins, lipids, and nucleic acids localized in drusen, much evidence supports an important role of oxidative stress in AMD pathogenesis. The retina is one of the highest oxygen-consuming tissues in the body, and the RPE is exposed to high levels of oxidative and photo-oxidative damage over a lifetime (Beatty et al. 2000). Increased production of reactive oxygen species is a proposed cellular insult from photo-oxidative damage. Lipofuscin (lipid-containing pigment granules associated with aging) and the lipofuscin retinoid fluorophore A2E (*N*-retinylidene-*N*-retinylethanolamine) are associated with AMD and are proposed to exert their harmful effects via production of reactive oxygen species and oxidative damage (Sparrow et al. 2002; Zhou et al. 2006). Despite the increasing threat of oxidative stress, ability of cells to detoxify reactive oxygen intermediates deteriorates with advancing age. Together, the deteriorating capacity to detoxify reactive oxygen species and the cumulative effects of oxidative stress are proposed to be a local insult contributing to disease (Beatty et al. 2000). This hypothesis is supported by studies suggesting that factors that increase oxidative stress exacerbate disease, while factors that ameliorate oxidative stress slow AMD progression (Bazan 2006; Group 2001; Tan et al. 2007). Finally, there is strong evidence for the importance of oxidative stress in vivo in AMD pathogenesis from several mouse mutant strains (Dong et al. 2009; Hollyfield et al. 2008; Imamura et al. 2006; Wong et al. 2007).

46.3 ER Stress and Oxidative Stress Interact

Protein folding leads to a net loss of reducing equivalents via disulfide bond formation. ER associated degradation (ERAD) is an important consumer of reducing equivalents because a large proportion of proteins (even under physiologic conditions) submit to degradation. Furthermore, protein secretion consumes cellular cysteine and depletes the cell of reducing equivalents. Thus, protein folding and subsequent degradation or secretion entails a net loss of reducing equivalents (Banhegyi et al. 2007). This is exacerbated when genetic mutations affect protein folding. Illegitimate disulfide bond formation, reduction/replacement by isomerization, and eventual ERAD all consume and further deplete cellular reducing equivalents. Oxidative stress in the ER contributes to endogenous peroxide generation in the cytosol and ER isomerases interact with glutathione that retro-translocates to the cytoplasm (Sevier and Kaiser 2008). Therefore, folding and secretion of proteins produces reactive oxygen species and illegitimate disulfide bond formation and subsequent ERAD of misfolded mutant proteins increases oxidative stress within cells (Sitia and Molteni 2004).

In normal protein folding, disulfide bonds are formed and broken as proteins are rearranged. Many chaperones are oxidoreductases with thiol groups that act as molecular switches for redox state and, thus, are sensitive to oxidative stress. In conditions of oxidative stress, the ratio of reduced/oxidized forms of chaperones available for normal protein folding is altered. Under these conditions there is illegitimate disulfide bond formation and stabilization of undesirable, intermediate conformations. Before misfolded proteins can be degraded, disulfide bonds must be reduced, however, excessive oxidation impedes disulfide bond reduction and inhibits ERAD. Thus, oxidative stress can inactivate chaperones, promote aberrant disulfide bond formation, promote stabilization of undesirable intermediates and inhibit degradation of misfolded proteins, which together cause ER stress (Banhegyi et al. 2007; Marciniak and Ron 2006).

46.4 ER and Oxidative Stress as Triggers for Inflammation and Disease

ER stress and oxidative stress lead to production of pro-inflammatory mediators including prostaglandins, leukotrines and tumor necrosis factor alpha (Hu et al.

2006) and de-repression of nuclear factor kappa B (Deng et al. 2004; Jiang et al. 2003). ER stress and oxidative stress can also activate systemic and local cascades directly implicated in AMD pathogenesis. C-reactive protein, and serum amyloid P are components of the systemic arm of the innate immune system, are localized to drusen, and are directly up-regulated by ER stress (Zhang et al. 2006). Moreover, local ER stress can lead to STAT3-dependent up regulation of vascular endothelial growth factor (a key molecular trigger for progression to CNV) (Zhang et al. 2006) and oxidative stress is shown in animal models to contribute to CNV (Dong et al. 2009).

There are relevant and important examples of ER/oxidative stress interacting and contributing to disease. Abnormally oxidized lipids in atherosclerotic plaques activate ER stress in endothelial cells and mediate a chronic inflammatory response. AMD and atherosclerosis are linked in epidemiological studies (Vingerling et al. 1995) and share risk factors including increased age, smoking, high fat diet and pathogen load. Both diseases have local extracellular deposits of abnormally oxidized molecules that precede chronic inflammation and there are striking similarities in the protein, lipid and cellular compositions between atherosclerotic plaques and drusen (de Boer et al. 2000; Hageman et al. 2001; 1999; Mullins et al. 2000; Suzuki et al. 2007). Importantly, mice immunized with an oxidization fragment of docosahexaenoic acid were shown to accumulate activated complement components in the outer retina and develop lesions resembling geographic atrophy (Hollyfield et al. 2008). This discovery and others (Wu et al. 2007) reveal a key link between oxidative damage, complement activation/de-repression, and retinal disease.

46.5 Future Experimental Approaches

Understanding the roles of ER stress and oxidative stress in AMD is important as these cellular processes represent pathways that could be targeted with small molecule therapeutics (Sauer et al. 2008). Studying retinal disease in mouse models with ER stress (via misfolded proteins or by other mechanisms) and in mutant animals that have misfolded proteins in combination with a reduced capacity to decrease oxidative stress ($Sod1^{-/-}$) or an impaired capacity to reduce ER stress (i.e. $Eif2a^{S51A}$) will contribute to testing this hypothesis. Bruch's membrane is an elaborate extracellular matrix. Extracellular matrix molecules are processed in the ER before secretion and represent strong candidate genes for ER stress-induced pathogenesis (Bateman et al. 2009). Conditionally expressed mutant alleles of extracellular matrix molecules can genetically dissect the relative contributions of RPE and choroid in the primary pathogenesis of disease. Understanding the primary location of the insult will determine necessary properties of potential therapeutics targeted at this mechanism (Fig. 46.1).

Fig. 46.1 Evidence supports that oxidative stress and complement activation/de-repression are common end stage pathways in AMD and each pathway is likely to have several genetic and environmental factors influencing it. We propose that ER stress, caused by misfolded proteins or other insults could be a primary tributary mechanism leading to initiation of AMD pathogenesis. Targeting these pathways with therapeutics could be an effective preventative therapy

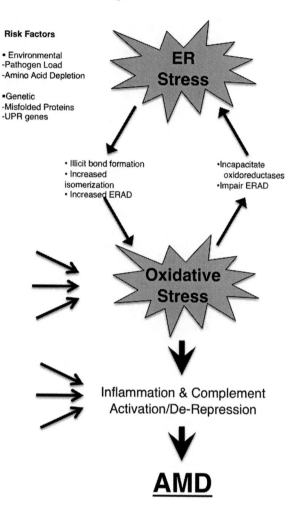

References

Banhegyi G, Benedetti A, Csala M et al (2007) Stress on redox. FEBS Lett 581:3634–3640

Bateman JF, Boot-Handford RP, Lamandé SR (2009) Genetic diseases of connective tissues: cellular and extracellular effects of ECM mutations. Nat Rev Genet 10:173–183

Bazan NG (2006) Survival signaling in retinal pigment epithelial cells in response to oxidative stress: significance in retinal degenerations. Adv Exp Med Biol 572:531–540

Beatty S, Koh H, Phil M et al (2000) The role of oxidative stress in the pathogenesis of age-related macular degeneration. Surv Ophthalmol 45:115–134

Cho E, Hung S, Willett WC et al (2001) Prospective study of dietary fat and the risk of age-related macular degeneration. Am J Clin Nutr 73:209–218

Crabb JW, Miyagi M, Gu X et al (2002) Drusen proteome analysis: an approach to the etiology of age-related macular degeneration. Proc Natl Acad Sci U S A 99:14682–14687

de Boer OJ, van der Wal AC, Becker AE (2000) Atherosclerosis, inflammation, and infection. J Pathol 190:237–243

Decanini A, Nordgaard C, Feng X et al (2007) Changes in select redox proteins of the retinal pigment epithelium in age-related macular degeneration. Am J Ophthalmol 143(4):607–615, e602

Deng J, Lu PD, Zhang Y et al (2004) Translational repression mediates activation of nuclear factor kappa B by phosphorylated translation initiation factor 2. Mol Cell Biol 24:10161–10168

Dong A, Xie B, Shen J et al (2009) Oxidative stress promotes ocular neovascularization. J Cell Physiol 219(3):544–552

Edwards AO, Ritter R, Abel KJ et al (2005) Complement factor H polymorphism and age-related macular degeneration. Science 308:421–424

Friedman E, Krupsky S, Lane A et al (1995) Ocular blood flow velocity in age-related macular degeneration. Ophthalmology 102:640–646

Group A-REDSR (2001) A randomized, placebo-controlled, clinical trial of high-dose supplementation with vitamins C and E, beta carotene, and zinc for age-related macular degeneration and vision loss: AREDS report no. 8. Arch Ophthalmol 119:1417–1436

Hageman GS, Anderson DH, Johnson LV et al (2005) A common haplotype in the complement regulatory gene factor H (HF1/CFH) predisposes individuals to age-related macular degeneration. Proc Natl Acad Sci U S A 102:7227–7232

Hageman GS, Luthert PJ, Victor Chong NH et al (2001) An integrated hypothesis that considers drusen as biomarkers of immune-mediated processes at the RPE-Bruch's membrane interface in aging and age-related macular degeneration. Prog Retin Eye Res 20:705–732

Hageman GS, Mullins RF, Russell SR et al (1999) Vitronectin is a constituent of ocular drusen and the vitronectin gene is expressed in human retinal pigmented epithelial cells. FASEB J 13:477–484

Haines JL, Hauser MA, Schmidt S et al (2005) Complement factor H variant increases the risk of age-related macular degeneration. Science 308:419–421

Hollyfield JG, Bonilha VL, Rayborn ME et al (2008) Oxidative damage-induced inflammation initiates age-related macular degeneration. Nat Med 14:194–198

Hu P, Han Z, Couvillon AD et al (2006) Autocrine tumor necrosis factor alpha links endoplasmic reticulum stress to the membrane death receptor pathway through IRE1alpha-mediated NF-kappaB activation and down-regulation of TRAF2 expression. Mol Cell Biol 26: 3071–3084

Imamura Y, Noda S, Hashizume K et al (2006) Drusen, choroidal neovascularization, and retinal pigment epithelium dysfunction in SOD1-deficient mice: a model of age-related macular degeneration. Proc Natl Acad Sci U S A 103:11282–11287

Javitt J (2003) Incidence of exudative age-related macular degeneration among elderly americans. Ophthalmology 110:1534–1539

Jiang HY, Wek SA, McGrath BC et al (2003) Phosphorylation of the alpha subunit of eukaryotic initiation factor 2 is required for activation of NF-kappaB in response to diverse cellular stresses. Mol Cell Biol 23:5651–5663

Kalayoglu MV, Bula D, Arroyo J et al (2005) Identification of Chlamydia pneumoniae within human choroidal neovascular membranes secondary to age-related macular degeneration. Graefes Arch Clin Exp Ophthalmol 243:1080–1090

Klaver CC, Assink JJ, van Leeuwen R et al (2001) Incidence and progression rates of age-related maculopathy: The Rotterdam Study. Invest Ophthalmol Vis Sci 42:2237–2241

Klaver CC, Wolfs RC, Assink JJ et al (1998) Genetic risk of age-related maculopathy. Population-based familial aggregation study. Arch Ophthalmol 116:1646–1651

Klein R, Klein BE, Linton KL (1992) Prevalence of age-related maculopathy. The Beaver Dam Eye Study. Ophthalmology 99:933–943

Klein R, Klein BE, Linton KL et al (1993) The Beaver Dam Eye Study: the relation of age-related maculopathy to smoking. Am J Epidemiol 137:190–200

Klein RJ, Zeiss C, Chew EY et al (2005) Complement factor H polymorphism in age-related macular degeneration. Science 308:385–389

Marciniak SJ, Ron D (2006) Endoplasmic reticulum stress signaling in disease. Physiol Rev 86:1133–1149

Mullins RF, Russell SR, Anderson DH et al (2000) Drusen associated with aging and age-related macular degeneration contain proteins common to extracellular deposits associated with atherosclerosis, elastosis, amyloidosis, and dense deposit disease. FASEB J 14:835–846

Sauer T, Patel M, Chan CC et al (2008) Unfolding the therapeutic potential of chemical chaperones for age-related macular degeneration. Expert Rev Ophthalmol 3:29–42

Seddon JM, Cote J, Rosner B (2003) Progression of age-related macular degeneration: association with dietary fat, transunsaturated fat, nuts, and fish intake. Arch Ophthalmol 121:1728–1737

Sevier C, Kaiser C (2008) Ero1 and redox homeostasis in the endoplasmic reticulum. Biochim Biophy Acta 1783:549–556

Shen JK, Dong A, Hackett SF et al (2007) Oxidative damage in age-related macular degeneration. Histol Histopathol 22:1301–1308

Sitia R, Molteni SN (2004) Stress, protein (mis)folding, and signaling: the redox connection. Sci STKE 239:e27

Sparrow JR, Zhou J, Ben-Shabat S et al (2002) Involvement of oxidative mechanisms in blue-light-induced damage to A2E-laden RPE. Invest Ophthalmol Vis Sci 43:1222–1227

Suzuki M, Kamei M, Itabe H et al (2007) Oxidized phospholipids in the macula increase with age and in eyes with age-related macular degeneration. Mol Vis 13:772–778

Tan JS, Wang J, Flood V et al (2007) Dietary antioxidants and the long-term incidence of age-related macular degeneration. The Blue Mountains Eye Study. Ophthalmology 115:334–341

Taylor HR, Muñoz B, West S et al (1990) Visible light and risk of age-related macular degeneration. Trans Am Ophthalmol Soc 88:163–173

Vingerling JR, Dielemans I, Bots ML et al (1995) Age-related macular degeneration is associated with atherosclerosis. The Rotterdam Study. Am J Epidemiol 142:404–409

Wong RW, Richa DC, Hahn P et al (2007) Iron toxicity as a potential factor in AMD. Retina 27:997–1003

Wu Z, Lauer T, Sick A et al (2007) Oxidative stress modulates complement factor H expression in retinal pigmented epithelial cells by acetylation of FOXO3. J Biol Chem 282:22414–22425

Zhang K, Shen X, Wu J et al (2006) Endoplasmic reticulum stress activates cleavage of CREBH to induce a systemic inflammatory response. Cell 124:587–599

Zhou J, Jang YP, Kim SR et al (2006) Complement activation by photooxidation products of A2E, a lipofuscin constituent of the retinal pigment epithelium. Proc Natl Acad Sci U S A 103:16182–16187

Chapter 47
Proteomic and Genomic Biomarkers for Age-Related Macular Degeneration

Jiayin Gu, Gayle J.T. Pauer, Xiuzhen Yue, Umadevi Narendra, Gwen M. Sturgill, James Bena, Xiaorong Gu, Neal S. Peachey, Robert G. Salomon, Stephanie A. Hagstrom, John W. Crabb, and The Clinical Genomic, and Proteomic AMD Study Group

Abstract Toward early detection of susceptibility to age-related macular degeneration (AMD), we quantified plasma carboxyethylpyrrole (CEP) oxidative protein modifications and CEP autoantibodies by ELISA in 916 AMD and 488 control donors. Mean CEP adduct and autoantibody levels were elevated in AMD plasma by ~60 and ~30%, respectively, and the odds ratio for both CEP markers elevated was ~3-fold greater in AMD than in control patients. Genotyping was performed for AMD risk polymorphisms associated with age-related maculopathy susceptibility 2 (*ARMS2*), high-temperature requirement factor A1 (*HTRA1*), complement factor H (*CFH*), and complement *C3*. The AMD risk predicted for those exhibiting elevated CEP markers and risk genotypes was 2- to 3-fold greater than the risk based on genotype alone. AMD donors carrying the ARMS2 and HTRA1 risk alleles were the most likely to exhibit elevated CEP markers. Receiver operating characteristic curves suggest that CEP markers alone can discriminate between AMD and control plasma donors with ~76% accuracy and in combination with genomic markers, provide up to ~80% discrimination accuracy. CEP plasma biomarkers, particularly in combination with genomic markers, offer a potential early warning system for predicting susceptibility to this blinding disease.

47.1 Introduction

A direct molecular link between oxidative damage and AMD was established by the finding that carboxyethylpyrrole (CEP), an oxidative protein modification generated from docosahexaenoate (DHA) – containing phospholipids, is elevated in Bruch's membrane and drusen from AMD patients (Crabb et al. 2002). Subsequently, CEP adducts as well as CEP autoantibodies were found to be elevated in plasma from

J.W. Crabb (✉)
Cole Eye Institute, Cleveland, OH, USA
e-mail: crabbj@ccf.org

R.E. Anderson et al. (eds.), *Retinal Degenerative Diseases*, Advances in Experimental Medicine and Biology 664, DOI 10.1007/978-1-4419-1399-9_47, © Springer Science+Business Media, LLC 2010

AMD donors (Gu et al. 2003a) and CEP adducts were found to stimulate neovascularization in vivo, suggesting a role in the induction of CNV (Ebrahem et al. 2006). From such observations, oxidative protein modifications were hypothesized to serve as catalysts of AMD pathology (Crabb et al. 2002; Gu et al. 2003a; Renganathan et al. 2008). Support for this hypothesis was provided by showing that mice immunized with CEP adducted mouse albumin develop a dry AMD-like phenotype (Hollyfield et al. 2008). While identified AMD susceptibility genes account for over half of AMD cases (Fritsche et al. 2008), many individuals carrying AMD risk genotypes may never develop the disease. Likewise, only a fraction of those diagnosed with early AMD progress to advanced stage disease with severe visual loss (AREDs 2001).

Toward the discovery of better methods to predict susceptibility to advanced AMD, we quantified CEP adducts and autoantibodies in over 1,400 plasma donors and also genotyped many of these donors for AMD risk polymorphisms in complement factor H (*CFH*) (Edwards et al. 2005; Hageman et al. 2005; Haines et al. 2005; Klein et al. 2005), complement *C3* (Maller et al. 2007; Yates et al. 2007), age-related maculopathy susceptibility 2 (*ARMS2*, also known as *LOC387715*) (Fritsche et al. 2008; Jakobsdottir et al. 2005; Maller et al. 2006; Rivera et al. 2005) and high-temperature requirement factor A1 (*HTRA1*) (Dewan et al. 2006; Yang et al. 2006). Here we review the results that demonstrate combined CEP proteomic and genomic biomarker measurements are more effective in predicting AMD than either method alone (Gu et al. 2009).

47.2 Methods

Clinically documented AMD and control blood donors were recruited from the Cole Eye Institute, Cleveland Clinic Foundation and the Eye Clinic, Louis Stokes Cleveland VA Medical Center. AMD disease progression was categorized based on fundus examination and patients were included in the study from AREDS AMD categories 2, 3 and 4 (AREDs, 2001). Nonfasting blood specimens were collected and plasma was prepared within 6 h and aliquotted to vials containing butylated hydroxytoluene and a protease inhibitor cocktail (Gu et al. 2003a), flushed with argon, quench-frozen in liquid nitrogen and stored at –80°C. DNA was isolated from blood using standard procedures. CEP adducts and CEP autoantibodies were measured by ELISA (Gu et al. 2003a) and Western blot analysis of plasma proteins from AMD and normal donors was performed as previously described (Crabb et al. 2002). AMD risk polymorphisms were genotyped in *HTRA1* (rs11200638 in the promoter region), *C3* (rs2230199 encoding a R102G interchange), and *CFH* (rs1061170 encoding a Y402H interchange) by restriction analysis. Those in *ARMS2* (*LOC387715* rs10490924 encoding a A69S interchange) were determined by direct DNA sequence analysis. Differences in plasma CEP adduct concentration and CEP autoantibody titer between control and AMD patients were evaluated using two sample t-tests in Minitab Release 15 (Minitab Inc., PA). To evaluate a relationship between CEP adducts and autoantibody titer with AMD susceptibility, a logistic regression model was fit with both variables as predictors of AMD using Proc Logistic in SAS 9.1 (SAS Institute Inc, Cary NC). Odds Ratios, c-statistics and p-values were determined based on log-transformed CEP marker concentrations. Validation of c-statistics was performed using 2000 bootstrap (random) resamplings and by 10-fold cross-validation. Sensitivity and specificity were calculated to maximize the sum of the two values using receiver operating characteristic (ROC) curves constructed with SAS 9.1 from the output of logistic regression analysis fit with either CEP adduct concentrations plus autoantibody titers, or homozygous risk genotype, or the combination of the CEP markers and the risk genotype. C-statistics and p-values comparing ROC curves were determined with SAS 9.1. For association analyses of combined effects of plasma CEP adducts and autoantibody titer with AMD risk genotypes, Odds ratios with 95% CI and Fisher Exact p-values were calculated with SAS 9.1 software.

47.3 Results

47.3.1 CEP Adducts and Autoantibodies Are Elevated in AMD Plasma

Plasma from a total of 488 control subjects and 916 AMD subjects were analyzed by ELISA, including 177 with early-stage dry AMD (category 2), 130 with mid-stage dry AMD (category 3) and 609 with advanced-stage AMD (category 4). Significantly higher mean levels of CEP adducts ($\sim$1.6x) and autoantibody titers ($\sim$1.3x) were found in AMD patients relative to control plasma ($p < 0.0001$). Plasma from all AMD categories exhibited elevated mean levels of CEP adducts and autoantibodies, with no significant difference between categories. Both CEP adduct and autoantibody levels were elevated above median control levels in 56% of AMD patients but in only 29% of control donors.

47.3.2 AMD Risk Based on CEP Biomarkers and Genotype

Genotyping of control ($n = 233$–404) and AMD ($n = 708$–788) patients for AMD risk polymorphisms associated with *ARMS2*, *HTRA1*, *CFH*, and *C3* allowed the risk for AMD to be estimated based on genotype alone and in combination with the CEP biomarker concentrations. Figure 47.1a shows that combining CEP measurements and genotype resulted in $\sim$2 to 3 folder higher odds ratios for AMD than from genotype alone. Sensitivity and specificity measures were determined with ROC curves from all AMD cases and controls for the CEP markers alone, the four genomic markers alone and the combined markers (Table 47.1). Calculated to maximize the sum of the two values, sensitivity ($\sim$73%) was greater for the CEP markers than for any of the genomic markers alone (31–60%) while specificity was greater for the

Table 47.1 Sensitivity and specificity of CEP markers and genomic markers

Markers alone	CEP	ARMS2	HTRA1	CFH	C3
Sensitivity (%)	73	31	37	60	36
Specificity (%)	65	94	89	77	86
C-statistic	0.76	0.62	0.63	0.69	0.62
95% CI	(0.73–0.79)	(0.58–0.67)	(0.58–0.68)	(0.64–0.73)	(0.57–0.66)
Joint effect of markers		CEP + ARMS2	CEP + HTRA1	CEP + CFH	CEP + C3
Sensitivity (%)		63	71	75	71
Specificity (%)		81	67	76	74
C-statistic		0.79	0.76	0.80	0.80
95% CI		(0.76–0.82)	(0.72–0.80)	(0.77–0.84)	(0.77–0.84)
P value		< 0.001	< 0.001	< 0.001	< 0.001

Sensitivity and specificity were determined from nonparametric ROC to maximize the sum of the two values and constructed from the output of logistic regression analysis fit with either CEP adduct concentrations plus autoantibody titers, or homozygous risk genotype, or the combination of the CEP biomarkers and the risk genotype. C-statistics, 95% CI and p-values comparing c-statistics derived from single and joint markers were determined with SAS 9.1. The c-statistic is a measure of the area under the ROC curve and the accuracy of the markers to discriminate between AMD cases and controls, with 1.0 equivalent to 100% accuracy and 0.5 equal to no discrimination. Combining the CEP and genomic markers significantly improved the c-statistics for all the genomic markers (Reproduced from Gu et al. 2009 with permission from The American Society for Biochemistry and Molecular Biology.)

genomic markers (77–94%). The combined markers exhibited 63–75% sensitivity and 67–81% specificity. The area under the ROC curves (c-statistics) were significantly greater ($p < 0.001$) for the combined markers (0.76–0.80) and CEP alone (0.76) than for the genomic markers alone (0.62–0.69).

Sensitivity and specificity were determined from nonparametric ROC to maximize the sum of the two values and constructed from the output of logistic regression analysis fit with either CEP adduct concentrations plus autoantibody titers, or homozygous risk genotype, or the combination of the CEP biomarkers and the risk genotype. C-statistics, 95% CI and p-values comparing c-statistics derived from single and joint markers were determined with SAS 9.1. The c-statistic is a measure of the area under the ROC curve and the accuracy of the markers to discriminate between AMD cases and controls, with 1.0 equivalent to 100% accuracy and 0.5 equal to no discrimination. Combining the CEP and genomic markers significantly improved the c-statistics for all the genomic markers. (Reproduced from Gu et al. 2009 with permission from The American Society for Biochemistry and Molecular Biology.)

47.3.3 The Association Between CEP Biomarkers and AMD Risk Genotypes

To probe for possible associations between CEP biomarker levels and AMD risk genotypes, we evaluated odds ratios for elevated CEP markers in the advanced

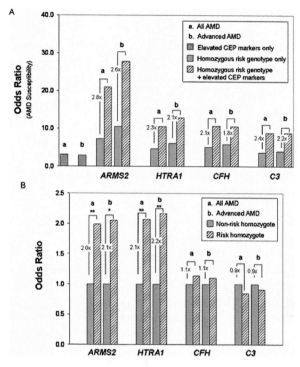

Fig. 47.1 AMD risk predicted by CEP markers and genotype. (**a**) Odds ratios for AMD risk based on elevated CEP markers only, genotype only (specific for the homozygous risk alleles *ARMS2*, *HTRA1*, *CFH* and *C3*), and joint effects of both are shown for all AMD and advanced AMD patients. (**b**) Odds ratio for both CEP markers to be elevated in AMD risk and non-risk homozygous genotypes are shown for all AMD or advanced AMD patients. Differences in CEP marker concentrations between homozygous risk and non-risk donors were statistically significant (**p < 0.01 and *p < 0.05, Fischer Exact Test) for *ARMS2* and *HTRA1* but not for *CFH* and *C3*. Odds ratios, 95% CI and *p*-values were determined with log-transformed CEP marker concentrations. (Reproduced from Gu et al. 2009 with permission from The American Society for Biochemistry and Molecular Biology.)

AMD cohort and in the entire AMD study population. The results (Fig. 47.1b) show ~2-fold significant increase in the odds ratios for elevated CEP markers over the non-risk genotype for AMD donors carrying homozygous risk alleles for *ARMS2* and *HTRA1* (*p* < 0.05), but not for *CFH* and *C3*. These results suggests that within the AMD population, individuals carrying the *ARMS2* or *HTRA1* homozygous risk genotypes, but not those carrying the *CFH* or *C3* risk genotypes, were more likely to exhibit elevated CEP markers than those carrying the non-risk alleles. These associations may be related to the sensitivity of the gene products to oxidative stress since *ARMS2* encodes a mitochondrial protein (Fritsche et al. 2008) and *HTRA1* encodes a heat shock serine protease activated by stress (Dewan et al. 2006; Yang et al. 2006).

47.4 Discussion

CEP protein modifications are generated by the reaction of an oxidation fragment derived uniquely from DHA-containing phospholipids, namely with 4-hydroxy-7-oxohept-5-enoic acid, with primary amino groups (e.g., protein ϵ-lysyl NH_2) (Gu et al. 2003a, b). DHA is highly oxidizable owing to its six double bond structure and furthermore, is abundant in retinal photoreceptor outer segments (Fliesler and Anderson 1983). The high oxygen tension and light in the retina provides a permissive environment for the production of oxidative post-translational modifications. Previously we found that rodents exposed to intense light accumulate elevated CEP adducts in the retina and elevated CEP adducts and autoantibodies in plasma (Gu et al. 2004; Renganathan et al. 2003). Other oxidative protein modifications accumulate in AMD ocular tissues, including for example, advanced glycation end products in the choriocapillaris, Bruch's membrane and CNV membranes (Handa et al. 1999; Ishibashi et al. 1998), and in RPE lipofuscin granules, nitrotyrosine, iso[4]levuglandin E_2-adducts and CEP (Ng et al. 2008).

This study shows that plasma CEP biomarker levels, in combination with genomic markers, can discriminate between AMD and control patients with up to ~80% accuracy and together proteomic and genomic biomarkers offer a potential early warning system for predicting AMD susceptibility. CEP biomarkers may also have utility in monitoring the efficacy of AMD therapeutics as CEP autoantibody titers appear to increase in direct proportion to the severity of RPE lesions in a mouse model of dry AMD (Hollyfield et al. 2008).

Acknowledgments This work was supported in part by US National Institute of Health grants EY015638, EY014239, GM21249, EY016072, BRTT 05–29 from the State of Ohio, a Foundation Fighting Blindness Center Grant, a Research to Prevent Blindness (RPB) Center Grant, a RPB Senior Investigator Award to JWC, a Steinbach Award to JWC, the VA Medical Research Service and the Cleveland Clinic Foundation. We thank Drs Joe G Hollyfield and Bela Anand-Apte for valuable discussions. The Clinical Genomic and Proteomic AMD Study Group was composed of the following individuals: David Barnhart OD[1], William J Dupps MD[1], Froncie A Gutman MD[1], Peter K Kaiser MD[1], Hilel Lewis MD[1,5], Richard E Gans MD[1,5], Bennie H Jeng MD[1], Gregory S Kosmorsky DO[1], Ronald R Krueger MD[1,5], Ann Laurenzi OD[1], Roger HS Langston, MD[1], Edward J Rockwood MD[1,5], William E Sax MD[1], Andrew P Schachat MD[1], Jonathan E Sears MD[1,5], Rishi Singh MD[1], Scott D Smith MD[1,5], Mindy Toabe OD[1], Elias I Traboulsi MD[1,5], Nadia Waheed MD[1], Steven E Wilson MD[1,5], and Stacia S. Yaniglos OD[4,6], Elisa Bala MD[1,4], Sonya Bamba MD[1], Sue Crowe BS[1], Patrice Nerone RN[1], Tiffany Ruez RN[1], and Ellen Simpson RN[1]. JWC is a consultant for Alcon Research Ltd and Allergan, Inc. and has received funding for this research from Merck & Co and Johnson and Johnson. JWC and RGS each have a license for CEP as an inventor with Frantz Biomarkers, LLC.

References

Age-Related Eye Disease Study Group (2001) A randomized, placebo-controlled, clinical trial of high-dose supplementation with vitamine C and E, beta carotene, and zinc for age-related macular degeneration and vision loss. Arch Ophthalmol 119:1417–1436
Crabb JW, Miyagi M, Gu X et al (2002) Drusen proteome analysis: an approach to the etiology of age-related macular degeneration. Proc Natl Acad Sci U S A 99:14682–14687

Dewan A, Liu M, Hartman S et al (2006) HTRA1 promoter polymorphism in wet age-related macular degeneration. Science 314:989–992

Ebrahem Q, Renganathan K, Sears J et al (2006) Carboxyethylpyrrole oxidative protein modifications stimulate neovascularization: implications for age-related macular degeneration. Proc Natl Acad Sci U S A 103:13480–13484

Edwards AO, Ritter R 3rd, Abel KJ et al (2005) Complement factor H polymorphism and age-related macular degeneration. Science 308:421–424

Fliesler SJ, Anderson RE (1983) Chemistry and metabolism of lipids in the vertebrate retina. Prog Lipid Res 22:79–131

Fritsche LG, Loenhardt T, Janssen A et al (2008) Age-related macular degeneration is associated with an unstable ARMS2 (LOC387715) mRNA. Nat Genet 40:892–896

Gu X, Meer SG, Miyagi M et al (2003a) Carboxyethylpyrrole protein adducts and autoantibodies, biomarkers for age-related macular degeneration. J Biol Chem 278:42027–42035

Gu J, Pauer GJT, Yue X et al (2009) Assessing susceptibility to age-related macular degeneration with proteomic and genomic biomarkers. Mol Cell Proteomics PMID: 19202148

Gu X, Renganathan K, Grimm C et al (2004) Rapid changes in retinal oxidative protein modifications induced by blue light. Invest Ophthalmol Vis Sci 45:E-abstract 3474

Gu X, Sun M, Gugiu B et al (2003b) Oxidatively truncated docosahexaenoate phospholipids: total synthesis, generation, and peptide adduction chemistry. J Org Chem 68:3749–3761

Hageman GS, Anderson DH, Johnson LV et al (2005) A common haplotype in the complement regulatory gene factor H (HF1/CFH) predisposes individuals to age-related macular degeneration. Proc Natl Acad Sci U S A 102:7227–7232

Haines JL, Hauser MA, Schmidt S et al (2005) Complement factor H variant increases the risk of age-related macular degeneration. Science 308:419–421

Handa JT, Verzijl N, Matsunaga H (1999) Increase in the advanced glycation end product pentosidine in Bruch's membrane with age. Invest Ophthalmol Vis Sci 40:775–779

Hollyfield JG, Bonilha VL, Rayborn ME et al (2008) Oxidative damage-induced inflammation initiates age-related macular degeneration. Nat Med 14:194–198

Ishibashi T, Murata T, Hangai M et al (1998) Advanced glycation end products in age-related macular degeneration. Arch Ophthalmol 116:1629–1632

Jakobsdottir J, Conley YP, Weeks DE et al (2005) Susceptibility genes for age-related maculopathy on chromosome 10q26. Am J Hum Genet 77:389–407

Klein RJ, Zeiss C, Chew EY et al (2005) Complement factor H polymorphism in age-related macular degeneration. Science 308:385–389

Maller JB, Fagerness JA, Reynolds RC et al (2007) Variation in complement factor 3 is associated with risk of age-related macular degeneration. Nat Genet 39:1200–1201

Maller J, George S, Purcell S et al (2006) Common variation in three genes, including a noncoding variant in CFH, strongly influences risk of age-related macular degeneration. Nat Genet 38:1055–1059

Ng KP, Gugiu B, Renganathan K et al (2008) Retinal pigment epithelium lipofuscin proteomics. Mol Cell Proteomics 7:1397–1405

Renganathan K, Ebrahem Q, Vasanji A et al (2008) Carboxyethylpyrrole adducts, age-related macular degeneration and neovascularization. Adv Exp Med Biol 613:261–267

Renganathan K, Sun M, Darrow R et al (2003) Light induced protein modifications and lipid oxidation products in rat retina. Invest Ophthalmol Vis Sci 44:E-abstract 5129

Rivera A, Fisher SA, Fritsche LG et al (2005) Hypothetical LOC387715 is a second major susceptibility gene for age-related macular degeneration, contributing independently of complement factor H to disease risk. Hum Mol Genet 14:3227–3236

Yang Z, Camp NJ, Sun H (2006) A variant of the HTRA1 gene increases susceptibility to age-related macular degeneration. Science 314:992–993

Yates JR, Sepp T, Matharu BK et al (2007) Complement C3 variant and the risk of age-related macular degeneration. N Engl J Med 357:553–561

Chapter 48
Impaired Intracellular Signaling May Allow Up-Regulation of CTGF-Synthesis and Secondary Peri-Retinal Fibrosis in Human Retinal Pigment Epithelial Cells from Patients with Age-Related Macular Degeneration

Piyush C. Kothary, Jaya Badhwar, Christina Weng, and Monte A. Del Monte

Abstract Age-related macular degeneration (AMD) is a major sight-threatening ocular disorder in the United States of America and the world, yet its etiology is not clearly understood, preventing the development of effective prevention or therapy. Connective tissue growth factor (CTGF) has been implicated in the pathological synthesis of peri-retinal fibrous tissue in patients with AMD. Very little is known about the mechanism of this interaction. In this study, the authors demonstrate that insulin like growth factor-1 (IGF-1) and glucose-stimulated CTGF production are not blocked by the MAP kinase pathway inhibitor, PD98059 in hRPE cells obtained from eyes of a patient with AMD in contrast to hRPE cells obtained from normal human eyes. This suggests that there may be abnormal CTGF synthesis regulation in AMD, which may play a role in fibrous peri-retinal membrane formation in patients with AMD-related proliferative vitreoretinopathy.

48.1 Introduction

The human retinal pigment endothelium (hRPE) is a single layer of cells located between the photoreceptors and Bruch's membrane. It is mitotically inactive in adult eyes. However, in some pathological states, it undergoes mitosis, cell division, and metaplasia. Growth factors have been implicated in inducing pathological proliferation and migration of hRPE cells (Kothary et al. 2001).

M.A. Del Monte (✉)
Department of Ophthalmology and Visual Sciences, University of Michigan/Kellogg Eye Center,
Ann Arbor, MI, USA
e-mail: madm@umich.edu

R.E. Anderson et al. (eds.), *Retinal Degenerative Diseases*, Advances in Experimental Medicine and Biology 664, DOI 10.1007/978-1-4419-1399-9_48, © Springer Science+Business Media, LLC 2010

Insulin like growth factor 1 (IGF 1) is a growth factor involved in control of proliferation of human retinal pigment epithelial (hRPE) cells (Spraul et al. 2000). Abnormal proliferation of hRPE cells has been shown to be present in the development of epiretinal membranes found in proliferative eye disease (Nagineni et al 2005). Lambooij et al. (2003) has shown that in eyes with choroidal neovascularization (CNV), IGF mRNA in the retina has the same distribution pattern as in normal retina. Further, IGF-1 and its receptor were co-localized in the normal human eye and in eyes with neovascular age-related macular degeneration (AMD), a disease that causes blindness. This suggests an autocrine function of IGF-I in the normal human retina as well as a possible role of abnormal regulation in the pathogenesis of neovascular AMD (Slomiany and Rosenzweig 2004). Abnormal IGF 1 synthesis, proliferation of hRPE cells, and hRPE cell migration to extracellular matrix (ECM) has also been implicated in the etiology of membrane formation in age related macular degeneration.

In addition, high concentrations of connective tissue growth factor (CTGF) correlate with increased intraocular fibrosis (Kuiper et al. 2006). CTGF was first identified as a 38-kDa cysteine-rich protein isolated from fibroblast conditioned culture media from human umbilical vein endothelial cells (Bradham et al. 1991). It is secreted by human vascular endothelial cells and is related to the SRC-induced immediate early gene product CEF-10. It was later found to stimulate the synthesis of extra-cellular matrix components and play a role in fibrosis.

Hyperglycemia is an independent risk factor that may contribute to the development of neovascularization via various signaling pathways (Khan and Chakrabarti 2007; Rosenthal et al. 2004). To investigate the role of CTGF in fibrotic peri-retinal membrane formation in patients with AMD-related proliferative vitreoretinopathy, we examined whether CTGF was regulated by high glucose and IGF-1 in in vitro cultured hRPE cells. We also exposed hRPE cells from an AMD patient and non-AMD patients to elevated glucose and IGF-1 in presence and absence of the ERK kinase inhibitor PD98059 (Zelivianski et al. 2003) to determine if the ERK kinase signaling pathway is involved in any changes detected.

48.2 Methods

48.2.1 Chemicals

IGF1 was purchased from Sigma Chemicals, St. Louis, MO. Anti-CTGF was purchased from R & D Systems, Minneapolis, MN. 3H-thymidine and 14C-Methionine were purchased from Amersham Corporation, Arlington Heights, IL. Ham's F-12 nutrient medium, Dulbecco's minimum essential media (DMEM), Hank's balanced salt solution, fetal bovine serum (FBS), penicillin, streptomycin and trypsin were purchased from GIBCO BRL, Gaithersburg, MD. PD98059 was purchased from Cell Signaling Technology, Beverly, MA.

48.2.2 *Establishment and Maintenance of hRPE Cell Cultures*

Primary cultures of hRPE cells were established from human eyes obtained from a patient with AMD and four without AMD as described previously (Kusaka et al. 1998; Kothary et al. 2001). Briefly, the anterior segment, vitreous and the retina of human eyes were surgically removed. The posterior segments were then washed with balanced salt solution, filled with papain (0.623 mg/ml in cystein/EDTA) and incubated for 1 h at 37°C. The Papain was aspirated and replaced with Ham's F-12 nutrient medium containing 15% FBS, 100 U/ml penicillin, 100 mg/ml streptomycin and 0.075% (wt/vol) sodium bicarbonate (medium-1). The now loosely adherent hRPE cells were detached by gentle brushing and hydrostatic pressure with a sterile fire polished Pasteur pipet. The cells were plated in 16-mm Primaria plates and incubated at 37°C in a 95% air/5% CO_2 incubator. The medium was changed every 3 days until the cells were confluent. Primary cultures were then washed with Hank's balanced salt solution and subcultured by trypsinization with 0.5 g/100 ml trypsin and 0.2 g/100 ml EDTA in Hank's normal salt solution (Sigma T-3924) at 37°C for 10 min. The cell suspension was centrifuged at $500 \times g$ and replated. The morphology of cells was examined daily by phase-contrast microscopy. For maintenance of cell lines, cells were plated in 75-mm flasks at density of 50,000 cells/flask. The medium was changed every three days until the cells were ready for trypsinization. Cells were counted by hemocytometer and viability was assessed by trypan blue exclusion.

48.2.3 *Cellular Proliferation*

Proliferation of cultured hRPE cells was determined by tritiated thymidine incorporation (3H-thy) and viable cell count by the trypan blue exclusion method as described previously (Kothary and Del Monte 2008). It showed that IGF-1 and fetal bovine serum are mitogenic and stimulate 3H-thy incorporation as well as increase in viable cell number of cultured hRPE cells obtained from the non-AMD control eyes as well as eyes from an AMD patient (Data not shown). This demonstrates that we have cell culture system that responds to biological stimuli and is suitable for intracellular signaling studies.

48.2.4 *Immunoprecipitation Assay*

To measure intracellular CTGF synthesis, hRPE cells were labeled by 14-C-Methionine and then treated with elevated glucose (hyperglycemia) and IGF-1 in the presence and absence of the ERK kinase inhibitor, PD98059, using the method described previously (Bitar et al. 1996; Kothary et al. 2006). hRPE cells were then lysed with zwittergent 3–12 and precipitated with antibody specific for CTGF.

48.2.5 Statistical Analysis

All values represent the % mean of control. Differences between two groups of data were tested by a Student 't' test. A $p < 0.05$ was used to assess significant differences between two groups.

48.3 Results

48.3.1 Effect of Glucose on 14C-CTGF Synthesis in hRPE Cells

Hyperglycemia (glucose $= 20$ mM) stimulated 14C-CTGF synthesis slightly in hRPE cells from control eyes obtained from Non-AMD patients and to a much greater extent in hRPE cells from a patient with AMD (Fig. 48.1).

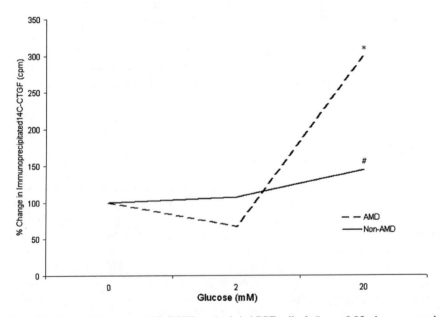

Fig. 48.1 Effect of glucose on 14C-CTGF synthesis in hRPE cells. *, #=$p < 0.05$ when compared with each other

48.3.2 Effect of IGF-1 on 14C-CTGF Synthesis in hRPE cells

IGF-1 (25 nM) stimulated 14C-CTGF synthesis minimally, if at all, in hRPE cells from eyes obtained of Non-AMD patients and to a much greater extent in hRPE cells from a patient with AMD (Fig. 48.2).

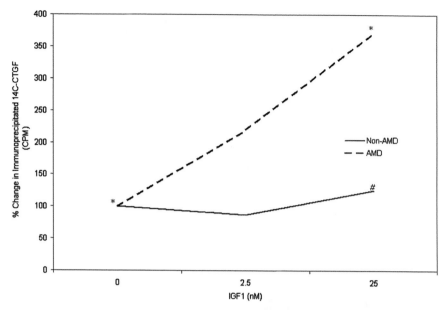

Fig. 48.2 Effect of IGF1 on 14C-CTGF synthesis in hRPE cells. *,#=$p < 0.05$ when compared with each other

48.3.3 Effect of PD98059 on Glucose Stimulated 14C-CTGF Synthesis in hRPE Cells

As shown in Fig. 48.3, elevated glucose (20 mM) stimulated 14C-CTGF synthesis only slightly in hRPE cells from Non-AMD control patients and to a much greater extent in hRPE cells from a patient with AMD, as seen in Fig. 48.1. However, PD98059 completely inhibited the glucose stimulated 14C-CTGF synthesis in Non-AMD patients. In addition, PD98059 (50 μM) only partially (but statistically significantly) inhibited glucose (20 mM) stimulation in hRPE cells from the AMD patient.

48.3.4 Effect of PD98059 on IGF-1 Stimulated 14C-CTGF Synthesis in hRPE Cells

As shown in Fig. 48.4, the IGF-1 (25 nM) stimulated 14C-CTGF synthesis in hRPE from AMD as well as Non-AMD patients, shown in Fig. 48.2, is significantly inhibited by PD98059 (50 μM) in hRPE from Non-AMD patients. However, PD98059 (50 μM) did not inhibit IGF-1 (25 mM) stimulated CTGF synthesis in hRPE cells from the AMD patient.

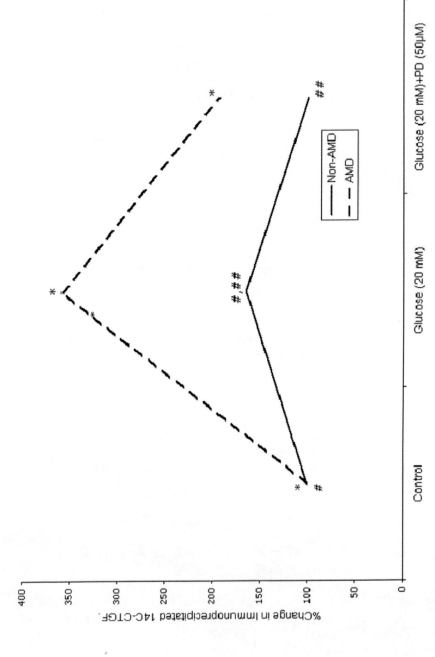

Fig. 48.3 Effect of PD98059 on glucose-stimulated 14C-CTGF synthesis. *,#,##= $p < 0.05$ when compared with each other

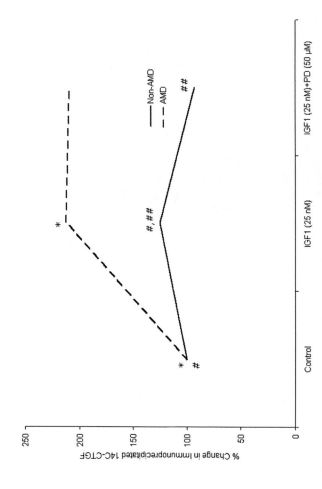

Fig. 48.4 Effect of PD98059 on IGF-1 stimulated 14C-CTGF synthesis. *,#,##= $p < 0.05$ when compared with each other

48.4 Discussion

The molecular mechanism for retinal fibro-genesis is unknown and thinking in this area is in a state of evolution. CTGF has been implicated in the pathogenesis of retinal fibro-genesis (Hinton et al. 2004). However, its signaling pathway in this system has not been elucidated. In the present study, we show that hyperglycemia and IGF-1 both stimulate CTGF synthesis, a proposed modulator of pathological retinal fibrosis, in cultured hRPE cells and this stimulation is inhibited the ERK pathway inhibitor, PD98059, in hRPE from control eyes but not in hRPE cells obtained from a patient with AMD.

Elevated glucose stimulates CTGF synthesis in a dose dependent manner in hRPE cells from AMD patients and to a lesser extent Non-AMD patients (Fig. 48.1). Hyperglycemia (20 mM glucose) stimulated CTGF synthesis was not completely blocked by the ERK inhibitor, PD98059 in hRPE cells from an AMD patient, while PD98059 completely blocked CTGF synthesis in hRPE cells Non-AMD patients (Fig. 48.3). Thus our data show that exposure of hRPE cells from Non-AMD patients to high glucose leads to an increase of CTGF expression, and the induction of CTGF by high glucose is mediated largely via ERK kinase pathway. However, exposure of hRPE cells from an AMD patient to high glucose leads to an increase of CTGF expression, and the induction of CTGF by high glucose is not completely blocked by ERK kinase pathway inhibitor.

To study the role of the ERK kinase signaling pathway in IGF-1 action, we exposed hRPE cells from an AMD patient and Non-AMD patients to increasing concentrations of IGF-1 and demonstrated that IGF-1 stimulates CTGF synthesis in dose dependent manner in hRPE cells from AMD as well as Non-AMD patients (Fig. 48.2). However, IGF-1 (25 nM) stimulated CTGF synthesis was not blocked by ERK inhibitor, PD98059, in hRPE cells from an AMD patient while PD98059 completely blocked CTGF synthesis in hRPE cells from Non-AMD patients (Fig. 48.4). Thus our data show that exposure of hRPE cells from Non-AMD patients to IGF-1 leads to an increase of CTGF expression, and the induction of CTGF by IGF-1 is mediated primarily via ERK kinase pathway. However, exposure of hRPE cells from an AMD patient to IGF-1 leads to an increase of CTGF expression, and the induction of CTGF by IGF-1 is not completely blocked by ERK kinase pathway inhibitor.

Our study demonstrates that normal hRPE cells produce CTGF via the ERK kinase signaling pathway. This result is consistent with the finding that ERK pathway mediates CTGF induction in fibroblasts (Blalock et al. 2003). In addition, our study also demonstrates that ERK pathways are impaired and there may be abnormal CTGF synthesis regulation in response to glucose and IGF-1 in hRPE cells a patient with AMD.

This differential response may play a role in the fibrotic peri-retinal membrane formation seen in patients with AMD-related proliferative vitreo-retinopathy. Our data supports the Shi-wen et al. (2000) postulation that the constitutive over expression of connective tissue growth factor may contribute directly to chronic, persistent fibrosis. In addition, these studies suggest that the source of elevated CTGF in AMD patients may be hRPE cells. In our studies of cultured hRPE cells from an AMD patient, we demonstrated that glucose and IGF-1 can induce abnormally elevated CTGF synthesis and anomalous regulatory pathways may be responsible. However, our in vitro studies cannot exclude that in vivo leakage of CTGF from the circulation through the defective blood retinal barrier (Kuiper et al. 2006) may also play a role.

In summary, our study has demonstrated that glucose and IGF-1 stimulation of CTGF synthesis in hRPE cells is mediated via ERK signaling. Impaired ERK signaling in hRPE cells in an AMD patient may result in abnormal synthesis of CTGF, which may play a role in the fibrotic peri-retinal membrane formation seen in AMD-related proliferative vitreo-retinopathies

Acknowledgments The authors thank Angela Joy Verkade for her assistance in preparing this chapter. This research was funded by the Skillman Foundation.

References

Bitar KN, Kothary S, Kothary PC (1996) Somatostatin inhibits bombesin-stimulated GI-protein via its own receptor in rabbit colonic smooth muscle cells. Pharm Exp Ther 276:714–719

Blalock TD, Duncan MR, Varela JC et al (2003) Connective tissue growth factor expression and action in human corneal fibroblast cultures and rat corneas after photorefractive keratectomy. Invest Ophthalmol Vis Sci 44:1879–1887

Bradham DM, Igarashi A, Potter RL et al (1991) Connective tissue growth factor: a cysteine-rich mitogen secreted by human vascular endothelial cells is related to the SRC-induced immediate early gene product CEF-10. J Cell Biol 114:1285–1294

Hinton DR, Spee C, He S et al (2004) Accumulation of NH(2)-terminal fragment of connective tissue growth factor in the vitreous of patients with proliferative diabetic retinopathy. Diabetes Care 27:758–764

Khan ZA, Chakrabarti S (2007) Cellular signaling and potential new treatment targets in diabetic retinopathy. Exp Diabetes Res 2007:31867–31879

Kothary PC, Del Monte MA (2008) A possible impaired signaling mechanism in human retinal pigment epithelial cells from patients with macular degeneration. Recent Adv Retin Degeneration 613:269–275

Kothary PC, Lahiri R, Kee L et al (2006) Pigment epithelium-derived growth factor inhibits fetal bovine serum stimulated vascular endothelial growth factor synthesis in cultured human retinal pigment epithelial cells. Retin Degenerative Dis 572:513–518

Kothary PC, Singal P, Patel P et al (2001) Influence of octoreotide (SMS) on intracellular pathways. Proceedings of World Congress Neuroinformatics 2:341–348

Kuiper EJ, De Smet MD, Van Meurs JC et al (2006) Association of connective tissue growth factor with fibrosis in vitreoretinal disorders. Arch Ophthalmol 124:1457–1462

Kusaka K, Kothary PC, Del Monte MA (1998) Modulation of basic fibroblast growth factor effect by retinoic acid in cultured retinal pigment epithelium. Curr Eye Res 17:524–530

Lambooij AC, Karel HM, Dicky J et al (2003) Insulin-like growth factor-1 and its receptor in neovascular age-related macular degeneration. Invest Ophthalmol Vis Sci 44:2192–2198

Nagineni CN, Kutty V, Detrick B et al (2005) Expression of PDGF and their receptors in human retinal pigment epithelial cells and fibroblasts: regulation by TGF. J Cell Physiol 203: 35–43

Rosenthal R, Wohlleben H, Malek G et al (2004) Insulin-like growth factor-1 contributes to neovascularization in age-related macular degeneration. Biochem Biophys Res Commun 323:1203–1208

Shi-wen X, Pennington D, Holmes A et al (2000) Autocrine overexpression of CTGF maintains fibrosis: RDA analysis of fibrosis genes in systemic sclerosis. Exp Cell Res 259:213–224

Slomiany MG, Rosenzweig SA (2004) IGF-1 induced VEGF and IGFBP-3 secretion correlates with increased HIF-1 expression and activity in retinal pigment epithelial cell line D407. Opthamol Vis Sci 45:2838–2847

Spraul CW, Kaven C, Amann J et al (2000) Effect of insulin-like growth factors 1 and 2, and glucose on the migration and proliferation of bovine retinal pigment epithelial cells in vitro. Ophthalmic Res 32:244–248

Zelivianski S, Spellman M, Kellerman M et al (2003) ERK inhibitor PD98059 enhances docetaxel-induced apoptosis of androgen-independent human prostate cancer cells. Int J Cancer 107: 478–485

Chapter 49
PPAR Nuclear Receptors and Altered RPE Lipid Metabolism in Age-Related Macular Degeneration

Goldis Malek, Peng Hu, Albert Wielgus, Mary Dwyer, and Scott Cousins

Abstract The pathophysiology of 'early' dry age-related macular degeneration (ARMD), characterized by the accumulation of lipid and protein-rich sub-retinal deposits remains largely unknown. Accumulation and dysregulated turnover of lipids as well as extracellular matrix (ECM) molecules in sub-retinal pigment epithelial (RPE) deposits and Bruch's membrane, itself an ECM, play a role in ARMD. Epidemiological studies have shown an increased risk for the disease associated with higher dietary intake of long chain poly-unsaturated fatty acids (LCPUFA) and specifically more so for n-6 versus n-3 fatty acids. PUFAs are membrane targets of lipid peroxidation and natural ligands for the nuclear receptors, peroxisome proliferator activated receptors (PPAR). Here we investigated the expression of genes involved in lipid metabolism and expression of the three isoforms of PPARs in an immortalized cell line of human RPE cells (ARPE19) in the presence or absence of fatty acids.

49.1 Introduction

Age-related macular degeneration (ARMD) is the leading cause of visual impairment in the Western world. It is a late on-set progressive degeneration involving the photoreceptors, neurosensory retina, Bruch's membrane, and the choriocapillaris. At the center of the disease is changes and degeneration of the retinal pigment epithelial cells (RPE). Clinically, ARMD progresses in different stages. Early or dry is characterized by the accumulation of lipid and protein rich extracellular deposits under the RPE including drusen, basal linear deposits and basal laminar deposits (Curcio and Millican 1999) collectively referred to as sub-RPE deposits. Geographic

G. Malek (✉)
Department of Ophthalmology, Duke University, Durham, NC, USA
e-mail: gmalek@duke.edu

R.E. Anderson et al. (eds.), *Retinal Degenerative Diseases*, Advances in Experimental Medicine and Biology 664, DOI 10.1007/978-1-4419-1399-9_49,
© Springer Science+Business Media, LLC 2010

atrophy is characterized by RPE atrophy and late or wet/exudative ARMD is characterized by endothelial invasion and pathological neovascularization under the retina (Bird et al. 1995; Green 1999). Though treatment options for the wet form of the disease are currently available and to some extent successful, there hasn't been any breakthrough in identification of drugs that directly target the sub-RPE deposit formation found in 85–90% of total ARMD patients living with this burden (Klein et al. 2007). Therefore, it is critical to further our understanding of the molecular and biological mechanisms that contribute to drusen formation.

49.1.1 Current Hypotheses Surrounding Sub-RPE Deposit Formation

The pathogenesis of dry ARMD is still poorly understood. Various epidemiologic risk factors have generated specific hypotheses. These include: *aging and RPE lysosomal failure* evident by accumulation of metabolic waste and lipofuscin formation; *family history/genetics* including risk associations with polymorphisms of CFH, LOC387715/ARMS2, HrtA-1, APOE, VEGF, MMP-9, and the mitochondrial gene MTND2*LHON4917G (4917G) (Schmidt et al. 2002; Edwards et al. 2005; Fiotti et al. 2005; Hageman et al. 2005; Haines et al. 2005; Klein et al. 2005; Yang et al. 2006; Ross et al. 2007; Canter et al. 2008); *chronic oxidative injury and inflammation* for which both the retina and RPE are particularly vulnerable due to the high levels of cumulative irradiation they are exposed to overtime and the composition of long chain polyunsaturated fatty acids (PUFA) which can be easily oxidized; and, *lipid dysregulation and accumulation* in RPE cells, Bruch's membrane and sub-RPE deposits. Modifiable risks associated with ARMD include smoking and diet. Though the stimulus for drusen formation is unknown, much of its content has been revealed by histochemistry, immunohistochemistry and proteomics (Crabb et al. 2002) to be composed of esterified and unesterified cholesterol, apolipoproteins (Malek et al. 2003; Curcio et al. 2005), vitronectin (Hageman et al. 1999), inflammatory proteins such as amyloid P, C5, CFH, C5b-9 (Hageman et al. 2001; Anderson et al. 2002; Johnson et al. 2002; Anderson et al. 2004), crystallins, calcium and many others.

49.1.2 Long Chain Poly-Unsaturated Fatty Acids (LCPUFA) are Associated with ARMD Risk

Fatty acids are not only a source of energy but also essential to physiological cell functions working as modulators of cellular signaling and metabolism, signal transduction, cell growth, differentiation, and membrane lipid composition. The significance of PUFAs are highlighted by the findings that altered levels of PUFA and their metabolites are quite common in obesity, atherosclerosis and cancer (B.M Forman, PNAS, 1997). Humans lack the $\Delta 15$ and 12 desaturase enzymes to de novo synthesize essential fatty acids, which are particularly rich in PUFAs, therefore they are dependent on dietary sources of these compounds (Sampath and Ntambi 2005). Depending on the position of the first double bond from the methyl end of the carbon chain, PUFAs are subdivided into n-6 (linoleic and arachidonic acids) and n-3 (linolenic, eicosapentanoic and docosahexanoic acid). Epidemiological studies have concluded that there is an inverse relationship between dietary intake of n-3 PUFA and risk of developing ARMD (SanGiovanni et al. 2007, 2008), a relationship also reported in atherosclerosis, cancer, Alzheimer's disease and diabetes. It is important to note that the pro-inflammatory nature of PUFAs and their propensity to lipid peroxidation is determined by both the n-6/n-3 PUFA ratio and the total PUFA content of tissue. Within the cell, PUFAs are natural ligands for nuclear receptors called peroxisome proliferator activated receptors (PPARs).

49.1.3 Peroxisome Proliferator Activated Receptors (PPARs) are Expressed in ARPE19 Cells

Peroxisome proliferator-activated receptors (PPARs), members of the steroid/thyroid nuclear receptor superfamily, are transcription factors activated by fatty acids and their derivatives. They are widely expressed and known to stimulate enlargement of peroxisomes, which contain a variety of oxidative metabolic processes such as beta-oxidation enzymes. After binding to endogenous ligands such as fatty acids/low density lipoproteins (LDL) or synthetic agonists, PPARs heterodimerize with another nuclear receptor, retinoid X receptor (RXR). This PPAR/RXR obligate heterodimer then binds to specific DNA response elements (PPRE) consisting of a direct repeat of the consensus hexameric motif AGGTCA interspaced by a single nucleotide, initiating DNA transcription and upregulation of specific PPAR genes. Functionally, they modulate the activity of genes involved in many processes including lipid homeostasis, glucose regulation, immune regulation, cell differentiation, inflammation, wound healing and have been associated with ischemia, cancer, systemic diseases such as atherosclerosis and diabetes, and age-related neurodegenerative diseases that share pathogenic mechanisms with ARMD including Alzheimer's disease (Kersten et al. 2000). In fact, PPARs and their high affinity synthetic agonists (fibrates and TZDs) have been marketed for hypercholesterolemia and type 2 Diabetes mellitus (Kersten et al. 2000; Olefsky and Saltiel 2000).

At least three isoforms of PPARs have been identified, alpha-α, delta-δ (also known as beta or NUC1) and gamma-γ, with the subtypes overlapping in activity, function and location. Currently there is no consensus as to the overall combined function of PPARs. PPAR-α is highly expressed in the liver, heart, muscle and kidney, as well as in cells of the arterial wall, while PPAR-γ is expressed at high levels in white adipose tissue, where it activates adipocyte differentiation, as well as foam cells, activated macrophages that play a major role in the pathogenesis of atherosclerosis (Chawla et al. 2001; Chinetti et al. 2001; Moore et al. 2001). PPAR-δ is ubiquitously expressed in various tissues and is one of the key regulators of energy

Fig. 49.1 Protein (**a**) and
RNA (**b**) expression of three
PPAR isoforms in extracts of
human cultured ARPE19
cells

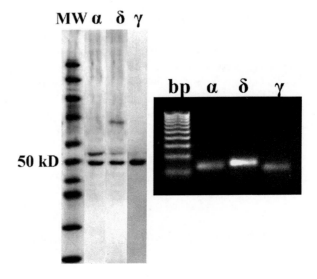

homeostasis in skeletal muscle. We have found that all three isoforms of PPARs
are expressed in an immortalized human RPE cell line (ARPE19; Fig. 49.1a, b).
Furthermore, robust PPAR-α, -β and -γ DNA binding activity in nuclear fractions of
ARPE19 was seen using a PPAR transcription factor assay (Cayman Chemical-data
not shown)

49.2 LcPUFA Regulates Gene Expression in ARPE19 Cells

49.2.1 Purpose and Methods

To obtain an overview of PUFA-regulated genes in ARPE19 cells, relevant to lipid
metabolism, we grew ARPE19 cells (ATCC) in media supplemented with 20 μM
PUFAs [n-6: arachidonic acid (AA) or n-3: docosahexanoic acid (DHA)] or 1% FBS
supplemented DMEM/F12 media for over 3 weeks and post-confluence. PUFA and
vehicle treated cells were harvested and total RNA was isolated using Qiagen micro
RNeasy kit. Total RNA was reverse transcribed using the iScript cDNA synthesis kit
(BioRad). Lipid-pathway focused gene expression kit (SABiosciences) along with
real-time PCR was used to evaluate 80 genes in RPE cells. Quantitative PCR was
performed using the BioRad icycler Realtime PCR system using cDNA, appropriate
primers and iQ SYBR Green Supermix detection reagent. The expression data were
normalized to 3 different housekeeping genes.

49.2.2 Results

Chronic lipid loading of ARPE19 cells with AA or DHA at concentrations of
greater than 50 μM was toxic to the cells (data not shown). Amongst the 80 genes

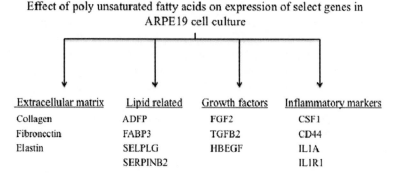

Fig. 49.2 Polyunsaturated fatty acids regulate gene expression in ARPE19 cells. These genes can broadly be categorized as extracellular matrix molecules, genes involved in lipid sequestration, synthesis and metabolism, inflammatory-related genes and growth factors

examined 18 were upregulated and 11 were downregulated with a 1.5-fold or greater difference between either PUFA treated group versus control. PUFAs were seen to differentially regulate lipid-related, extracellular matrix (ECM), inflammatory and growth factor genes (Fig. 49.2).

PUFA feeding of cells resulted in upregulation of genes implicated in atherosclerosis such as Selectin P-ligand (SELPLG) and adipogenic genes including adipose differentiation-related protein (ADRP). ADRP is a ubiquitously expressed protein, found in the highest levels in adipose tissue. Its expression is increased in cells under conditions that increase lipid accumulation and triacylglycerol synthesis. Another gene of interest is TGFβ which was also detected at higher levels in PUFA treated cells. Overproduction of TGFβ may stimulate production of ECMs such as collagen, fibronectin and elastin as seen in wound healing (Sime 2008). PPRE, the location on genes to which the PPAR-RXR heterodimer binds to in order to initiate gene transcription, is not located in the promoter of ECM, supporting the idea that intermediary gene(s) may be involved in this pathway.

49.2.3 Discussion

Lipid dysregulation plays a role in the pathogenesis of ARMD, a disease characterized in part by alterations in the content and composition of extracellular matrix. We believe that this altered matrix has the ability to promote further deposit formation and potentially neovascularization. Lower dietary intake of n-3 PUFAs is associated with decreased risk for progression of ARMD. PUFAs have been shown to affect gene expression through at least three different nuclear receptors; PPAR, liver X receptor and hepatocyte nuclear factor-4 (Sampath and Ntambi 2005). Nuclear PPARs in RPE cells are constitutively activated by lipids from adjacent photoreceptors and diet and have a detectable baseline activity. Following PUFA treatment we found elevated levels of ADRP, a ubiquitously expressed protein increased in cells under conditions of lipid sequestration as well several other genes involved in lipid metabolism which are currently under investigation. We also looked at the effects of PUFAs on ECM expression, since they accumulate in Bruch's membrane and sub-RPE deposits in ARMD. Since the promoter of ECMs lack a PPRE, it is unlikely that PUFA-ligand activated PPARs 'directly' stimulate ECM regulation, rather it would involve intermediary molecules such as TGFβ or PAI (plasminogen activator inhibitor), which have been shown to regulate ECM production in the lung and liver (Arteel 2008). Specifically, PAI has been shown to inhibit ECM breakdown suggesting that a potential mechanism by which PPARs influence ECM production could be through TGFβ which stimulates an increase in PAI, decreasing ECM degradation, resulting in an overall increase of ECM.

Altered activated states of the three isoforms of PPARs support the evolutionary notion of PPARs as a solution to the 'hypoxia-lipid' conundrum as proposed by Nunn et al. (2007) where 'the ability to store and burn fat is essential for survival, but is a "double-edged sword", as fats are potentially highly toxic'. Some evidence exists demonstrating PPAR-γ may be a potential player in late neovascular ARMD, in which concomitant with RPE degeneration, the underlying choriocapillaris becomes less fenestrated, impairing transport of macromolecules, such as oxygen, between the retina and choroidal blood supply. This hypoxia may in part stimulate neovascularization through VEGF. Murata and colleagues have shown that PPAR-γ not only may be a downstream inhibitor of VEGF, but also intravitreal treatment of murine eyes after laser induced CNV with synthetic agonists resulted in smaller sized lesions and less leakage compared to placebo (Murata et al. 2000). Our long term goals are to understand how dietary and or elevated locally produced lipids contribute to the pathology of sub-RPE deposit formation in ARMD. Studies on the role of the individual PPAR isoforms and their activation state following dietary insult in ARPE19, as a potential link in progression of dry ARMD, are ongoing.

Acknowledgments This work was supported by a grant from the International Retinal Research Foundation and Research to Prevent Blindness.

References

Anderson DH, Mullins RF et al (2002) A role for local inflammation in the formation of drusen in the aging eye. Am J Ophthalmol 134(3):411–431

Anderson DH, Talaga KC et al (2004) Characterization of beta amyloid assemblies in drusen: the deposits associated with aging and age-related macular degeneration. Exp Eye Res 78(2): 243–256

Arteel GE (2008) New role of plasminogen activator inhibitor-1 in alcohol-induced liver injury. J Gastroenterol Hepatol 23(Suppl 1):S54–S59

Bird AC, Bressler NM et al (1995) An international classification and grading system for age-related maculopathy and age-related macular degeneration. The International ARM Epidemiological Study Group. Surv Ophthalmol 39(5):367–374

Canter JA, Olson LM et al (2008) Mitochondrial DNA polymorphism A4917G is independently associated with age-related macular degeneration. PLoS ONE 3(5):e2091

Chawla A, Boisvert WA et al (2001) A PPAR gamma-LXR-ABCA1 pathway in macrophages is involved in cholesterol efflux and atherogenesis. Mol Cell 7(1):161–171

Chinetti G, Fruchart JC et al (2001) Peroxisome proliferator-activated receptors (PPARs): nuclear receptors with functions in the vascular wall. Z Kardiol 90(Suppl 3):125–132

Crabb JW, Miyagi M et al (2002) Drusen proteome analysis: an approach to the etiology of age-related macular degeneration. Proc Natl Acad Sci U S A 99(23):14682–14687

Curcio CA, Millican CL (1999) Basal linear deposit and large drusen are specific for early age-related maculopathy. Arch Ophthalmol 117(3):329–339

Curcio CA, Presley JB et al (2005) Esterified and unesterified cholesterol in drusen and basal deposits of eyes with age-related maculopathy. Exp Eye Res 81(6):731–741

Edwards AO, Ritter R 3rd et al (2005) Complement factor H polymorphism and age-related macular degeneration. Science 308(5720):421–424

Fiotti N, Pedio M et al (2005) MMP-9 microsatellite polymorphism and susceptibility to exudative form of age-related macular degeneration. Genet Med 7(4):272–277

Green WR (1999) Histopathology of age-related macular degeneration. Mol Vis 5:27

Hageman GS, Anderson DH et al (2005) A common haplotype in the complement regulatory gene factor H (HF1/CFH) predisposes individuals to age-related macular degeneration. Proc Natl Acad Sci U S A 102(20):7227–7232

Hageman GS, Luthert PJ et al (2001) An integrated hypothesis that considers drusen as biomarkers of immune-mediated processes at the RPE-Bruch's membrane interface in aging and age-related macular degeneration. Prog Retin Eye Res 20(6):705–732

Hageman GS, Mullins RF et al (1999) Vitronectin is a constituent of ocular drusen and the vitronectin gene is expressed in human retinal pigmented epithelial cells. FASEB J 13(3):477–484

Haines JL, Hauser MA et al (2005) Complement factor H variant increases the risk of age-related macular degeneration. Science 308(5720):419–421

Johnson LV, Leitner WP et al (2002) The Alzheimer's A beta-peptide is deposited at sites of complement activation in pathologic deposits associated with aging and age-related macular degeneration. Proc Natl Acad Sci U S A 99(18):11830–11835

Kersten S, Desvergne B et al (2000) Roles of PPARs in health and disease. Nature 405(6785):421–424

Klein R, Klein BE et al (2007) Fifteen-year cumulative incidence of age-related macular degeneration: the Beaver Dam Eye Study. Ophthalmology 114(2):253–262

Klein RJ, Zeiss C et al (2005) Complement factor H polymorphism in age-related macular degeneration. Science 308(5720):385–389

Malek G, Li CM et al (2003) Apolipoprotein B in cholesterol-containing drusen and basal deposits of human eyes with age-related maculopathy. Am J Pathol 162(2):413–425

Moore KJ, Fitzgerald ML et al (2001) Peroxisome proliferator-activated receptors in macrophage biology: friend or foe? Curr Opin Lipidol 12(5):519–527

Murata T, He S et al (2000) Peroxisome proliferator-activated receptor-gamma ligands inhibit choroidal neovascularization. Invest Ophthalmol Vis Sci 41(8):2309–2317

Nunn AV, Bell J et al (2007) The integration of lipid-sensing and anti-inflammatory effects: how the PPARs play a role in metabolic balance. Nucl Recept 5(1):1

Olefsky JM, Saltiel AR (2000) PPAR gamma and the treatment of insulin resistance. Trends Endocrinol Metab 11(9):362–368

Ross RJ, Bojanowski CM et al (2007) The LOC387715 polymorphism and age-related macular degeneration: replication in three case-control samples. Invest Ophthalmol Vis Sci 48(3):1128–1132

Sampath H, Ntambi JM (2005) Polyunsaturated fatty acid regulation of genes of lipid metabolism. Annu Rev Nutr 25:317–340

SanGiovanni JP, Chew EY et al (2007) The relationship of dietary lipid intake and age-related macular degeneration in a case-control study: AREDS Report No. 20. Arch Ophthalmol 125(5):671–679

SanGiovanni JP, Chew EY et al (2008) The relationship of dietary omega-3 long-chain polyunsaturated fatty acid intake with incident age-related macular degeneration: AREDS Report No. 23. Arch Ophthalmol 126(9):1274–1279

Schmidt S, Klaver C et al (2002) A pooled case-control study of the apolipoprotein E (APOE) gene in age-related maculopathy. Ophthalmic Genet 23(4):209–223

Sime PJ (2008) The antifibrogenic potential of PPARgamma ligands in pulmonary fibrosis. J Investig Med 56(2):534–538

Yang Z, Camp NJ et al (2006) A variant of the HTRA1 gene increases susceptibility to age-related macular degeneration. Science 314(5801):992–993

Chapter 50
The Pathophysiology of Cigarette Smoking and Age-Related Macular Degeneration

S. S. Ni Dhubhghaill, M.T. Cahill, M. Campbell, L. Cassidy, M.M. Humphries, and P. Humphries

Abstract Age-related macular degeneration (AMD) is the most common form of visual impairment, in people over 65, in the Western world. AMD is a multifactorial disease with genetic and environmental factors influencing disease progression. Cigarette smoking is the most significant environmental influence with an estimated increase in risk of 2- to 4-fold. Smoke-induced damage in AMD is mediated through direct oxidation, depletion of antioxidant protection, immune system activation and atherosclerotic vascular changes. Moreover, cigarette smoke induces angiogenesis promoting choroidal neovascularisation and progression to neovascular AMD. Further investigation into the effects of cigarette smoke through in vitro and in vivo experimentation will provide a greater insight into the pathogenesis of age-related macular degeneration.

50.1 Introduction

Age-related macular degeneration (AMD) is a progressive, degenerative eye condition affecting the central (macular) portion of the retina (Gehrs 2006), and is the leading cause of visual impairment in people over 65 in the Western world (Klein 2007). With aging populations, the prevalence and incidence of this disease are increasing, resulting in increased debilitation and social burden.

Clinically AMD may be classified as either atrophic or neovascular. Atrophic AMD is the commonest form, affecting approximately 85% of persons with AMD (Klein 1997). It is characterized by retinal pigment epithelium cell layer (RPE) abnormalities, drusen (collections of extracellular debris beneath the RPE), and in some cases retinal pigment epithelial detachment (RPED). Geographic atrophy (GA) is an advanced form of atrophic AMD involving widespread atrophy of the RPE, inducing apoptosis of overlying photoreceptors and subsequent exposure of choroidal vessels.

S.S. Ni Dhubhghaill (✉)
The Ocular Genetics Unit, Department of Genetics, Trinity College Dublin, Dublin 2, Ireland
e-mail: nidhubs@tcd.ie

R.E. Anderson et al. (eds.), *Retinal Degenerative Diseases*, Advances in Experimental Medicine and Biology 664, DOI 10.1007/978-1-4419-1399-9_50,
© Springer Science+Business Media, LLC 2010

Neovascular AMD typically occurs in areas of atrophic AMD and is characterised by the infiltration of choroidal neovascularisation (CNV) through Bruch's membrane towards the neural retina. These new choroidal vessels are fragile and may result in multiple complications – haemorrhage, retinal detachment, retinal atrophy and disciform scarring resulting in rapid visual loss (Schmidt-Erfurth 2007). CNV is likely a response to tissue injury and similar in nature to the granular tissue of the generalised wound healing response (Donoso et al. 2006).

50.2 Cigarette Smoking as a Risk Factor for AMD

50.2.1 AMD and Cigarette Smoke

The aetiology of AMD is complex, involving interactions between genetic and environmental risk factors. Cigarette smoking is the most significant environmental risk factor contributing to the development of AMD (Thornton et al. 2005). Smoking increases the risk of developing AMD 2- to 4-fold and passive smokers are also at an increased risk (Lois et al. 2008). Cigarette smoke further affects AMD by promoting progression from atrophic to neovascular AMD (Chakravarthy et al. 2007). This may occur up to ten years earlier in smokers than in non-smokers (Mitchell et al. 2002). Cessation reduces the risk of developing AMD and progression to neovascular AMD (Khan et al. 2006) and for every 1,000 smokers that successfully quit, there would be 48 fewer cases of macular degeneration with 12 fewer cases of blindness (Hurley et al. 2008).

50.2.2 Cigarette Smoke Constituents

Cigarette smoke is separated into two phases, a gas phase and a tar phase based on passage through a standard filter (Church and Pryor 1985). With each cigarette, smokers consume over 4,000 different compounds (Hoffmann et al. 1997). Therefore it is unlikely that cigarette smoke exerts its pathological effects through a single biochemical pathway. Though the consequences of ocular exposure to the full range of cigarette smoke constituents are not yet known, it is thought that oxidative damage, vascular and inflammatory changes play key roles in the pathogenesis of AMD (U.S. Department of Health and Human services CfDCaP et al. 2004).

50.3 Oxidative Stress

50.3.1 Oxidative Damage in AMD

The RPE layer is exposed to high levels of oxidative damage from both the retina and the systemic circulation (Beatty et al. 2000). It has been hypothesized that cumulative oxidative damage to the RPE contributes to the development and progression of atrophic AMD (Beatty et al. 2000; Cai et al. 2000) and without the metabolic support of the RPE, overlying photoreceptors undergo apoptosis. This hypothesis is supported clinically by the modest benefits of antioxidant therapy in dry AMD (AREDS 2000).

Two single nucleotide polymorphisms (SNPs) Loc387715/ARMS2 and A4917G in mitochondrial DNA have been linked to AMD (Canter et al. 2008). It is plausible that the structural protein changes conferred by these SNPs impair the ability of the mitochondrion to process oxidative stresses. Thus, oxidative damage to mitochondrial DNA leading to RPE apoptosis may be a key step in the initiation of AMD (Sharma et al. 2008).

Mice exposed to chronic cigarette smoke display RPE apoptosis and Bruch membrane alterations which can be attributed to oxidative damage (Fujihara et al. 2008). Moreover, chronic smoke exposure in mice yields basal laminar deposits reminiscent of drusen (Espinosa-Heidmann et al. 2006).

50.3.2 Reactive Oxygen Species in Cigarette Smoke

Cigarette smoke contains $>10^{15}$ free radicals per inhalation (Church and Pryor 1985) and numerous other chemicals that may be metabolized into reactive oxygen intermediates. These oxidants in cigarette smoke can pass through the alveolar walls and enter the circulation (Yamaguchi et al. 2006). Plasma markers of lipid peroxidation are increased after smoking confirming that smoke derived radicals pass into the circulation with the potential to exert widespread systemic effects (Frei et al. 1991).

50.3.3 Acrolein-Induced Oxidative Stress

In addition to directly generating short-lived reactive oxygen species, cigarette smoke contains a number of more stable components that inflict oxidative damage. Acrolein is an unsaturated aldehyde found in the gas phase of cigarette smoke in quantities of 3–220 μg per cigarette (Faroon et al. 2008). It is capable of exerting an oxidant-mediated damage, inducing protein modifications and promoting the formation of advanced glycation end-products (AGEPs) and advanced lipid end products (ALEPs) (Kirkham et al. 2003). RPE cells exposed to acrolein show a decrease in viability and mitochondrial membrane potential due to oxidative stress (Jia et al. 2007).

50.3.4 Cadmium-Induced Oxidative Stress

In humans, the main source of cadmium intake is through cigarette smoke (Bernhard et al. 2005). Plasma and retinal levels of cadmium are significantly higher in

smokers than non-smokers (Bernhard et al. 2006). Cadmium accumulates preferentially in the RPE and choroid (Wills et al. 2008) and may contribute to the
development of AMD through an increase in reactive oxygen species. Cadmium
exposure reduces viability and membrane integrity of cultured RPE cells and this
damage was likely oxidative (Wills et al. 2008). Interestingly, cadmium has been
found at increased concentrations in the urine of smokers and non-smokers with
AMD supporting a role for cadmium in the pathogenesis of AMD (Eric et al.
2007).

50.4 Cigarette Smoke Depletion of Antioxidant Protection

50.4.1 Systemic Antioxidant Mechanisms

Several systems exist to protect against oxidant-mediated cellular damage. Diet
derived antioxidant vitamins B, C and E provide protection by reacting with radicals
terminating oxidation cascades. Cigarette smoke depletes plasma concentrations of
vitamin C, E and carotenoids (Chow et al. 1986; Alberg 2002; Panda et al. 1999;
Bruno and Traber 2006) and supplementation of antioxidants inhibits cigarette
smoke induced oxidative damage in vivo (Panda et al. 2000).Acute cigarette
smoke exposure also reduces the levels of endogenous circulating anti-oxidant
molecules. Glutatione, cysteine, methylumbellifere glucuronide and ferrodxidase
are all reduced in serum after smoke exposure (Moriarty et al. 2003; Van der Vaart
et al. 2004). Enzymes that degrade reactive molecules and generate endogenous
antioxidants such as superoxide dismutase (SOD), catalase and glutathione peroxidase are also crucial in cellular defense against oxidative damage. Distuption of
superoxide dismutase in mice results in drusen-like deposits in the eye, and SOD
knock-out animals have been used as a model of dry-AMD (Edwards and Malek
2007).

50.4.2 Local Ocular Antioxidants

Carotenoids are present in a large concentration in the macula giving it a yellowish
appearance and providing protection from oxidative damage (Loane et al. 2008).
Reduced levels of macular pigments have been associated with AMD, due to the
loss of this antioxidant protective capacity (O'Connell et al. 2006). Supplementary
therapy with dietary macular pigments may offset this damage and reduce disease
progression in macular degeneration. Cigarette smoking has been shown to reduce
macular pigment (Hammond et al. 1996) and, by compromising local antioxidant
protection, may promote AMD.

50.5 Non-oxidative Chemical Damage by Cigarette Smoke

50.5.1 Nicotine

Of the numerous constituents of cigarette smoke, nicotine is the only known ingredient to possess addictive properties. Nicotine promotes angiogenesis in vitro (Heeschen et al. 2001) and in vivo (Suner et al. 2004) and these biological effects can be applied to AMD. Angiogenesis is likely due to a nicotine-induced increase in expression of Vascular Endothelial Growth Factor (VEGF) in endothelial cells (Conklin et al. 2002). A nicotine-induced increase of VEGF could account for the expedited progression to neovascular AMD seen in smokers.

Nornicotine, a metabolite of nicotine catalyses the metabolism of retinoids to all-E-retinal which can lead to the accumulation of lipofuscin, a constituent of drusen, in RPE cells (Brogan et al. 2005). Nicotine also exerts a vasoconstrictive action via α-adrenergic stimulation which may impair blood flow through the choroid (Zhu and Parmley 1995).

50.5.2 Polycyclic Aromatic Hydrocarbons

Polycyclic aromatic hydrocarbons (PAH) have been linked to the toxicity of cigarette smoke through vascular and carcinogenic effects in cardiovascular and respiratory disease (Ambrose and Barua 2004). Benzo[a]pyrene is a PAH found in cigarette smoke and that damages nuclear and mitochondrial DNA in bovine RPE (Patton et al. 2002) through the formation of a reactive epoxide. Benzo(e)pyrene is a related polycyclic aromatic hydorcarbon molecule cause caspase mediated cell apoptosis of human RPE cells (Sharma et al. 2008) perhaps through the generation of similar epoxides.

50.6 Inflammation

50.6.1 Inflammation and AMD

Drusen deposits in atrophic AMD contain evidence of chronic low grade inflammation supporting the hypothesis that inflammation is central in pathogenesis of AMD (Anderson et al. 2002). The complement cascade may be central this process. A number of genetic risk factors associated with AMD are involved in the activation and regulation of the complement pathway and thus far, SNPs in complement components C3, CFH, C2 and Factor B have been implicated in the pathogenesis of AMD (Haines et al. 2005; Gold et al. 2006; Yates et al. 2007).

Inflammatory mediators also govern the progression from atrophic to neovascular AMD. Depletion of macrophages in a laser-induced animal model of CNV inhibits the immune response and the subsequent neovascularization (Espinosa-Heidmann et al. 2003).

50.6.2 Cigarette Smoke and Complement Pathway

Cigarette smoke can directly activate C3, a key component in the Alternative complement pathway (Kew et al. 1985) as well as reduce serum levels of CFH, a circulating inhibitor of complement activation. It is possible therefore that complement-related genetic risk factors and cigarette smoke-induced complement activation act synergistically to promote inflammation in AMD.

50.6.3 Cigarette Smoke and Other Inflammatory Mediators

Cigarette smoke is also associated with a state of systemic chronic low-grade inflammation (Yanbaeva et al. 2007). Leukocyte and neutrophil concentrations are elevated in the blood of smokers (Van der Vaart et al. 2004; Solberg et al. 1998). Human monocytes are activated by cigarette smoke in vitro through oxidant-mediated pathways (Walters et al. 2005) indicating that the oxidative stress and immunological hyposhteses of AMD aetiology may not be mutually exclusive.

50.7 Vascular Changes

The vascular model of AMD provides an alternative hypothesis for the aetiology of AMD (Friedman 2000). This model postulates that the initial changes in AMD occur in the choroidal vasculature in a process analogous to atherosclerosis. Cigarette smoke exacerbates atherosclerotic changes in the coronary arteries (Ambrose and Barua 2004), oxidizes cholesterol and low-density lipoproteins (Mahfouz et al. 1995), and activates platelets promoting aggregation (Tonga et al. 2008). Smoke also induces blood vessel constriction through α-adrenergic receptor activation. In vivo, animals exposed to chronic cigarette smoke display significantly increased choroidal vascular resistance (Bettman et al. 1958). A decrease in choroidal circulation may impair the clearance of debris from the RPE and lead to the depositions in the Bruch membrane seen in AMD (Friedman 2004).

Cigarette smoke exposure significantly alters the branching pattern and extracellular matrices of proliferating vessels (Melkonian et al. 1999). These vessels were accompanied by a higher number of fibroblasts than unexposed controls. Thus smoke may further compromise the infiltrating vessels in CNV membranes.

50.8 Conclusions

Age-related macular degeneration is a disease of multifactorial aetiology with both genetic and environmental influences. Cigarette smoke is the most significant environmental factor known. This highly potent toxin causes oxidative stress, promotes inflammation and induces vascular changes. Further assessment of the

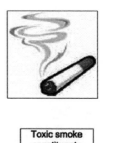

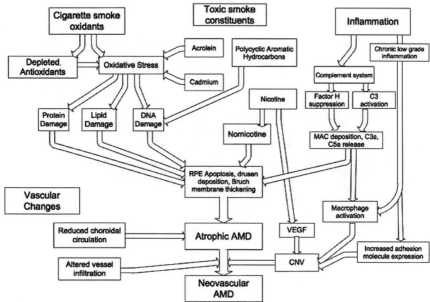

Fig. 50.1 Cigarette smoke-mediated influences in the pathophysiology of AMD

effects of smoke in vitro and in vivo is required to fully understand its role in the pathophysiology of AMD (Fig. 50.1).

Acknowledgments This work is supported by the Research Foundation of the Royal Victoria Eye and Ear Hospital, Dublin and the Irish Research Council for Science Engineering and Technology (IRCSET).

References

AREDS (2000) The age-related eye disease study: a clinical trial of zinc and antioxidants – AREDS report no. 2. J Nutr 130(5S Suppl):1516S–1519S

Alberg AJ (2002) The influence of cigarette smoking on circulating concentrations of antioxidant micronutrients. Toxicology 180:121–137

Ambrose JA, Barua RS (2004) The pathophysiology of cigarette smoking and cardiovascular disease. J Am Coll Cardiol 43:1731–1737

Anderson DH, Mullins RF, Hageman GS et al (2002) A role for local inflammation in the formation of drusen in the aging eye. Am J Ophthalmol 134:411–431

Beatty S et al (2000) The role of oxidative stress in the pathogenesis of age-related macular degeneration. Surv Ophthalmol 45(2):115–134

Bernhard D, Rossmann A, Henderson B et al (2006) Increased serum cadmium and strontium levels in young smokers: effects on arterial endothelial cell gene transcription. Arterioscler Thromb Vasc Biol 26:833–838

Bernhard D, Rossmann A, Wick G (2005) Metals in cigarette smoke. IUBMB Life 57(12):805–809

Bettman JW, Fellows V, Chao P (1958) The effect of cigarette smoking on the intraocular circulation. AMA Arch Ophthalmol 59(4):481–488

Brogan AP, Dickerson TJ et al (2005) Altered retinoid homeostasis catalyzed by a nicotine metabolite: implications in macular degeneration and normal development. PNAS 102(30): 10433–10438

Bruno RS, Traber MG (2006) Vitamin E biokinetics, oxidative stress and cigarette smoking. Pathophysiology 13:143–149

Cai J, Nelson KC et al (2000) Oxidative damage and protection of the RPE. Prog Eye Res 19(2):205–221

Canter JA, Olson LM, Spencer K et al (2008) Mitochondrial DNA polymorphism A4917G is independently associated with age-related macular degeneration. PLoS ONE 3(5):e2091

Chakravarthy U, Augood C, Bentham GC et al (2007) Cigarette smoking and age-related macular degeneration in the EUREYE study. Ophthalmology 114(6):1157–1163

Chow CK, Thacker RR, Changchit C et al (1986) Lower levels of vitamin C and carotenes in plasma of cigarette smokers. J Am Coll Nutr 5(3):305–312

Church DF, Pryor WA (1985) Free-radical chemistry of cigarette smoke and its toxicological implications. Environ Health Perspect 64:111–126

Conklin BS, Zhao W et al (2002) Nicotine and cotinine up-regulate vascular endothelial growth factor expression in endothelial cells. Am J Pathol 160(2):413–418

Donoso LA et al (2006) The role of inflammation in the pathogenesis of age-related macular degeneration. Surv Ophthalmol 51(2):137–152

Edwards AO, Malek G (2007) Molecular genetics of AMD and current animal models. Angiogenesis 10:119–132

Eric JC, Good JA, Butz JA et al (2007) Urinary cadmium and age-related macular degeneration. Am J Ophthalmol 144(3):414–418

Espinosa-Heidmann DG, Suner IJ et al (2003) Macrophage depletion diminishes lesion size and severity in experimental choroidal neovascularisation. IOVS 44:3586–3592

Espinosa-Heidmann DG, Suner IJ et al (2006) Cigarette smoke-related oxidants and the development of sub-RPE deposits in an experimental animal model of dry AMD. IOVS 47: 729–737

Faroon O, Roney N, Taylor J et al (2008) Acrolein environmental levels and potential for human exposure. Toxicol Ind Health 24:543

Frei B, Forte TM et al (1991) Gas phase oxidants of cigarette smoke induce lipid peroxidation and changes in lipoprotein properties in human blood plasma. Biochem J 277:133–138

Friedman E (2000) The role of the atherosclerotic process in the pathogenesis of age-related macular degeneration. Am J Ophthalmol 130(5):658–663

Friedman E (2004) Update of the vascular model of AMD. Br J Ophthalmol 88:160–161

Fujihara M, Nagai N, Sussan T et al (2008) Chronic cigarette smoke causes oxidative damage and apoptosis to retinal pigmented epithelial cells in mice. PLoS ONE 3(9):e3119

Gehrs KM (2006) Age-related macular degeneration – emerging pathogenic and therapeutic concepts. Ann Med 38:450–471

Gold B, Merriam JE, Zernant J et al (2006) Variation in factor B (BF) and complement component 2 (C2) genes is associated with age-related macular degeneration. Nat Genet 38(4):458–462

Haines JL et al (2005) Complement factor H variant increases the risk of age-related macular degeneration. Science 308:419–421

Hammond BR, Wooten BR, Snodderly DM (1996) Cigarette smoking and retinal carotenoids: implications for age-related macular degeneration. Vision Res 36(18):3003–3009

Heeschen C, Jang JJ et al (2001) Nicotine stimulates angiogenesis and promotes tumor growth and atherosclerosis. Nat Med 7(7):833–839

Hoffmann D, Djordjevic MV, Hoffmann I (1997) The changing cigarette. Prev Med 26:427–434

Hurley SF, Matthews JP, Guymer RH (2008) Cost-effectiveness of smoking cessation to prevent age-related macular degeneration. Cost Eff Resour Alloc 6(18):1–10

Jia L, Liu Z et al (2007) Acrolein, a toxicant in cigarette smoke, causes oxidative damage and mitochondrial dysfunction in RPE cells: protection by (R)-a-Lipoic acid. IOVS 48:339–348

Kew RR et al (1985) Cigarette smoke can activate the alternative pathway in vitro by modifying the third component of complement. J Clin Invest 75:1000–1007

Khan JC et al (2006) Smoking and age-related macular degeneration: the number of pack years of cigarette smoking is a major determinant of risk for both geographic atrophy and choroidal neovascularization. Br J Ophthalmol 90:75–80

Kirkham PA, Spooner G et al (2003) Cigarette smoke triggers macrophage adhesion and activation: role of lipid peroxidation products and scavenger receptor. Free Radic Biol Med 35(7):697–710

Klein R (1997) The five-year incidence and progression of age-related maculopathy: the Beaver Dam Eye Study. Ophthalmology 104:7–21

Klein R (2007) Overview of progress in the epidemiology of age-related macular degeneration. Ophthalm Epidem 14(4):184–187

Loane E, Kelliher C, Beatty S et al (2008) The rational and evidence base for a protective role of macular pigment in age-related maculopathy. Br J Ophthalmol 92(9):1163–1168

Lois N, Abdelkader E, Reglitz K et al (2008) Environmental tobacco smoke exposure and eye disease. Br J Ophthalmol 92:1304–1310

Mahfouz MM, Hulea SA, Kummerow FA (1995) Cigarette smoke increases cholesterol oxidation and lipid peroxidation of low-density lipoprotein and decreases its binding to the hepatic receptor in vitro. J Environ Pathol Toxicol Oncol 14(3–4):181–192

Melkonian G, Le C et al (1999) Normal patterns of angiogenesis and extracellular matrix deposition in chick chorioallantoic membranes are disrupted by mainstream and sidestream smoke. Toxicol Appl Pharmacol 163:26–37

Mitchell P, Wang JJ et al (2002) Smoking and the 5-year incidence of age-related maculopathy: the Blue Mountains Eye Study. Arch Ophthalmol 120(10):1357–1363

Moriarty SE, Shah JH, Lynn M et al (2003) Oxidation of glutathione and cysteine in human plasma associated with smoking. Free Radic Biol Med 35(12):1582–1588

O'Connell E, Neelam K, Nolan J et al (2006) Macular carotenoids and age-related maculopathy. Ann Acad Med Singapore 35(11):821–830

Panda K, Chattopadhyay R et al (1999) Vitamin C prevents cigarette smoke induced oxidative damage of proteins and increased proteolysis. Free Radic Biol Med 27(9/10):1064–1079

Panda K, Chattopadhyay R et al (2000) Vitamin C prevents cigarette smoke-induced oxidative damage in vivo. Free Radic Biol Med 29(2):115–124

Patton WP, Routledge MN et al (2002) Retinal pigment epithelial cell DNA is damaged by exposure to benzo[a]pyrene, a constituent of cigarette smoke. Exp Eye Res 74:513–522

Schmidt-Erfurth UM (2007) Management of neovascular age-related macular degeneration. Prog Ret Eye Res 26:437–451

Sharma A, Neekhra A, Gramajo AL et al (2008) Effects of Benzo(e)Pyrene, a toxic component of cigarette smoke, on human retinal pigment epithelial cells in vitro. Invest Ophthalmol Vis Sci 49:5111–5117

Solberg Y et al (1998) The association between cigarette smoking and ocular diseases. Surv Ophthalmol 42(6):535–547

Suner IJ, Espinosa-Heidmann DG et al (2004) Nicotine increases size and severity of experimental choroidal neovascularization. IOVS 45:311–317

Thornton J et al (2005) Smoking and age-related macular degeneration: a review of association. Eye 19:935–944

Tonga AR, Latina V, Orlando R et al (2008) Cigarette smoke inhibits adenine nucleotide hydrolysis by human platelets. Platelets 19(7):537–542

U.S. Department of Health and Human services CfDCaP, National Centre for Chronic Disease Prevention and Health Promotion, and Office on Smoking and Health (2004) The health consequences of smoking; a report of the Surgeon General Atlanta, GA

Van der Vaart H, Timens W, Ten Hacken NHT (2004) Acute effects of cigarette smoke on inflammation and oxidative stress: a review. Thorax 59:713–721

Walters M, Paul-Clark MJ et al (2005) Cigarette smoke activates human monocytes by an oxidant-AP-1 signaling pathway: implications for steroid resistance. Mol Pharmacol 68:1343–1353

Wills NK, Sadagopa Ramanujam VM, Chang J et al (2008) Cadmium accumulation in the human retina: effects of age, gender, and cellular toxicity. Exp Eye Res 86:41–51

Yamaguchi Y, Nasu F et al (2006) Oxidants in the gas phase of cigarette smoke pass through the lung alveolar wall and raise systemic oxidative stress. J Pharmacol Sci 103:275–282

Yanbaeva DG, Dentener MA, Creutzberg EC et al (2007) Systemic effects of smoking. Chest 131(5):1557–1566

Yates JRW, Sepp T et al (2007) Complement C3 variant and the risk of age-related macular degeneration. NEJM 357:553–561

Zhu B, Parmley WW (1995) Hemodynamic and vascular effects of active and passive smoking. Am Heart J 130:1270–1275

Chapter 51
Oxidative Stress and the Ubiquitin Proteolytic System in Age-Related Macular Degeneration

Scott M. Plafker

Abstract AMD is a leading cause of irreversible vision loss in people over 60 years of age. Although the pathogenesis of this disease is multifactorial, clinical studies have revealed that oxidative damage is a significant etiological factor. The ubiquitin proteolytic system (UPS) plays a major cytoprotective role in the retina. It accomplishes this largely by degrading oxidatively-damaged proteins to prevent their toxic accumulation. In this review, we discuss numerous features of the UPS in the retina and propose various ways that components of the UPS can be harnessed for therapeutic intervention in AMD. We discuss published work describing the distribution of various UPS enzymes in different retinal cell types and present new findings describing the localization of the class III ubiquitin conjugating enzymes. These enzymes are functional homologues of a pair of yeast enzymes that mediate the degradation of misfolded and oxidatively-damaged proteins. We also discuss recent work showing that only newly synthesized proteins which have incurred oxidative damage are targeted for degradation by the UPS whereas the turnover of oxidatively-damaged, long-lived proteins is largely unchanged. Additionally, we review recent work describing how polyubiquitylation influences the sorting of damaged proteins into one of two novel intracellular compartments. Finally, we discuss how the UPS modulates the stability and activity of Nrf2, the major anti-oxidant transcription factor in the retina.

51.1 Oxidative Stress and Age-Related Macular Degeneration

AMD is a leading cause of irreversible vision loss in people over 60 years of age. The pathogenesis of this disease is multifactorial and appears to involve a combination of environmental, metabolic, and genetic inputs. Morphological changes and

S.M. Plafker (✉)
University of Oklahoma Health Sciences Center, Oklahoma City, OK, 73104, USA
e-mail: scott-plafker@ouhsc.edu

R.E. Anderson et al. (eds.), *Retinal Degenerative Diseases*, Advances in Experimental Medicine and Biology 664, DOI 10.1007/978-1-4419-1399-9_51,
© Springer Science+Business Media, LLC 2010

disruptions to the numerous cell types in the macular region accompany the onset and progression of AMD. Among the cells and structures that become altered are the retinal pigment epithelium (RPE), the photoreceptors, the choriocapillaris, and Bruch's membrane. The two types of AMD, wet and dry, are distinguishable. Wet (or exudative) AMD is characterized by neovascularization in the choriocapillaris and fluid leakage in the subretinal macular region whereas the hallmark of dry (or atrophic) AMD is degeneration of photoreceptors and the RPE monolayer. Both types are characterized by irregular and/or loss of pigmentation from the RPE. In addition, although dry AMD is more prevalent, it can progress to the wet form thus putting the patient at risk for more severe vision loss (all reviewed in Nowak 2006).

Oxidative stress is widely held to be a significant pathological factor in AMD progression. Clinical evidence supporting this comes from numerous studies, most notably, the Age-Related Eye Disease Study (AREDS) (2001). This study showed that high doses of anti-oxidants and zinc slowed wet AMD progression and vision loss. Biochemical evidence implicating oxidative stress stems from the observation that the toxic, lipid-rich, granules that become deposited between the RPE monolayer and Bruch's membrane are largely composed of oxidized proteins and lipids and are a hallmark of AMD pathology. These aggregates grow in size to become drusen and trigger a cascade of pro-inflammatory processes involving the complement system, acute phase proteins, and cytokines. This in turn promotes new blood vessel formation, fluid leakage, and macular scarring, leading to visual loss (reviewed in Ehrlich et al. 2008). Compelling experimental evidence that oxidative damage is a root cause of AMD comes from recent work by Hollyfield et al. (2008). These investigators demonstrated that major pathological hallmarks of dry AMD could be reconstituted in mice immunized with carboxyethylpyrrole (CEP)-derivatized albumin. CEP is a unique oxidation product of docosahexaenoic acid, the major polyunsaturated fatty acid in the photoreceptor outer segments of most vertebrates (Benolken et al. 1973). Importantly, CEP is adducted to proteins in drusen deposits (Crabb et al. 2002) and CEP-adducted protein levels are elevated in the plasma of AMD patients (Gu et al. 2003).

51.2 The Ubiquitin Proteolytic System (UPS) and Oxidative Stress in the Retina

Ubiquitin (Ub) is a highly conserved, 76 amino acid polypeptide that gets post-translationally attached to target proteins by the coordinated actions of a Ub-activating enzyme (E1), a Ub-conjugating enzyme (E2), and a Ub protein ligase (E3) (Fig. 51.1). Ub is first activated in an ATP-dependent manner by the E1. The activated Ub is then transferred to the active site cysteine of an E2 in a transesterification reaction. A third enzymatic component, an E3 protein ligase, cooperates with the E2 to transfer Ub to substrates. Substrate selection and specificity are conferred primarily through the pairing of particular E2–E3 combinations. After transfer of the first Ub to a target lysine, subsequent Ubs are attached sequentially to a lysine

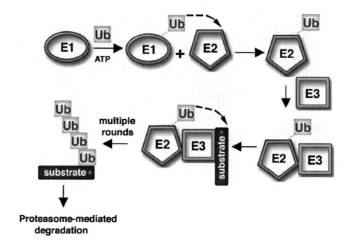

Fig. 51.1 Cartoon of the enzyme cascade that attaches Ub to substrates. The types of enzymes that cooperate to transfer Ub to substrates are illustrated. Of note, E3 ligases can be single polypeptides or alternatively, multi-subunit complexes

of the previously added Ub. When lysine 48 is utilized for polyUb chain assembly, the resulting polyUb structure signals delivery of the modified target to the 26S proteasome, a macromolecular assembly of proteases, for destruction. In contrast, polyUb chains constructed through other lysines (e.g., K63) of Ub typically result in non-proteolytic outcomes. Protein targets can also be regulated in non-proteolytic ways by monoubiquitylation. Balance in the Ub system is achieved by a set of deubiquitylating isopeptidases that cleave Ub off of substrates (reviewed in Fang and Weissman 2004).

Efforts to characterize the UPS in the retina have revealed that multiple retinal cell types have distinct subsets of UPS components. For example, four different Ub conjugating enzymes ($E2_{14 K}$, $E2_{20 K}$, $E2_{25 K}$, and $E2_{35 K}$) have been identified in bovine rod outer segments (Obin et al. 1996). PGP 9.5, a Ub carboxy-terminal hydrolase, is only present in retinal ganglion and horizontal cells (Bonfanti et al. 1992), but the Ub hydrolase, UCH-L3, is enriched in photoreceptor inner segments (Sano et al. 2006). We have observed that a subset of highly conserved Ub conjugating enzymes, the class III E2s, are differentially expressed in the mouse retina (Fig. 51.2). These three enzymes are functional homologues of a pair of yeast E2s, Ubc4 and Ubc5, that play essential roles in mediating the degradation of misfolded and oxidatively-damaged proteins (Kaganovich et al. 2008; Matuschewski et al. 1996; Medicherla and Goldberg 2008). The mouse versions of these enzymes are called UbcM2, UbcM3, and UBE2E2, and each is identical to its human counterpart. These enzymes are distinguished from one another by unique N-terminal extensions of 40–60 residues (Matuschewski et al. 1996).

To analyze the distribution of the class III E2s in the retina, we raised rabbit polyclonal antibodies against the unique N-terminal extensions and labeled

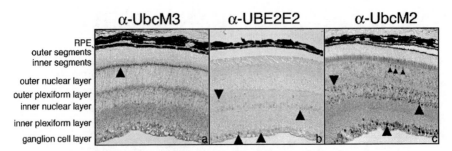

Fig. 51.2 Differential expression of class III E2s in the mouse eye. Paraffin-embedded sections from 8-month old SvEv129 mice were immunolabeled with the indicated antibodies. The *black arrowheads* highlight specific labeling in each panel. Serial sections from the same eye were labeled individually with each antibody

paraffin-embedded eye sections from 8-month old, SvEv129 mice. a-UbcM2 immunolabeling was most prominent in ganglion cells (Fig. 51.2, panel c) as well as the inner nuclear layer. In addition, a subpopulation of photoreceptors was labeled (Fig. 51.2, panel c, small arrowheads) as were the nuclei in the RPE layer. a-UbcM3 yielded a punctate pattern of immunolabeling at the interface between the inner and outer segments of the photoreceptors (Fig. 51.2, panel a). We speculate that this may represent labeling of Mueller cells. a-UBE2E2 faintly but specifically immunolabeled retinal ganglion cells and a subpopulation of nuclei of the inner nuclear layer (Fig. 51.2, panel b). Retinal substrates for the abovementioned UPS enzymes remain to be determined.

The retina is exquisitely susceptible to oxidative damage due to its robust oxygen consumption, exceptionally high content of polyunsaturated fatty acids, and exposure to bright light. Collectively, these factors create an environment of redox flux in which proteins, DNA, and lipids become oxidatively damaged. Removal and/or reversal of these oxidatively damaged biomolecules is required to prevent the toxicity that can result from their accumulation. Such accumulation is a hallmark of numerous neurodegenerative disorders including AMD (reviewed in Sas et al. 2007). Recent work has shed new light on the mechanisms by which cells process, sequester, and eliminate misfolded and aggregated proteins. In an elegant series of experiments using both yeast (i.e., *S. cerevisiae*) and mammalian cells, two novel, cellular 'compartments' for sequestering misfolded proteins were characterized (Kaganovich et al. 2008). One is a juxtanuclear quality control compartment, named JUNQ, which is enriched with chaperone proteins and proteasomes. This inclusion accumulates soluble misfolded proteins that can either be processed for Ub-dependent degradation or alternatively, refolded. In contrast, insoluble, aggregated proteins are sequestered in an inclusion termed the IPOD (insoluble protein deposit). The IPOD is localized peripherally (perivacuolar in yeast) and accumulates non-diffusing aggregates that cannot be salvaged. Numerous autophagic marker proteins co-localize with the IPOD. Importantly, the IPOD is the site of accumulation of disease-associated, amyloidogenic proteins such as prion proteins and Huntington's protein. Intriguingly, polyubiquitylation is a critical factor in determining the solubility of a misfolded protein and thus whether the protein gets sorted to the JUNQ or the IPOD. These findings imply that the UPS could potentially be harnessed (e.g., over-expression of particular UPS enzymes) to direct oxidatively damaged and misfolded proteins to the JUNQ for destruction and thereby decrease the kinetics with which toxic aggregates accumulate in IPODs within the retinal cells of AMD patients.

The UPS plays a primary role in destroying misfolded and damaged proteins (e.g., oxidant-induced) and this function is conserved from yeast to man (reviewed in Ross and Pickart 2004). Multiple lines of evidence implicate a critical function for the UPS in countering oxidative stress in the retina. The Taylor laboratory has had a long-standing interest in the interplay between oxidative stress and the UPS in various ocular tissues. These investigators have produced a body of work supporting the notion that the UPS selectively degrades oxidatively damaged proteins in the retina and lens and that inhibition of the UPS, either by pharmacological means or with mutant Ub, leads to the deleterious accumulation of oxidized proteins (e.g., Dudek et al. 2005; Shang et al. 2001).

Despite the widely held notion that the UPS indiscriminately disposes of oxidatively damaged proteins to prevent their toxic accumulation, Medicherla and Goldberg have recently demonstrated that in *S. cerevisiae*, only newly synthesized proteins that have incurred oxidative damage are targeted for degradation by the UPS. In contrast, the turnover of oxidatively-damaged, long-lived proteins ($\geq$ 60 min post-synthesis) is largely unchanged (Medicherla and Goldberg 2008). The authors interpret these findings to indicate that nascently-synthesized proteins which undergo oxidative damage are prevented from folding properly and this unfolding, and/or denaturation, is what triggers their degradation by the UPS. In contrast, because 'older' proteins are already in their final conformation and in complexes with their binding partners, oxidative damage does not drive their unfolding. The 'older' proteins are thus more resistant to being denatured by oxidants and subsequently less susceptible to degradation by the UPS. It remains to be determined whether this scenario holds true for human cells but if so, it could provide new insights into the etiology of AMD and other neurodegenerative disorders. For example, it implies that the protein aggregates that accumulate in AMD patients are derived mainly from newly-synthesized, oxidant-damaged proteins. As a corollary, it suggests that enhancing the capacity of the UPS to degrade this class of compromised proteins may be a legitimate therapeutic strategy for treating AMD. Therefore, it should be a high priority to validate the findings of Medicherla and Goldberg in mammalian retinas and also to determine the fate of oxidatively-damaged 'older' proteins, many of which are likely being inactivated, though not denatured, in the highly oxidizing environment of the retina.

51.3 The UPS and the Cytoprotective Transcription Factor, Nrf2

Not only does the UPS mediate the degradation of misfolded and damaged proteins, but it also functions to counter the deleterious effects of oxidative stress in other ways. Perhaps most importantly for the retina is the role that the UPS plays in regulating the stability of nuclear-factor-E2-related factor 2 (**Nrf2**). Nrf2 is a critical anti-oxidant transcription factor that binds to a cis-acting regulatory element, called the antioxidant response element (ARE), embedded in the promoters of phase 2 genes. Phase 2 genes encode detoxification enzymes and other factors responsible for eliminating reactive oxygen species (ROS). Thus, in response to an oxidative stress, Nrf2 induces the expression of an anti-oxidant defense system that re-establishes redox homeostasis (all reviewed in Li and Kong 2009).

The degradation of Nrf2 by the UPS is directly coupled to cellular redox state (Nguyen et al. 2003). That is, in the absence of an oxidative insult, Nrf2 is constitutively destroyed by the UPS. Oxidative stress, however, arrests this degradation, and the stabilized Nrf2 is now able to translocate into the nucleus and induce phase 2 gene transcription (Fig. 51.3). This control of Nrf2 stability can be readily observed in vivo by comparing the steady levels of Nrf2 in the presence and absence of either a proteasome inhibitor (e.g., MG132) or chemical inducers of oxidative stress (e.g., tert-butylhydroquinone (tBHQ)) (Fig. 51.4). Nrf2 degradation during redox homeostasis is mediated by a specific UPS E3 ligase called CUL3[Keap1] (Kobayashi et al. 2004). CUL3[Keap1] is comprised of three core proteins–cullin 3 (CUL3), Keap1, and ROC1 (Fig. 51.5). CUL3 is a scaffold. Through its C-terminal domain, it binds the RING-finger protein, ROC1. ROC1 recruits and coordinates an Ub-charged E2 into the complex. The N-terminal domain of CUL3 binds the substrate adaptor, Keap1.

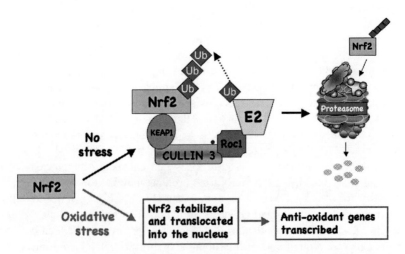

Fig. 51.3 The stability and activity of Nrf2 are redox-sensitive. Nrf2 is constitutively degraded by CUL3[Keap1] and the 26S proteasome in the absence of stress but is stabilized in response to oxidative stress. Stabilized Nrf2 induces the expression of a battery of anti-oxidant genes

Fig. 51.4 Nrf2 stability is
controlled by cellular redox
status and by the UPS. a-Nrf2
western blot demonstrating
that endogenous Nrf2 in
RPE-1 cells is stabilized by
oxidative stress (TBHQ) or
by proteasome inhibition
(MG132). ETOH and DMSO
are the vehicles for TBHQ
and MG132, respectively.
The *asterisk* marks a
non-specific band

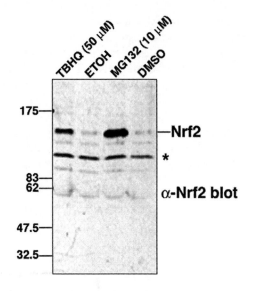

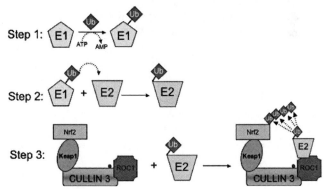

Fig. 51.5 Nrf2 ubiquitylation is mediated by the multi-subunit E3 ligase CUL3^{Keap1}. Step 1: Ub
is activated by the E1 enzyme in an ATP-dependent manner. Step 2: The activated Ub is transferred
to an E2 enzyme. Step 3: The Ub-charged E2 is recruited to the ROC1 component of CUL3^{Keap1}
and directly transfers Ub to Nrf2. Nrf2 is recruited to CUL3^{Keap1} by the Keap1 substrate adaptor.
The small ball on CUL3 is Nedd8, a Ub-like protein that regulates the activity of CUL3-based E3
ligases

Keap1, in turn, recruits Nrf2 into the complex. Ub-modified Nrf2 is subsequently
degraded by the 26S proteasome. The capacity of CUL3^{Keap1} to conjugate polyUb
chains to Nrf2 is regulated by a small Ub-like modifier called Nedd8. Nedd8 is
covalently attached and then removed from CUL3 by a dedicated set of enzymes
and this dynamic cycling is required for Nrf2 ubiquitylation (all reviewed in Bosu
and Kipreos 2008).

Strategies to potentiate the cytoprotective activity of Nrf2 have centered on
stabilizing the transcription factor by repressing CUL3^{Keap1} function. CUL3^{Keap1}

repression in vivo can be accomplished through multiple mechanisms all of which culminate in the dissociation of the Keap1:Nrf2 complex from CUL3. The best characterized of these mechanisms is predicated on modifying redox-sensitive cysteine residues within Keap1 (Dinkova-Kostova et al. 2002; Levonen et al. 2004). In particular, Cys151 of Keap1 has been definitively shown to function as a redox sensor that mediates the binding of Keap1 to CUL3 (Eggler et al. 2007; Zhang et al. 2004). Current models support the notion that oxidant-induced modification of Cys151 dissociates Keap1:CUL3 binding and results in Nrf2 stabilization. As predicted for a redox sensor, mutation of this cysteine to serine blocks the capacity of Keap1 to detect alterations in intracellular redox status and to promote the dissociation of Keap1:Nrf2 from CUL3 in response to oxidative stress (Zhang and Hannink 2003; Zhang et al. 2004). Thus, Nrf2 is not efficiently stabilized in cells expressing Keap1 (C151S) following an oxidative insult (Yamamoto et al. 2008). This same cysteine is also targeted by the dietary anti-oxidant, sulforaphane, an isothiocyanate found in broccoli and other cruciferous vegetables (Zhang et al. 2004). In this way, sulforaphane-modified Keap1 functionally mimics an oxidant stress and results in the stabilization and activation of Nrf2 in homeostatic cells.

The central role of Nrf2 in protecting and preserving retinal health and function has been revealed through recent studies exploring the therapeutic potential of sulforaphane. Sulforaphane administration has been demonstrated to protect against photoreceptor degeneration in rodent models of experimental light stress (e.g., Tanito et al. 2005; Kong et al. 2007). In addition, the Talalay laboratory (the discoverers of sulforaphane) (Zhang et al. 1992) has shown that the compound can protect cultured retinal pigment epithelial cells from photooxidative damage (Gao and Talalay 2004). These studies and others support the idea that sulforaphane could have potential clinical utility in preventing and/or slowing the progress of retinal degeneration in AMD patients. Furthermore, they provide a rationale for further pursuing strategies to enhance Nrf2 stabilization by manipulating the UPS. Unlike dietary anti-oxidants, which require high doses, do not specifically target the retina, and require frequent administration, ocular gene therapy-based approaches targeting particular UPS enzymes in either the RPE or photoreceptors could potentially overcome these shortcomings and greatly advance efforts to prevent AMD and/or retard its progression.

References

AREDS (2001) A randomized, placebo-controlled, clinical trial of high-dose supplementation with vitamins C and E, beta carotene, and zinc for age-related macular degeneration and vision loss: AREDS Report No. 8. Arch Ophthalmol 119:1417–1436

Benolken RM, Anderson RE, Wheeler TG (1973) Membrane fatty acids associated with the electrical response in visual excitation. Science 182:1253–1254

Bonfanti L, Candeo P, Piccinini M et al (1992) Distribution of protein gene product 9.5 (PGP 9.5) in the vertebrate retina: evidence that immunoreactivity is restricted to mammalian horizontal and ganglion cells. J Comp Neurol 322:35–44

Bosu DR, Kipreos ET (2008) Cullin-RING ubiquitin ligases: global regulation and activation cycles. Cell Div 3:7

Crabb JW, Miyagi M, Gu X et al (2002) Drusen proteome analysis: an approach to the etiology of age-related macular degeneration. Proc Natl Acad Sci U S A 99:14682–14687

Dinkova-Kostova AT, Holtzclaw WD, Cole RN et al (2002) Direct evidence that sulfhydryl groups of Keap1 are the sensors regulating induction of phase 2 enzymes that protect against carcinogens and oxidants. Proc Natl Acad Sci U S A 99:11908–11913

Dudek EJ, Shang F, Valverde P et al (2005) Selectivity of the ubiquitin pathway for oxidatively modified proteins: relevance to protein precipitation diseases. FASEB J 19:1707–1709

Eggler AL, Luo Y, van Breemen RB et al (2007) Identification of the highly reactive cysteine 151 in the chemopreventive agent-sensor Keap1 protein is method-dependent. Chem Res Toxicol 20:1878–1884

Ehrlich R, Harris A, Kheradiya NS et al (2008) Age-related macular degeneration and the aging eye. Clin Interv Aging 3:473–482

Fang S, Weissman AM (2004) A field guide to ubiquitylation. Cell Mol Life Sci 61:1546–1561

Gao X, Talalay P (2004) Induction of phase 2 genes by sulforaphane protects retinal pigment epithelial cells against photooxidative damage. Proc Natl Acad Sci U S A 101:10446–10451

Gu X, Meer SG, Miyagi M et al (2003) Carboxyethylpyrrole protein adducts and autoantibodies, biomarkers for age-related macular degeneration. J Biol Chem 278:42027–42035

Hollyfield JG, Bonilha VL, Rayborn ME et al (2008) Oxidative damage-induced inflammation initiates age-related macular degeneration. Nat Med 14:194–198

Kaganovich D, Kopito R, Frydman J (2008) Misfolded proteins partition between two distinct quality control compartments. Nature 454:1088–1095

Kobayashi A, Kang MI, Okawa H et al (2004) Oxidative stress sensor Keap1 functions as an adaptor for Cul3-based E3 ligase to regulate proteasomal degradation of Nrf2. Mol Cell Biol 24:7130–7139

Kong L, Tanito M, Hung Z et al (2007) Delay of photoreceptor degeneration in tubby mouse by sulforaphane. J Neurochem 101(4):1041–1052

Levonen AL, Landar A, Ramachandran A et al (2004) Cellular mechanisms of redox cell signalling: role of cysteine modification in controlling antioxidant defences in response to electrophilic lipid oxidation products. Biochem J 378:373–382

Li W, Kong AN (2009) Molecular mechanisms of Nrf2-mediated antioxidant response. Mol Carcinog 48:91–104

Matuschewski K, Hauser HP, Treier M et al (1996) Identification of a novel family of ubiquitin-conjugating enzymes with distinct amino-terminal extensions. J Biol Chem 271:2789–2794

Medicherla B, Goldberg AL (2008) Heat shock and oxygen radicals stimulate ubiquitin-dependent degradation mainly of newly synthesized proteins. J Cell Biol 182:663–673

Nguyen T, Sherratt PJ, Huang HC et al (2003) Increased protein stability as a mechanism that enhances Nrf2-mediated transcriptional activation of the antioxidant response element. Degradation of Nrf2 by the 26 S proteasome. J Biol Chem 278:4536–4541

Nowak JZ (2006) Age-related macular degeneration (AMD): pathogenesis and therapy. Pharmacol Rep 58:353–363

Obin MS, Jahngen-Hodge J, Nowell T et al (1996) Ubiquitinylation and ubiquitin-dependent proteolysis in vertebrate photoreceptors (rod outer segments). Evidence for ubiquitinylation of Gt and rhodopsin. J Biol Chem 271:14473–14484

Ross CA, Pickart CM (2004) The ubiquitin-proteasome pathway in Parkinson's disease and other neurodegenerative diseases. Trends Cell Biol 14:703–711

Sano Y, Furuta A, Setsuie R et al (2006) Photoreceptor cell apoptosis in the retinal degeneration of Uchl3-deficient mice. Am J Pathol 169:132–141

Sas K, Robotka H, Toldi J et al (2007) Mitochondria, metabolic disturbances, oxidative stress and the kynurenine system, with focus on neurodegenerative disorders. J Neurol Sci 257:221–239

Shang F, Nowell TR Jr, Taylor A (2001) Removal of oxidatively damaged proteins from lens cells by the ubiquitin-proteasome pathway. Exp Eye Res 73:229–238

Tanito M, Masutani H, Kim YC, Nishikawa M, Ohira A, Yodoi J (2005) Sulforaphane induces thioredoxin through the antioxidant-responsive element and attenuates retinal light damage in mice. Invest Ophthalmol Vis Sci 46(3):979–987

Yamamoto T, Suzuki T, Kobayashi A et al (2008) Physiological significance of reactive cysteine residues of Keap1 in determining Nrf2 activity. Mol Cell Biol 28:2758–2770

Zhang DD, Hannink M (2003) Distinct cysteine residues in Keap1 are required for Keap1-dependent ubiquitination of Nrf2 and for stabilization of Nrf2 by chemopreventive agents and oxidative stress. Mol Cell Biol 23:8137–8151

Zhang DD, Lo SC, Cross JV et al (2004) Keap1 is a redox-regulated substrate adaptor protein for a Cul3-dependent ubiquitin ligase complex. Mol Cell Biol 24:10941–10953

Zhang Y, Talalay P, Cho CG et al (1992) A major inducer of anticarcinogenic protective enzymes from broccoli: isolation and elucidation of structure. Proc Natl Acad Sci U S A 89:2399–2403

Chapter 52
Slit-Robo Signaling in Ocular Angiogenesis

Haoyu Chen, Mingzhi Zhang, Shibo Tang, Nyall R. London, Dean Y. Li, and Kang Zhang

Abstract Slit-Robo signaling was firstly discovered as a major repellent pathway at the midline of the central nervous system. Intense investigation found that this pathway also plays an important role in other biological process including angiogenesis. Robo4 is the vascular endothelial cell specific member of Robo family. It was found that Slit-Robo signaling can inhibit endothelial cell migration, tube formation and vascular permeability. Slit-Robo signaling also plays an important role in embryonic and tumor angiogenesis. In animal model of ocular angiogenesis, addition of Slit inhibited laser induced choroidal neovascularization, oxygen induced retinopathy and VEGF induced retinal permeability in a Robo4 dependent manner. Recent data demonstrates that Robo1 and Robo4 form a heterodimer in endothelial cells, The role of this heterodimer in counteracting VEGF signaling is unknown. Further investigation is required to better understand Slit-Robo signaling and develop novel therapy for angiogenesis.

52.1 Ocular Angiogenesis

Angiogenesis, the growth of new blood vessels from pre-existing vessels, is an important biological process involved in several physiologic and pathological conditions. These include development of embryo vasculature, would healing, female reproductive cycling, tumor growth and metastasis, ischemic cardiovascular diseases, ocular disorders and so on. The eye is an optic transparent organ, which allows in vivo observation of retina and choroid with the assistant of some optic instruments. Therefore, the eye provides a valuable model to study angiogenesis

H. Chen (✉)
Joint Shantou International Eye Center, Shantou University and the Chinese University of Hong Kong, North Dongxia Road, Shantou, 515041 China; Moran Eye Center, University of Utah, Salt Lake City, Utah 84112 USA
e-mail: drchenhaoyu@gmail.com

R.E. Anderson et al. (eds.), *Retinal Degenerative Diseases*, Advances in Experimental Medicine and Biology 664, DOI 10.1007/978-1-4419-1399-9_52,
© Springer Science+Business Media, LLC 2010

(Campochiaro and Hackett 2003). Development of retinal vasculature is an example of physiological angiogenesis. Pathological angiogenesis or neovascularization may occur in several ocular tissues, such as cornea, iris, anterior chamber angle, retina and choroid, and usually result in severe vision impairment even blindness.

Age-related macular degeneration (AMD) is one of the leading causes of irreversible blindness in developed countries (Friedman et al. 2004). The prevalence of AMD in the developing world such as China is increasing as well (Zou et al. 2005). Among two clinical types, wet AMD usually results in more severe vision loss due to neovascularization of choroid by breakthrough of Bruch's membrane to sub subretinal or sub retinal pigment epithelium space, hemorrhage and eventually fibrous formation. Diabetic retinopathy (DR) is the most common cause of legal blindness in working-age United States adults and accounts for 10% of new blindness at all ages (Varma et al. 2007). The most severe type of DR, proliferative diabetic retinopathy (PDR) is characterized by retinal neovascularization, eventually vitreoretinal hemorrhage, tractional retinal detachment and vision loss. Macular edema is a clinical syndrome related to retinal or choroidal neovascularization. It occurs when fluid and proteins accumulated at macular region secondary to the leakage of inner or outer blood-retina barrier.

The imbalance of angiogenic and anti-angiogenic factors is the major mechanism of angiogenesis. Vascular endothelial growth factor (VEGF) is the most potent angiogenic factor and anti-VEGF therapy has been successfully showed inhibiting tumor and macular degeneration (Rosenfeld et al. 2006). However, more and more novel signaling pathways have been discovered by intense investigation. These findings help us better understand the pathogenesis of angiogenesis and provide novel therapeutic targets.

52.2 Slit-Robo Signaling in Axon Guidance

The nerve fibers and blood vessels follow parallel routes in peripheral tissues. For example, in the retina, the relationships between retinal blood vessel and ganglion cell axons are accompanied by each other in a radial orientation (Gariano and Gardner 2005). More importantly, the pattern of growth of nerve fiber and blood vessel are similar too. During development, there is a special structure at the distal tip of neuron axon called growth cone, which can dynamically extend filopodia to explore repulsive or attractive guidance cues in the spatial environment, interpret these signals and direct the growth of axon. Similarly, there is specialized endothelial cell, termed tip cell, covers the distal end of vascular sprouts. Tip cells dynamically form filopodial extension and recognize signals at surrounding cells and the matrix environment (Adams 2006). Based on the structure and functional similarity, it is suggested that the signals controlling axon pathfinding may also control endothelial tip cell guidance and angiogenic sprouting of blood vessels. There are several examples of these pathways, including Ephrins-Eph receptors, Semaphorins-Neuropilins, Netrins-UNC5 and Slit-Robo.

The *Slit* and *Robo* gene was first identified from Drosophila melanogaster. There are three family members of Slit identified till now, Slit1, Slit2 and Slit3. The Slits are large, secreted multidomain glycoproteins including leucine-rich repeats, EGF-like repeats, laminin G domain, and C-terminal cysteine-rich knot (Rothberg et al. 1990). Robo is the receptor of Slit, and there are four Robo family members identified so far, Robo1, Robo2, Robo3 and Robo4. Robo is a single-pass transmembrane receptor with an extracellular region containing immunoglobulin (Ig) domains and fibronectin type III repeats, and an intracellular tail composed of conserved motifs (CC0, CC1, CC2, and CC3) (Kidd et al. 1998).

Slit-Robo signaling was first discovered as a major repellent pathway at the midline of the central nervous system. Activation of Slit-Robo signaling triggers changesin cytoskeletal structure within the growth cone and results in axon repulsion (Li et al. 1999). With extensive investigation, many other Robo-dependent Slit functions were discovered, including axon branching and migration of neurons, migration of leucocytes and inflammation, migration of endothelial cells, development of the lung and kidney, tumor angiogenesis and metastasis (Hohenester et al. 2006). We will discuss the role of Slit-Robo signaling in angiogenesis in detail below.

52.3 Slit-Robo Signaling in Angiogenesis

The endothelial cell specific Robo family member, called Robo4 or magic round-about, was firstly identified using a bioinformatic strategy. Robo4 has similar domains in cytoplasmic region and transmembrane domain with other Robo members. However, there are only two IgG and two fibronectin domains in the ligand-binding region of Robo4, which is quite different from the five IgG and three fibronectin domains of the other Robo family members (Huminiecki et al. 2002). It was reported that Robo4 bind to Slit2 in immunoprecipitation and immunofluorescence, despite its unique extracellular domain structure (Park et al. 2003).

In vitro studies showed that Robo4 expressed specific in endothelial cells but not in neural, vascular smooth muscle cells or other types of cell (Huminiecki et al. 2002; Jones et al. 2008), while Robo1, Robo2, Robo3 did not express in human microvascular endothelial cell (HMVEC) (Park et al. 2003). In vivo, Robo4 expressed specifically in embryonic vasculature and predominantly in adult vasculature (Park et al. 2003). Further investigation revealed that Robo4 expression was limited to stalk cells but not tip cells in the developing retinal vasculature (Jones et al. 2008). The expression of Robo4 was upregulated by hypoxia in endothelial cells (Huminiecki et al. 2002) and mice retina (Jones et al. 2008). Robo4 is also over expressed in tumors endothelial cells compared to normal adult endothelial cells in numerous solid tumors (Huminiecki et al. 2002; Seth et al. 2005).

There is controversy on the function of Slit-Robo signaling in endothelial cells and angiogenesis. It was reported that the endothelial cell migration induced by VEGF or Human Embryonic Kidney 293 cells conditioned media was inhibit by Slit-myc conditioned media while the proliferation was not affected. The inhibitory effect of Slit-myc conditioned media on HMVEC migration is blocked by depleting the conditioned media with either N-Robo1 or anti-myc antibody (Park et al. 2003). In another study, endothelial cell migration induced by VEGF, fibroblast growth factors (FGF) or fetal bovine serum was inhibited by transfection of Robo4 but not soluble Robo4. The migration effect of VEGF was also inhibited by external addition of Slit2 and rescued by addition of soluble Robo4 (Seth et al. 2005). It was also reported that recombinant N terminal cleavage of Slit2 prevented the platelet-derived growth factor (PDGF)-stimulated migration of vascular smooth muscle cells (Liu et al. 2006). Endothelial cell migration, tube formation and permeability induced by VEGF have been found to be inhibited by Slit2 and the inhibitory effects were lost in *Robo4* knockout endothelial cells (Jones et al. 2008). These finding suggested that Slit-Robo signaling is an inhibitor of angiogenesis. However, it was also reported that Slit-Robo signaling has pro-angiogenic effects and blockage of Slit-Robo signaling can inhibit angiogenesis. Recombinant Slit2 protein was reported to attract endothelial cells and promote tube formation in a Robo1-dependent manner (Wang et al. 2003). It was also reported that soluble Robo4 inhibited VEGF- and FGF-stimulated endothelial cell migration and endothelial proliferation in vitro, inhibited tube formation in the rat aortic ring assay *Ex vivo* and angiogenesis in the rodent subcutaneous sponge model in vivo (Suchting et al. 2005).

The role of Robo4 in embryonic angiogenesis was studied in zebrafish. Both overexpression and knockdown of zebrafish *Robo4* resulted in asynchronous intersomitic vessel (ISV) sprouting, culminating in a reduction and misdirection of the intersomitic vessels. The vascular phenotype in *Robo4* knockdown was rescued by human Robo4 expression (Bedell et al. 2005). In another report, injection of zebrafish Robo4 disrupted ISVs sprouting from dorsal aorta. Furthermore, angioblasts isolated from Robo4 embryos showed movement that resemble cells actively searching for guidance and continue rolling in a nondirectional manner (Kaur et al. 2008).

A role for Slit-Robo signaling in tumor angiogenesis has also been reported. Robo4 expression was increased on tumor vessels of brain, colon, breast, kidney, and bladder. Further histological studies found that the expression of Robo4 was upregulated in site of active angiogenesis (Huminiecki et al. 2002; Seth et al. 2005). Deletion or epigenetic modification of the Slit–Robo genes has been identified in the progression of numerous cancers (Dallol et al. 2002; Narayan et al. 2006). Blockade of Slit2 activity in tumor bearing mice through overexpression of RoboN or addition of a monoclonal antibody that blocks Robo1–Slit binding gave reduced tumor microvessel densities and tumor masses (Wang et al. 2003).

52.4 Slit-Robo Signaling in Ocular Angiogenesis

In the mouse retina, Robo4 is expressed specifically in vascular endothelial cells, which was detected by immunohistochemistry. While Slit2 expression was detected in cells near the retinal blood vessels. In oxygen induced retinopathy mice model, the expression of Robo4 was up-regulated while the other *Robo* or *Slit* genes were not (Jones et al. 2008).

Three mice models were setup to investigate the roles of Slit-Robo signaling in ocular angiogenesis. Laser-induced choroidal neovascularization, which mimics age-related macular degeneration, is commonly used to study choroidal angiogenesis in the mouse. Intravitreal administration of Slit2 reduced choroidal neovascularization in wild type mice; however, the effect was lost in *Robo4* null mice. Oxygen induced retinopathy is the most common used animal model for retinal neovascularization that mimics the ischemia-induced angiogenesis observed in proliferative diabetic retinopathy and retinopathy of prematurity. Similarly, intravitreal administration of recombinant Slit2 markedly reduced area of isolectin labeled retinal neovascularization and of FITC-dextran leakage from retinal vasculature in wild type but not in *Robo4* null mice. The third model used is VEGF induced retinal permeability which mimics macular edema. Similarly, intravitreal administration of recombinant Slit2 markedly reduced leakage of Evans blue from retinal vasculature in wild type mice. This effect was not observed in *Robo4* null mice. These finding suggested that Slit-Robo Signaling can inhibit ocular angiogenesis in Robo4 dependent pattern. Considering the expression of robo4 on stalk cells but not tip cells, Slit-Robo signaling may provides a tonic pathway that stabilized ocular blood vessels (Jones et al. 2008).

52.5 Signaling Pathway of Slit-Robo System in Angiogenesis

There is controversy on the Slit-Robo binding in vascular system. Overexpressed human Slit2 coimmunoprecipitated with Robo4, indicating direct binding of Slit2 to Robo4 (Park et al. 2003). Overexpression of Robo4 blocked migration of endothelial cells towards VEGF and FGF and that this effect was dependent on Slit2 binding to the extracellular domain of Robo4 (Seth et al. 2005). The inhibitory effects of Slit2 on endothelial cells and ocular angiogenesis are dependent on Robo4 and loss in *Robo4* null mice (Jones et al. 2008). These results suggested that Robo4 is a receptor for Slit2 on endothelial cells. However, it was also reported that Robo1 forms a heterodimeric complex with Robo4. Robo1 is essential for Robo4-mediated filopodia induction (Sheldon et al. 2009). Robo1 and Robo4 interact and share molecules such as Slit2, Mena and Vilse, a Cdc42-GAP (Kaur et al. 2008).

Since Slit-Robo signaling play important role in cell migration in both neuron and endothelial cells, the signaling pathway of Slit-Robo1 in neuron may also provides cue for downstream signaling of Slit-Robo4 in endothelial cell. The intracellular signaling that regulates the actin cytoskeleton is a good candidate of the downstream signaling of Slit-Robo. Robo4 can bind the Mena, an actin regulatory protein, suggesting that Robo4, like Robo1, can control cell movement by locally remodel the actin cytoskeleton (Park et al. 2003). Addition of Slit2 to endothelial cells led to the inhibition of FAK phosphorylation (Seth et al. 2005). Robo4 knockdown endothelial cells show up regulation of Rho small guanosine triphos-phatase (GTPase). Zebrafish Robo4 rescues both Rho GTPase homeostasis and serum reduced chemotaxis in Robo4 knockdown cells. In addition, this study mech-anistically implicates IRSp53 in the signaling nexus between activated Cdc42 and Mena, both of which are involved with Robo4 signaling in endothelial cells (Kaur et al. 2008).

VEGF and PDGF signaling are key pathways in angiogenesis; therefore it is nec-essary to test the interaction of Slit-Robo signaling with VEGF and PDGF signaling. Treatment of endothelial cells with Slit2 reduced VEGF-165 stimulated phosphory-lation of the Src family of nonreceptor tyrosine kinases and Src-dependent activation of the Rho family small GTPase Rac1 (Jones et al. 2008). Recombinant N terminal cleavage of Slit2 prevented PDGF-mediated activation of GTPase Rac1 and for-mation of lamellipodia in smooth muscle cells, both of which are involved in cell motility (Liu et al. 2006).

52.6 Perspective

Slit-Robo signaling has been shown to play an important role in angiogenesis including ocular angiogenesis. The application of Slit can inhibit ocular angio-genesis in disease models and counteract the ability of VEGF in mice. However, controversy exists still whether it is pro-angiogenic or anti-angiogenic signaling The details of Slit-Robo signaling are not fully understood, as well as how these signaling events affect the role of Slit-Robo signaling in pathogenesis of ocular angiogenesis. Therefore, more investigation is required to better understand the role of Slit-Robo in angiogenesis and develop novel therapeutic approaches for ocular angiogenesis diseases like age related macular degeneration, diabetic retinopathy and macular edema.

Acknowledgments We thank the following support to HC: Kaisi Funds at Sun Yat-sen University, JSIEC Starting grants; to ST: National Key Science and Technology Project from 'Tenth Five-Year Plan' of China, National Natural Science Foundation of China; to KZ: National Institutes of Health Grants R01EY14428, R01EY14448, P30EY014800, and GCRCM01-RR00064, Foundation Fighting Blindness, the Macular Vision Research Foundation, Veterans Affairs Merit Award, and Research to Prevent Blindness to NRL: the Ruth L. Kirschstein National Research Service Award.

References

Adams RH (2006) Nerve cell signposts in the blood vessel roadmap. Circ Res 98:440–442
Bedell VM, Yeo SY, Park KW et al (2005) roundabout4 is essential for angiogenesis in vivo. Proc Natl Acad Sci U S A 102:6373–6378
Campochiaro PA, Hackett SF (2003) Ocular neovascularization: a valuable model system. Oncogene 22:6537–6548
Dallol A, Forgacs E, Martinez A et al (2002) Tumour specific promoter region methylation of the human homologue of the Drosophila Roundabout gene DUTT1 (ROBO1) in human cancers. Oncogene 21:3020–3028

Friedman DS, O'Colmain BJ, Munoz B et al (2004) Prevalence of age-related macular degeneration in the United States. Arch Ophthalmol 122:564–572

Gariano RF, Gardner TW (2005) Retinal angiogenesis in development and disease. Nature 438:960–966

Hohenester E, Hussain S, Howitt JA (2006) Interaction of the guidance molecule slit with cellular receptors. Biochem Soc Trans 34:418–421

Huminiecki L, Gorn M, Suchting S et al (2002) Magic roundabout is a new member of the roundabout receptor family that is endothelial specific and expressed at sites of active angiogenesis. Genomics 79:547–552

Jones CA, London NR, Chen H et al (2008) Robo4 stabilizes the vascular network by inhibiting pathologic angiogenesis and endothelial hyperpermeability. Nat Med 14:448–453

Kaur S, Samant GV, Pramanik K et al (2008) Silencing of directional migration in roundabout4 knockdown endothelial cells. BMC Cell Biol 9:61

Kidd T, Brose K, Mitchell KJ et al (1998) Roundabout controls axon crossing of the CNS midline and defines a novel subfamily of evolutionarily conserved guidance receptors. Cell 92:205–215

Li HS, Chen JH, Wu W et al (1999) Vertebrate slit, a secreted ligand for the transmembrane protein roundabout, is a repellent for olfactory bulb axons. Cell 96:807–818

Liu D, Hou J, Hu X et al (2006) Neuronal chemorepellent Slit2 inhibits vascular smooth muscle cell migration by suppressing small GTPase Rac1 activation. Circ Res 98:480–489

Narayan G, Goparaju C, Arias-Pulido H et al (2006) Promoter hypermethylation-mediated inactivation of multiple Slit-Robo pathway genes in cervical cancer progression. Mol Cancer 5:16

Park KW, Morrison CM, Sorensen LK et al (2003) Robo4 is a vascular-specific receptor that inhibits endothelial migration. Dev Biol 261:251–267

Rosenfeld PJ, Brown DM, Heier JS et al (2006) Ranibizumab for neovascular age-related macular degeneration. N Engl J Med 355:1419–1431

Rothberg JM, Jacobs JR, Goodman CS et al (1990) Slit: an extracellular protein necessary for development of midline glia and commissural axon pathways contains both EGF and LRR domains. Genes Dev 4:2169–2187

Seth P, Lin Y, Hanai J et al (2005) Magic roundabout, a tumor endothelial marker: expression and signaling. Biochem Biophys Res Commun 332:533–541

Sheldon H, Andre M, Legg JA et al (2009) Active involvement of Robo1 and Robo4 in filopodia formation and endothelial cell motility mediated via WASP and other actin nucleation-promoting factors. FASEB J 23:513–522

Suchting S, Heal P, Tahtis K et al (2005) Soluble Robo4 receptor inhibits in vivo angiogenesis and endothelial cell migration. FASEB J 19:121–123

Varma R, Macias GL, Torres M et al (2007) Biologic risk factors associated with diabetic retinopathy: the Los Angeles Latino Eye Study. Ophthalmology 114:1332–1340

Wang B, Xiao Y, Ding BB et al (2003) Induction of tumor angiogenesis by Slit-Robo signaling and inhibition of cancer growth by blocking Robo activity. Cancer Cell 4:19–29

Zou HD, Zhang X, Xu X et al (2005) Prevalence study of age-related macular degeneration in Caojiadu blocks, Shanghai. Zhonghua Yan Ke Za Zhi 41:15–19

Part V
Animal Models of Retinal Degeneration

Chapter 53
Evaluation of Retinal Degeneration in P27KIP1 Null Mouse

Yumi Tokita-Ishikawa, Ryosuke Wakusawa, and Toshiaki Abe

Abstract

Purpose: p27kip1 is well-known as a cell cycle inhibitor and also plays an important role for cell differentiation. We hypothesized that if we caused retinal degeneration in a p27(–/–) mouse, then the appropriate method of restoration may be different from that of wild mice and therefore suggest a therapeutic methodology for retinal regeneration.

Methods: Histological and electrophysiological (ERG) examination was performed on p27(–/–) mice retina. We injected N-methy-N-nitrosourea (MNU) to induce retinal degeneration. BrdU was used to identify the dividing cells in the retina.

Results: Thicker retina were observed in the p27(–/–) mice when compared to those of the p27(–/+) mice or wild type mice. Almost all retinal layers were thick and optic nerves were also enlarged. A statistically significant decrease of a and b waves amplitudes of ERG was observed in p27(–/–) mice when compared to those of the other mice. BrdU and nestin positive cells were present at the outer nuclear layer with no difference between p27(–/–) and wild type mice after MNU injection.

Conclusion: p27(–/–) mice showed thicker retina and less retinal function than those of other mice. The MNU-induced retinal degeneration in p27(–/–) mice closely resembled the reaction of the other mice with no retinal regeneration observed in our experimental condition.

T. Abe (✉)

Division of Clinical Cell Therapy, School of Medicine, Tohoku University, 1-1 Seiryomachi Aobaku, Miyagi, Sendai 980-8574 Japan

e-mail: to-shi@oph.med.tohoku.ac.jp

R.E. Anderson et al. (eds.), *Retinal Degenerative Diseases*, Advances in Experimental Medicine and Biology 664, DOI 10.1007/978-1-4419-1399-9_53, 467
© Springer Science+Business Media, LLC 2010

53.1 Introduction

Inherited retinal degeneration or age-related macular degeneration can lead to severe ocular damage and to an extremely negative prognosis. Although many new approaches have been tried, the effectiveness of these treatments is far from satisfactory for patients. Neuronal regeneration is one of the targets for the treatment of retinal degeneration. Although the retina of warm-blooded vertebrates are believed to be incapable of neural regeneration, many authors have accumulated evidence that suggests the ability of some cells in the retina to re-enter their cell cycle, then differentiate and proliferate (Fischer et al. 2001). Neuronal differentiation is tightly regulated by various factors (Ohnuma et al. 2003). Cyclin-dependent kinases (CDKs) inhibitors have been suggested as playing an important role in neural differentiation via a cell cycle arrest-independent mechanism (Joseph et al. 2003) and p27kip1 is one of these CDK inhibitor molecules (Cunningham et al. 2001). We hypothesized that p27kip1 null (p27(–/–)) mice may show different reactions during retinal degeneration when compared to those of wild mice and that this difference will lead to some new insights for regenerative therapy for retinal degeneration.

53.2 Materials and Methods

53.2.1 Animals and Biosafety

The procedure used complied strictly with the Association for Research in Vision and Ophthalmology (ARVO) Statement for the Use of Animals in Ophthalmic and Vision Research. p27(–/–) mice were kindly provided from Keiko Nakayama (Professor, Division of Developmental Genetics, Tohoku University Graduate School of Medicine).

53.2.2 MNU-Induced Retinal Degeneration

N-methyl-N-nitrosourea (MNU; Sigma-Aldrich), a direct-acting alkylating agent, was dissolved in saline solution containing 0.05% acetic acid and was administered intraperitoneally (60 mg/kg body weight) (Nambu et al. 1997).

53.2.3 Electroretinography

A ganzfeld stimulator was used to stimulate the eyes and a data acquisition system (Universal Testing and Analysis System-Electrophysiology 3000; UTAS-E 3000: LKC Technologies, Inc., Gaithersburg, MD) was used to record the Electroretinography (ERG).

53.2.4 Histological Examination and Immunohistochemistry

Hematoxylin-eosin (H-E) staining, BrdU incorporation and immunohistochemistry for nestin was performed.

53.3 Results

53.3.1 Fundus Examination and Histology of the Retina

Fundus examination showed an enlargement of the size of the optic nerve head and the size of the retinal vessels around the optic disc (Fig. 53.1a and b). Histological examination showed thicker retina in p27(–/–) (Fig. 53.1c) mice when compared to those of p27(–/+) (not shown) or wild type (Fig. 53.1d) mice. The thicker layers were observed in almost all layers in the retina.

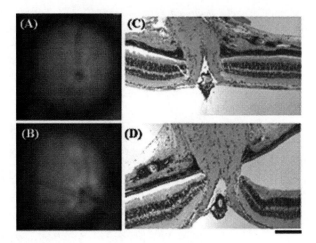

Fig. 53.1 Fundus photograph and histological examination. Fundus photograph ((**a**) and (**b**)) and histology ((**c**) and (**d**)) show enlargement of optic nerve head and thicker retina in p27(–/–) mice. Bars indicated 100 μm

53.3.2 ERG

When we performed ERG, statistically significant decreases of a and b waves amplitudes were observed in p27(–/–) mice when compared to those of wild mice (Table 53.1). These findings were clearer in 12 month-old mice than in 3 month-old mice.

Table 53.1 The results of electroretinography are shown

	3 M	
	a-wave (μV)	b-wave (μV)
Wild	128.4±48.1	363.1±88.3
p27–/–	108.3±40.5	304.7±89.1
P	0.115	0.029
	12 M	
	a-wave (μV)	b-wave (μV)
Wild	112.3±17.8	264.0±37.0
p27–/–	73.6±30.6	166.3±63.4
P	0.010	0.009

53.3.3 BrdU Incorporation

MNU injection showed retinal degeneration similar to that reported by others (Fig. 53.2a and b) (Nambu et al. 1997). We found that the degree of retinal degeneration seemed almost the same between p27(–/–) and wild type mice. When we examined BrdU incorporation, BrdU positive cells were observed at the ONL (Fig. 53.2c and d). Although we did not perform quantitative analysis, there seemed to be no difference between wild and p27(–/–) mice.

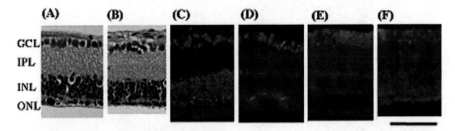

Fig. 53.2 BrdU incorporation and immunohistochemistry of nestin 3 M after MNU injection BrdU positive cells were observed at the ONL ((**a**): wild mice, (**b**) p27(–/–)). Nestin immunoreactivity was observed at inner retinal layer and outer plexiform layer. ((**c**) wild mice, (**d**) p27(–/–) mice). (**e**) and (**f**) show H-E finding, respectively

53.3.4 Immunohistology of Nestin

Although we did not perform quantification, nestin-like immunoreactivity seemed to show no differences between p27(–/–) and wild type mice (Fig. 53.2e and f).

53.4 Discussion

Acute damage stimulates Müller glia to re-enter the cell cycle, and induce expression of CASH-1, Pax6 and Chx10, transcription factors expressed by embryonic retinal progenitors. Fischer and coworker reported that, in response to damage, Müller glia was a potential source of neural regeneration (Fischer et al. 2001). Cdk inhibitors have been reported to stop cell-cycle activity during development and in maintaining cells in a terminally differentiated state, demonstrating a cell-selective expression pattern in various organs (Nakayama et al. 1996). When we performed histological examination, we found thick retina and optic nerves in p27kip1 (–/–) mice. These results may demonstrate the failure of the retina to differentiate. Interestingly, mice with thick retina did not show a normal response by ERG examination, even though each cell in the retina seemed to be normal. The results may relate to other reports that mice homozygote for p27 mutation had severe hearing loss and their organ of Corti exhibited an increase in the number of inner and outer hair cells (Kanzaki et al. 2006). These results may show that adequate cell differentiation and normal cell number is important for normal retinal function.

When we generated retinal degeneration by MNU injection, as was reported previously (Nambu et al. 1997), although we found retinal degeneration, we could not find any differences between p27(–/–) and wild mice. When we examined the BrdU incorporation and nestin expression in the retina, we also could not find any differences between p27(–/–) and control wild mice. These results may show that under our experimental condition, the suppression of cell cycle molecules p27kip1 on its own may not induce retinal regeneration.

In conclusion, the CDKs inhibitor, p27(–/–) itself may induce retinal abnormalities, both histologically and electrophysiologically. However, p27(–/–) itself did not induce retinal regeneration in our experimental condition.

References

Cunningham JJ et al (2001) Cyclin-dependent kinase inhibitors in the development of the central nervous system. Cell Growth Differ 12:387–396

Fischer AJ et al (2001) Muller glia are a potential source of neural regeneration in the postnatal chicken retina. Nat Neurosci 4:247–252

Joseph B et al (2003) p57(Kip2) cooperates with Nurr1 in developing dopamine cells. Proc Natl Acad Sci U S A 100:15619–15624

Kanzaki S et al (2006) p27(Kip1) deficiency causes organ of Corti pathology and hearing loss. Hear Res 214:28–36

Nakayama K et al (1996) Mice lacking p27(Kip1) display increased body size, multiple organ hyperplasia, retinal dysplasia, and pituitary tumors. Cell 85:707–720

Nambu H et al (1997) Morphologic characteristics of N-methyl-N-nitrosourea-induced retinal degeneration in C57BL mice. Pathol Int 47:377–383

Ohnuma S et al (2003) Neurogenesis and the cell cycle. Neuron 40:199–208

Chapter 54
Differences in Photoreceptor Sensitivity to Oxygen Stress Between Long Evans and Sprague-Dawley Rats

Vicki Chrysostomou, Jonathan Stone, and Krisztina Valter

Abstract

Purpose: To examine the susceptibility of photoreceptors to hyperoxic stress in two rat strains, the pigmented Long Evans (LE) and the albino Sprague-Dawley (SD).

Methods: Adult LE and SD rats were exposed to hyperoxia (75% oxygen) for 14 days. Retinas were assessed for electroretinogram (ERG) responses, cell death, and expression of a retinal stress factor.

Results: In the LE strain, exposure to hyperoxia significantly reduced amplitudes of rod a-wave, rod b-wave and cone b-wave components of the ERG, and caused a 55-fold increase in photoreceptor cell death rates, and an upregulation of GFAP expression. In the SD strain, hyperoxic exposure had no measurable effect on the ERG response of rods or cones, and resulted in a modest (5-fold) increase in the rate of photoreceptor cell death.

Conclusions: In LE and SD strains, hyperoxia induces cell death specific to photoreceptors. The effect is an order of magnitude more severe in the pigmented LE strain suggesting a strong genetic component to oxygen sensitivity, as reported previously between the albino Balb/C and pigmented C57BL/6 strains of mice.

54.1 Introduction

It has long been known that hyperoxia is specifically toxic to photoreceptors (Noell 1955). Elevation of the partial pressure of oxygen in the retina results in photoreceptor degeneration that increases as a function of time (Yamada et al. 1999; Okoye et al. 2003; Geller et al. 2006) and oxygen concentration (Wellard et al. 2005). The vulnerability of photoreceptors to hyperoxia is a result of the unique architecture of oxygen delivery to the outer retina. The outer retina lacks intrinsic blood vessels;

V. Chrysostomou (✉)
Research School of Biological Sciences, The Australian National University, Canberra, Australia
e-mail: vicki.chrysostomou@anu.edu.au

R.E. Anderson et al. (eds.), *Retinal Degenerative Diseases*, Advances in Experimental Medicine and Biology 664, DOI 10.1007/978-1-4419-1399-9_54,
© Springer Science+Business Media, LLC 2010

oxygen diffuses to photoreceptors from choroidal vessels located behind the retinal pigment epithelium (RPE). Presumably because the choroidal vessels lie external to the photoreceptors that they serve, the flow of blood through the choroid is not regulated in response to levels of oxygen or other local metabolic factors (Chan-Ling and Stone 1993; Stone et al. 1999). As a consequence, photoreceptors, unlike most other tissues in the body, are poorly protected against fluctuations of oxygen.

Although all photoreceptors have a pre-determined vulnerability to hyperoxia due to the retinal architecture, the degree of this vulnerability appears to differ between strains of mouse. Photoreceptors in the adult pigmented C57BL/6 J mouse strain are relatively vulnerable to hyperoxia, while those in the albino BALB/cJ, C57BL/6–c$^{2 J}$ and A/J strains are relatively resistant (Yamada et al. 1999; Walsh et al. 2004; Smit-McBride et al. 2007). These strain-dependent differences suggest a genetic basis for photoreceptor sensitivity to oxygen stress and, recently, a strong determinant for the A/J–C57BL/6 difference has been localized to chromosome 6 (Smit-McBride et al. 2007).

To date, the vulnerabilities of different adult rat strains to oxygen stress have not been explored. However, work in the neonatal rat suggests that, like the mouse, there are strain-dependent differences to oxygen stress. Pigmented Dark Agouti, Hooded Wistar and Brown Norway rats are more vulnerable to oxygen-induced retinopathy than albino Sprague-Dawley, Fischer 344, Wistar-Furth and Lewis rats (Gao et al. 2002; van Wijngaarden et al. 2005). Using formal backcross analysis, the genetic basis of the Dark Agouti-Fischer 344 difference has been modeled using an autosomal dominant pattern of inheritance (van Wijngaarden et al. 2007).

Here, we test the impact of hyperoxia on photoreceptors in the mature retina of two rat strains; the pigmented Long Evans (LE) and the albino Sprague-Dawley (SD).

54.2 Methods

54.2.1 Animal Strains and Oxygen Exposure

All procedures were in accordance with the ARVO Statement for the Use of Animals in Ophthalmic and Vision Research. Pigmented Long Evans (LE) and albino Sprague-Dawley (SD) rats aged 90–150 days were used. All animals were born, raised and exposed to hyperoxia in dim cyclic illumination (12 h 5 lux/12 h dark). Animals were exposed to hyperoxia (75% oxygen) for 14 days by placing litter boxes inside a plexiglass chamber in which the oxygen concentration was controlled by a feedback system (OxyCycler, Biospherix).

54.2.2 Electroretinography

Animals were dark-adapted overnight and prepared for recording in dim red illumination as described previously (Chrysostomou et al. 2008). Following previous reports, (Nixon et al. 2001), responses to a standard test flash (44.5 cds/m^2) were considered to be 'mixed' with contributions from rods and cones. Responses to the test flash preceded, by 400 msec, by a conditioning flash (12 cds/m^2) were considered those of cones. By subtracting the cone response from the 'mixed' response, the rod response was isolated. The standard flash stimulus was sufficient to elicit saturated a-wave and b-wave responses.

54.2.3 Immunohistochemistry and TUNEL Labeling

Enucleated eyes were fixed, processed, cryoembedded and cryosectioned as described previously (Chrysostomou et al. 2008). Immunohistochemical labelling of retinal cryosections was performed using antibodies specific for glial fibrillary acidic protein (GFAP). Retinal cryosections were labeled using the TUNEL technique to identify the fragmentation of DNA characteristic of apoptosis.

54.3 Results

54.3.1 Rod and Cone Components of the ERG after Hyperoxia

Full field ERG responses were recorded in LE and SD adult rats before and after 14 days exposure to hyperoxia. In the pigmented LE strain, exposure to hyperoxia for 14 days significantly ($P<0.05$) reduced the amplitude of rod a-wave (Fig. 54.1a), rod b-wave (Fig. 54.1b) and cone b-wave (Fig. 54.1c) components of the ERG, by 29, 46 and 49% respectively. In the albino SD strain the effect of hyperoxic exposure on the ERG was much less marked, and did not reach statistical significance for any of these three ERG components (Figs. 54.1a–c).

54.3.2 Impact of Hyperoxia on the Rate of Photo receptor Death

In both strains, 14 days hyperoxic exposure increased the frequency of TUNEL+ cells in the retina; the increases were confined to the outer nuclear layer (data not shown). In the LE strain, hyperoxia resulted in a 55-fold increase in the frequency of TUNEL+ cells. By contrast, the same hyperoxic exposure resulted in a much smaller (5-fold) increase in TUNEL labeling of SD photoreceptors (Fig. 54.2a). Hyperoxia-induced DNA damage to LE and SD photoreceptors was not uniform across the retina. Photoreceptors in the peripheral retina were relatively unaffected, and there was a strong concentration of TUNEL+ cells in the central retina (Fig. 54.2b).

54.3.3 Impact of Hyperoxia on GFAP Expression

In normoxic LE and SD retinas, GFAP expression was confined to astrocyte cell bodies and processes at the inner surface of the retina (left panels of Figs. 54.3a and b). After 14 days hyperoxic exposure, GFAP was prominent in radially-oriented

Fig. 54.1 ERG responses were recorded in LE and SD rats before (normoxia) and immediately after (hyperoxia) 14 days exposure to 75% oxygen. Exposure to hyperoxia significantly reduced the amplitudes of rod (**a,b**) and cone (**c**) components of the ERG in the LE but not the SD strain of rat. Histograms show mean ± SEM (*n*=7). * *P* < 0.05 using a student's *t*-test

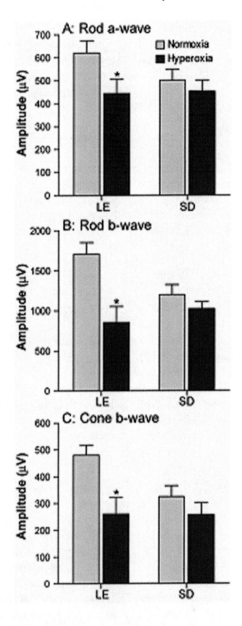

Müller cell processes in the LE retina (right panel of Fig. 54.3a). Raised GFAP expression was most prominent in the central LE retina, co-localising with areas of high TUNEL labeling. In the SD retina, hyperoxic exposure had no effect on GFAP expression (right panel of Fig. 54.3b).

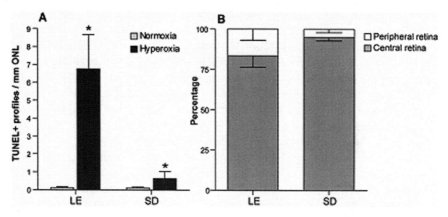

Fig. 54.2 Frequency and distribution of TUNEL+ profiles in LE and SD retinas after hyperoxic exposure. (**a**) Hyperoxia-induced increases in TUNEL+ profiles were much greater in the LE retina than the SD retina. (**b**) In both strains, TUNEL+ profiles were more common in the central retina than the peripheral retina (200 μm from the retinal edge) after hyperoxia. Histograms show mean ± SEM (n=5). * $P < 0.01$ using a student's t-test

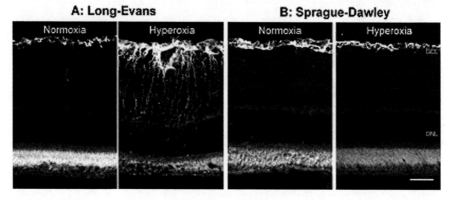

Fig. 54.3 Expression of the stress-inducible factor GFAP in LE and SD retinas after hyperoxic exposure. Immunoreactivity for GFAP was markedly upregulated in the LE (**a**) but not the SD (**b**) retina after 14 days hyperoxic exposure. All images are taken from the central retina. GCL, ganglion cell layer; ONL, outer nuclear layer. Scale bar = 20 μm

54.4 Discussion

In the retinas of both LE and SD strains of rat, hyperoxia induced cell death specific to photoreceptors. Quantitatively, the photoreceptor death induced by hyperoxia was an order of magnitude higher in the LE strain, in which hyperoxia also reduced rod and cone components of the ERG and upregulated the expression of a stress-inducible protein (GFAP) by Müller cells.

'Oxygen phenotypes', such as that described here for the rat, may provide a useful basis for identification of the genes that determine photoreceptor vulnerability to oxygen stress, and of the mechanisms involved. The regulation of oxygen vulnerability has been localised to chromosome 6 in the mouse, using the C57BL/6 (vulnerable) and A/J (resistant) phenotypes (Smit-McBride et al. 2007). The present results show that genetically-determined variations in oxygen susceptibility are not unique to the mouse. They may therefore play a role in human retinal dystrophies, since the partial depletion of photoreceptors is known to cause irreversible and progressive hyperoxia of the outer layers of the retina. This rise has been demonstrated in three models of retinal degeneration; the RCS rat (Yu et al. 2000), the P23H-3 rat (Yu et al. 2004) and the Abyssinian cat (Padnick-Silver et al. 2006).

There may be an association between ocular pigmentation and susceptibility of photoreceptors to oxygen stress. Using a backcross analysis, van Wijngaarden and colleagues (2007) found that the trait for susceptibility to oxygen-induced retinopathy in Dark Agouti and Fischer 334 rats was associated with pigmentation. Other studies that have exposed either the neonatal (Gao et al. 2002; van Wijngaarden et al. 2005) or adult (Yamada et al. 1999; Walsh et al. 2004; Smit-McBride et al. 2007) rodent retina to hyperoxia, show a similar trend: albino mice (BALB/cJ, C57BL/6-c^{2J}, A/J) and rats (SD, Fischer 344, Wistar–Furth, Lewis) are more resistant to oxygen stress than pigmented mice (C57BL/6 J) and rats (Dark Agouti, Hooded Wistar, Brown Norway). The current findings from LE and SD retinas also fit this pattern.

Ocular pigmentation includes high concentrations of melanin within melanosomes of RPE cells. The biological effect of RPE melanin is not completely understood; both protective and cytotoxic roles have been described. Melanins are efficient antioxidants, able to scavenge free radicals, quench electronically excited states, inhibit lipid peroxidation and chelate metal ions (Dunford et al. 1995; Rozanowska et al. 1999; Zhang et al. 2000; Ye et al. 2003). However, aged, photolysed or oxidized melanosomes lose their antioxidant properties and become increasingly able to generate reactive oxygen species (Burke et al. 2007; Zadlo et al. 2007; Zareba et al. 2007). High oxygen levels may also trigger the conversion of melanin from antioxidant to pro-oxidant thus making photoreceptors in pigmented retinas more vulnerable to oxygen stress than those in albino retinas.

References

Burke JM, Henry MM, Zareba M et al (2007) Photobleaching of melanosomes from retinal pigment epithelium: I. Effects on protein oxidation. Photochem Photobiol 83:920–924

Chan-Ling T, Stone J (1993) Retinopathy of prematurity: origins in the architecture of the retina. Prog Retin Eye Res 12:155–178

Chrysostomou V, Stone J, Stowe S et al (2008) The status of cones in the rhodopsin mutant P23H-3 retina: light-regulated damage and repair in parallel with rods. Invest Ophthalmol Vis Sci 49:1116–1125

Dunford R, Land EJ, Rozanowska M et al (1995) Interaction of melanin with carbon- and oxygen-centered radicals from methanol and ethanol. Free Radic Biol Med 19:735–740

Gao G, Li Y, Fant J et al (2002) Difference in ischemic regulation of vascular endothelial growth factor and pigment epithelium-derived factor in brown norway and Sprague-Dawley rats contributing to different susceptibilities to retinal neovascularization. Diabetes 51:1218–1225

Geller S, Krowka R, Valter K et al (2006) Toxicity of hyperoxia to the retina: evidence from the mouse. Adv Exp Med Biol 572:425–437

Nixon PJ, Bui BV, Armitage JA et al (2001) The contribution of cone responses to rat electroretinograms. Clin Exp Ophthalmol 29:193–196

Noell WK (1955) Visual cell effects of high oxygen pressures. Fed Proc 14:107–108

Okoye G, Zimmer J, Sung J et al (2003) Increased expression of brain-derived neurotrophic factor preserves retinal function and slows cell death from rhodopsin mutation or oxidative damage. J Neurosci 23:4164–4172

Padnick-Silver L, Kang Derwent JJ, Giuliano E et al (2006) Retinal oxygenation and oxygen metabolism in Abyssinian cats with a hereditary retinal degeneration. Invest Ophthalmol Vis Sci 47:3683–3689

Rozanowska M, Sarna T, Land EJ et al (1999) Free radical scavenging properties of melanin interaction of eu- and pheo-melanin models with reducing and oxidising radicals. Free Radic Biol Med 26:518–525

Smit-McBride Z, Oltjen SL, Lavail MM et al (2007) A strong genetic determinant of hyperoxia-related retinal degeneration on mouse chromosome 6. Invest Ophthalmol Vis Sci 48:405–411

Stone J, Maslim J, Valter-Kocsi K et al (1999) Mechanisms of photoreceptor death and survival in mammalian retina. Prog Retin Eye Res 18:689–735

van Wijngaarden P, Brereton HM, Coster DJ et al (2007) Genetic influences on susceptibility to oxygen-induced retinopathy. Invest Ophthalmol Vis Sci 48:1761–1766

van Wijngaarden P, Coster DJ, Brereton HM et al (2005) Strain-dependent differences in oxygen-induced retinopathy in the inbred rat. Invest Ophthalmol Vis Sci 46:1445–1452

Walsh N, Bravo-Nuevo A, Geller S et al (2004) Resistance of photoreceptors in the C57BL/6-c2J, C57BL/6 J, and BALB/cJ mouse strains to oxygen stress: evidence of an oxygen phenotype. Curr Eye Res 29:441–447

Wellard J, Lee D, Valter K et al (2005) Photoreceptors in the rat retina are specifically vulnerable to both hypoxia and hyperoxia. Visual Neurosci 22:222–229

Yamada H, Yamada E, Hackett SF et al (1999) Hyperoxia causes decreased expression of vascular endothelial growth factor and endothelial cell apoptosis in adult retina. J Cell Physiol 179: 149–156

Ye T, Simon JD, Sarna T (2003) Ultrafast energy transfer from bound tetra(4-N,N,N,N-trimethylanilinium) porphyrin to synthetic dopa and cysteinyldopa melanins. Photochem Photobiol 77:1–4

Yu D-Y, Cringle SJ, Su E-N et al (2000) Intraretinal oxygen levels before and after photoreceptor loss in the RCS rat. Invest Ophthalmol Vis Sci 41:3999–4006

Yu D-Y, Cringle S, Valter K et al (2004) Photoreceptor death, trophic factor expression, retinal oxygen status, and photoreceptor function in the P23H rat. Invest Ophthalmol Vis Sci 45: 2013–2019

Zadlo A, Rozanowska MB, Burke JM et al (2007) Photobleaching of retinal pigment epithelium melanosomes reduces their ability to inhibit iron-induced peroxidation of lipids. Pigment Cell Res 20:52–60

Zareba M, Sarna T, Szewczyk G et al (2007) Photobleaching of melanosomes from retinal pigment epithelium: II. Effects on the response of living cells to photic stress. Photochem Photobiol 83:925–930

Zhang X, Erb C, Flammer J et al (2000) Absolute rate constants for the quenching of reactive excited states by melanin and related 5,6-dihydroxyindole metabolites: implications for their antioxidant activity. Photochem Photobiol 71:524–533

Chapter 55
Retinal Degeneration in a Rat Model of Smith-Lemli-Opitz Syndrome: Thinking Beyond Cholesterol Deficiency

Steven J. Fliesler

Abstract Smith-Lemli-Opitz Syndrome (SLOS) is a recessive hereditary disease caused by a defect in the last step in cholesterol biosynthesis – the reduction of the Δ7 double bond of 7-dehydrocholesterol (7DHC) – resulting in the abnormal accumulation of 7DHC and diminished levels of Chol in all bodily tissues. Treatment of rats with AY9944 – a drug that inhibits the same enzyme that is genetically defective in SLOS (i.e., DHCR7, 3β-hydroxysterol-Δ7-reductase) – starting in utero and continuing throughout postnatal life, provides a convenient animal model of SLOS for understanding the disease mechanism and also for testing the efficacy of therapeutic intervention strategies. Herein, the biochemical, morphological, and electrophysiological hallmarks of retinal degeneration in this animal model are reviewed. A high-cholesterol diet partially ameliorates the associated visual function deficits, but not the morphological degeneration. Recent studies using this model suggest that the disease mechanism in SLOS goes well beyond the initial cholesterol pathway defect, including global metabolic alterations, lipid and protein oxidation, and differential expression of hundreds of genes in multiple ontological gene families. These findings may have significant implications with regard to developing more optimal therapeutic interventions for managing SLOS patients.

55.1 Introduction

Cholesterol is a ubiquitous lipid constituent in all mammalian cells and tissues. In the plasma membrane of most higher eukaryotic cells, cholesterol typically accounts for 30–50 mol% of the total lipid (reviewed in: Yeagle 1985). It is no mere quirk

S.J. Fliesler (✉)
Veterans Administration Western New York Healthcare System, and the Department of Ophthalmology and Biochemistry, University at Buffalo (State University of New York), Buffalo, NY 14215, USA
e-mail: fliesler@buffalo.edu

R.E. Anderson et al. (eds.), *Retinal Degenerative Diseases*, Advances in Experimental Medicine and Biology 664, DOI 10.1007/978-1-4419-1399-9_55,
© Springer Science+Business Media, LLC 2010

of fate that cholesterol, as opposed to literally thousands of other possible sterols, is
the overwhelmingly dominant, if not sole, resident sterol in such cells and tissues.
Other sterols do not seem to provide the essential features requisite to promote and
preserve normal cellular structure, function, and viability (reviewed in: Demel and
DeKruyff 1976; Bloch 1989). Perhaps the most clear-cut evidence for the essential role that cholesterol plays in human biology is the existence of a group of
devastating, often lethal, hereditary human diseases that involve specific, genetically determined defects in the enzymes responsible for cholesterol biosynthesis
(reviewed in: Porter 2003). While each of these diseases has a distinct phenotype,
they all involve dysmorphologies as well as profound defects in the development
and function of the nervous system. The first and best described of these diseases,
as well as the most common, is Smith-Lemli-Opitz Syndrome (SLOS) (Smith et al.
1964; reviewed in: Porter 2008). The primary biochemical defect in SLOS involves
the enzyme DHCR7 (3β-hydroxysterol-Δ7-reductase; EC1.3.1.21), which converts
7-dehydrocholesterol (7DHC) to cholesterol (Fig. 55.1) (reviewed in: Correa-Cerro
and Porter 2005). Over a hundred disease-causing mutations in the DHCR7 gene,

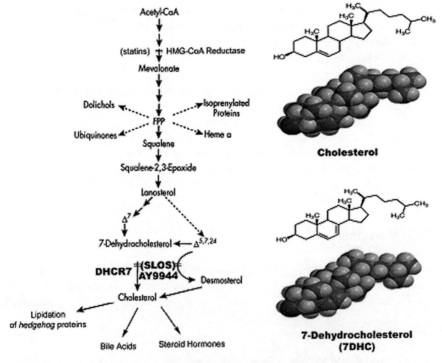

Fig. 55.1 The cholesterol pathway, indicating the defective biochemical reaction in Smith-
Lemli-Opitz Syndrome (SLOS), normally catalyzed by DHCR7 (3β-hydroxysterol-Δ7-reductase),
and the site at which AY9944 inhibits the pathway. The chemical structures of cholesterol and 7-dehydrocholesterol (7DHC) are shown. FPP, farnesylpyrophosphate; $\Delta^{5,7,24}$, 7-
dehydrodesmosterol

spread throughout its 9 exons, have been discovered (reviewed in: Yu and Patel 2005), and the spectrum of disease severity is quite broad, from mild to lethal.

Despite decades of study, the biological roles of cholesterol in the retina have yet to be fully elucidated. In the course of our studies of cholesterol biosynthesis and metabolism in the retina (reviewed in: Fliesler and Keller 1997; Fliesler 2002), we asked two fundamental questions: (1) What are the consequences of depleting the retina of its endogenous cholesterol, with regard to its development, structure, and function; and (2) Can sterols other than cholesterol support the normal development, structure and function of the retina? Given the information provided above, we reasoned that disrupting cholesterol biosynthesis should have significant and deleterious consequences on retinal development, histological and ultrastructural organization, and electrophysiological function. Herein, we show that these expectations were born out, using a pharmacologically induced rat model of SLOS.

55.2 The AY9944 Rat Model of SLOS: Biochemical Findings

Studies performed in the 1960s (reviewed in: Gofflot 2002) demonstrated that treatment of rodents (mice and rats) with inhibitors of cholesterol biosynthesis had profound effects on embryogenesis and early postnatal development. One of these inhibitors was AY9944 (*trans*-1,4-bis(2-chlorobenaminomethyl)cyclohexane dihydrochloride), a relatively selective inhibitor of DHCR7 (Dvornik et al. 1963; Givner and Dvornik 1965), the same enzyme as is defective in SLOS (see Fig. 55.1). With the elucidation in 1993–1994 of the link between defective cholesterol biosynthesis and SLOS, it became evident that treatment of rodents with such inhibitors could yield a model of SLOS (Xu et al. 1995; Kolf-Clauw et al. 1996). Typically, however, those rodent models tended not to be viable for more than a few days to a week.

Since the neural retina in rats and mice develops over the course of the first four postnatal weeks, we refined and optimized the conditions and dosage of administering AY9944 in Sprague-Dawley rats to yield a SLOS model that reproduced the biochemical hallmarks of the human disease (i.e., markedly elevated 7DHC levels and reduced cholesterol levels in all tissues) while also maintaining viability for at least three postnatal months (Fliesler et al. 1999, 2004, 2007). Figure 55.2 shows an example of a typical reverse-phase HPLC chromatogram of nonsaponifiable lipids extracted from the retinas of 1-month-old AY9944-treated (Fig. 55.2a) and control rats (Fig. 55.2b). In this case, the 7DHC/cholesterol mole ratio in the treated animal's retina was almost 4:1, whereas in the control it's zero, since 7DHC is not normally present at appreciable steady-state levels in the retina. The rats are maintained on a cholesterol-free diet, such that their only source of sterols is that derived biogenically via de novo synthesis. The key to improved viability is not to expose the fetuses to AY9944 within the first gestational week, to provide a low dosage of AY9944 during gestation, either by feeding the pregnant dams chow containing 1 mg AY9944 per 100 g chow (Fliesler et al. 1999, 2004) or by continuously infusing them with a sterile, PBS-buffered solution of AY9944 (0.37 mg/kg/day; at

Fig. 55.2 Reverse-phase
HPLC chromatogram of
retinal nonsaponifiable lipids
from a 1-month old
AY9944-treated rat (*left
panel*) and an age-matched
control rat (*right panel*). Note
the dominance of 7DHC and
the markedly lower level of
cholesterol (denoted by the
asterisk) in the treated
sample, whereas cholesterol
is the only detectable sterol in
the control. Detection by UV
absorbance at 205 nm (A205)

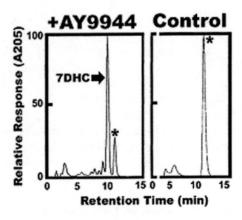

2.5 µL/h) via an Alzet[®] osmotic pump (Fliesler et al. 2007), and injecting the pups (typically three times per week) subcutaneously with buffered AY9944 solution (25–30 mg/kg). Under the conditions of our studies, the 7DHC/cholesterol mole ratio typically is >5:1 in both serum and liver within the first postnatal month of exposure to AY9944, and can reach values of >11:1 by three months postnatal. This biochemical hallmark exceeds that of even the most severely affected SLOS patients (Tint et al. 1995). In the case of the retina, by three months of AY9944 treatment the 7DHC/cholesterol mole ratio is typically >5:1; hence, there is a progressive increase in the relative amount of 7DHC in retina, from 1 to 3 months.

55.3 Retinal Degeneration in the SLOS Rat Model: Histology and Ultrastructure

The histological changes in the retina that occur as a function of postnatal age in the AY9944-induced SLOS rat model have been presented in detail elsewhere (Fliesler et al. 1999, 2004) and are summarized in Fig. 55.3. About the first postnatal day (P1) the cells of the retina, with the exception of the ganglion cell layer (GCL), are still not yet differentiated and the retina of AY9944-treated rats (Fig. 55.3a) appears virtually identical to that of an age-matched control (not shown). Subsequently, up to about the first postnatal month, the retinal undergoes maturation and the histological organization and appearance of the retina in AY9944-treated rats (P33, Fig. 55.3b) again is essentially equivalent to those of age-matched control rats (not shown). However, by about the second postnatal month, the number of pyknotic nuclei in the outer nuclear layer (ONL; i.e., photoreceptors) dramatically increases, and the thickness of the ONL and photoreceptor outer segment (OS) layer is noticeably reduced in AY9944-treated rats (P69, Fig. 55.3c), relative to age-matched controls (not shown). By 10–12 postnatal weeks, the ONL and POS layer show further, marked reductions (P93, Fig. 55.3d). Quantitative morphometric analysis (Fliesler

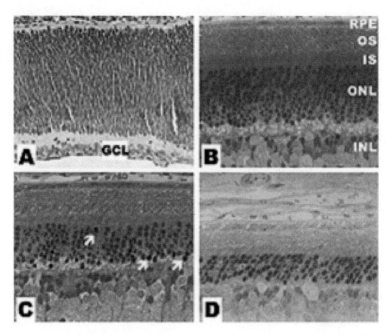

Fig. 55.3 Histology of the retina in the SLOS (AY9944-treated) rat model as a function of post-natal development. (**a**) Postnatal day (P) 1; (**b**) P33; (**c**) P69; (**d**) P92. *Arrows* (panel C) indicate pyknotic nuclei in the photoreceptor layer. Note progressive thinning of the outer segment (OS) layer and outer nuclear layer (ONL) with age. GCL, ganglion cell layer; INL, inner nuclear layer; IS, inner segment layer; RPE, retinal pigment epithelium

et al. 2004) has shown that, on average, the OS layer thickness is reduced by nearly a third (30–35%) while ONL thickness is reduced by 20–25%, relative to controls, by three postnatal months of treatment, and the degeneration is fairly symmetrical across the vertical meridian.

Ultrastructurally, rod outer segments in the SLOS rat model, while shortened relative to age-matched controls after one postnatal month (Fliesler et al. 1999), appear otherwise normal, even after three postnatal months when retinal degeneration has progressed significantly (Fliesler et al. 2004). However, the RPE is decidedly abnormal, compared to controls, by three postnatal months in AY9944-treated rats (Fig. 55.4). The RPE cytoplasm becomes grossly congested with phagosomes (ingested tips of shed outer segment membranes), lipid droplets, and a variety of membranous inclusion bodies, regardless of what time of day tissue specimens are prepared. [Normally, such material is largely cleared from the RPE cytoplasm within the first 1–2 h after light onset in animals maintained in cyclic light.] That said, the polarity of the RPE cells appears relatively normal, with well-extended apical villi and mitochondria lined up proximal to the basal infoldings of the RPE plasma membrane. Given the large load of ingested ROS tips and accumulation of phagosomes in the SLOS rat RPE, one might expect the A2E levels to be substantially elevated,

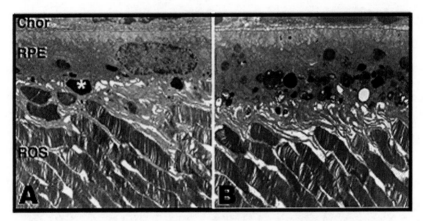

Fig. 55.4 Ultrastructure of the neural retina and RPE in a three-month old control rat (**a**) and in an age-matched SLOS rat (**b**). Note the substantial congestion of the RPE with phagosomes (denoted by *asterisk*) and other densely-staining membranous inclusions in the SLOS rat retina, compared to the control. The general ultrastructural appearance of rod outer segments (ROS) in both panels is comparable. Chor, choroid

relative to controls. However, preliminary studies (J.R. Sparrow and S.J. Fliesler, unpublished) indicate this is not the case. Regardless, given the pathological condition of the RPE and the severely shortened ROS in this model, one would predict that visual function should be substantially compromised. That turns out to be true (see below).

55.4 Retinal Degeneration in the SLOS Rat Model: Electrophysiological Deficits

Within the first postnatal month, retinal function in the SLOS rat model is robust, with scotopic (rod) ERG amplitudes being at least as great, if not greater than, those of age-matched controls, although the implicit times for the scotopic b-waves are greater (response timing more sluggish) than in controls (Fliesler et al. 1999). However, by 3 months of AY9944 treatment, both rod and cone ERG amplitudes are significantly reduced and photoresponse timing is delayed, compared to controls (Fliesler et al. 2004). In addition, both rod sensitivity (S) and maximal photoresponse (R_{mP3}) values are reduced about 2-fold, relative to age-matched controls. These findings correlate well with the histological and ultrastructural observations (see above), and indicate that there is progressive visual dysfunction in the SLOS rat model, both with regard to phototransduction efficiency as well as postreceptor signal transmission. Importantly, these findings are consistent with the rod (Elias et al. 2003) and cone (A.B. Fulton, personal communication) functional deficits observed in SLOS patients.

55.5 Effects of Feeding a High-Cholesterol Diet

Interestingly, feeding a high (2%, by wt.) cholesterol diet can yield marked improvements particularly in the cone ERG responses (Fliesler et al. 2007): photopic b-wave amplitudes are increased nearly 2-fold, approaching normal levels, and b-wave timing is also significantly improved (although still not normal). The effects of the high cholesterol diet on the rod system, however, are far less pronounced, although there is substantial improvement in both a- and b-wave implicit times. Notably, dietary cholesterol supplementation in the SLOS rat model actually results in near normalization of the steady-state levels of cholesterol in the retina by three postnatal months, while also significantly lowering the 7DHC levels (by about 30%), such that the 7DHC/cholesterol mole ratio is reduced by 3-fold, compared to age-matched SLOS rats fed cholesterol-free chow (Fliesler et al. 2007). Despite this, however, histological degeneration of the retina is not spared, although there is a substantial (and statistically significant) reduction in the number of pyknotic photoreceptor nulei in the retinas of cholesterol-fed SLOS rats compared to those maintained on a cholesterol-free diet.

55.6 Perspective: Thinking Beyond the Cholesterol Deficiency in SLOS

While the standard of care for managing SLOS patients is cholesterol supplementation therapy (reviewed in: Porter 2008), the efficacy of this approach is quite variable and, typically, minimal. Indeed, the above findings suggest that while restoring cholesterol levels in the retina is helpful, there's something missing in the treatment regimen that prevents full rescue of retinal structure and visual function. We propose that, although cholesterol deficiency caused by a defect in DHCR7 is the *primary* (initiating) cause of the disease, SLOS involves *secondary* defects in non-sterol metabolic pathways as well as additional biochemical changes.

Using the SLOS rat model, we've shown that there is a dramatic and progressive loss of docosahexaenoic acid (DHA, 22:6n-3) in whole retinas (Ford et al. 2008) and ROS membranes (Boesze-Battaglia et al. 2008), compared to age-matched controls. As expected, such dramatic alterations in membrane fatty acid composition cause profound perturbations in ROS membrane fluidity (Boesze-Battaglia et al. 2008), which undoubtedly reduces the efficiency of phototransduction (as reflected in the scotopic a-wave parameters). The presence of lipid hydroperoxides (LPO) in SLOS rat retinas, at levels comparable to those observed in photodamaged rats, has been demonstrated (Richards et al. 2006), and the LPO levels increase dramatically when SLOS rats are exposed to intense constant light, correlating with the extent of histological damage observed in the retina under such conditions (Vaughan et al. 2006). Furthermore, preliminary reports have indicated the oxidative modification of retinal proteins with reactive aldehydes that are end-products derived from oxidative degradation of both n-3 and n-6 fatty acids (Fliesler et al. 2006). Such proteins modifications are known to compromise protein structure and function and have been implicated in various diseases that involve oxidative stress (reviewed in Negre-Salvayre et al. 2008). Curiously, rhodopsin (the overwhelmingly dominant ROS membrane protein) somehow evades such modifications (Fliesler et al. 2006). In addition, initial DNA microarray analysis has revealed that hundreds of genes are differentially expressed in retinas of SLOS rats, compared to age-matched controls (Siddiqui et al. 2007, 2008), with the number and types of differentially expressed genes correlating well with the time course of retinal degeneration. Notably, among the affected gene families are those associated with oxidative stress and regulation of cell death.

Given the evidence for oxidation of both lipids and proteins in the SLOS rat model, in addition to the expected sterol pathway modifications, we suggest that future development of therapeutic interventions for clinical management of SLOS patients should include antioxidants in addition to cholesterol supplementation. Determining which antioxidants to use, the dosage, timing, and formulation with cholesterol will be challenging. The SLOS rat model described herein offers an excellent test system with which to evaluate the efficacy of these various factors in advance of randomized clinical testing in human patients.

Acknowledgments The author thanks the following collaborators for their significant contributions to the studies briefly summarized herein: Robert E. Anderson, Kathleen Boesze-Battaglia, R. Steven Brush, Deborah Ferrington, David Ford, Rebecca Kapphahn, Drake Mitchell, Barbara Nagel, Neal Peachey, Michael Richards, Akbar Siddiqui, and Dana Vaughan. This work was supported, in part, by U.S.P.H.S. (NEI/NIH) grant EY007361, by a departmental Challenge Grant and a Senior Scientific Investigator Award from Research to Prevent Blindness, and by a grant from the March of Dimes.

References

Bloch K (1989) Sterol structure and function. Steroids 53(3–5):261–270

Boesze-Battaglia K, Damek-Poprawa M, Mitchell DC et al (2008) Alteration of retinal rod outer segment membrane fluidity in a rat model of Smith-Lemli-Opitz syndrome. J Lipid Res 49(7):1488–1499

Correa-Cerro LS, Porter FD (2005) 3beta-Hydroxysterol delta7-reductase and the Smith-Lemli-Opitz syndrome. Mol Genet Metab 84(2):112–126

Demel RA, DeKruyff B (1976) The function of sterols in membranes. Biochim Biophys Acta 457(2):109–132

Dvornik D, Kraml M, Dubuc J et al (1963) A novel mode of inhibition of cholesterol biosynthesis. J Am Chem Soc 85:3309

Elias ER, Hansen RM, Irons M et al (2003) Rod photoreceptor responses in children with Smith-Lemli-Opitz syndrome. Arch Ophthalmol 121(12):1738–1743

Fliesler SJ (2002) Effects of cholesterol biosynthesis inhibitors on retinal development, structure, and function. In: Fliesler SJ (ed) Sterols and oxysterols: chemistry, biology and pathobiology. Research Signpost, Kerala, India, 77–109

Fliesler SJ, Kapphahn BJ, Ferrington DA et al (2006). Rhodopsin resists oxidative modification by PUFA-derived aldehydes and nitrosylation during light- and metabolically-induced retinal degenerations. Abstract, Annual Meeting, Association for Research in Vision and Ophthalmology (ARVO), Ft. Lauderdale, FL, May, 2006 [on CD-ROM]

Fliesler SJ, Keller RK (1997) Isoprenoid metabolism in the vertebrate retina. Int J Biochem Cell Biol 29(6):877–894

Fliesler SJ, Peachey NS, Richards MJ et al (2004) Retinal degeneration in a rodent model of Smith-Lemli-Opitz syndrome: electrophysiological, biochemical, and morphological features. Arch Ophthalmol 122(8):1190–2000

Fliesler SJ, Richards MJ, Miller C-Y, Peachey NS (1999) Marked alteration of sterol metabolism and composition without compromising retinal development or function. Invest Ophthalmol Vis Sci 40:1792–1801

Fliesler SJ, Vaughan DK, Jenewein EC et al (2007) Partial rescue of retinal function and sterol steady-state in a rat model of Smith-Lemli-Opitz syndrome. Pediatr Res 61:273–278

Ford DA, Monda JK, Brush RS et al (2008) Lipidomic analysis of the retina in a rat model of Smith-Lemli-Opitz syndrome: alterations in docosahexaenoic acid content of phospholipid molecular species. Neurochem 105(3):1032–1047

Givner ML, Dvornik D (1965) Agents affecting lipid metabolism – XV. Biochemical studies with the cholesterol synthesis inhibitor AY-9944 in young and mature rats. Biochem Pharmacol 14:611–619

Gofflot F (2002) Defects in cholesterol biosynthesis and abnormal embryonic development. In: Fliesler SJ (ed) Sterols and oxysterols: chemistry, biology, and pathobiology. Research Signpost, Trivandrum, India, 47–76

Kolf-Clauw M, Chevy F, Wolf C et al (1996) Inhibition of 7-dehydrocholesterol reductase by the teratogen AY9944: a rat model for Smith-Lemli-Opitz syndrome. Teratology 54:115–125

Negre-Salvayre A, Coatrieux C, Inggueneau C, Salvayre R (2008) Advanced lipid peroxidation end products in oxidative damage to proteins. Potential role in diseases and therapeutic prospects for the inhibitors. Br J Pharmacol 53(1):6–20

Porter FD (2003) Human malformation syndromes due to inborn errors of cholesterol synthesis. Curr Opin Pediatr 15:607–613

Porter FD (2008) Smith-Lemli-Opitz syndrome: pathogenesis, diagnosis and management. Eur J Hum Genet 16(5):535–541

Richards MJ, Nagel BA, Fliesler SJ (2006) Lipid hydroperoxide formation in the retina: correlation with retinal degeneration and light damage in a rat model of Smith-Lemli-Opitz syndrome. Exp Eye Res 82:538–541

Siddiqui AM, Richards MJ, Fliesler SJ (2007) Global differential and temporal transcriptional profiling of retinas from AY9944-treated (SLOS) vs. control rats. Abstract, Annual Meeting, Association for Research in Vision and Ophthalmology (ARVO), Ft. Lauderdale, FL, May, 2007 [on CD-ROM]

Siddiqui AM, Wassif CA, Porter FD et al (2008) A systems-level approach to temporal transcriptional profiling of retinas in a rat model of Smith-Lemli-Opitz syndrome. Abstract, Annual Meeting, Association for Research in Vision and Ophthalmology (ARVO), Ft. Lauderdale, FL, May, 2008 [on CD-ROM]

Smith DW, Lemmli L, Opitz JM (1964) A newly recognized syndrome of multiple congenital anomalies. J Pediatr 64:210–217

Tint GS, Salen G, Batta AK et al (1995) Correlation of severity and outcome with plasma sterol levels in variants of the Smith-Lemli-Opitz syndrome. J Pediatr 127(1):82–87

Vaughan DK, Peachey NS, Richards MJ et al (2006) Light-induced exacerbation of retinal degeneration in a rat model of Smith-Lemli-Opitz syndrome. Exp Eye Res 82:496–504

Xu G, Salen G, Shefer S et al (1995) Reproducing abnormal cholesterol biosynthesis as seen in the Smith-Lemli-Opitz syndrome by inhibiting the conversion of 7-dehydro-cholesterol to cholesterol in rats. J Clin Invest 95:76–81

Yeagle PL (1985) Cholesterol and the cell membrane. Biochim Biophys Acta 822(3–4):267–287

Yu H, Patel SB (2005) Recent insights into the Smith-Lemli-Opitz syndrome. Clin Genet 68(5):383–391

Chapter 56
Do Calcium Channel Blockers Rescue Dying Photoreceptors in the *Pde6b*[rd1] Mouse?

Peter Barabas, Carolee Cutler Peck, and David Krizaj

Abstract Retinitis pigmentosa (RP) is a genetically heterogeneous set of blinding diseases that affects more than a million people worldwide. In humans, ~5–8% of recessive and dominant RP cases are caused by nonsense mutations in the *Pde6b* gene coding for the ß-subunit of the rod photoreceptor cGMP phosphodiesterase 6 (PDE6-ß). The study of the disease has been greatly aided by the *Pde6b*[rd1] *(rd1)* mouse model of RP carrying a null PDE6ß allele. Degenerating *rd1* rods were found to experience a pathological increase in intracellular calcium concentration ('Ca overload') when they enter the apoptotic process at postnatal day 10. A 1999 study suggested that the Ca^{2+} channel antagonist D-*cis* diltiazem delays the kinetics of *rd1* rod degeneration, conferring partial rescue of scotopic vision. Subsequent reports were mixed: whereas several studies failed to replicate the original results, others appeared to confirm the neuroprotective effects of Ca^{2+} channel antagonists such as diltiazem, nilvadipine and verapamil. We discuss the discrepancies between the results of different groups and suggest plausible causes for the discordant results. We also discuss potential involvement of recently identified Ca^{2+}-dependent mechanisms that include protective calcium ATPase mechanisms, ryanodine and IP3 calcium stores, and store operated channels in *Pde6b*[rd1] neurodegeneration.

56.1 Introduction

Retinitis pigmentosa (RP), a genetically heterogeneous set of blinding diseases affecting more than a million people worldwide, derives its name from an accumulation of pigment clusters in the neural retina. Early symptoms associated with the main rod-cone dystrophy variants include night blindness and loss of peripheral

D. Krizaj (✉)
Department of Ophthalmology and Visual Sciences, Moran Eye Center, University of Utah School of Medicine, Salt Lake City, UT 84132, USA
e-mail: david.krizaj@hsc.utah.edu

The authors Peter Barabas and Carolee Cutler Peck equally contributed to this work.

R.E. Anderson et al. (eds.), *Retinal Degenerative Diseases*, Advances in Experimental Medicine and Biology 664, DOI 10.1007/978-1-4419-1399-9_56,

vision, followed by eventual loss of central vision. One of the best-characterized forms of recessive RP in humans is caused by a nonsense mutation in the gene coding for the β subunit of the rod photoreceptor cGMP phosphodiesterase 6 (PDE6b) that has been linked to 5–8% cases of RP (McLaughlin et al. 1995). The essential features of photoreceptor degeneration in human RP have been replicated in rodent models, which can be studied over much shorter time frames. The $Pde6b^{rd1}$ ($rd1$) mouse model carries a recessive nonsense mutation in PDE6b (reviewed in Farber 1995). The mutation is characterized by rapid degeneration of rods beginning at late stages of photoreceptor differentiation, which in turn triggers apoptosis of cones. By P90, virtually all photoreceptors have disappeared (Carter-Dawson et al. 1978; Punzo et al. 2009) except ~3% of cone perikarya in the dorsal retina (Jimenez et al. 1996). While gene therapy and pharmacological treatments have been attempted to ameliorate photoreceptor degeneration in RP models, a significant bottleneck for developing treatment has occurred due to the large number of different genes that lead to RP (>46; www.sph.uth.tmc.edu/Retnet/) and the apparent inconsistency of pharmacological studies focused on treating RP. Hopes for a possible restorative pharmacological intervention were kindled by the report that D-cis-diltiazem – an antagonist of voltage-activated Ca^{2+} channels which is commonly used as a cardio-protectant – partially rescues $rd1$ photoreceptors (Frasson et al. 1999). Suppression of Ca^{2+} pathways that orchestrate apoptotic cascades in rods and cones promised to deliver a general therapeutic strategy that could be applied to treating recessive retinal degenerations. Subsequent reports appeared to confirm (Read et al. 2002; Sanges et al. 2006) or repudiate (Pawlyk et al. 2002; Bush et al. 2000) the basic findings of the Frasson study. The aim of this paper is to review the literature, explore potential mechanisms involved in $Pde6b^{rd1}$ neurodegeneration in the light of recent findings on Ca^{2+} signaling in vertebrate photoreceptors and explore the possibilities offered by the pharmacological approach to prevention of photoreceptor degeneration.

56.1.1 The Pde6b^{rd1} Mouse and Increased [cGMP]

The $Pde6b^{rd1}$ ($rd1$) mouse phenotype was first identified in a Harvard albino mouse strain and subsequently found in wild and laboratory mice across the United States and Europe (e.g., Pittler and Baehr 1991; Pittler et al. 1993). The mutation is associated with a nonfunctional rod-specific PDE6 gene located on the mouse chromosome 5. Every mouse strain with the $rd1$ gene carries a murine leukemia provirus integrated into the first intron, combined with a point mutation which introduces a stop codon in exon 7 (Farber 1995; Huang et al. 1995). At P10, 33% of mRNA is transcribed in $Pde6b^{rd1}$ rods (Viczian et al. 1992), however, the message is not expressed, presumably due to nonsense-mediated decay of PDEb6 mRNA and/or instability of the truncated PDE6b peptide (Bowes et al. 1990; W. Baehr, personal communication). Loss of the β subunit completely eliminates function of the PDE complex which consists of a catalytic dimer (non-identical α and β subunits) and two inhibitory γ subunits. PDE malfunction affects both amplitude and kinetics of the photocurrent and results in cGMP, Na^+ and Ca^{2+} overloads within $rd1$ cells (Farber 1995).

Although it is clear that *rd1* phenotype is caused by mutated PDE6, the causal relationship between abnormally high [cGMP] and apoptosis is still not well understood. cGMP content in the *Pde6b^rd1* retina increases days before signs of degeneration become apparent, reaching its maximum around the eye opening when rod degeneration is at its peak (Farber and Lolley 1974). Early signs of *rd1* expression in photoreceptors such as retarded growth of OS and IS are seen 4–8 days after birth (Sanyal and Bal 1973). Swelling of rod mitochondria and appearance of vacuoles in the IS occur at P8 (Farber and Lolley 1974). While cellular integrity and thickness of P10 *rd1* ONL is comparable to the WT, OS disks show signs of disruption, chromatin is fragmented and the P10 increase in TUNEL-positive outer nuclear layer (ONL) cells is followed by rapid degeneration of rods by P14. At P18-P21, rods are gone, leaving a single row of cone perikarya (Carter-Dawson et al. 1978) and a total loss of image-forming vision by P40.

56.1.2 Calcium Regulation and Overload in the Photoreceptor Inner Segment

Rod photoreceptors are formed by two compartments, the OS and the IS, that communicate through a thin nonmotile cilium. PDE6 in the wild type retina is located in the OS whereas the pro-apoptotic cascades are confined to the IS. *Pde6b^rd1* retinas express a rudimentary OS, hence it is not clear whether a messenger mechanism transmits a 'degenerate and die' message from the OS to the IS and/or the entire holoenzyme complex remains 'stuck' in the IS. Such a messenger could be the metabolic stress caused by depletion of ATP expended to combat excessive Na^+ and Ca^{2+} influx or ER stress caused by accumulation of proteins in the ER. An alternative, which is not mutually exclusive, is that the signal is mediated by elevated $[Ca^{2+}]$ itself as Ca^{2+} regulates all aspects of photoreceptor function, including degeneration (Krizaj and Copenhagen 2002; Szikra and Krizaj 2009).

There is little doubt that degenerating photoreceptors experience Ca^{2+} overload. Elevated cytosolic Ca^{2+} concentrations in *rd1* rods have been measured directly with Ca^{2+} indicator dyes and indirectly by observing compensatory changes in Ca^{2+}-dependent proteins. Around P10, $[Ca^{2+}]i$ elevations are observed in acutely dissociated *rd1* rods and in cultured *rd1* explants (Doonan et al. 2005; Sanges et al. 2006), accompanied by upregulated CaM kinase II and migration of phosducins and associated $Gt_{\beta 1\gamma 1}$ subunits (Donovan and Cotter 2002; Hauck et al. 2005) whereas the calpain inhibitor calpastatin is strongly downregulated (Paquet-Durand et al. 2006). Other parallel signs of Ca^{2+}-dependent changes in *rd1* rods include prominent increases in m and µ calpain proteases, cleavage of caspases-3 and -12, AIF (apoptosis-inducing factor; Sharma and Rohrer 2004). Mitochondria are depolarized by excess Ca^{2+} (Doonan et al. 2005), possibly leading to activation of the permeability transition pore (He et al. 2000) and translocation of AIF and caspase 12 into the nucleus (Sanges et al. 2006). Another Ca^{2+} store, the endoplasmic reticulum (ER), activates pro-apoptotic Bid, Bax, PERK, IRE1α and ATF4 pathways (Lin et al. 2007). Given that *rd1* rods experience an enormous degree of ER stress due to the traffic jam of proteins normally destined for the OS, it is very likely that there is a concomitant malfunction of SERCA-mediated Ca^{2+} sequestration and ryanodine & IP3 receptor mediated release of ER Ca^{2+} (see below).

In early 1990s, Mark Tso's group at the University of Illinois showed that flunarizine but not nimodipine protects photoreceptors stressed by exposure to strong light. While nimodipine (a dihydropyridine) is a specific L-type channel antagonist (Li et al. 1991), the diphenylpiperazine flunarizine is a non-specific antagonist of Ca^{2+} channels (Edward et al. 1991). Two L-type antagonists -D-*cis*-diltiazem and verapamil – were however found to inhibit photoreceptor degeneration in the *Drosophila rdbB* mutant (Sahly et al. 1992) and to confer partial protection on *Pde6b^{rd1}* photoreceptors (Frasson et al. 1999; Takano et al. 2004; Sanges et al. 2006). These studies initiated interest in pharmacological approach to protecting vision through management of Ca^{2+} overloads.

56.2 D-*cis*-diltiazem and Neuroprotection in the Retina

The dihydropyridine diltiazem is a competitive antagonist of L-type calcium channels with an IC_{50} of ~5 μM (Koch and, Kaupp 1985). The D-*cis* stereoisomer is the active compound in several commonly used prescription drugs. Three other L-type blockers, verapamil, nilvadipine, nimodipine and nifedipine are also designated for human use.

The first important study using D-*cis* diltiazem was performed by Serge Picaud's group in Strasbourg and published in Nature Medicine in 1999 (Frasson et al. 1999). The protocol involved intraperitoneal (IP) injections of D-*cis*-diltiazem two times a day, starting at P9, reaching a daily dose of 54 mg per kg body weight, a dose ~6-fold higher than the maximal allowed human daily dose (<1 mg/kg 4 times daily; Bush et al. 2000). Retinal wholemounts and slices were labeled with an antibody against rhodopsin and outcomes were measured indirectly via the scotopic ERG b-wave which showed a remaining b-wave (~20 μV) in 4 out of 10 animals treated at P36. Though the amplitude was small (compared to ~800 μV in wild type eyes), this result was highly significant as the *rd1* scotopic b-wave is basically flat around P21 (Pawlyk et al. 2002). Additionally, the diltiazem-treated cohort at P36 had ~18,600 surviving rods, a 2- to 3-fold increase compared to 7,500 rods in non-treated animals; a modest protective effect on cone survival was also observed. These early results prompted a clinical study which found that diltiazem, supplemented with vitamin E, improves vision in human RP patients (Pasantes-Morales et al. 2002).

56.2.1 Criticism of the Frasson Study

The immediate concern voiced by Tso was that the rhodopsin antibody used by Frasson et al. might have depicted ongoing rod degeneration rather than healthy, 'protected', cells (Edward and Tso 2000). Several groups, which attempted to replicate the original study using D-*cis*-diltiazem in different models of RP degeneration, reported mostly discouraging results. A histological + ERG study by Sieving's group found no significant rescue in the P23H rat that carries a dominant negative opsin mutation (Bush et al. 2000). A follow-up study using the same methodology in the *rcd1* dog that also carries a stop codon in its PDE6b gene found no neuroprotection (Pearce-Kelling et al. 2001). Yamazaki et al. (2002), Fox et al. (2003) and Takano et al. (2004) observed no effect of D-*cis* diltiazem on $Pde6b^{rd1}$ rods after treating P9 mice for 7 days with 1 mg/ml diltiazem (i.e., at ~50 times lower dose than the Frasson study). Finally, Pawlyk et al. (2002), using a different *rd1* strain, found no significant differences in a double blind study that reproduced the original study conditions. There were no changes in rhodopsin and cone (S and M) opsin immunoreactivity nor were changes observed in the ERG, leading the authors to conclude 'there is no compelling rationale for testing D-*cis*-diltiazem (Cardizem, Hoechst-Marion Roussel) as a possible treatment for RP.'

56.2.2   Subsequent Evidence Shows L-Type Channels Are Involved in Degeneration

As D-*cis* diltiazem in the Frasson study only partially (~50%) blocked L-type channels, a stronger effect would be expected with full channel block. A subsequent study found that elimination of the β_2 subunit of the L-type calcium channel results in degeneration at a (delayed) rate similar to that in the Frasson study (Read et al. 2002). A 40% increase in the number of surviving cells at P21 was observed in $Pde6b^{rd1}$ $^{-}\beta_2$ KO animals, directly and unambiguously confirming involvement of L-type channels in *rd1* degeneration. Subsequently, Sanges et al. (2006) showed that the D-*cis* stereoisomer blocked Ca^{2+} overload, resulting in a decreased number of TUNEL-positive *rd1* rods. Translocation of AIF and caspase-12 to the nucleus of remaining rods was inhibited, confirming the effectiveness of D-*cis* diltiazem in retinal *rd1* explants.

Nilvadipine, an L-type antagonist often used in Japan, was effective in decreasing photoreceptor cell loss in the RCS rat (Yamazaki et al. 2002), $Pde6b^{rd1}$ (Takano et al. 2004), and *rds* mice (Takeuchi et al. 2008). The effect of nilvadipine vs the lack of effect seen with diltiazem treatment was ascribed to greater permeability of dihydropyridines vs benzothiazepins (Takano et al. 2004). Surprisingly, while nilvadipine appeared to preserve photoreceptor structure, it had no effect on ERG b-wave amplitudes. Microarray analysis after nilvadipine treatment showed downregulation of proapoptotic genes coding for caspase-3, -9, and -14 as well as ADP-ribosyl cyclase, the product of which acts as an allosteric modulator of the ryanodine receptor (RyR). RyR itself, a major cellular mediator of calcium-induced calcium release in Photoreceptor ER (Krizaj and Copenhgen, 2002), was upregulated (Takano et al. 2004), implicating Ca^{2+} stores in *rd1* degeneration.

D-*cis*-diltiazem inhibits not only L-type calcium channels, but also CNG channels and vice versa, the L-*cis* isomer inhibits L-type channels with an IC_{50}

$\sim$ 75 μM (Koch and Kaupp 1985). A slight advantage of L-*cis* over the D-*cis* isomer was suggested for retinas treated with zaprinast (Vallazza-Deschamps et al. 2005) or lead (Fox et al. 2003). In conclusion, while elimination of L-type-mediated Ca^{2+} entry delays, but does not prevent, *rd1* rod degeneration, the accumulated evidence supports the notion that Ca^{2+} overload mediated by some type of Ca^{2+} channel potentiates degeneration.

56.3 Other Players May Be Involved

The ineffectiveness of L-type channel blockade in rat and dog might have been due to drug dosing and accessibility issues (some dihydropyridines are notoriously difficult to get into solution let alone across the blood-brain barrier). Alternatively, the rhodopsin mutation in the P23H mutant and the *Mertk* mutation in the RCS rat may involve different degeneration mechanisms unrelated to Ca^{2+} influx. A final possibility is that Ca^{2+} regulation in degenerating photoreceptors involves players that were not directly affected by L-type and/or CNG channel antagonists.

Edward et al. (1991) hinted at the contribution of IP3-sensitive intracellular Ca^{2+} stores localized in the ER. Indeed, suppression of Ca^{2+} sequestration into the ER kills differentiating photoreceptors (Linden et al. 1999; Chiarini et al. 2003), presumably due to global suppression of mRNA translation that occurs in cells with depleted Ca^{2+} stores (Brostrom and Brostrom 2003). Conversely, at P10-P12, Ca^{2+} overload in *rd1* cells coincides with peak expression of pro-apoptotic ER markers such as caspase-12, phospho-pancreatic ER kinase (p-PERK), phospho-eukaryotic initiation factor 2α (p-eIF2α) and glucose-regulated protein-78 (GRP78/BiP) (Yang et al. 2007, Lin et al. 2007), possibly resulting in augmentation of the untranslated protein response (UPR). This suggests that a critical junction for preventing Ca^{2+}-mediated apoptosis might be Ca^{2+} stores and/or store-operated channels rather than L-type/CNG channels.

Store-operated channels belonging to different canonical TRPC classes are prominently expressed in rods and cones (Szikra et al. 2008; Krizaj et al. 2008a) together with their activators, STIM1 proteins (Szikra et al. 2009). TRPCs play an increasingly recognized role in generating Ca^{2+} overloads that drive calpains, implicated in both apoptosis (Marasa et al. 2006; Shan et al. 2008) and neuroprotection (Bollimuntha et al. 2006; Yamamoto et al. 2007). In normal retinas, Ca^{2+} influx through these channels is likely to serve a neuroprotective function by preventing pathological decreases in $[Ca^{2+}]$ in cells exposed to saturating light, which when prolonged was shown to trigger photoreceptor degeneration (Leconte and Barnstable 2000; Woodruff et al. 2003). TRPC transcription and expression is dramatically affected in *Pde6b^{rd1}* degeneration together with upregulated expression of the major protective PMCA1 calcium transporters (Krizaj and Copenhagen 2002; Krizaj et al. 2008b). This suggests that *rd1* rods are battling Ca^{2+} overload by upregulation of endogenous Ca^{2+} clearance mechanisms. It remains to be seen whether upregulation of these ATPases prolongs rod survival. In summary, the *Pde6b^{rd1}* mouse model has greatly facilitated studies of retinal degeneration caused by defects in expression and function of PDE6. This degeneration is intimately associated with chronic elevation in $[Ca^{2+}]i$ which has a causal role in activating pro-apoptotic pathways within the inner segment. The conflicting interpretations of pharmacological effects may stem partly from lack of drug specificity and partly from our lack of a comprehensive understanding of Ca^{2+} regulation and trafficking in the photoreceptor IS. Successful therapeutic interventions will depend on our understanding of signaling pathways involved in the degeneration process.

Acknowledgments This work was supported by the Knights Templar Eye Foundation, International Retina Research Foundation, Moran TIGER award, the NIH (EY13870), Foundation Fighting Blindness and an unrestricted grant from Research to Prevent Blindness to the Moran Eye Institute. We thank Dr. Wolfgang Baehr for helpful comments. Dr. Barabas wishes to thank Dr. Julianna Kardos and the Chemical Research Center of the Hungarian Academy of Sciences for support.

References

Bollimuntha S, Ebadi M, Singh BB (2006) TRPC1 protects human SH-SY5Y cells against salsolinol-induced cytotoxicity by inhibiting apoptosis. Brain Res 1099:141–149

Bowes C, Li T, Danciger M et al (1990) Retinal degeneration in the rd mouse is caused by a defect in the beta subunit of rod cGMP-phosphodiesterase. Nature 347:677–680

Brostrom MA, Brostrom CO (2003) Calcium dynamics and endoplasmic reticular function in the regulation of protein synthesis: implications for cell growth and adaptability. Cell Calcium 34:345–363

Bush RA, Kononen L, Machida S et al (2000) The effect of calcium channel blocker diltiazem on photoreceptor degeneration in the rhodopsin Pro213His rat. Invest Ophthalmol Vis Sci 41:2697–2701

Carter-Dawson LD, LaVail MM, Sidman RL (1978) Differential effect of the rd mutation on rods and cones in the mouse retina. Invest Ophthalmol Vis Sci 17:489–498

Chiarini LB, Leal-Ferreira ML, de Freitas FG et al (2003) Changing sensitivity to cell death during development of retinal photoreceptors. J Neurosci Res 74:875–883

Donovan M, Cotter TG (2002) Caspase-independent photoreceptor apoptosis in vivo and differential expression of apoptotic protease activating factor-1 and caspase-3 during retinal development. Cell Death Differ 9:1220–1231

Doonan F, Donovan M, Cotter TG (2005) Activation of multiple pathways during photoreceptor apoptosis in the rd mouse. Invest Ophthalmol Vis Sci 46:3530–3538

Edward DP, Lam TT, Shahinfar S et al (1991) Amelioration of light-induced retinal degeneration by a calcium overload blocker. Flunarizine. Arch Ophthalmol 109:554–562

Edward DP, Tso MO (2000) Rod photoreceptor rescue or degeneration. Nat Med 6:116

Farber DB (1995) From mice to men: the cyclic GMP phosphodiesterase gene in vision and disease. The Proctor Lecture. Invest Ophthalmol Vis Sci 36:263–275

Farber DB, Lolley RN (1974) Cyclic guanosine monophosphate: elevation in degenerating photoreceptor cells of the C3H mouse retina. Science 186:449–451

Fox DA, Poblenz AT, He L et al (2003) Pharmacological strategies to block rod photoreceptor apoptosis caused by calcium overload: a mechanistic target-site approach to neuroprotection. Eur J Ophthalmol 13(Suppl 3):S44–S56

Frasson M, Sahel JA, Fabre M et al (1999) Retinitis pigmentosa: rod photoreceptor rescue by a calcium-channel blocker in the rd mouse. Nat Med 5:1183–1187

Hauck SM, Ekström PA, Ahuja-Jensen P et al (2005) Differential modification of phosducin protein in degenerating rd1 retina is associated with constitutively active Ca^{2+}/calmodulin kinase II in rod outer segments. Mol Cell Proteomics 5:324–336

He L, Poblenz AT, Medrano CJ et al (2000) Lead and calcium produce rod photoreceptor cell apoptosis by opening the mitochondrial permeability transition pore. J Biol Chem 275: 12175–12184

Jiménez AJ, García-Fernández JM, González B et al (1996) The spatio-temporal pattern of photoreceptor degeneration in the aged rd/rd mouse retina. Cell Tissue Res 284:193–202

Koch KW, Kaupp UB (1985) Cyclic GMP directly regulates a cation conductance in membranes of bovine rods by a cooperative mechanism. J Biol Chem 260:6788–6800

Krizaj D, Huang H, Cutler-Peck C et al (2008b) Calcium signaling in rod and cone photoreceptor degeneration. Proc. XIIIth International Symposium on Retinal Degeneration, Sept 18–23, 2008; Emeishan, China

Krizaj D, Morgans CW, Thoreson WH et al (2008a) TRPC6 modulates cone signals in the vertebrate retina. Proc. FASEB, Snowmass, CO

Leconte L, Barnstable CJ (2000) Impairment of rod cGMP-gated channel alpha-subunit expression leads to photoreceptor and bipolar cell degeneration. Invest Ophthalmol Vis Sci 41: 917–926

Li JP, Edward DP, Lam TT et al (1991) Nimodipine, a voltage-sensitive calcium channel antagonist, fails to ameliorate light-induced retinal degeneration in rat. Res Commun Chem Pathol Pharmacol 72:347–352

Lin JH, Li H, Yasumura D et al (2007) IRE1 signaling affects cell fate during the unfolded protein response. Science 318:944–949

Linden R, Rehen SK, Chiarini LB (1999) Apoptosis in developing retinal tissue. Prog Retin Eye Res 18:133–165

Marasa BS, Rao JN, Zou T et al (2006) Induced TRPC1 expression sensitizes intestinal epithelial cells to apoptosis by inhibiting NF-kappaB activation through Ca^{2+} influx. Biochem J 397: 77–87

McLaughlin ME, Ehrhart TL, Berson EL et al (1995) Mutation spectrum of the gene encoding the beta subunit of rod phosphodiesterase among patients with autosomal recessive retinitis pigmentosa. Proc Natl Acad Sci U S A 92:3249–3253

Paquet-Durand F, Azadi S, Hauck SM et al (2006) Calpain is activated in degenerating photoreceptors in the rd1 mouse. J Neurochem 96:802–814

Pasantes-Morales H, Quiroz H, Quesada O (2002) Treatment with taurine, diltiazem, and vitamin E retards the progressive visual field reduction in retinitis pigmentosa: a 3-year follow-up study. Metab Brain Dis 17(3):183–197

Pawlyk BS, Li T, Scimeca MS et al (2002) Absence of photoreceptor rescue with D-*cis*-diltiazem in the rd mouse. Invest Ophthalmol Vis Sci 43:1912–1915

Pearce-Kelling SE, Aleman TS, Nickle A et al (2001) Calcium channel blocker D-*cis*-diltiazem does not slow retinal degeneration in the PDE6B mutant rcd1 canine model of retinitis pigmentosa. Mol Vis 7:42–47

Pittler SJ, Keeler CE, Sidman RL, Baehr W (1993) PCR analysis of DNA from 70-year-old sections of rodless retina demonstrates indentity with the mouse rd defect. Proc Natl Acad Sci U S A 90:9616–9619

Punzo C, Kornacker K, Cepko CL (2009) Stimulation of the insulin/mTOR pathway delays cone death in a mouse model of retinitis pigmentosa. Nat Neurosci 12:44–52

Read DS, McCall MA, Gregg RG (2002) Absence of voltage-dependent calcium channels delays photoreceptor degeneration in rd mice. Exp Eye Res 75:415–420

Sahly I, Bar Nachum S, Suss-Toby E et al (1992) Calcium channel blockers inhibit retinal degeneration in the retinal-degeneration-B mutant of Drosophila. Proc Natl Acad Sci U S A 89:435–439

Sanges D, Comitato A, Tammaro R et al (2006) Apoptosis in retinal degeneration involves cross-talk between apoptosis-inducing factor (AIF) and caspase-12 and is blocked by calpain inhibitors. Proc Natl Acad Sci U S A 103:17366–17371

Sanyal S, Bal AK (1973) Comparative light and electron microscopic study of retinal histogenesis in normal and rd mutant mice. Z Anat Entwicklungsgesch 142:219–238

Shan D, Marchase RB, Chatham JC (2008) Overexpression of TRPC3 increases apoptosis but not necrosis in response to ischemia-reperfusion in adult mouse cardiomyocytes. Am J Physiol Cell Physiol 294:C833–C841

Sharma AK, Rohrer B (2004) Calcium-induced calpain mediates apoptosis via caspase-3 in a mouse photoreceptor cell line. J Biol Chem 279:35564–35572

Szikra T, Cusato K, Thoreson WB et al (2008) Depletion of calcium stores regulates calcium influx and signal transmission in rod photoreceptors. J Physiol 586:4859–4875

Szikra T, Krizaj D (2009) Calcium signals in inner segments of photoreceptors. In: Tombran-Tink J, Barnstable C (eds) The visual transduction cascade: basic and clinical principles, Jumana Press, Totowa, NJ, pp 197–223

Szikra T, Barabas P, Bartoletti TM, Huang W, Akopian A, Thoreson WB, Krizaj D (2009) Calcium homeostasis and cone signaling are regulated by interactons between calcium stores and plasma membrane ion channels. PLoS One 4(8):e6723

Takano Y, Ohguro H, Dezawa M et al (2004) Study of drug effects of calcium channel blockers on retinal degeneration of rd mouse. Biochem Biophys Res Commun 313:1015–1022

Takeuchi K, Nakazawa M, Mizukoshi S (2008) Systemic administration of nilvadipine delays photoreceptor degeneration of heterozygous retinal degeneration slow (rds) mouse. Exp Eye Res 86:60–69

Vallazza-Deschamps G, Cia D, Gong J et al (2005) Excessive activation of cyclic nucleotide-gated channels contributes to neuronal degeneration of photoreceptors. Eur J Neurosci 22:1013–1022

Viczian A, Sanyal S, Toffenetti J et al (1992) Photoreceptor-specific mRNAs in mice carrying different allelic combinations at the rd and rds loci. Exp Eye Res 54:853–860

Woodruff ML, Wang Z, Chung HY et al (2003) Spontaneous activity of opsin apoprotein is a cause of Leber congenital amaurosis. Nat Genet 35:158–164

Yamamoto S, Wajima T, Hara Y et al (2007) Transient receptor potential channels in Alzheimer's disease. Biochim Biophys Acta 1772:958–967

Yamazaki H, Ohguro H, Maeda T et al (2002) Preservation of retinal morphology and functions in royal college surgeons rat by nilvadipine, a $Ca^{(2+)}$ antagonist. Invest Ophthalmol Vis Sci 43:919–926

Yang LP, Wu LM, Guo XJ et al (2007) Activation of endoplasmic reticulum stress in degenerating photoreceptors of the rd1 mouse. Invest Ophthalmol Vis Sci 48:5191–5198

Chapter 57
Effect of PBNA on the NO Content and NOS Activity in Ischemia/Reperfusion Injury in the Rat Retina

Liangdong Li, Zhihua Huang, Hai Xiao, Xigui Chen, and Jing Zeng

Abstract

Objective: To investigated the effect of Polygonum Bistorta L. n-butyl Alcohol (PBNA) extract on the NO content and NOS activity in ischemia/reperfusion (I/R) injury in the rat retina.

Methods: The model of retinal I/R injury in SD rats was made by reperfusion for 1 h after occlusion of common carotid artery (CCA) for 1 h. The rats were randomly divided into four groups: control group, retinal I/R injury group, low-dosage PBNA treated group and high-dosage treated PBNA group. The control group was injected with 1 ml/kg NS through sublingual vein after CCA was dissociated. Other groups were treated with normal saline or PBNA before occlusion of CCA. After occlusion of CCA for 1 h following reperfusion for 1 h, blood was collected and serum was separated to determine the contents of NO, the activity of T-NOS, iNOS and eNOS.

Result: (1) The contents of NO in I/R group showed lower values than in control group ($P<0.001$) and low-dosage PBNA treated group ($P<0.05$). (2) The activities of T-NOS in both low-dosage PBNA group and high-dosage group increased, compared with I/R group ($P<0.01$). (3) The activity of serum iNOS in I/R group increased compared with control group ($P<0.05$) and low-dosage PBNA treated group evidently ($P<0.05$). (4) The activity of serum eNOS in I/R group decreased compared with control group ($P<0.05$), both low-dosage ($P<0.05$) and high-dosage PBNA ($P<0.01$) treated group markedly.

Conclusion: The date suggest that PBNA have a therapeutic effect on retinal ischemia/reperfusion injury by increasing the activities of T-NOS and eNOS, decreasing the activity of iNOS, elevating the content of NO, enhancing the Anti-oxidation and expanding the blood vessel.

J. Zeng (✉)
Pharmaceutic College, Gannan Medical University, Ganzhou, Jiangxi Province 341000, China
e-mail: zengjing61@hotmail.com

R.E. Anderson et al. (eds.), *Retinal Degenerative Diseases*, Advances in Experimental
Medicine and Biology 664, DOI 10.1007/978-1-4419-1399-9_57,
© Springer Science+Business Media, LLC 2010

57.1 Introduction

Retinal ischemia/reperfusion (I/R) injury is a clinical common ischemic optical disease, led to frequently by the occlusion of retinal vessels induced by the embolism of central retinal vein and artery, acute angle-closure glaucoma and retinopathy. In many patients, retina was seriously injured and visual function was further injured after the reperfusion followed occlusion. multiple factors such as Ca^{2+} overloading (Torin et al. 2000), free radical (Pannicke et al. 2005), the over release of exitotoxicitic amino acids (Kwon et al. 2005; Dijk et al. 2004), Inflammatory reaction (Sanchez et al. 2003), retinal nerve cell apoptosis (Oz et al. 2005), the changes of content of NO and activity of NOS (Cheon et al. 2003; Hangai et al. 1996), play roles in retinal I/R injury which can grow blind and can led to irreversible visual loss if treatment is not given promptly. So, it is very important to research on some effective new drugs to treat the retinal I/R injury.

Polygonum Bistora L, which is the dry rhizoma of Polygonaceae Plants, has the effects of clearing heat and eliminating dampness, relieving convulsion, detumescence and relieving pain. Extracts from Polygonum Bistora L were extracted by different solvents in turns: 95% alcohol, ligarine, acetic ether and n-butanol, and the n-butanol extracts were called Polygonum Bistorla L. n-Butyl Alcohol Extract (PBNA) which major reconstituents were ligustrin, quercetin-3-rutinoside, catechin and Mururin A (Liu et al. 2006). Our previous study showed that PBNA can expand blood vessels and protect heart muscle from ischemia (Li et al. 2007; Ye et al. 2006). To learn whether PBNA has a beneficial effect on retinal I/R injury, in this study we investigated the effect of PBNA on retina and the change of the content of NO and the activity of NOS and their relation in I/R injury by occlusion of common carotid artery.

57.2 Materials and Methods

57.2.1 Animals and Reagents

Sprague Dawley (SD) rats (male, 250~280 g, age: 8~10 weeks) were obtained from Jiangxi traditional Chinese medical college and maintained in the Center of Laboratory Animal Resources at Gannan medical college.

PBNA supplied by Shenyang Pharmaceutical University was dissolved in double distillation Water and 0.22 μm filtered. Kits of NO, T-NOS, iNOS and eNOS were provided by Nanjing Jiancheng Bioengineering Corporation.

57.2.2 Induction of Retinal I/R

Twenty-four rats were divided into four groups randomly: control group (sham operation), retinal I/R injury group, low-dosage PBNA treated group and high-dosage treated PBNA group. Retinal I/R injury were induced by reperfusion followed occlusion of common carotid artery. Rats were anesthetized by peritoneal injection of 350 mg/kg 10% chloral hydrate. Sterilize the skin with 75% alcohol and made a midline incision in the ventral surface of the neck. Dissected muscles and lamina praetrachealis, to expose and isolate the comman carotid artery (CCA), and then occlude it with a clip. To make retinal ischemia sure, the pupils were dilated and fluorescence fundus angiography (FFA) were performed. After occlusion for 60 min, unclamp the clip and FFA were performed again to make sure the restoration of blood supply. Repeat all the steps for the sham operation group, except for occluding the common carotid artery. 1 ml/kg NS was injected through sublingual vein after CCA was dissociated in control group. Other groups were treated with normal saline, low-dosage PBNA (0.3 mg/kg) or high-dosage PBNA (1 mg/kg) through sublingual vein respectively before occlusion of CCA.

57.2.3 Detection of MDA and NO Concentration, SOD and GSH-PX Activity

After 60 min reperfusion, collect blood by abdominal caval vein. The supernatants were collected by centrifugation at 3,000 r/min at 4°C for 10 min and were stored at −80°C. NO content was determined using Nitrate Reductase method, the activities of T-NOS, iNOS and eNOS were measured by chromatometry.

57.2.4 Statistical Analysis

All experimental data are expressed as means ± SEM. Statistical comparisons between the control and treatment groups were carried out using one-way analysis of variance (ANOVA) followed by Newman-Keuls *post-hoc* test. Probability levels of 0.05 or smaller were used for reporting statistical significance.

57.3 Results

57.3.1 Effect of PBNA on Serum NO Content in Retinal I/R Injury

Serum.NO content in I/R group showed a significant higher value than in the control group ($P<0.001$). Serum NO content rose in group treated with low-dosage PBNA ($P<0.05$) (Fig. 57.1).

57.3.2 Effect of PBNA on T-NOS Activity in Retinal I/R Injury

In both groups of low-dosage and high-dosage PBNA treated, T-NOS activities increased ($P<0.01$) (Fig. 57.2).

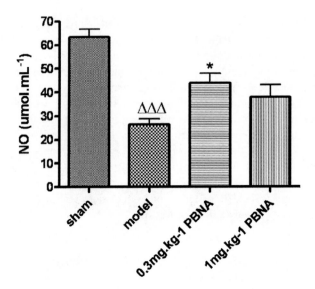

Fig. 57.1 Concentration of NO in serum

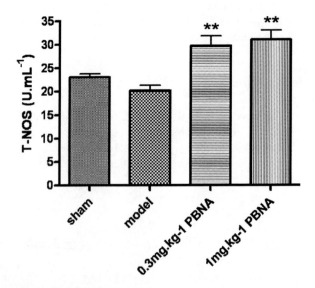

Fig. 57.2 Activity of T-NOS in serum

57.3.3 *Effect of PBNA on iNOS Activity in Retinal I/R Injury*

Serum iNOS activity in I/R group increased compared with control group ($P<0.05$), and declined after low-dosage PBNA treated ($P<0.05$) (Fig. 57.3).

Fig. 57.3 Activity of iNOS
in serum

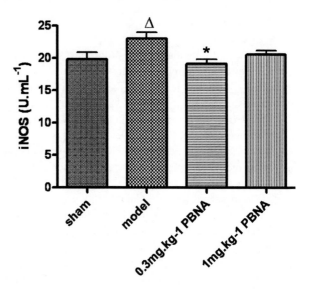

57.3.4 Effect of PBNA on Serum eNOS Activity in Retinal I/R Injury

Serum iNOS activity in I/R group was lower obviously than control group ($P<0.05$) and grew higher in groups treated with both low-dosage and high-dosage PBNA ($P<0.05$, $P<0.01$) (Fig. 57.4).

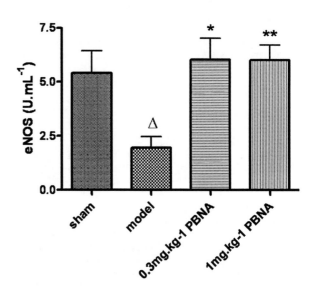

Fig. 57.4 Activity of eNOS
in serum

57.4 Discussion

Studies showed that some cells could not restore normal structure and physiological functions after retinal ischemia for 60 min, that is ischemia caused irreversible cell death, which was one of the cause of visual loss in patient with retinal ischemia.

Nitric oxide (NO) is a free radical that plays a variety of roles in the pathophysiology of many diseases (Stewart et al. 1994). It is synthesized by three isoforms of NO synthase (NOS): neuronal (nNOS), endothelial (eNOS), and inducible (iNOS) isoforms; the former two share enzymatic characteristic and are termed constitutive isoforms (cNOS) (Marietta 1994). All isoforms have been shown to be present or inducible in neural retina (Chakravarthy et al. 1995; Hangai et al. 1996). Hangai et al. (1996) suggested that the express of iNOS mRNA increased obviously during ischemic in rats and get to a peak at 2 h. iNOS mRNA mainly expressed in the heterophil granulocyte infiltrated in retina by hybridization in situ. It suggested that NO induced by iNOS in leucocyte could be one of the factors involving in retinal I/R injury. Masanori et al. (1999) found that after ischemia ended, eNOS mRNA initially decreased until 6 h, then increased to a peak at 12 h, and decreased progressively beyond 24 h until the final measurement at 96 h of reperfusion. While Cheon et al. (2003) suggest that an increase in eNOS expression could be associated with the degenerative changes in the ischemic retina.

Our study showed that serum NO content declined, serum iNOS activity increased and serum eNOS activity in I/R group, which was consistent with the reports of Masanori and Hangai. The results could be turned over by treating with PBNA.

This suggested that PBNA has a therapeutic effect on retina ischemia/reperfusion injury probability for the reason that it could increase the activity of T-NOS and eNOS, decrease the activity of iNOS, raise the content of NO, enhance the Antioxidation and expand the blood vessel.

Acknowledgments This work was supported by Nature Science Fund of Jiangxi Province (NO. 2008GZY0068) and Science research plan from department of Education of Jiangxi Province (NO. [2006] 252).

References

Chakravarthy U, Stitt AW, McNallyJ et al (1995) Nitric oxide synthase activity and expression in retinal capillary endothelial cells and pericytes. Curr Eye Res 14:285–294
Cheon EW, Park CH, Kang SS et al (2003) Change in endothelial nitric oxide synthase in the rat retina following transient ischemia. Neuroreport 14(3):329–333
Dijk F, Kraal-Muller E, KamphuisW (2004) Ischemia-induced changes of AMPA-type glutamate receptor subunit expression pattern in the rat retina: a real-time quantitative PCR study. Invest Ophthalmol Vis Sci 45:330–341
Hangai M, Miyamoto K, Hiroi K et al (1999) Roles of constitutive nitric oxide synthase in postischemic rat retina. Invest Ophthalmol Vis Sci 40:450–458
Hangai M, Yoshimura N, Hiroi K et al (1996) Inducible nitricoxide synthase in retinal ischemia-reperfusion injury. Exp Eye Res 63:501–509

Kwon YH, Rickman DW, Baruah S et al (2005) Vitreous and retinal amino acid concentrations in experimental central retinal artery occlusion in the primate. Eye 19:455–463

Li L, Li X, Huang Z et al (2007) Effects of PBNA on the contraction of rabbit thoracic aorta in vitro. Pharmacol Clinics Chinese Mater Med 23:53–54

Liu X, Li WW, Sheng K et al (2006) Studies on the chemical constituents of the n-BuOH extract of Polygonum Bistorta L. J Shenyang Pharmaceut Univ 23:16–18

Marietta MA (1994) Nitric oxide synthase: aspects concerning structure and catalysis. Cell 8: 927–930

Oz O, Gurelik G, Akyurek N et al (2005) A short duration transient ischemia induces apoptosis in retinal layers: an experimental study in rabbits. Eur J Ophthalmol 15:233–238

Pannicke T, Uckermann O, Iandiev I et al (2005) Altered membrane physiology in Muller glial cells after transient ischemia of the rat retina. Glia 50:1–11

Sanchez RN, Chan CK, Garg S et al (2003) Interleukin-6 in retinal ischemia reperfusion injury in rats. Invest Ophthalmol Vis Sci 44:4006–4011

Stewart AG, Phan LH, Grigoriadis G (1994) Physiological and pathophysiological roles of nitric oxide. Microsurgery 15:693–702

Torin N, Akaike A, Yasuyoshi H et al (2000) Lomerizine, a Ca^{2+} channel blocker, reduces glutamate induced neurotoxicity and ischemia reperfusion damage in rat retina. Exp Eye Res 70:475–484

Ye H, Wang X, Huang Z et al (2006) The protective effect of Polygonum Bistora L. n-Butyl alcohol extract on myocardial ischemia. Lishizhen Med Mater Med Res 17:907–909

Chapter 58
Recent Insights into the Mechanisms Underlying Light-Dependent Retinal Degeneration from *X. Laevis* Models of Retinitis Pigmentosa

Orson L. Moritz and Beatrice M. Tam

Abstract We have recently developed transgenic *X. laevis* models of retinitis pigmentosa based on the rhodopsin P23H mutation in the context of rhodopsin cDNAs derived from several different species. The mutant rhodopsin in these animals is expressed at low levels, with levels of export from the endoplasmic reticulum to the outer segment that depend on the cDNA context. Retinal degeneration in these models demonstrates varying degrees of light dependence, with the highest light dependence coinciding with the highest ER export efficiency. Rescue of light dependent retinal degeneration by dark rearing is in turn dependent on the capacity of the mutant rhodopsin to bind chromophore. Our results indicate that rhodopsin chromophore can act in vivo as a pharmacological chaperone for P23H rhodopsin, and that light-dependent retinal degeneration caused by P23H rhodopsin is due to reduced chromophore binding.

Retinitis pigmentosa (RP) is a multigenic disorder involving progressive loss of visual function. Symptoms develop in childhood or early adulthood, including night blindness and progressive loss of peripheral vision (tunnel vision), and often progress to complete blindness (Berson 1993). Rhodopsin is the gene most frequently involved in autosomal dominant RP, accounting for a quarter of cases (Sohocki et al. 2001). Rhodopsin is comprised of the G-protein coupled receptor rod opsin and the covalently bound chromophore 11-cis retinal, and is the major protein of the rod outer segment (ROS). Light absorption causes chromophore isomerization, initiating visual transduction, which is quickly suppressed by rhodopsin phosphorylation, binding of arrestin, and dissociation of photoisomerized chromophore (Lamb and Pugh 2006).

O.L. Moritz (✉)
Department of Ophthalmology and Visual Sciences, UBC/VGH Eye Care Centre, 2550 Willow Street, Vancouver, BC, V5Z 3N9, Canada
e-mail: olmoritz@interchange.ubc.ca

R.E. Anderson et al. (eds.), *Retinal Degenerative Diseases*, Advances in Experimental Medicine and Biology 664, DOI 10.1007/978-1-4419-1399-9_58,
© Springer Science+Business Media, LLC 2010

There is significant anecdotal and experimental evidence indicating that light exposure modulates disease severity in some forms of RP. Several instances of variable phenotype in related patients suggest environmental influences, and several lines of evidence indicate that the retina is asymmetrically affected in patients with specific mutations, with the lower retina (which receives greater illumination from overhead lighting) more seriously affected. Furthermore, several animal models of RP harboring rhodopsin mutations similar to those found in RP patients have retinal degeneration (RD) with some degree of light dependence. This includes mouse models based on the rhodopsin mutation T17M, a dog model with a T4R mutation, rats harboring the P23H mutation, and drosophila expressing P23H rhodopsin. (For review of this literature, see Paskowitz et al. 2006). The P23H mutation is the most common cause of autosomal dominant RP in North America, where it is linked to 10% of cases (Sohocki et al. 2001).

The cell death pathways relevant to RP remain largely uncharacterized. However, in the case of light-dependent RD associated with rhodopsin mutations, it seems plausible that the mechanisms of visual transduction mechanisms would be involved. However, this is largely unsupported by cell culture studies. In cultured epithelial cells, the majority of RP-causing rhodopsin mutations cause defects in biosynthesis and transport (Kaushal and Khorana 1994; Sung et al. 1991). Most RP-causing mutations, including P23H, are partly or completely retained in the ER of cultured cells (Kaushal and Khorana 1994). These mutants bind chromophore and activate transducin poorly. Thus, it is difficult to resolve how a misfolded protein that is retained or degraded in the ER by quality control mechanisms could inappropriately activate visual transduction. The confusion is further complicated by the finding that mice are partially protected from RD by knockout of transducin (Samardzija et al. 2006), and that P23H rhodopsin is present in the ROS of transgenic mice and rats (Ablonczy et al. 2000; Olsson et al. 1992).

Recently, we and others have addressed these questions using amphibian models of RP (Tam and Moritz 2006, 2007; Zhang et al. 2008). Our results suggest that ER export of mutant P23H rhodopsin is a light sensitive process, thereby reconciling several apparent discrepancies between systems. We utilized certain properties of transgenic X. laevis to address questions that would be intractable in other transgenic models. Primary transgenic X. laevis are relatively easy to generate, and their retinal photoreceptors are large and easily imaged. Furthermore, many antibodies raised against mammalian rhodopsins do not cross-react with endogenous X. laevis rhodopsin. These properties allowed us to compare expression levels and intracellular localizations (particularly ER retention) between a variety of different mutant rhodopsins in-vivo, as well as the light sensitivities of the resulting RDs.

We compared P23H rhodopsin transgenes based on an epitope tagged X. laevis cDNA, and bovine, mouse and human cDNAs, while Zhang et al. examined untagged X. laevis P23H rhodopsin (Tam and Moritz 2006, 2007; Zhang et al. 2008). All forms of P23H rhodopsin express at low levels. Because RD occurs at expression levels significantly below endogenous rhodopsin (even at the level of mRNA) this argues for a gain-of-function mechanism of cell death (Zhang et al. 2008). Furthermore, examination of the intracellular distributions of the mutant proteins revealed that they do not efficiently exit the ER, suggesting a folding or stability defect (Tam and Moritz 2006, 2007). In addition, there are subtle differences in localization between variants. In particular, bovine P23H rhodopsin has a greater propensity to escape the ER and arrive at the ROS (Tam and Moritz 2007), while *X. laevis* P23H rhodopsin is almost exclusively restricted to the ER (Tam and Moritz 2006). However, bovine P23H rhodopsin expression levels are still low when compared to wildtype bovine rhodopsin.

Interestingly, the propensity for small quantities of mutant rhodopsin to escape the ER correlates strongly with the propensity for RD to be rescued by dark rearing. RD caused by the bovine P23H rhodopsin transgene is extremely light dependent, while other RDs are less light dependent (human P23H) or light independent (epitope tagged *X. laevis* P23H) (Tam and Moritz 2006, 2007). This suggests that light acts directly on P23H rhodopsin, rather than causing a general change in cell physiology. Any effects of light such as up-regulation of pro-apoptotic genes are secondary to a direct effect on mutant rhodopsin. Interestingly, in contrast to our results, Zhang et al. (2008) found RD caused by *X. laevis* P23H rhodopsin to be light dependent. Our transgenes differed only in that we used conservative changes to introduce epitope tags in the rhodopsin sequence. These changes appear to be responsible for the differences in our results.

The correlation of light dependent RD with ROS localization of P23H rhodopsin suggests that visual transduction through mutant rhodopsin might contribute to cell death. To test this, we blocked signal transduction using a P23H/K296R double mutant (K296R is a non-signaling rhodopsin mutant (Cohen et al. 1993)). We did not find significant rescue of RD, although we did observe a trend (Tam and Moritz 2007). This is analogous to experiments in which transducin knockout background partially rescued RD in P23H transgenic mice (Samardzija et al. 2006), although in our case, only signal transduction through P23H rhodopsin was blocked. Thus, our results do not contradict those of Samardzija et al. (2006) rather, both experiments demonstrate that visual transduction is not responsible for cell death, but may modulate the process.

Although P23H/K296R-induced RD tends to be less severe than P23H-induced RD in bright cyclic light (1,700 lux), the K296R mutation blocks rescue of RD by dark rearing, i.e. in dim light or darkness K296R exacerbates RD (Tam and Moritz 2007). The K296R mutation not only prevents signal transduction, but also prevents chromophore binding (Cohen et al. 1993). Thus, the rescue mechanism associated with dark rearing is blocked by preventing chromophore binding. This suggests the experiments of Noorwez et al. (2004), in which biosynthesis of P23H rhodopsin is enhanced by 11-cis retinal.

Under dark rearing conditions, the proportion of P23H rhodopsin delivered to the ROS increases significantly for animals expressing human and bovine P23H rhodopsin (Tam and Moritz 2007), suggesting that chromophore binding improves ER exit efficiency. In fact, for bovine P23H rhodopsin, the expression level under dark rearing conditions approached levels obtained with wildtype bovine rhodopsin.

Unexpectedly, western blots demonstrated precise removal of at least 23 amino acids from the N-terminus of bovine P23H rhodopsin (Tam and Moritz 2007).

Furthermore, antibodies directed at N- and C-terminal epitopes produced distinct labeling patterns for human P23H, but not wildtype, rhodopsins. The N-terminal epitope was abundant in the ER and dramatically absent from ROS, while the C-terminal epitope was abundant in ROS, and less prominent in ER (Fig. 58.1). This suggests that the N-terminus was cleaved from the majority of P23H rhodopsin transported from the ER to the ROS. In fact, similarly truncated products have been reported in cell culture studies (Noorwez et al. 2004), and transgenic mice (Jin, Heth and Roof 1995). Because this proteolysis occurs within the secretory pathway, it is distinct from ER quality control mechanisms for removing and degrading mis-folded proteins, which involve retrotranslocation to the cytoplasm and proteolytic degradation by the proteosome. Truncated P23H rhodopsin clearly remains in the secretory pathway and is transported to the ROS. This activity therefore resembles ER resident proteases such as gamma secretase or signal peptidase.

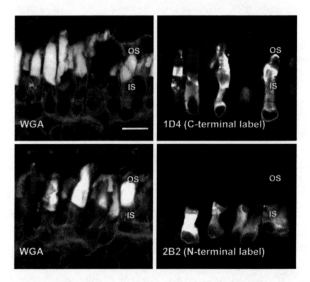

Fig. 58.1 ER retention and N-terminal cleavage of P23H rhodopsin. Sections of *X. laevis* retina expressing human P23H rhodopsin were labeled with wheat germ agglutinin (WGA, *left panels*), or anti-mammalian rhodopsin antibodies (*right panels*). The antibody epitopes are located in the C-terminus (1D4, *top right*) or N-terminus (2B2, *bottom right*). Note the labeling of inner segments (IS), consistent with ER retention of the P23H rhodopsin, and the lack of outer segment (OS) labeling by 2B2, consistent with truncation of the N-terminus of P23H rhodopsin in the secretory pathway. Bar = 20 μM

Truncated P23H rhodopsin is found in greatest abundance in retinas expressing bovine P23H rhodopsin, and is essentially absent from retinas expressing *X. laevis* P23H rhodopsin. Thus, between gene constructs, the light dependence of RD also correlates with the extent of P23H rhodopsin truncation (Tam and Moritz 2007). However, for a given transgene, dark rearing does not significantly increase the ratio of cleaved to full length P23H rhodopsin. Thus, dark rearing does not rescue RD

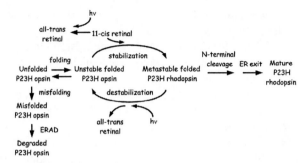

Fig. 58.2 Proposed mechanisms by which light influences P23H rhodopsin biosynthesis. Newly synthesized unfolded P23H opsin may either fold or misfold, and misfolded P23H opsin is subject to ER associated degradation (ERAD). Folded P23H opsin is unstable, but is stabilized by chromophore binding (P23H rhodopsin). P23H rhodopsin is likely to exit the ER, while P23H opsin is likely to unfold, increasing the likelihood of misfolding and ERAD. ER exit is inefficient in the presence of light (hν), either due to a reduction in chromophore supply (*top*) or conversion of rhodopsin to opsin, resulting in increased unstable opsin, increased misfolded opsin, ER stress, and cell death. ER exit of P23H rhodopsin may be further enhanced by N-terminal cleavage. However, this step is not light dependent. (Not shown: presumably P23H opsin may also exit the ER)

by increasing the rate of N-terminal truncation, although differences in truncation efficiency could explain differences in the extent of rescue between different P23H rhodopsin genotypes (Fig. 58.2).

On the basis of these findings, we propose a mechanism for the light dependence of RD in which export of P23H rhodopsin from the ER is more efficient in the dark due to increased binding of light-sensitive chromophore (Fig. 58.2). 11-cis retinal likely stabilizes P23H against unfolding prior to ER exit, or may facilitate the kinetics of a rate limiting step in folding. Furthermore, ER exit may be further facilitated by N-terminal cleavage. Differences in the thermodynamic stabilities of P23H rhodopsins or the efficiency of N-terminal cleavage may underlie the species-dependent variation in rescue of RD by dark rearing. In support of this hypothesis, it has long been known that rhodopsin is considerably more thermodynamically stable than opsin (Hubbard 1958).

These results support the hypothesis that certain RP phenotypes are influenced by light exposure, and suggest that it may be possible to restore rhodopsin biosynthesis (to some extent) by protection from light in these patients. Furthermore, our results also imply that therapy with 11-cis retinal analogues suggested by other authors (Govardhan and Oprian 1994; Noorwez et al. 2003) may be a means of treating certain forms of RP.

These results largely resolve the discrepancies between in-vivo and cell culture studies. The models provide complementary insight: a single rhodopsin mutant may have a defect in biosynthesis *or* be correctly folded and transported, with the tipping point dependent on the cDNA used to construct the transgene, chromophore availability, and light intensity. Cell culture studies will provide a useful system for identifying mechanisms to enhance rhodopsin folding, and animal models will provide a means for testing these mechanisms in-vivo.

Many other disorders are associated with protein misfolding and ER retention (Schroder and Kaufman 2005). In many cases, ER exit can be promoted by ligands or small molecules (pharmacological chaperones). For example, p-glycoprotein mutants can be rescued by the substrate cyclosporine A, CFTR can be rescued by corr-2b, and a hERG potassium channel mutant can be rescued by channel blockers. P23H rhodopsin provides yet another example. In fact, many retinal dystrophies are caused by defective biosynthesis of proteins; for example, misfolding mutations of peripherin/rds, ABCA4, and ELOVL4 (Grayson and Molday 2005) are associated with retinal dystrophies, and could be rescued by similar mechanisms. Indeed, higher-order assembly of the digenic RP-associated peripherin/rds mutant L185P requires co-expression of its interaction partner rom-1 (Goldberg and Molday 1996). Even where no ligand is known, it may be possible to identify ligands by screening, or based on structural data.

Our understanding of the mechanisms underlying rescue of RD by dark rearing is incomplete. We lack an explanation for the rescuing effects of disruption of signal transduction (observed in mice and suggested in *X. laevis*). Additionally, the specific role of N-terminal cleavage needs to be addressed. One can envision mechanisms by which cleavage could promote ER exit, as the mutant residue and both N-linked glycosylation sites are removed. ER quality control mechanisms involving retention and surveillance of glycosylated proteins by lectin chaperones are well documented (Schroder and Kaufman 2005). Is eliminating glycosylation or removal of the P23H residue a key event in rescue? Does cleavage represent a cause or consequence of ER exit? What is the protease? Is promoting truncation another approach to RP therapy?

Most importantly, we must identify the mechanisms relevant to human disease. In 1980, a small clinical trial of light deprivation of two RP patients of unreported genotype showed no significant benefits (Berson 1980). A great deal of information has accumulated since these studies were conducted, and it may soon be appropriate to revisit this approach in trials directed at genetic subsets of RP.

References

Ablonczy Z, Knapp DR, Darrow R et al (2000) Mass spectrometric analysis of rhodopsin from light damaged rats. Mol Vis 6:109–115

Berson EL (1980) Light deprivation and retinitis pigmentosa. Vision Res 20(12):1179–1184

Berson EL (1993) Retinitis pigmentosa. The Friedenwald Lecture. Invest Ophthalmol Vis Sci 34(5):1659–1676

Cohen GB, Yang T, Robinson PR et al (1993) Constitutive activation of opsin: influence of charge at position 134 and size at position 296. Biochemistry 32(23):6111–6115

Goldberg AF, Molday RS (1996) Defective subunit assembly underlies a digenic form of retinitis pigmentosa linked to mutations in peripherin/rds and rom-1. Proc Natl Acad Sci U S A 93(24):13726–13730

Govardhan CP, Oprian DD (1994) Active site-directed inactivation of constitutively active mutants of rhodopsin. J Biol Chem 269(9):6524–6527

Grayson C, Molday RS (2005) Dominant negative mechanism underlies autosomal dominant Stargardt-like macular dystrophy linked to mutations in ELOVL4. J Biol Chem 280(37): 32521–32530

Hubbard R (1958) The thermal stability of rhodopsin and opsin. J Gen Physiol 42(2):259–280

Jin J, Heth CA, Roof DJ (1995) P23H mutant human opsin in transgenic murine retina: truncation of N-terminus and lack of glycosylation. Invest Ophthalmol Vis Sci 36(4):S424

Kaushal S, Khorana HG (1994) Structure and function in rhodopsin. 7. Point mutations associated with autosomal dominant retinitis pigmentosa. Biochemistry 33(20):6121–6128

Lamb TD, Pugh EN Jr (2006) Phototransduction, dark adaptation, and rhodopsin regeneration the proctor lecture. Invest Ophthalmol Vis Sci 47(12):5137–5152

Noorwez SM, Kuksa V, Imanishi Y et al (2003) Pharmacological chaperone-mediated in vivo folding and stabilization of the P23H-opsin mutant associated with autosomal dominant retinitis pigmentosa. J Biol Chem 278(16):14442–14450

Noorwez SM, Malhotra R, McDowell JH et al (2004) Retinoids assist the cellular folding of the autosomal dominant retinitis pigmentosa opsin mutant P23H. J Biol Chem 279(16):16278–16284

Olsson JE, Gordon JW, Pawlyk BS et al (1992) Transgenic mice with a rhodopsin mutation (Pro23His): a mouse model of autosomal dominant retinitis pigmentosa. Neuron 9(5):815–830

Paskowitz DM, LaVail MM, Duncan JL (2006) Light and inherited retinal degeneration. Br J Ophthalmol, 90(8):1060–1066

Samardzija M, Wenzel A, Naash M et al (2006) Rpe65 as a modifier gene for inherited retinal degeneration. Eur J Neurosci 23(4):1028–1034

Schroder M, Kaufman RJ (2005) The mammalian unfolded protein response. Annu Rev Biochem 74:739–789

Sohocki MM, Daiger SP, Bowne SJ et al (2001) Prevalence of mutations causing retinitis pigmentosa and other inherited retinopathies. Hum Mutat 17(1):42–51

Sung CH, Schneider BG, Agarwal N et al (1991) Functional heterogeneity of mutant rhodopsins responsible for autosomal dominant retinitis pigmentosa. Proc Natl Acad Sci U S A 88(19):8840–8844

Tam BM, Moritz OL (2006) Characterization of rhodopsin P23H-induced retinal degeneration in a *Xenopus laevis* model of retinitis pigmentosa. Invest Ophthalmol Vis Sci 47(8):3234–3241

Tam BM, Moritz OL (2007) Dark rearing rescues P23H rhodopsin-induced retinal degeneration in a transgenic *Xenopus laevis* model of retinitis pigmentosa: a chromophore-dependent mechanism characterized by production of N-terminally truncated mutant rhodopsin. J Neurosci 27(34):9043–9053

Zhang R, Oglesby E, Marsh-Armstrong N (2008) *Xenopus laevis* P23H rhodopsin transgene causes rod photoreceptor degeneration that is more severe in the ventral retina and is modulated by light. Exp Eye Res 86(4):612–621

Chapter 59
A Hypoplastic Retinal Lamination in the Purpurin Knock Down Embryo in Zebrafish

Mikiko Nagashima, Junichi Saito, Kazuhiro Mawatari, Yusuke Mori, Toru Matsukawa, Yoshiki Koriyama, and Satoru Kato

Abstract Recently, we cloned a photoreceptor-specific purpurin cDNA from axotomized goldfish retina. In the present study, we investigate the structure of zebrafish purpurin genomic DNA and its function during retinal development. First, we cloned a 3.7-kbp genomic DNA fragment including 1.4-kbp 5′-flanking region and 2.3-kbp full-length coding region. In the 1.4-kbp 5′-upstream region, there were some cone-rod homeobox (crx) protein binding motifs. The vector of the 1.4-kbp 5′-flanking region combined with the reporter GFP gene showed specific expression of this gene only in the photoreceptors. Although the first appearance time of purpurin mRNA expression was a little bit later (40 hpf) than that of crx (17–24 hpf), the appearance site was identical to the ventral part of the retina. Next, we made purpurin or crx knock down embryos with morpholino antisense oligonucleotides. The both morphants (purpurin and crx) showed similar abnormal phenotypes in the eye development; small size of eyeball and lacking of retinal lamination. Furthermore, co-injection of crx morpholino and purpurin mRNA significantly rescued these abnormalities. These data strongly indicate that purpurin is a key molecule for the cell differentiation during early retinal development in zebrafish under transcriptional crx regulation.

59.1 Introduction

Purpurin is originally discovered as a retina-specific secretory protein in developing chick retina (Schubert and LaCorbiere 1985). In retinal cell culture, purpurin has cell adhesive and survival effects (Schubert et al. 1986). Recently we found that purpurin was a trigger molecule for optic nerve regeneration in adult goldfish retina (Matsukawa et al. 2004). Following optic nerve transection, the level of purpurin mRNA rapidly increased in the photoreceptor cells 2–5 days and then

S. Kato (✉)
Department of Molecular Neurobiology, University of Kanazawa, Kanazawa 920-8640, Japan
e-mail: satoru@med.kanazawa-u.ac.jp

R.E. Anderson et al. (eds.), *Retinal Degenerative Diseases*, Advances in Experimental Medicine and Biology 664, DOI 10.1007/978-1-4419-1399-9_59,
© Springer Science+Business Media, LLC 2010

rapidly decreased by 10 days. Application of recombinant purpurin protein promoted neurite outgrowth from adult goldfish retinal explant culture (Matsukawa et al. 2004). During zebrafish retinal development, purpurin mRNA appeared in the ventral part of the retina at 40 hours post fertilization (hpf). The expression was located in the photoreceptor cells at 3–5 days after fertilization (dpf) and decreased by 10 dpf (Tanaka et al. 2007). Purpurin protein was secreted into all retinal layers. In the present study, we aimed to investigate the structure of purpurin genomic DNA and its function during the early stage of zebrafish retinal development. At first, we cloned 3.7-kbp genomic DNA fragment which included 1.4-kbp 5′-flanking region and 2.3-kbp of full-length of coding region of purpurin from zebrafish genomic DNA library. Purpurin gene had 6 exons and 5 introns. Secondly, we characterized 1.4-kbp 5′-flanking region. Transgenic zebrafish embryos injected with a constructed DNA of 1.4-kbp promoter region and GFP reporter gene showed photoreceptor specific expression of GFP. This region contained some cone-rod homeobox (crx) protein binding motifs, which found in promoter region of several photoreceptor-specific genes. Finally, we made purpurin and crx knock down zebrafish embryos by injection of morpholino antisense oligonucleotides. Phenotypes of these morphant (purpurin and crx) were very similar, small size of eyeball and lacking of differentiated retinal lamination. The role of purpurin during the early development of zebrafish retina and its transcriptional regulation by crx were thus discussed.

59.2 Materials and Methods

59.2.1 Experimental Animals

Zebrafish (*Danio rerio*) were reared in a water tanks at 28°C with a 12:12 h light-dark cycle. Fertilized embryos were collected after natural spawning, and were kept in embryo medium containing 0.003% phenylthiourea.

59.2.2 Screening of Genomic DNA for Zebrafish Purpurin

An amplified zebrafish brain genomic DNA library in the Lambda FixII/XhoI partial Fill-in vector (Stratagene Inc.) was screened with radiolabeled cDNA derived from zebrafish purpurin cDNA. *Escherichia coli* cells (XL-1 Blue MRN) were infected with recombinant phages, and 1.0×10^6 phage plaques were screened. After hybridization with ^{32}P-labeled cDNA probes, duplicate filters were washed four times and exposed to X-ray films. Positive plaques were then selected three times. The nucleotide sequences of the obtained genomic DNA clones on both strands were determined using a dye terminator kit and Ampli *Tag*DNA polymerase (Applied Biosystems) on a DNA sequencer (ABIPRISM 310 Genetic Analyzer; Applied Biosystems).

59.2.3 Construction of the pur-GFP Reporter Vector

The purpurin promoter-GFP (pur-GFP) vector was composed of 1.4-kbp 5′-flanking region of zebrafish purpurin genomic DNA and pAcGFP 1-1 vector (Clontech). A 1428-bp 5′-flanking region of zebrafish purpurin genomic DNA was generated by PCR (forward primer: 5′-TGG CAA TAA AGC TCG ACG TA-3′; reverse primer: 5′-GTG GTT CTC CAC AAG GCT GT-3′). The 1428-bp fragment was cloned into pGEM-T Easy vector (Promega), and subsequently excised by ApaI/SacI digestion, and ligated into the corresponding sites of the pAcGFP 1-1 vector. The linearized pur-GFP vector was injected into one-cell stage of zebrafish embryos.

59.2.4 Morpholino and Microinjections

Morpholinos were obtained from Gene Tools. Purpurin morpholino was composed of MO1: 5′-TCA CAA AGC ATA CAA CAT ACC CTC T-3′. Crx gene morpholino was composed of 5′-ATG TAG GAC ATC ATT CTT GGG ACG G-3′ (Shen and Raymond 2004). A standard morpholino (5′-CCT CTT ACC TCA GTT ACA ATT TAT A-3′) was used as control. The morpholinos were diluted in distilled water at 0.5 mM in 0.1% phenol red, and were microinjected into 1–2 cell stage of embryos.

59.2.5 In Situ Hybridization

Whole mount in situ hybridization was performed as previously described (Sugitani et al. 2006) with a slight modification. In brief, embryos fixed and stored in 100% methanol at −20 °C were rehydrated, acetylated, and permeabilized with 10 μg/ml proteinase K at room temperature for 20–30 min. After refixation in 4% paraformaldehyde solution, embryos were prehybridized in hybridization buffer for 30 min. Hybridization was performed with 100 ng of probe in 200 μl hybridization solution overnight at 70°C. On the next day, the embryos were washed and treated with 20 mg/ml RNase at 37°C for 30 min. To detect the signals, the samples were incubated with alkaline phosphatase-conjugated anti-DIG antibody (Roche) overnight at 4°C. Visualization of the signals was done using tetrazolium-bromo-4 chloro-3-indolyl-phosphate (Roche).

59.2.6 RNA Isolation, RT-PCR and mRNA Synthesis

Total RNA was isolated from 30 embryos at 3 dpf using Sepasol-RNA I super (Nacalai tesque). RT-PCR was performed using Reverse Transcriptase XL (AMV) (TaKaRa) and TaKaRa LA Taq (TaKaRa). Primer sequences (exon 1 forward primer: 5′-CAT TCA TTC AGG ACA TCA TC-3′; exon 5 reverse primer:

5′-GCC ATG CAG ATC TCA TCT TG-3′; mRNA forward primer: 5′-GGA TCC TAC ACT ACT AAA ACC-3′; mRNA reverse primer: 5′-TGA TGC ACA CAT GCA CCT CTA-3′) were designed from the zebrafish purpruin sequences (GenBank accession no. AB242211). For mRNA synthesis, PCR product was ligated into pGEM-T easy vector (Promega). The linearized DNA was transcribed to 5′-capped purpurin mRNA with 3′ poly A tail using a mMESSAGE mMACHINE T7 Ultra Kit (Ambion).

59.3 Results

59.3.1 Isolation and Characterization of Zebrafish Purpurin Gene

To investigate transcriptional mechanism of purpurin gene, we cloned genomic DNA for purpurin from zebrafish genomic DNA library using the full-length zebrafish purpurin cDNA probe. We obtained 7 positive clones after three times screening from 1×10^6 phage plaques. One of these clones was sequenced and was a 3.7-kbp genomic DNA fragment which was composed of 1.4-kbp 5′-flanking region and 2.3-kbp full-length coding region. The sequence data were registered in GenBank under accession no. AB242211. The structure of the 3.7-kbp genomic DNA is shown in Fig. 59.1a. The purpurin gene had 6 exons and 5 introns. Exon 1 was 62-bp, exon 2 was 118-bp, exon 3 was 137-bp, exon 4 was 113-bp, exon 5 was 213-bp and exon 6 was 197-bp in length. Intron 3 was 1057-bp, and the others were 97-124-bp in length. The initial codon ATG was located in exon 2, and the stop codon TAA was located in exon 6. A presumed TATA box was positioned at −54-bp upstream from the transcriptional start site +1. A polyadenylation signal AATAA was positioned at +2314 in exon 6. To determine the promoter activity of the 1.4-kbp 5′-flanking region for retina specific expression, we constructed pur-GFP reporter vector (Fig. 59.1b). The pur-GFP vector was composed of the 1.4-kbp (−1,481 to −3) 5′-flanking region of zebrafish purpurin gene and pAcGFP1-1 vector. The linearized pur-GFP vector was injected into one cell stage of zebrafish embryos. Retinal sections at 5 dpf revealed that GFP expression was limited to the photoreceptor cells (Fig. 59.1c). GFP signal was also detected in pineal gland (data not shown). *In situ* hybridization study also showed purpurin mRNA expressed in the photoreceptor cells at 5 dpf (Fig. 59.1d). These results indicate that the 1.4-kbp 5′-flanking region of this genomic clone has regulatory site(s) for the photoreceptor-specific expression of purpurin gene.

59.3.2 Similar Phenotypes of Purpurin and Crx Morphant

The 1.4-kbp 5′-flanking regon contained three OTX (GATTA) motifs and four OTX-like (AATTA) motifs (Fig. 59.1a). These sequences are characterized as crx

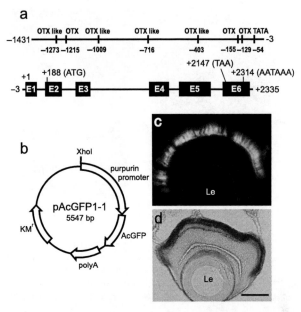

Fig. 59.1 The structure of purpurin gene and photoreceptor-specific expression of reporter gene. (**a**) Structures of 1.4-kbp 5′-flanking region and 2.3-kbp transcriptional region of the purpurin gene are shown in minimized length. The transcription start site is positioned at +1. The thin vertical bars in the 5′-promoter region show crx recognition motifs (three OTX and four OTX-like) and the TATA box. The black squares in the transcriptional region show the exons. The purpurin gene has 6 exons and 5 intorns. The translation start codon is within exon 2 and the stop codon is within exon 6. A polyadenylation signal AATAAA is positioned at +2314 of exon 6. (**b**) Construction of the pur-GFP reporter vector. (**c**) GFP expression in pur-GFP transgenic zebrafish at 5 dpf. (**d**) In situ hybridization study of purpurin mRNA at 5 dpf. Scale = 50 μm. Le: lens

recognition and binding motif in zebrafish and mammals (Kawamura et al. 2005). Crx is a photoreceptor-specific transcriptional factor, and the expression and the function of crx in the zebrafish retina are well studied by Raymond group (Liu et al. 2001; Shen and Raymond 2004). During zebrafish retinal development, crx mRNA first appears in ventral part of the retina at 17–24 hpf. At 52 hpf, the expression is expanded to the photoreceptor layer and the outermost inner nuclear layer. Knock down of crx gene using morpholino resulted in small size of eyeball and lacking of retinal lamination (Fig. 59.2b) compared to the control retina (Fig. 59.2a). During zebrafish retinal development, purpurin mRNA first appears in ventral part of the retina at 40 hpf and the expression is spread to the photoreceptor layer at 48–72 hpf (Tanaka et al. 2007). Knock down of purpurin gene using morpholino also resulted in small size of eyeball and lacking of retinal lamination (Fig. 59.2c). Similar phenotypes of purpurin and crx morphants are shown in Table 59.1.

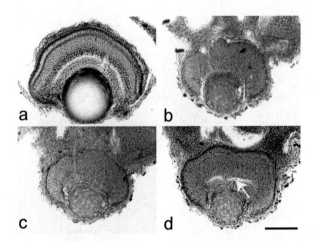

Fig. 59.2 Toluidine blue staining of control (**a**), crx morphant (**b**), purpurin morphant (**c**) and crx morphant co-injected with purpurin mRNA (**d**) retina at 3 dpf. (**a**) Retinal lamination is completely formed in the control retina at 3 dpf. (**b, c**) Crx or purpurin morphants do not show any retinal lamination at 3 dpf. (**d**) Injection of purpurin mRNA into the crx morphant rescues the small size of eyeball and lacking of retinal lamination. An *arrow* indicates the inner plexiform layer in (**d**). Scale bar = 50 μm

Table 59.1 Similar phenotypes of purpurin and crx morphant at 3 dpf

	Control embryo	Purpurin morphant	Crx morphant
Eye size	>230 μm	<200 μm	<200 μm
Retinal lamination	Completion	Lacking	Lacking
Cell differentiation			
Photoreceptor cells	+++	−	−
Bipolar cells	+++	−	−
Ganglion cells	+++	++	+[a]
Müller glial cells	+++	±	±[a]
Proliferative state	−	++	++
Cell death per retina	7.3 cells/	27.7 cells/	N/A
Visual function (5 dpf)	++	−	N/A

[a]Refer to Shen and Raymond (2004); N/A: not analyzed.

59.4 Rescuing Effect of Purpurin mRNA to the Crx Morphant

The most notable effect of purpurin or crx knock down is small eye and lacking of retinal lamination. Therefore, we tested effect of co-injection of purpruin mRNA and crx morpholino. In the control eye at 3 dpf, the size of eyeball was more than 230 μm and retinal lamination was complete (Table 59.1, Fig. 59.2a). In the crx morphant, about 80% of embryos showed small eyeball (<200 μm, Table 59.1) and lacking of retinal lamination (Fig. 59.2b). Co-injection of 0.5 mM crx morpholino and 44 ng/μl purpurin mRNA notably rescued these abnormal phenotypes (Fig. 59.2d).

59.5 Discussion

In this study, we demonstrated the possibility that crx is a transcriptional regulator for purpurin gene during early development of zebrafish retina; (1) Purpurin promoter region contained crx binding motifs. (2) The appearance time of crx mRNA was a little bit earlier than that of purpurin, and initial appearance site of both mRNAs was just identical. (3) Crx knock down embryos generated the small size of eyeball and lacking of retinal lamination as seen as in the purpurin morphant. (4) Injection of purpurin mRNA into crx morphant rescued these abnormalities. And our preliminary study showed that knock down of crx markedly reduced purpurin expression at 3 dpf, but not vise versa. Although it is still unclear that crx directly binds to the purpurin promoter region, crx might be a transcriptional factor for purpurin gene.

Crx is a member of *otx/otd* gene family of paired-like homeobox gene (Royet and Finkelstein 1995; Bally-cuif and Boncinelli 1997). In developing mouse retina, crx expression begins by day E 12.5 and peaks at day P 3 (Chen et al. 1997; Furukawa et al. 1997). The day E12.5 is approximately the time of cone cell genesis and the day P3 is near the time of maximal genesis of rod cells (Carter and LaVail 1979). In mice homozygous for targeted null mutation of crx, photoreceptors fail to form outer segment and eventually become degenerative (Furukawa et al. 1999). Mutations in human crx gene have been identified in three kinds of photoreceptor degeneration diseases (cone-rod dystrophy, retinitis pigmentosa and Leber congenital amaurosis) (Freund et al. 1997; Sohocki et al. 1998; Silva et al. 2000). Therefore, crx is essential for differentiation and maintenance of photoreceptors in mammals. In contrast, zebrafish crx regulates retinal neurogenesis, not only photoreceptor cells but also inner retinal cells. There is many photoreceptor specific genes regulated by crx, such as rhodopsin, arrestin, phosdusin and cGMP phosphodiesterase (Livesey et al. 2000; Zhu and Craft 2000; Pittler et al. 2004). However they are all involved in photo-signal transduction. The secreted purpurin protein might act as a retinol binding protein or an adhesive molecule for cell differentiation. Although mammalian purpurin is not yet identified, we propose that fish purpurin offers a solving cue for photoreceptor degeneration and the determination of cell fate in the retinal development.

References

Bally-cuif L, Boncinelli E (1997) Transcriptional factors and head formation in vertebrates. Bioessays 19:127–135

Carter DL, LaVail MM (1979) Rods and cones in the mouse retana. II. Autoradiographic analysis of cell generation using tritiated thymidine. J Comp Neurol 188:263–272

Chen S, Wang QL, Nie Z et al (1997) Crx, a novel Otx-like paired-homeodomain protein, binds to and transactivates photoreceptor cell-specific genes. Neuron 19:1017–1030

Freund CL, Gregory-Evans CY, Furukawa T et al (1997) Cone-rod dystrophy due to mutations in a novel photoreceptor-specific homeobox gene (CRX) essential for maintenance of the photoreceptors. Cell 91:543–553

Furukawa T, Morrow EM, Cepko CL (1997) Crx, a novel otx-like homeobox gene, shows photoreceptor-specific expression and regulates photoreceptor differentiation. Cell 91:531–541

Furukawa T, Morrow EM, Li T et al (1999) Retinopathy and attenuated circadian entrainment in Crx-deficient mice. Nat Genet 23:466–470

Kawamura S, Takeshita K, Tsujimura T et al (2005) Evolutionarily conserved and divergent regulatory sequences in the fish rod opsin promoter. Comp Biochem Physiol B Biochem Mol Biol 141:391–399

Liu Y, Shen Y, Test JS et al (2001) Isolation and characterization of a zebrafish homologue of the cone rod homeoboxi gene. Invest Ophthalmol Vis Sci 42:481–487

Livesey FJ, Furukawa T, Steffen MA et al (2000) Microarray analysis of the transcriptional network controlled by the photoreceptor homeobox gene Crx. Curr Biol 10:301–310

Matsukawa T, Sugitani K, Mawatari K et al (2004) Role of purpurin as a retinol-binding protein in goldfish retina during the early stage of optic nerve regeneration: its priming action on neurite outgrowth. J Neurosci 24:8346–8353

Pittler SJ, Zhang Y, Chen S et al (2004) Functional analysis of the rod photoreceptor cGMP phosphodiesterase alpha-subunit gene promoter: Nrl and Crx are required for full transcriptional activity. J Biol Chem 279:19800–19807

Royet J, Finkelstein R (1995) Pattern formation in Drosophila head development: the role of the orthodenticle homeobox gene. Development 121:3561–3572

Schubert D, LaCorbiere M (1985) Isolation of an adhesion-mediating protein from chick neural retina adherons. J Cell Biol 101:1071–1077

Schubert D, LaCorbiere M, Esch F (1986) A chick neural retina adhesion and survival molecule is a retinol-binding protein. J Cell Biol 102:2295–2301

Shen YC, Raymond PA (2004) Zebrafish cone-rod (crx) homeobox gene promotes retinogenesis. Dev Biol 269:237–251

Silva E, Yang JM, Li Y et al (2000) A CRX null mutation is associated with both Leber congenital amaurosis and a normal ocular phenotype. Invest Ophthalmol Vis Sci 41:2076–2079

Sohocki MM, Sullivan LS, Mintz-Hittner HA et al (1998) A range of clinical phenotypes associated with mutations in CRX, a photoreceptor transcription-factor gene. Am J Hum Genet 63: 1307–1315

Sugitani K, Matsukawa T, Koriyama Y et al (2006) Upregulation of retinal transglutaminase during the axonal elongation stage of goldfish optic nerve regeneration. Neuroscience 142:1081–1092

Tanaka M, Murayama D, Nagashima M et al (2007) Purpurin expression in the zebrafish retina during early development and after optic nerve lesion in adults. Brain Res 1153:34–42

Zhu X, Craft CM (2000) Modulation of CRX transactivation activity by phosducin isoforms. Mol Cell Biol 20:5216–5226

Chapter 60
Functional Changes in Inner Retinal Neurons in Animal Models of Photoreceptor Degeneration

Theresa Puthussery and W. Rowland Taylor

Abstract Retinitis Pigmentosa (RP) refers to a heterogeneous group of inherited disorders that result in the death of rod and cone photoreceptors. There is now abundant evidence to suggest that inner retinal neurons, particularly the bipolar and horizontal cells, undergo significant morphological changes and changes in neurotransmitter receptor expression in response to photoreceptor degeneration. Some of these alterations could impact the choice and success of intervention strategies for these conditions, and it is therefore necessary to understand the timing and nature of any functional deficits resulting from degenerative changes. This paper will review the evidence for functional alterations in the inner retina in animal models of (RP), with particular emphasis on the bipolar and ganglion cells.

60.1 Introduction

Retinitis Pigmentosa comprises a large group of inherited disorders that result in the progressive degeneration of rod, and subsequently cone, photoreceptors. It was initially believed that photoreceptors were exclusively affected by the condition, since the thickness of the inner nuclear layer appears unchanged even at late stages in the degenerative process. It is now well established that the second order neurons, the bipolar and horizontal cells, undergo dramatic morphological changes in the outer plexiform layer in response to photoreceptor death, showing extensive dendritic retraction and remodelling (Strettoi and Pignatelli 2000; Gargini et al. 2007). Moreover, there is evidence for cell body migration, in the case of rod bipolar cells (Gargini et al. 2007), and changes in expression of neurotransmitter receptors (see Marc et al. (2003) for detailed review). Careful quantification has revealed that some

T. Puthussery (✉)
Department of Ophthalmology, Casey Eye Institute, Oregon Health & Science University, Portland, OR, USA
e-mail: puthusse@ohsu.edu

R.E. Anderson et al. (eds.), *Retinal Degenerative Diseases*, Advances in Experimental Medicine and Biology 664, DOI 10.1007/978-1-4419-1399-9_60,
© Springer Science+Business Media, LLC 2010

apoptosis of inner retinal neurons, including rod bipolar cells and horizontal cells, does occur at late stages in the degenerative process (Strettoi and Pignatelli 2000; Gargini et al. 2007). It is critical to understand the timing and functional ramifications of these changes, since they may impact the choice and eventual success of treatment strategies. This review will discuss the evidence for functional alterations in the inner retina in animal models of retinal degeneration, with particular emphasis on neurons of the 'through' pathway, the bipolar and ganglion cells.

60.2 Bipolar Cell Function in Retinal Degeneration

Numerous strategies that show promise for the treatment of RP are contingent on the normal functioning of bipolar cells. For example, Maclaren et al. (2006) showed that photoreceptor precursor cells could be successfully transplanted and integrated into a degenerated mouse retina, however, the success of such an approach most likely relies on the normal functioning of bipolar cells at the time of transplantation. A detailed knowledge of the timing of bipolar cell functional changes would also be critical for appropriate design of retinal implants, targeting of gene-therapy to photoreceptors or the incorporation of photosensitive channels into bipolar cells themselves (Lagali et al. 2008). In this section, we will summarise what is known about the localisation and function of glutamate receptors on bipolar cells in the degenerating retina.

60.2.1 Glutamate Receptors of Bipolar Cells in the Normal and Degenerating Retina

In darkness, glutamate is released from photoreceptors and activates glutamate receptors that are tightly localized to the dendritic tips of the bipolar cells. There are two functionally distinct types of bipolar cells that respond with opposite polarities depending on the type of glutamate receptors expressed. ON bipolar cells (including rod bipolar cells) express the sign-inverting metabotropic glutamate receptor, mGluR6 (Nakajima et al. 1993). Activation of this receptor activates a G-protein coupled cascade that leads to the closure of an as yet unidentified cation-permeable channel, thereby hyperpolarising the cell (Slaughter and Miller 1985). In contrast, OFF cone bipolar cells express sign-conserving ionotropic glutamate receptors of the α-amino-3-hydroxyl-5-methyl-4-isoxazole-propionate (AMPA)/kainate type that are depolarised in response to glutamate.

Alterations in the localisation and expression of mGluR6 receptors have been described in a variety of animal models of retinal degeneration using immuno-histochemistry. In mouse models such as the *rd1* (Strettoi and Pignatelli 2000), *rd10* (Gargini et al. 2007; Puthussery et al. 2009; Barhoum et al. 2008) and *crx* knockout (Pignatelli et al. 2004), there is evidence for progressive down-regulation of mGluR6 protein with advancing rod photoreceptor degeneration. In addition to down-regulation, the residual mGluR6 is mislocalised and forms clusters on the cell somata and axons. Similar changes occur in rat models such as the P23H (Cuenca et al. 2004), S334ter (Seiler et al. 2008) and RCS rat (Cuenca et al. 2005; Pinilla et al. 2007), however, the somatic mislocalisation of mGluR6 is more uniform and marked than in mouse models. Interestingly, the patterns of mGluR6 mislocalisation in the degenerating rat and mouse retinas appear to mimic the immature patterns of localisation seen in the respective species during early retinal development (Nomura et al. 1994; Ueda et al. 1997).

Whilst deafferentation clearly results in the down regulation of mGluR6 receptors in ON bipolar cells, the expression of ionotropic glutamate receptors in the outer plexiform layers seems to be maintained, or possibly even up-regulated, in response to photoreceptor death. Our laboratory evaluated the expression of the AMPA receptor subunits GluR1, GluR2 and GluR4 at varying stages of degeneration in the *rd10* mouse. Using immunohistochemistry, we showed robust expression of all three receptor subunits, even after complete degeneration of cone photoreceptors (Puthussery et al. 2009). These data are further supported by gene expression studies that have shown the up-regulation of GluR1, GluR3 and GluR4 during and after the peak period of photoreceptor degeneration in the *rd1* mouse (Namekata et al. 2006). Moreover, changes in flip-to-flop alternative splicing of the GluR1 receptor have been reported (Namekata et al. 2006), and given the expression of this receptor by OFF bipolar cells (Hack et al. 2001), it is feasible that this could lead to altered AMPA receptor kinetics in these cells. Increased protein expression of GluR1 has also been described in the *rdta* mouse (Liu et al. 2001).

60.2.2 Evidence for Bipolar Cell Dysfunction

60.2.2.1 Rod Bipolar Cells

To date, few studies have used single-cell electrophysiology to assay bipolar cell function during photoreceptor degeneration. In the *rd1* retina, Varela et al. (2003) recorded glutamate responses from enzymatically dissociated rod bipolar cells at 4–8 weeks of age. They showed that only one of 13 cells responded to glutamate puffed onto the dendrites. Since it has been shown that the rod-to-rod bipolar cell synapse does not develop normally in the *rd1* mouse (Blanks et al. 1974), it is unclear whether the observed functional deficits are due to developmental anomalies or are a secondary consequence of photoreceptor degeneration. More recently, Barhoum et al. (2008) evaluated rod bipolar cell responses to exogenously applied glutamate in a slice preparation of the *rd10* retina at postnatal day 60, a time after complete degeneration of rod photoreceptors. They demonstrated that *wild-type* and *rd10* retinas were similar in that ~50% of RBCs responded to puff application of glutamate, with no significant difference in the response amplitudes between the two groups. This is a surprising finding, given the very marked down-regulation of the mGluR6 at P60 in the *rd10* retina.

Recently, our laboratory has taken advantage of an approach originally described by Nawy (2004) to pharmacologically simulate light stimulation in ON bipolar cells in slice preparations of the degenerating retina. The group III metabotropic glutamate receptor agonist L-AP4 is applied to retinal slices to activate the mGluR6 receptors and simulate the high receptor occupancy that occurs due to glutamate release in the dark-adapted retina. We then simulate a light flash by pressure ejection of high concentrations of the mGluR6 antagonist CPPG onto the bipolar cell dendrites. The CPPG rapidly displaces the AP4 and generates an inward current that shows remarkably similar magnitude and kinetics to a true light response. Using this approach, we have found that rod bipolar cells in the *rd10* retina show progressive alterations in mGluR6 currents, with decreased response amplitudes and alterations in kinetics in the early stages of degeneration (postnatal day 20), and near complete loss of rod bipolar cell responses by postnatal day 45 (Puthussery et al. 2009). While these results conflict with those of Barhoum et al. (2008) who found that mGluR6 responses were unchanged in the degenerated retina, they accord more closely with the dramatic loss in mGluR6 expression evident from the immunohistochemical findings.

The dysfunction of rod bipolar cells during retinal degeneration has also been suggested from electroretinography studies. The b-wave of the electroretinogram (ERG) is known to reflect the activity of ON-bipolar cells (Stockton and Slaughter 1989; Green and Kapousta-Bruneau 1999) and the rod contribution to the b-wave can be isolated using stimulus parameters that exploit the temporal or chromatic properties of the rods. Gargini et al. (2007) recorded ERGs in the *rd10* mouse using light stimuli in which the mean luminance was sinusoidally modulated over a range of temporal frequencies in an effort to better isolate changes in b-wave kinetics. They showed that deficits in the b-wave were detectable as early as P18, and suggested that changes in bipolar cell function occur even in the early stages of photoreceptor degeneration. However, since the ERG is produced by a chain of events, it is not possible to determine where the deficit arises, be it by reduced efficiency of presynaptic signalling in the rods, or by post-synaptic alterations in rod bipolar cells, such as a reduced expression of mGluR6 receptors.

Another approach that has been employed to assess bipolar cell function during progression of retinal degeneration is the use of the organic cation 1-amino-4-guanidobutane (agmatine) to map the activity of discrete cell populations in vivo and in vitro (Marc et al. 2005). Agmatine is believed to enter cells through open cation channels, including ionotropic glutamate receptors that are activated by AMPA, kainate or NMDA as well as the unidentified cation channel downstream of the mGluR6 receptor. Immunohistochemical analysis with agmatine selective antibodies is used to assay cell activity under a variety of conditions.

Marc et al. (2007) showed that intravitreal injection of agmatine, followed by a 45 min period in mesopic light, results in the uptake of agmatine into a large proportion of rod bipolar cells in the wild-type retina. However, when the rodless coneless (*rdcl*) mutant mouse was examined under the same conditions, virtually no bipolar cells had any agmatine signal, suggesting permanent closure of the mGluR6-gated ion channel (Marc et al. 2003). This result is surprising, since mGluR6 activation closes the cation channels, and therefore the loss of glutamatergic input from photoreceptors should open mGluR6-gated channels and produce agmatine uptake. Thus, these findings suggest either that an alternate source of glutamate drives channel closure or, more likely, that the mGluR6-gated cation channels are either absent, or not opened, due to disturbances in the transduction pathway in the *rdcl* mouse.

These same techniques have been used to evaluate kainate receptor activity in a human RP retina (Marc et al. 2007), and in the P347L rhodopsin transgenic rabbit (Jones et al. 2008). These studies revealed an unexpectedly high number of activated bipolar cells and it was suggested that this was most likely due to aberrant expression of iGluRs by rod bipolar cells. Although there is some evidence for gene expression of iGluRs by rod bipolar cells in the normal retina (Hughes 1997), to date, there has been no functional evidence to confirm this. Our laboratory recently investigated the sensitivity of rod bipolar cells to kainate/AMPA puff application in the *wt* and *rd10* retina and found no evidence for iGluR-activated currents (Puthussery et al. 2009).

In summary, these data suggest that photoreceptor degeneration results in the loss of glutamate sensitivity in the rod bipolar cells that correlates with a loss of expression of the mGluR6 receptor.

60.2.2.2 Cone Bipolar Cells

Whole-cell patch clamp recordings from our laboratory indicate that ON cone bipolar cells show alterations in mGluR6-gated currents after death of cone photoreceptors (Puthussery et al. 2009). In contrast, OFF bipolar cells may remain responsive to glutamate agonists even after complete cone degeneration. Using patch-clamp electrophysiology on retinal slices from 6-month-old *rd10* retina, we demonstrated robust inward currents in OFF bipolar cells when the glutamate agonists AMPA and kainate were puffed onto the dendrites. Marc et al. (2007) showed loss of KA driven agmatine entry into OFF bipolar cells in two rapidly progressing cone-decimating models of RP, the *rdcl* mouse and the *hrhoG* mouse. However, in regions of the *hrhoG* mutant mouse and also in a human retina where some residual, grossly deconstructed cone photoreceptors remained, KA could still drive agmatine entry into OFF bipolar cells suggesting that focal cone survival could spare local iGluR function. In our electrophysiology studies, we saw no immunohistochemical evidence for residual cones in the six-month old *rd10* retina, although it is possible that cones were missed if the proteins used to identify them were no longer expressed after degeneration.

60.3 Ganglion Cell Function in Retinal Degeneration

Restoration of visual function in the late-stages of retinal degeneration requires the survival and function of the retinal ganglion cells. Examination of human patients reveals that after photoreceptor degeneration, the ganglion cells survive long after visual function is lost, and this has prompted efforts to restore vision by targeting retinal ganglion cells for stimulation either electrically, via prosthetic retinal implants, or by genetic techniques that render the ganglion cells, or their presynaptic cells light sensitive. Genetic expression of the photo-sensitive channels, channelrhodopsin (Bi et al. 2006) and melanopsin (Lin et al. 2008) in ganglion cells has resulted in behaviourally detectable visual responses in mouse models, and shows particular promise for future therapies.

The utility of mouse models in aiding the development of such treatment strategies lies in the similarity with the human diseases. In this regard, the most widely studied mouse model, the *rd1* mouse, is problematic since photoreceptor apoptosis commences before the retina is fully developed, and therefore developmental and degenerative changes are confounded. Nonetheless, recent studies of the *rd1* mouse have shown that, similar to the human condition, the retinal ganglion cells survive and, unlike bipolar cells, retain normal morphology and central projections after complete photoreceptor degeneration (Mazzoni et al. 2008). Analysis of the electrophysiological properties of the ganglion cells in the *rd1* mouse by two groups (Margolis and Detwiler 2007; Stasheff 2008) found that in the degenerated retina the majority of ganglion cells were rhythmically active due to oscillatory excitatory and inhibitory inputs from bipolar and amacrine cells. Such spontaneous discharge demonstrates that the ganglion cells are functionally viable, and that the presynaptic cells are capable of generating potent synaptic drive. However, a potential complication is that a high level of spontaneous discharge in the ganglion cells would degrade the output from RD retinas, which had been rendered light sensitive either genetically or prosthetically, since many of the action potentials in the ganglion cells would not be correlated with the visual stimulus. On the other hand, it is possible that the spontaneous discharge of ganglion cells diminishes in treated retinas that receive light-evoked inputs. For example, the *rd1* model that was rendered light-sensitive by introducing channelrhodopsin-2 into the bipolar cells, did not appear to generate high levels of spontaneous discharge in the ganglion cells (Lagali et al. 2008).

The origins of the oscillations, which arise within the presynaptic circuitry are unknown, and as others have noted (Stasheff 2008), they may represent developmental anomalies that arise due to the early onset of photoreceptor degeneration. In this respect, the *rd1* model may not be a good proxy for human RP and it will be important to examine the structure and function of ganglion cells in other mouse models. The *rd10* model, with its delayed onset of degeneration would be a good candidate.

Currently the outlook is very encouraging for the development of treatments for retinal degenerations, but it will be essential to further develop sensitive assays to evaluate the timing and extent of inner retinal dysfunction. This will be required not only to appropriately target intervention strategies, but also to evaluate the success of those treatments. Further work is also needed to investigate the nature of functional changes across a range of animal models of retinal degeneration.

References

Barhoum R, Martinez-Navarrete G, Corrochano S et al (2008) Functional and structural modifications during retinal degeneration in the rd10 mouse. Neuroscience 155:698–713

Bi A, Cui J, Ma YP et al (2006) Ectopic expression of a microbial-type rhodopsin restores visual responses in mice with photoreceptor degeneration. Neuron 50:23–33

Blanks JC, Adinolfi AM, Lolley RN (1974) Photoreceptor degeneration and synaptogenesis in retinal-degenerative (rd) mice. J Comp Neurol 156:95–106

Cuenca N, Pinilla I, Sauve Y et al (2004) Regressive and reactive changes in the connectivity patterns of rod and cone pathways of P23H transgenic rat retina. Neuroscience 127:301–317

Cuenca N, Pinilla I, Sauve Y et al (2005) Early changes in synaptic connectivity following progressive photoreceptor degeneration in RCS rats. Eur J Neurosci 22:1057–1072

Gargini C, Terzibasi E, Mazzoni F et al (2007) Retinal organization in the retinal degeneration 10 (rd10) mutant mouse: a morphological and ERG study. J Comp Neurol 500:222–238

Green DG, Kapousta-Bruneau NV (1999) A dissection of the electroretinogram from the isolated rat retina with microelectrodes and drugs. Vis Neurosci 16:727–741

Hack I, Frech M, Dick O et al (2001) Heterogeneous distribution of AMPA glutamate receptor subunits at the photoreceptor synapses of rodent retina. Eur J Neurosci 13:15–24

Hughes TE (1997) Are there ionotropic glutamate receptors on the rod bipolar cell of the mouse retina? Vis Neurosci 14:103–109

Jones BW, Marc RE, Terasaki H et al (2008) Computational molecular phenotyping and excitation mapping in the P347L rhodopsin transgenic rabbit model of retinitis pigmentosa. IOVS 49:ARVO E-Abstract 2986

Lagali PS, Balya D, Awatramani GB et al (2008) Light-activated channels targeted to ON bipolar cells restore visual function in retinal degeneration. Nat Neurosci 11:667–675

Lin B, Koizumi A, Tanaka N et al (2008) Restoration of visual function in retinal degeneration mice by ectopic expression of melanopsin. Proc Natl Acad Sci U S A 105:16009–16014

Liu LO, Laabich A, Hardison A et al (2001) Expression of ionotropic glutamate receptors in the retina of the rdta transgenic mouse. BMC Neurosci 2:7

MacLaren RE, Pearson RA, MacNeil A et al (2006) Retinal repair by transplantation of photoreceptor precursors. Nature 444:203–207

Marc RE, Jones BW, Anderson JR et al (2007) Neural reprogramming in retinal degeneration. Invest Ophthalmol Vis Sci 48:3364–3371

Marc RE, Jones BW, Watt CB et al (2003) Neural remodeling in retinal degeneration. Prog Retin Eye Res 22:607–655

Marc RE, Kalloniatis M, Jones BW (2005) Excitation mapping with the organic cation AGB2+. Vision Res 45:3454–3468

Margolis DJ, Detwiler PB (2007) Different mechanisms generate maintained activity in ON and OFF retinal ganglion cells. J Neurosci 27:5994–6005

Mazzoni F, Novelli E, Strettoi E (2008) Retinal ganglion cells survive and maintain normal dendritic morphology in a mouse model of inherited photoreceptor degeneration. J Neurosci 28:14282–14292

Nakajima Y, Iwakabe H, Akazawa C et al (1993) Molecular characterization of a novel retinal metabotropic glutamate receptor mGluR6 with a high agonist selectivity for L-2-amino-4-phosphonobutyrate. J Biol Chem 268:11868–11873

Namekata K, Okumura A, Harada C et al (2006) Effect of photoreceptor degeneration on RNA splicing and expression of AMPA receptors. Mol Vis 12:1586–1593

Nawy S (2004) Desensitization of the mGluR6 transduction current in tiger salamander ON bipolar cells. J Physiol 558:137–146

Nomura A, Shigemoto R, Nakamura Y et al (1994) Developmentally regulated postsynaptic localization of a metabotropic glutamate receptor in rat rod bipolar cells. Cell 77:361–369

Pignatelli V, Cepko CL, Strettoi E (2004) Inner retinal abnormalities in a mouse model of Leber's congenital amaurosis. J Comp Neurol 469:351–359

Pinilla I, Cuenca N, Sauve Y et al (2007) Preservation of outer retina and its synaptic connectivity following subretinal injections of human RPE cells in the Royal College of Surgeons rat. Exp Eye Res 85:381–392

Puthussery T, Gayet-Primo J, Pandey S et al (2009) Differential loss and preservation of glutamate receptor function in bipolar cells in the rd10 mouse model of retinitis pigmentosa. Eur J Neurosci 29:1533–1542

Seiler MJ, Thomas BB, Chen Z et al (2008) BDNF-treated retinal progenitor sheets transplanted to degenerate rats: improved restoration of visual function. Exp Eye Res 86:92–104

Slaughter MM, Miller RF (1985) Characterization of an extended glutamate receptor of the on bipolar neuron in the vertebrate retina. J Neurosci 5:224–233

Stasheff SF (2008) Emergence of sustained spontaneous hyperactivity and temporary preservation of OFF responses in ganglion cells of the retinal degeneration (rd1) mouse. J Neurophysiol 99:1408–1421

Stockton RA, Slaughter MM (1989) B-wave of the electroretinogram. A reflection of ON bipolar cell activity. J Gen Physiol 93:101–122

Strettoi E, Pignatelli V (2000) Modifications of retinal neurons in a mouse model of retinitis pigmentosa. Proc Natl Acad Sci U S A 97:11020–11025

Ueda Y, Iwakabe H, Masu M et al (1997) The mGluR6 5′ upstream transgene sequence directs a cell-specific and developmentally regulated expression in retinal rod and ON-type cone bipolar cells. J Neurosci 17:3014–3023

Varela C, Igartua I, De la Rosa EJ et al (2003) Functional modifications in rod bipolar cells in a mouse model of retinitis pigmentosa. Vision Res 43:879–885

Chapter 61
Photoreceptor Cell Degeneration in *Abcr*$^{-/-}$ Mice

Li Wu, Taka Nagasaki, and Janet R. Sparrow

Abstract Mice harboring a null mutation in *Abca4/Abcr* serve as a model of autosomal recessive Stargardt disease. Consistent with the human retinal disorder, deficiency in Abcr is associated with substantial accumulations of lipofuscin pigments in retinal pigment epithelial (RPE) cells. To observe for photoreceptor cell degeneration in these mutant mice, outer nuclear layer (ONL) thickness was measured at 200 μm intervals superior and inferior to the optic nerve head. ONL width in *Abcr*$^{-/-}$ mouse was reduced at 8–9 month and 11 and 13 months relative to *Abcr*$^{+/+}$ mice; thinning was more pronounced centrally and in superior retina. The numbers of photoreceptor nuclei spanning the width of the outer nuclear layer were also reduced. No evidence of age-related ONL thinning was observed in *Abcr*$^{+/+}$ mice at these ages. We conclude that albino *Abcr*$^{-/-}$ mice exhibit progressive photoreceptor cell loss that is detectable at 8 months of age and that has worsened by 11 and 13 months of age. The measurement of ONL thickness is an established approach to assessing photoreceptor cell integrity and can be used in preclinical studies using *Abcr*$^{-/-}$ mice.

61.1 Introduction

Mutations in *ABCA4* (*ABCR*), the gene encoding the photoreceptor-specific ATP-binding cassette transporter (Sun et al. 1999), are responsible for some types of inherited retinal degeneration including an autosomal recessive form of retinitis pigmentosa, recessive cone-rod dystrophy and recessive Stargardt disease (Klevering et al. 2004; Maugeri et al. 2000; Shroyer et al. 2001). All of these inherited blinding disorders are characterized by excessive accumulations of autofluorescent lipofuscin in retinal pigment epithelial (RPE) cells. This disease feature is replicated in

J.R. Sparrow (✉)
Department of Ophthalmology, Columbia University, New York, NY 10032, USA
e-mail: jrs88@columbia.edu

R.E. Anderson et al. (eds.), *Retinal Degenerative Diseases*, Advances in Experimental Medicine and Biology 664, DOI 10.1007/978-1-4419-1399-9_61,
© Springer Science+Business Media, LLC 2010

the *Abcr* null mutant mouse (Weng et al. 1999) wherein levels of the lipofuscin fluorophores A2E and isoA2E are increased several fold (Kim et al. 2004, 2007; Mata et al. 2001; Weng et al. 1999). Even greater increases in another lipofuscin pigment all-*trans*-retinal dimer-phosphatidylethanolamine (atRAL dimer-PE) are observed (Kim et al. 2007). Characterization of the *Abcr*$^{-/-}$ mouse retina also revealed delayed dark adaptation, increased levels of all-*trans*-retinal and elevated phosphatidylethanolamine (Weng et al. 1999). Although at 6 months of age, the numbers of photoreceptor nuclei were found not to be diminished (Mata et al. 2001), it was recently reported that in 11 month old *Abcr*$^{-/-}$ mice fed both control and vitamin A supplemented diet, the numbers of rows of nuclei across the outer nuclear layer was reduced as compared to wild-type mice (Radu et al. 2008).

Several therapeutic strategies aimed at alleviating vision loss in recessive Stargardt disease have been tested in *Abcr*$^{-/-}$ mice. These approaches include vector-based gene therapies (Kong et al. 2008) and the administration of compounds that limit the visual cycle including isotretinoin (Radu et al. 2003), an inhibitor of 11-*cis*-retinol dehydrogenase; the retinoid analog fenretinide that lowers serum vitamin A (Radu et al. 2005); and compounds that target RPE65 (Maeda et al. 2008; Maiti et al. 2006). In these pre-clinical studies quantitation of A2E served as the therapeutic outcome measure.

Although HPLC quantitation of the lipofuscin pigment A2E serves as an objective measure of therapeutic efficacy, additional endpoint measures are desirable. Since the measurement of outer nuclear layer thickness is a widely accepted approach to assessing photoreceptor cell integrity (Lavail et al. 1987; Michon et al. 1991), we have undertaken to compare outer nuclear layer (ONL) thickness in age-matched albino *Abcr*$^{-/-}$ and *Abcr*$^{+/+}$ mice, homozygous for the Leu-450 allele of Rpe65.

61.2 Methods

61.2.1 Animals and Rearing

Albino *Abca4/Abcr* null mutant mice homozygous for Rpe65-Leu450, were generated and genotyped for the *Abcr* null mutation and Rpe65-Leu450Met variant by PCR-amplification of tail DNA as previously reported (Kim et al. 2004). For Rpe65, digestion of the 545-bp product with *Mwo*I restriction enzyme (New England Biolabs), yielded 180- and 365-bp fragments if the sequence corresponded to Leu-450; Met-450 was associated with the undigested 545-bp band; and heterozygous mice exhibited all 3 bands. *Abcr*$^{-/-}$ and *Abcr*$^{+/+}$ mice were raised under 12-h on-off cyclic lighting with in-cage illuminance of 30–80 lux. Mice were anaesthetized and perfused with 4% paraformaldehyde in phosphate buffered saline. Following enucleation, eyes were immersed in 4% paraformaldehyde for 24 h at 4°C. The proposed research involving animals has been approved by the Institutional Animal Care and Use Committee (IACUC).

61.2.2 Measurement of Outer Nuclear Layer Thickness

Sagittal 6-mm paraffin serial sections of murine retina were prepared and stained with hematoxylin and eosin. Microscopic images were acquired and analyzed using a digital imaging system (Leica Microsystems; Leica Application suite; Welzlar, Germany). For measurement of ONL thickness, two to three sections through the optic nerve head of the left eyes were imaged with a 10 X objective. ONL thickness was measured at 200 μm intervals superior and inferior to the edge of the optic nerve head along the vertical meridian; ONL width in pixels was converted to microns (1 pixel: 0.92 μm) and data from the three sections were averaged. For groups of $Abcr^{-/-}$ and $Abcr^{+/+}$ mice at each age, mean ONL thickness at each position along the vertical meridian was plotted as a function of eccentricity from the optic nerve head (Mittag et al. 1999; Tanito et al. 2005). Values were compared by unpaired t-test or one-way analysis of variance (ANOVA) as appropriate, and significance was assessed at the 0.05 level (GraphPad Software Inc, La Jolla CA).

61.2.3 Counting Photoreceptor Nuclei

The numbers of nuclei extending across the width of the ONL were determined in superior hemiretina at a fixed distance of 600 μm from the edge of the optic disc. Counting was performed using a digital image obtained from one section per eye photographed with a 63 X objective. Three lines were drawn (5 μm apart) at this position and nuclei traversed by the line were counted by 2 individuals, one of whom was masked to mouse age and genotype. Nuclei counts obtained by the 2 individuals along the three lines were averaged to give a value for each eye. Values were compared by unpaired t-test.

61.3 Results

We probed for evidence of photoreceptor cell degeneration in $Abcr^{-/-}$ mice at ages 5 months, 8–9 months, 11 and 13 months using standard morphological methods based on measurement of ONL thickness. Shown in Fig. 61.1 are representative images of hematoxylin and eosin stained superior central retinas obtained with a 10 X objective; images captured at higher magnification (40 X objective) are in the insets. A difference in ONL width between $Abcr^{-/-}$ and $Abcr^{+/+}$ retina was visible at 8–9 months of age (Fig. 61.1).

ONL thicknesses were plotted as a function of distance in 200 μm intervals superior and inferior to the optic nerve head in the vertical plane. Examination of ONL measurements in $Abcr^{+/+}$ at 5 months, 8–9 months (mean age 8.2 months) and 12 months of age revealed that these measurements did not vary as a function of these ages (one-way ANOVA, $p > 0.05$) (Fig. 61.2). Conversely, in $Abcr^{-/-}$ mice at 8–9

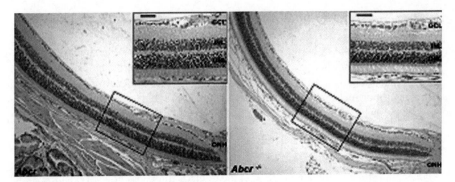

Fig. 61.1 Representative light micrographs of *Abcr*$^{+/+}$ and *Abcr*$^{-/-}$ mouse retinas. Images of inferior hemisphere along the vertical meridian; age 9 months. Insets, higher magnification images obtained in the regions indicated. ONH, optic nerve head; GCL, ganglion cell layer; INL, inner nuclear layer; ONL, outer nuclear layer. Magnification bar, 50 μm

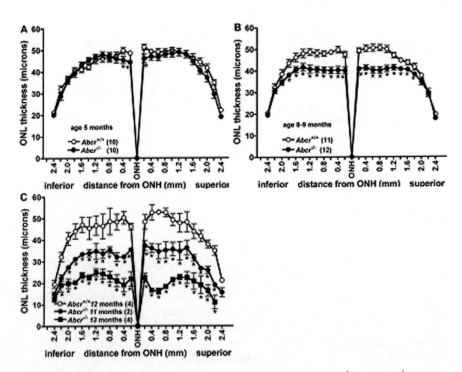

Fig. 61.2 Quantification of outer nuclear layer (ONL) thickness in *Abcr*$^{+/+}$ and *Abcr*$^{-/-}$ mice at age 5 month (**a**), 8–9 months (**b**) and 11–13 months (**c**). Measurements are plotted as a function of distance from the optic nerve head (ONH) in the inferior and superior hemispheres. Mean ± SEM; numbers of mice presented in *parentheses*

months (mean age 8.5 months) a decrease in ONL thickness was observed, the thinning being most noticeable in central retina. For example, comparison of $Abcr^{-/-}$ and $Abcr^{+/+}$ mice at 8–9 months of age revealed a 15–20% reduction in ONL thickness, 0.2–1.0 mm superior and inferior to ONH ($p < 0.05$) (Fig. 61.2). In $Abcr^{-/-}$ mice at 11 months of age, the difference in ONL thickness was further accentuated, there being a 23–36% decrease at eccentricities of 0.2–1.0 mm in $Abcr^{-/-}$ relative to $Abcr^{+/+}$ mice ($p < 0.05$) (Fig. 61.2). At 8–9 months of age, the degenerative changes were slightly more distinct in superior retina as compared to inferior retina, the reduction in the inferior hemiretina ranging from 15 to 19%, while the decrease in superior hemiretina was 17–20%. In $Abcr^{-/-}$ mice aged 13 months, the thinning of ONL in superior retina was clearly more pronounced, decreases in the 0.2–1.0 mm zones being 54–69% superiorly and 48–62% inferiorly when compared to $Abcr^{+/+}$ mice (age 12 months). Statistically significant differences ($p < 0.05$) between $Abcr^{+/+}$ and $Abcr^{-/-}$ mice in terms of ONL thickness were observed at 5 months of age only at 0.2 and 0.4 mm from the ONH inferiorly and 0.2 mm superiorly (Fig. 61.2).

Measurements of ONL thickness agreed with the counts of nuclei spanning the width of the ONL. The numbers of nuclei at 5 months of age in $Abcr^{-/-}$ mice were not significantly different than in $Abcr^{+/+}$ mice ($Abcr^{+/+}$: 9.8 ± 0.24; $Abcr^{-/-}$: 9.6 ± 0.33, mean $\pm$ SEM; $p > 0.05$). Conversely at 8–9 months, the mean number of nuclei in $Abcr^{-/-}$ mice was reduced by 22% relative to $Abcr^{+/+}$ ($Abcr^{+/+}$: 9.5 ± 0.25; $Abcr^{-/-}$: 7.4 ± 0.39, mean $\pm$ SEM; $p < 0.05$).

61.4 Discussion

The $Abcr^{-/-}$ mouse is notable for exhibiting an excessive accumulation of the bis-retinoid pigments that constitute the lipofuscin of RPE cells (Kim et al. 2004; 2007; Weng et al. 1999). By morphometric analysis of ONL thickness combined with counting of photoreceptor cell nuclei spanning the ONL, we have demonstrated that albino $Abcr^{-/-}$ mice display photoreceptor cell loss that is clearly detectable at 8 months of age and that has worsened by 12 and 13 months of age. Thinning of the ONL was more marked in the superior hemisphere of retina. The amassing of RPE lipofuscin to pronounced levels in $Abcr^{-/-}$ mice precedes the loss of photoreceptor cells; for instance by 3 months of age, A2E levels in the mutant mice are approximately 5-fold greater than in $Abcr^{+/+}$ mice (Kim et al. 2007). Indeed it is potentially significant that by 8 months of age, A2E levels appear to reach a plateau.

As compared to some other mouse models of retinal degeneration, the loss of photoreceptors in the $Abcr^{-/-}$ mice occurred with later onset. For instance, mice expressing the P23H substitution in rhodopsin, a mutation prevalent in human autosomal dominant retinitis pigmentosa, exhibit substantial reduction in ONL thickness, even at 2 months of age (Naash et al. 1993). Mice carrying a naturally occurring autosomal recessive mutation in $Rpe65$ ($Rpe65^{rd12}$) develop a retinal degeneration that is considered to be slowly progressing, yet even then, ONL width is reduced by 30–40% at age 6–7 months of age (Pang et al. 2005; Redmond et al. 1998).

In the present study ONL thicknesses in $Abcr^{+/+}$ mice were consistent with previous reports (Kurth et al. 2007); moreover, we did not observe an age-related thinning of ONL in $Abcr^{+/+}$ mice examined between 5 and 12 months. Consistent with this, most studies of wild-type mice have reported age-related photoreceptor cell loss only after 1 year of age. For example, ONL thickness measurements were reported to be the same at 2, 4, 6 and 12 months of age in BALB/cJ, C57BL/6 and C57BL/6-C^{2J} mice (Bravo-Nuevo et al. 2004; Li et al. 2001), while another study described a 40% decline in rows of photoreceptor nuclei between 2 and 17 months of age (BALB/c mice) (Gresh et al. 2003). Similarly, screening of several in-bred laboratory strains of mice, including BALB/cJ, BALB/cByJ, A/J, NZW/LacJ and 129P3/J, revealed normal retinal morphology at 10–12 months of age but noticeable ONL thinning by 22–24 months (Chang 2008). On the other hand, Danciger et al. presented ONL thickness data that reflected a decline of approximately 6 μm between 6 and 12 months of age in BALB/c mice (Danciger et al. 2003).

In conclusion, we suggest that two measures of therapeutic efficacy are available for preclinical studies of recessive Stargardt disease utilizing the $Abcr^{-/-}$ mouse: HPLC quantitation of RPE lipofuscin fluorophores such as A2E and ONL thickness measurement. Both approaches are also translatable to non-invasive endpoint measures in human clinical trials – analysis of fundus autofluorescence in human subjects serves as a measure of RPE lipofuscin while segmentation of the outer retinal complex [ORC: thickness of ONL, inner segments (IS) and outer segments (OS)] in OCT images of the human eye is akin to ONL thickness measurements in mice.

Acknowledgments This work was supported by National Institutes of Health Grant EY12951 (to JRS), a gift from Dr. Gertrude Neumark Rothschild and a grant from Research to Prevent Blindness to the Department of Ophthalmology. JRS is the recipient of a Research to Prevent Blindness Senior Investigator Award.

References

Bravo-Nuevo A, Walsh N, Stone J (2004) Photoreceptor degeneration and loss of retinal function in the C57BL/6-C2J mouse. Invest Ophthalmol Vis Sci 45:2005–2012

Chang B (2008) Age-related eye disease. In: Chalupa LM, Williams RW (eds), Eye, retina and visual system of the mouse, The MIT Press, Cambridge, MA, pp 581–590

Danciger M, Lyon J, Worrill D et al (2003) A strong and highly significant QTL on chromosome 6 that protects the mouse from age-related retinal degeneration. Invest Ophthalmol Vis Sci 44(6):2442–2449

Gresh J, Goletz PW, Crouch RK et al (2003) Structure-function analysis of rods and cones in juvenile, adult, and aged C57BL/6 and Balb/c mice. Vis Neurosci 20:211–220

Kim SR, Fishkin N, Kong J et al (2004) The Rpe65 Leu450Met variant is associated with reduced levels of the RPE lipofuscin fluorophores A2E and iso-A2E. Proc Natl Acad Sci U S A 101(32):11668–11672

Kim SR, Jang YP, Jockusch S et al (2007) The all-trans-retinal dimer series of lipofuscin pigments in retinal pigment epithelial cells in a recessive Stargardt disease model. Proc Natl Acad Sci U S A 104:19273–19278

Klevering BJ, Maugeri A, Wagner A et al (2004) Three families displayinng the combination of Stargardt's disease with cone-rod dystrophy or retinitis pigmentosa. Ophthalmology 111: 546–553

Kong J, Kim SR, Binley K et al (2008) Correction of the disease phenotype in the mouse model of Stargardt disease by lentiviral gene therapy. Gene Ther 15:1311–1320

Kurth I, Thompson DA, Rüther K et al (2007) Targeted disruption of the murine retinal dehydrogenase gene Rdh12 does not limit visual cycle function. Mol Cell Biol 27:1370–1379

LaVail MM, Gorrin GM, Repaci MA et al (1987) Genetic regulation of light damage to photoreceptors. Invest Ophthalmol Vis Sci 28:1043–1048

Li C, Cheng M, Yang H et al (2001) Age-related changes in the mouse outer retina. Optom Vis Sci 78:425–430

Maeda A, Maeda T, Golczak M et al (2008) Retinopathy in mice induced by disrupted all-trans-retinal clearance. J Biol Chem 283:26684–26693

Maiti P, Kong J, Kim SR et al (2006) Small molecule RPE65 antagonists limit the visual cycle and prevent lipofuscin formation. Biochem 45:852–860

Mata NL, Tzekov RT, Liu X et al (2001) Delayed dark adaptation and lipofuscin accumulation in *Abcr*^{+/−} mice: implications for involvement of *ABCR* in age-related macular degeneration. Invest Ophthalmol Vis Sci 42:1685–1690

Maugeri A, Klevering BJ, Rohrschneider K et al (2000) Mutations in the ABCA4 (ABCR) gene are the major cause of autosomal recessive cone-rod dystrophy. Am J Hum Genet 67(4):960–966

Michon JJ, Li ZL, Shioura N et al (1991) A comparative study of methods of photoreceptor morphometry. Invest Ophthalmol Vis Sci 32:280–284

Mittag TW, Bayer AU, LaVail MM (1999) Light-induced retinal damage in mice carrying a mutated SOD I gene. Exp Eye Res 69:677–683

Naash MI, Hollyfield JG, Al-Ubaidi MR et al (1993) Simulation of human autosomal dominant retinitis pigmentosa in transgenic mice expressing a mutated murine opsin gene. Proc Natl Acad Sci U S A 90:5499–5503

Pang JJ, Chang B, Hawes NL et al (2005) Retinal degeneration 12 (rd12): a new, spontaneously arising mouse model for human Leber congenital amaurosis (LCA). Mol Vis 11:152–162

Radu RA, Han Y, Bui TV et al (2005) Reductions in serum vitamin A arrest accumulation of toxic retinal fluorophores: a potential therapy for treatment of lipofuscin-based retinal diseases. Invest Ophthalmol Vis Sci 46:4393–4401

Radu RA, Mata NL, Nusinowitz S et al (2003) Treatment with isotretinoin inhibits lipofuscin and A2E accumulation in a mouse model of recessive Stargardt's macular degeneration. Proc Natl Acad Sci U S A 100(8):4742–4747

Radu RA, Yuan Q, Hu J et al (2008) Accelerated accumulation of lipofuscin pigments in the RPE of a mouse model for ABCA4-mediated retinal dystrophies following vitamin A supplementation. Invest Ophthalmol Vis Sci 49:3821–3829

Redmond TM, Yu S, Lee E et al (1998) Rpe65 is necessary for production of 11-*cis*-vitamin A in the retinal visual cycle. Nat Genet 20:344–351

Shroyer NF, Lewis RA, Yatsenko AN et al (2001) Null missense *ABCR* (*ABCA4*) mutations in a family with Stargardt disease and retinitis pigmentosa. Invest Ophthalmol Vis Sci 42: 2757–2761

Sun H, Molday RS, Nathans J (1999) Retinal stimulates ATP hydrolysis by purified and recon-stituted ABCR, the photoreceptor-specific ATP-binding cassette transporter responsible for Stargardt disease. J Biol Chem 274(12):8269–8281

Tanito M, Elliot MH, Kotake Y et al (2005) Protein modifications by 4-hydroxynonenal and 4-hydroxyhexenal in light-exposed rat retina. Invest Ophthalmol Vis Sci 46:3859–3868

Weng J, Mata NL, Azarian SM et al (1999) Insights into the function of Rim protein in photore-ceptors and etiology of Stargardt's disease from the phenotype in Abcr knockout mice. Cell 98(1):13–23

Chapter 62
Investigating the Mechanism of Disease in the RP10 Form of Retinitis Pigmentosa

Catherine J. Spellicy, Dong Xu, Garrett Cobb, Lizbeth Hedstrom, Sara J. Bowne, Lori S. Sullivan, and Stephen P. Daiger

Abstract Retinitis pigmentosa (RP) is a disease characterized by its vast heterogeneity. Many genes are associated with RP, and the disease causing mutations identified in these genes are even more numerous. To date there are 15 genes that cause autosomal dominant RP (adRP) alone. The role of some of these genes, while complex and not completely understood, is somewhat intuitive in that they are involved in pathways such as phototransduction. However, the role of other genes in retinal disease is not as predictable due to their ubiquitous function and/or expression. One such gene is inosine monophosphate dehydrogenase 1 (IMPDH1) IMPDH1 is a gene involved in de novo purine synthesis and is ubiquitously expressed. IMPDH1 mutations account for 2% of all adRP cases and are a rare cause of Leiber Congenital Amaurosis. Despite its ubiquitous expression missense mutations in this gene cause only retinal degeneration. This paradox of tissue specific disease in the presence of ubiquitous expression has only recently begun to be explained. We have shown in a recent study that novel retinal isoforms of IMPDH1 exist and may account for the tissue specificity of disease. We have gone on to characterize these retinal isoforms both in our laboratory and in collaboration with Dr. Lizbeth Hedstrom's laboratory at Brandeis University (Waltham, MA) in order to understand more about them. We believe that through clarifying the mechanism of disease in RP10 we will be equipped to consider treatment options for this disease.

62.1 Introduction

Mutations in inosine monophosphate dehydrogenase 1 (IMPDH1) cause autosomal dominant retinitis pigmentosa (adRP) (Bowne et al. 2002; Kennan et al. 2002) and are also a rare cause of Leber congenital amaurosis (LCA) (Bowne et al.

S.P. Daiger (✉)
The University of Texas Health Science Center Houston, Human Genetics Center, 1200 Herman Pressler, Houston TX, 77030, USA
e-mail: stephen.p.daiger@uth.tmc.edu

R.E. Anderson et al. (eds.), *Retinal Degenerative Diseases*, Advances in Experimental Medicine and Biology 664, DOI 10.1007/978-1-4419-1399-9_62, © Springer Science+Business Media, LLC 2010

2006b). Although it was recently discovered that IMPDH1 is involved in adRP, the functional properties of IMPDH1 have been known since at least the 1950s (e.g. Magasanik et al. 1957). Despite the fact that the IMPDH1 enzyme has been, historically, well studied, the question remains – why do mutations in IMPDH1 cause retinal disease? Our research, and data reported by other groups, suggests several hypotheses.

62.2 Retinitis Pigmentosa

Retinitis pigmentosa (RP) is the most common heritable retinopathy affecting approximately 1 in 3,700 individuals worldwide (Haim 2002). RP is a disease characterized by progressive constriction of visual fields via apoptosis of the rod photoreceptor cells. Patients affected with RP are often left legally or completely blind due to this process (Heckenlively and Daiger 2002).

RP shows phenotypic, genetic, and allelic heterogeneity. The phenotype of RP is heterogeneous in that individuals in the same family and/or even the same sibship may have different symptoms despite carrying an identical genetic mutation. Phenotypic heterogeneity in RP may be attributed to modifying factors and/or environmental factors that have yet to be identified (Daiger, Shankar et al. 2006). Mutations causing autosomal dominant (adRP), autosomal recessive (arRP) or X-linked RP (xlRP) have been identified in a total of 31 genes, with another 9 loci implicated by linkage (http://www.sph.uth.tmc.edu/RetNet) Within these disease-associated genes there may be one or many disease-causing alleles. Approximately 60% of dominant mutations can be identified at this time (Sullivan et al. 2006a, b; Daiger et al. 2007; Gire et al. 2007; Bowne et al. 2008), therefore additional disease-causing genes and/or mutations remain to be found.

62.3 RP10 – Disease Caused by Mutations in IMPDH1

In 2002 our laboratory discovered that missense mutations in the IMPDH1 gene cause adRP (Bowne et al. 2002; Kennan et al. 2002). The IMPDH1 gene is located on chromosome 7q32.1 and accounts for approximately 2.5% of all adRP cases (Bowne et al. 2006b; Sullivan et al. 2006a). In addition to adRP, rare dominant-acting mutations in IMPDH1 cause a congenital form of blindness known as Leber congenital amaurosis or LCA (Bowne et al. 2006). Disease-causing variants in IMPDH1 are mainly missense mutations, the most common of which is the Asp226Asn mutation accounting for about 2% of adRP cases in the United States alone (Wada et al. 2005). The phenotype resulting from IMPDH1 mutations tends to be severe with early onset and rapid progression, sometimes also presenting with cystoid macular edema (CME) (Kozma et al. 2005; Schatz et al. 2005; Wada et al. 2005).

62.4 IMPDH Structure and Function

IMPDH is enzymatically active in the homotetramer state. Each IMPDH monomer is composed of an eight-stranded alpha/beta barrel structure that performs the enzymatic function, and a flanking subdomain that is composed of two cystathionine β-synthase-like regions, called CBS domains (Carr et al. 1993).

IMPDH is part of a highly conserved class of enzymes found in both prokaryotes and eukaryotes (Senda and Natsumeda 1994). It functions in the de novo purine synthesis pathway. Specifically, IMPDH catalyzes the rate-limiting step of guanine nucleotide synthesis by converting inosine 5′-monophosphate (IMP) to xanthosine 5′-monophosphate (XMP) with the concomitant reduction of nicotinamide adenine dinucleotide (NAD^+) (Hedstrom 1999). XMP can go on to be converted to guanine monophosphate (GMP) by GMP synthetase (Fig. 62.1).

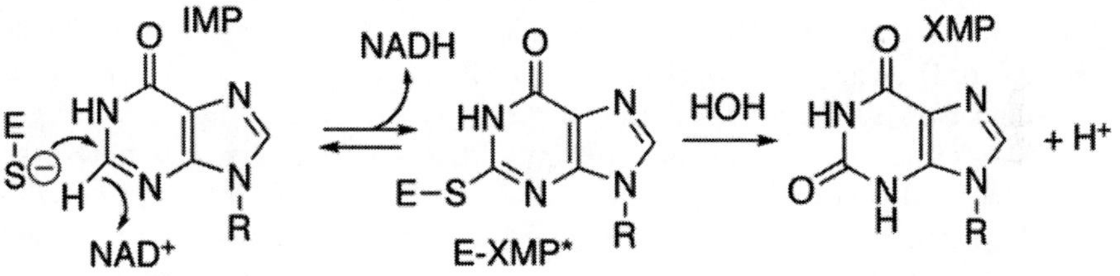

Fig. 62.1 Chemical reaction catalyzed by the inosine monophosphate dehydrogenase (IMPDH) enzyme. IMPDH functions in de novo guanine nucleotide synthesis by converting inosine 5′-monophosphate (IMP) to xanthosine 5′-monophosphate (XMP) with the concomitant reduction of nicotinamide adenine dinucleotide (NAD^+) (Hedstrom 1999). Figure produced by Dr. Lizbeth Hedstrom, Brandeis University (Waltham, MA)

Mammals have two homologues of the IMPDH gene, IMPDH1 and IMPDH2, which upon translation are 84% identical in humans (Natsumeda et al. 1990). Human IMPDH1 is located on chromosome 7q32.1 and human IMPDH2 is located on chromosome 3p21.2 (Glesne et al. 1993; Gu et al. 1994). The IMPDH isozymes are indistinguishable in enzymatic activity (Carr et al. 1993) but have different inhibitory properties (Hager et al. 1995). Research shows that IMPDH1 and IMPDH2 are differentially expressed between tissues (Natsumeda et al. 1990; Jain et al. 2004). Our analysis using SAGE methodology shows that IMPDH1 mRNA is exceptionally abundant in the retina; the abundance of IMPDH1 in the retina is approximately ten times the average levels found elsewhere in the body, perhaps indicating that retinal tissue has a unique requirement for IMPDH1. IMPDH2 mRNA is scarce in retinal tissue but more abundant elsewhere in the body (Bowne et al. 2006a). Indeed, research shows that the majority of the GTP in mouse retina is produced by IMPDH1, not IMPDH2 or the salvage pathway (Aherne et al. 2004).

62.5 IMPDH Binds Single Stranded Nucleic Acids

In 2004 Dr. Lizbeth Hedstrom's lab at Brandeis University, Waltham MA, showed that IMPDH proteins bind single-stranded nucleic acids with nanomolar (physiological) affinity (McLean et al. 2004). The binding occurs via the CBS domains and IMPDH appears to bind about 100 bp of single-stranded polynucleotides. The nucleic acid binding activity does not inhibit function of the enzyme, and if the CBS domains are removed from the protein, nucleic acid binding function is ablated.

The majority of the adRP and LCA-associated mutations reside in or near the IMPDH1 CBS domains in the protein structure (Mortimer and Hedstrom 2005; Bowne et al. 2006). To test the effect of the adRP/LCA-associated mutations on the nucleic acid binding activity of IMPDH1 several recombinant proteins were produced. Recombinant wild type IMPDH1 was produced in a typical bacterial system, and IMPDH1 proteins with the following missense mutations were also produced: Arg224Pro, Val268Ile, Asp226Asn, Arg105Trp, Thr116Met, Asn198Lys, and His372Pro (Bowne et al. 2002; Kennan et al. 2002; Bowne et al. 2006b). Two additional genetic variants were tested that are known to be benign, Ala285Thr and His296Arg (Bowne et al. 2006b). When adRP mutations are 'knocked in' to the recombinant IMPDH1 protein, the kinetic parameters of the enzyme are unchanged, however the nucleic acid binding property of the protein is altered in most cases (Mortimer and Hedstrom 2005; Bowne et al. 2006b). Binding affinity for ssDNA was decreased in all the known pathogenic mutations by a factor ranging from 7 to 32. In addition, some of the pathogenic variants bound an increased portion of the random pool of ssDNA. As expected, the non-pathogenic variants did not differ significantly from the wild type enzyme in either measure (Mortimer and Hedstrom 2005; Bowne et al. 2006b). These data suggest that IMPDH1 has a unique function that involves binding single stranded nucleic acids.

62.6 Retinal Isoforms of IMPDH1

Although alternate starts of transcription, and thus alternate transcripts of IMPDH1 were previously identified, only one protein was known to be produced from these transcripts (Gu and Mitchell 1997). This traditionally-studied form of IMPDH1 is referred to as 'canonical IMPDH1' or IMPDH1 (514) IMPDH1 (514) results from the transcription and translation of exons 1-14, excluding exon 13b (see genomic structure, Fig. 62.2a) Upon translation, the IMPDH1 (514) protein is 514 amino acids in length and predicted to be 55.6 kD in molecular weight.

In 2006 our laboratory discovered that retinal-specific isoforms of IMPDH1 exist (Bowne et al. 2006). A series of experiments using human and mouse retinal cDNA were performed to identify the predominant IMPDH1 transcript in the retinal tissue in these species and results showed several novel mRNA transcripts. These novel transcripts result from both alternate splicing events and alternate starts of transcription and translation. Results showed that exon A is transcribed in retina and is

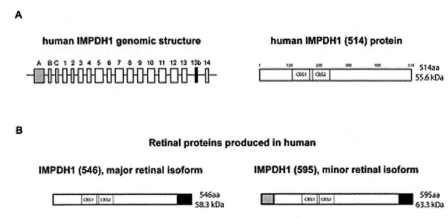

Fig. 62.2 (**a**) Genomic structure of IMPDH1 in humans and the 'canonical' IMPDH1 (514) protein. The 'canonical' IMPDH1 (514) protein results from translation of exons 1-14. (**b**) Retinal-specific isoforms of IMPDH1 in human. The *black* portion of the proteins represents the amino acid sequence resulting from the addition of exon 13b in the spliced transcript. The *grey* portion of the protein represents the sequence resulting from the addition of exon A in the spliced transcript. IMPDH1 (546) is the most abundant isoform found in human retina and results from the translation of exons 1-14 and exon 13b. The less abundant isoform in human retina is IMPDH1 (595) which is translated from exons 1-14 and exons A and 13b. CBS1 and CBS2 illustrate the approximate location of the cystathionine β-synthase-like (CBS) domains in the proteins

spliced, in frame, directly to exon 1, leading to a novel protein sequence at the N terminus upon translation. In addition, the data showed that a novel 17 bp exon exists between exons 13 and 14, exon 13b. Exon 13b causes a frame shift in transcription that abolishes the stop codon, and leads to a novel protein sequence at the C terminus, as well. Exon 13b was present in almost all the retinal transcripts analyzed (Bowne et al. 2006a).

There are two predominant transcripts present in human and mouse retina. One transcript includes exons 1 through 14, but also contains exons A and 13b. The other most abundant transcript in human and mouse retina also includes exons 1 through 14 and exon 13b, but not exon A (Fig. 62.2b) (Bowne et al. 2006a). Upon translation these two transcripts result in proteins that are referred to as '1+13b' or IMPDH1 (546), and 'A+13b' or IMPDH1 (595), respectively. The names IMPDH1 (546) and IMPDH1 (595), based on the amino acid lengths of the retinal isoforms, will be the nomenclature used here.

We also performed experiments to characterize the IMPDH1 (546) and (595) isoforms in other species. Retinal tissues from several mammalian species, including sheep, dog, mouse, cow, pig, rat, and human, were analyzed by western blot for the various IMPDH1 protein isoforms. Antibodies specific to each IMPDH1 isoform were used to visualize the proteins in each species. These data show that the retinal isoforms of IMPDH1 are not only transcribed but also translated in the retina of human and in all other species tested. Secondly, the relative abundances of the two retinal proteins are different among the species observed, with humans being different from all the rest. Specifically, data showed that in most species IMPDH1 (595) is the most abundant isoform. In pig and sheep the isoforms appear to be equal in abundance, and human is unique in that IMPDH1 (546) is the abundant isoform. Lastly, the sizes of the retinal isoforms differ slightly between species (Spellicy et al. 2007). This indicates there may be slight sequence differences and/or post-translational modifications between species.

Despite the fact that IMPDH1 (514) is ubiquitously expressed in the body, disease resulting from IMPDH1 mutations is limited strictly to the retina. The discovery of the retinal isoforms of IMPDH1 provides a possible explanation for this long-standing mystery – that the mechanism of disease is specific to the retinal isoforms and therefore does not manifest in other tissues.

62.7 Kinetic and Nucleic Acid Binding Properties of Retinal IMPDH1

In collaboration with Dr. Hedstrom's laboratory we repeated the kinetic and nucleic acid binding experiments using the retinal isoforms of IMPDH1. Measuring NAD^+ production as an indicator of enzyme activity we showed that the IMPDH1 (546) and IMPDH1 (595) are able to convert IMP to XMP with kinetic parameters similar to that of IMPDH1 (514) Cellular localization experiments were also performed in vivo for both retinal isoforms and showed a distribution identical to IMPDH1 (514) (Xu et al. 2008).

Nucleic acid binding studies were performed using radiolabeled single-stranded nucleic acids and two different membranes to measure nucleic acid affinity of the proteins (hybond, which binds free nucleic acids, and nitrocellulose, which binds protein and protein-nucleic acid complexes) The ratio of free and bound single-stranded nucleotides was used to calculate the affinity of IMPDH (546) and IMPDH1 (595) for polynucleotides (McLean et al. 2004; Mortimer and Hedstrom 2005; Bowne et al. 2006b; Xu et al. 2008). Interestingly, the retinal isoforms of IMPDH1 failed to bind polynucleotides almost completely (Xu et al. 2008). However, recent research from Dr. Hedstrom's laboratory shows that IMPDH1 (595) and (546) both associate with polyribosomes translating RNA in bovine retina. In addition, inclusion of the Asp226Asn mutation in either of these protein isoforms inhibits the interaction, sometimes completely (Mortimer et al. 2008). It is possible that the additional protein sequence at the C terminus of the protein blocks this activity, or that another protein component is needed in vivo to potentiate this interaction.

62.8 Conclusion

Elucidating the mechanism of retinal disease in RP10 presents a formidable task. Many questions remain about the function of IMPDH1 as it relates specifically to the retina. Strides have been made towards starting to address these questions; discovery of the retinal-specific isoforms may help explain the tissue specificity of disease, and data suggest that retinal IMPDH1 may have a novel function in RNA transcription, translation, or stabilization. We are optimistic that these novel findings are a first step in understanding retinal disease caused by IMPDH1 mutations.

References

Aherne A, Kennan A et al (2004) On the molecular pathology of neurodegeneration in IMPDH1-based retinitis pigmentosa. Hum Mol Genet 13(6):641–650

Bowne S, Liu Q et al (2006) Why do mutations in the ubiquitously expressed housekeeping gene IMPDH1 cause retina-specific photoreceptor degeneration?. Invest Ophthalmol Vis Sci 47(9):3754–3765

Bowne S, Sullivan L et al (2002a) Mutations in the inosine monophosphate dehydrogenase 1 gene (IMPDH1) cause the RP10 form of autosomal dominant retinitis pigmentosa. Hum Mol Genet 11(5):559–568

Bowne S, Sullivan L et al (2006) Spectrum and frequency of mutations in IMPDH1 associated with autosomal dominant retinitis pigmentosa and leber congenital amaurosis. Invest Ophthalmol Vis Sci 47(1):34–42

Bowne S, Sullivan L et al (2008b) Mutations in the TOPORS gene cause 1% of autosomal dominant retinitis pigmentosa. Mol Vis 14:922–927

Carr S, Papp E et al (1993) Characterization of human type I and type II IMP dehydrogenases. J Biol Chem 268(36):27286–27290

Daiger S, Bowne S et al (2007) Perspective on genes and mutations causing retinitis pigmentosa. Arch Ophthalmol 125(2):151–158

Daiger S, Shankar S et al (2006) Genetic factors modifying clinical expression of autosomal dominant RP. Adv Exp Med Biol 572:3–8

Gire A, Sullivan L et al (2007) The Gly56Arg mutation in NR2E3 accounts for 1–2% of autosomal dominant retinitis pigmentosa. Mol Vis 13:1970–1975

Glesne D, Collart F et al (1993) Chromosomal localization and structure of the human type II IMP dehydrogenase gene (IMPDH2). Genomics 16(1):274–277

Gu J, Kaiser-Rogers K et al (1994) Assignment of the human type I IMP dehydrogenase gene (IMPDH1) to chromosome 7p31.3-p32. Genomics 24(1):179–181

Gu J, Mitchell B (1997) Regulation of the human inosine monophosphate dehydrogenase type I gene: utilization of alternative promoters. J Biol Chem 272:4458–4466

Hager P, Collart F et al (1995) Recombinant human inosine monophosphate dehydrogenase type I and type II proteins. Biochem Pharmacol 49(9):1323–1329

Haim M (2002) The epidemiology of retinitis pigmentosa in Denmark. Acta Ophthalmol Scand 233:1–34

Heckenlively J, Daiger S (2002) In: Rimoin DL, Connor JM, Pyeritz RE, Korf BR (eds), Emery and Rimoin's principals and practices of medical genetics, 4th edn. Churchill Livingston, London, pp 3555–3593

Hedstrom L (1999) IMP dehydrogenase: mechanism of action and inhibition. Curr Med Chem 6:545–560

Jain J, Almquist S et al (2004) Regulation of inosine monophosphate dehydrogenase type I and type II isoforms in human lymphocytes. Biochem Pharmacol 67:767–776

Kennan A, Aherne A et al (2002) Identification of an IMPDH1 mutation in autosomal dominant retinitis pigmentosa (RP10) revealed following comparative microarray analysis of transcripts derived from retinas of wild-type and Rho$^{-/-}$ mice. Hum Mol Genet 11(5):547–558

Kozma P, Hughbanks-Wheaton D et al (2005) Phenotypic characterization of a large family with RP10 autosomal-dominant retinitis pigmentosa: an Asp226Asn mutation in the IMPDH1 gene. Am J Ophthalmol 140(5):858–867

Magasanik B, Moyed H et al (1957) Enzymes essential for the biosynthesis of nucleic acid guanine; inosine 5′-phosphate dehydrogenase of aerobacter aerogenes. J Biol Chem 226(1):339–350

McLean J, Hamaguchi N et al (2004) Inosine 5′-monophosphate dehydrogenase binds nucleic acids in vitro and in vivo. Biochem J 379:243–251

Mortimer S, Hedstrom L (2005) Autosomal dominant retinitis pigmentosa mutations in inosine 5′-monophosphate dehydrogenase type I disrupt nucleic acid binding. Biochem J 390(Pt 1): 41–47

Mortimer S, Xu D et al (2008) IMP dehydrogenase type 1 associates with polyribosomes translating Rhodopsin RNA. J Biol Chem 283(52):36354–36360

Natsumeda Y, Ohno S et al (1990) Two distinct cDNAs for human IMP dehydrogenase. J Biol Chem 265(9):5292–5295

Schatz P, Ponjavic V et al (2005) Clinical phenotype in a Swedish family with a mutation in the IMPDH1 gene. Ophthalmic Genet 26(3):119–124

Senda M, Natsumeda Y (1994) Tissue-differential expression of two distinct genes for human IMP dehydrogenase (E.C.1.1.1.205). Life Sci 54(24):1917–1926

Spellicy C, Daiger S et al (2007) Characterization of retinal inosine monophosphate dehydrogenase 1 in several mammalian species. Mol Vis 13:1866–1872

Sullivan L, Bowne S et al (2006a) Prevalence of disease-causing mutations in families with autosomal dominant retinitis pigmentosa: a screen of known genes in 200 families. Invest Ophthalmol Vis Sci 47(7):3052–3064

Sullivan L, Bowne S et al (2006b) Genomic rearrangements of the PRPF31 gene account for 2.5% of autosomal dominant retinitis pigmentosa. Invest Ophthalmol Vis Sci 47(10):4579–4588

Wada Y, Sandberg M et al (2005) Screen of IMPDH1 gene among patients with dominant retinitis pigmentosa and clinical features associated with the most common mutation, Asp226Asn. Invest Ophthalmol Vis Sci 46(5):1735–1741

Xu D, Cobb G et al (2008) Retinal isoforms of inosine 5′-monophosphate dehydrogenase type 1 are poor nucleic acid binding proteins. Arch Biochem Biophys 472:100–104

Chapter 63
Congenital Stationary Night Blindness in Mice – A Tale of Two *Cacna1f* Mutants

N. Lodha, S. Bonfield, N.C. Orton, C.J. Doering, J.E. McRory, S.C. Mema, R. Rehak, Y. Sauvé, R. Tobias, W.K. Stell, and N.T. Bech-Hansen

Abstract

Background: Mutations in *CACNA1F*, which encodes the $Ca_v1.4$ subunit of a voltage-gated L-type calcium channel, cause X-linked incomplete congenital stationary night blindness (CSNB2), a condition of defective retinal neurotransmission which results in night blindness, reduced visual acuity, and diminished ERG b-wave. We have characterized two putative murine CSNB2 models: an engineered null-mutant, with a stop codon (*G305X*); and a spontaneous mutant with an ETn insertion in intron 2 of *Cacna1f* (*nob2*).

Methods: *Cacna1f*^{G305X}: Adults were characterized by visual function (photopic optokinetic response, OKR); gene expression (microarray) and by cell death (TUNEL) and synaptic development (TEM). *Cacna1f*^{nob2}: Adults were characterized by properties of *Cacna1f* mRNA (cloning and sequencing) and expressed protein (immunoblotting, electrophysiology, filamin [cytoskeletal protein] binding), and OKR.

Results: The null mutation in *Cacna1f*^{G305X} mice caused loss of cone cell ribbons, failure of OPL synaptogenesis, ERG b-wave and absence of OKR. In *Cacna1f*^{nob2} mice alternative ETn splicing produced $\sim90\%$ *Cacna1f* mRNA having a stop codon, but $\sim10\%$ mRNA encoding a complete polypeptide. *Cacna1f*^{nob2} mice had normal OKR, and alternatively-spliced complete protein had WT channel properties, but alternative ETn splicing abolished N-terminal protein binding to filamin.

Conclusions: $Ca_v1.4$ plays a key role in photoreceptor synaptogenesis and synaptic function in mouse retina. *Cacna1f*^{G305X} is a true knockout model for human CSNB2, with prominent defects in cone and rod function. *Cacna1f*^{nob2} is an incomplete knockout model for CSNB2, because alternative splicing in an ETn element

N. Lodha (✉)
Department Medical Genetics, Faculty of Medicine, University of Calgary, Calgary, Alberta T2N 4N1, Canada
e-mail: nlodha@ucalgary.ca

leads to some full-length $Ca_V1.4$ protein, and some cones surviving to drive photopic visual responses.

63.1 Introduction

The incomplete form of X-linked congenital stationary night blindness (iCSNB, CSNB2) is one of a heterogeneous group of human visual disorders due to defects in retinal neurotransmission, characterized by reduced function in rod and cone photoreceptor pathways (Miyake et al. 1986; Tremblay et al. 1995). The clinical features of CSNB2 are highly variable and may include reduced visual acuity, impaired night vision, refractive disorders, nystagmus and strabismus (Miyake et al. 1986; Boycott et al. 2000; Miyake 2002; Lodha et al. 2009). The full-field flash electroretinograms (ERGs) of CSNB2 patients reveal abnormal rod- and cone-system responses, indicating impairment of synaptic transmission from photoreceptors to bipolar cells.

CSNB2 is an X-linked recessive condition due to mutations in *CACNA1F*, the gene for the pore-forming α_{1F}-subunit of an L-type voltage-gated calcium channel, $Ca_V1.4$ (Bech-Hansen et al. 1998; Strom et al. 1998). Since $Ca_V1.4$ is the major mediator of transmitter release from rods and cones, it has been assumed that the impairment of synaptic transmission in CSNB2 is due to insufficiency of calcium currents through mutant $Ca_V1.4$ channels (Bech-Hansen et al. 1998; Strom et al. 1998; Baumann et al. 2004). To understand the pathophysiology of human CSNB2, we have characterized two murine CSNB2 models: an engineered null mutant with a stop codon at amino acid residue 305 (G305X: Cacna1f ^{G305X}; (Mansergh et al. 2005; Orton et al. 2007; Raven et al. 2008)), and a spontaneous mutant in which the insertion of a retrovirus-like early transposon (ETn) causes the production of abnormal Cacna1f-encoded transcripts and proteins mutant (nob2: Cacna1f ^{nob2}; (Chang et al. 2006; Bayley and Morgans 2007)). Here we describe further investigations of these two models and discuss insights that we have gained from such studies.

63.2 Methods

Previous reports have described our methods for immunofluorescence (Mansergh et al. 2005; Morgans et al. 2005; Chang et al. 2006; Raven et al. 2008), optokinetic response (OKR: Prusky and Douglas 2004; Bonfield et al. 2007; Umino et al. 2008), and flash electroretinography (ERG: Mansergh et al. 2005; Orton et al. 2007; Doering et al. 2008; Raven et al. 2008). In *G305X* mice, differences between gene expression in adult wild-type and mutant retinas were characterized by a retina-specific microarray (Orton et al. 2007), and effects of mutations on retinal development and synaptogenesis were assessed by the TUNEL method and caspase immunocytochemistry (putatively indicating apoptptosis) plus transmission electron microscopy (TEM) in P10-P28 mice (Orton et al. 2007; Raven et al. 2008). In adult *nob2* mice, mRNA was cloned and sequenced, expressed protein was characterized by immunoblotting for $Ca_V1.4/\alpha_{1F}$ and a pull-down assay for binding to filamin (a cytoskeletal protein), and the properties of wild-type and mutant $Ca_V1.4$ channels expressed in HEK cells were determined by patch-clamping (Doering et al. 2008).

63.3 Results

Although these models for CSNB2 are similar, they differ in several important respects:

Cacna1f^{G305X}: A loss-of-function mutation was created by inserting a self-excising Cre-lox-neocassette into exon 7 of *Cacna1f*, the murine orthologue of *CACNA1F* (Mansergh et al. 2005). Its scotopic ERG had an a-wave of marginally reduced amplitude and no post-receptoral b-wave and oscillatory potentials (Fig. 63.1a and b), while its photopic ERG (Fig. 63.1c), as well as visual evoked

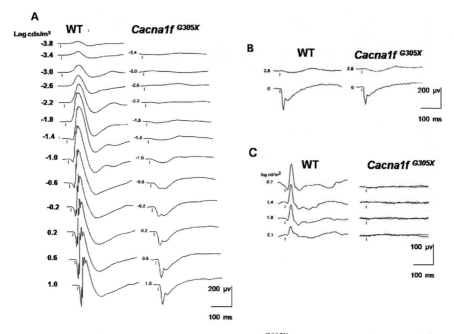

Fig. 63.1 Electroretinogram (ERG) findings in *Cacna1f*^{G305X} mice. (**a**) Scotopic ERG: Intensity-response series of scotopic electroretinograms in wild-type (*Cacna1f*^{WT}) and mutant mice (*Cacna1f*$^{G305X/G305X}$, *Cacna1f*$^{G305X/Y}$). In the *Cacna1f*^{G305X} mice, the ERG b-wave is absent, providing an electronegative configuration to the bright-flash responses. Oscillatory potentials (OPs) are also absent in mutant mice. Numbers at the left of individual recordings are stimulus intensity in log cd s/m. (**b**) Comparison of ERG responses between a *Cacna1f*^{G305X} mutant mouse and a wild-type animal with intravitreal injection of CoCl2. The bright-flash response after CoCl2 injection in the wild-type is identical to the one in the mutant, suggesting that the *Cacna1f*-mutant ERG response is mostly generated by photoreceptor activity. (**c**) Photopic ERG is undetectable in *Cacna1f*^{G305X} mice (modified from Mansergh et al. 2005)

potentials and multi-unit activities in the superior colliculus, were absent (Mansergh et al. 2005). Immunoreactive $Ca_V1.4$ protein was not detectable in the outer plexi-form layer (OPL), dendrites of second-order neurons sprouted into the photorecep-tor layer, and TEM showed a profound loss of photoreceptor synapses (Mansergh et al. 2005). Microarray of retina from affected males and females revealed marked reductions in expression of cone-specific genes (data not shown). Photopic spa-tial contrast-sensitivity (CS) functions for optokinetic responses (OptoMotry^{TM}) of wild-type controls were as described previously ((Prusky and Douglas 2004; Umino et al. 2008); Bonfield 2009), with optimal drift speed ~12 d/s, peak contrast sensitivity ~15 (threshold contrast ~ 6.5%) at spatial frequency (SF) 0.061–0.1 c/d, and acuity (highest SF for response at 100% contrast) >0.4 c/d. In contrast, affected G305X mice (Cacna1f $^{G305X/y}$ and Cacna1f $^{G305X/G305X}$) gave no optoki-netic response, while heterozygous females (Cacna1f $^{G305X/+}$) responded robustly

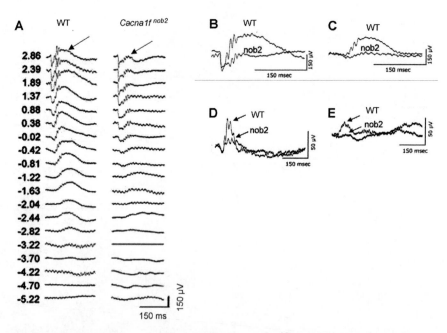

Fig. 63.2 Electroretinogram (ERG) findings in Cacna1f^{nob2} mice. (**a**) Scotopic ERG (dark adapted): Intensity-response series of scotopic electroretinograms in wild-type (Cacna1f^{WT}) and mutant (Cacna1f^{nob2}) mice. Scotopic ERG b-wave is nearly absent in mutant mice at low inten-sity and appears at higher intensity, though with a reduced amplitude, providing an electronegative configuration to the bright-flash responses. The oscillatory potentials (OPs) are absent in mutant mice at low intensity, but are present at high intensity. (**b, c**) Details of scotopic ERG at intensities 1.89 log cd/m^2 (**b**) and –0.81 log cd/m^2 (**c**). Wild type and mutant ages nearly P52. The b-wave and OP can be elicited, especially at higher luminance and their amplitude increases with increasing stimulus intensity. (**d, e**) Photopic ERG (light-adapted). (**d**: high intensity of 1.89 log cd/m^2; **e**: low intensity of 0.38 log cd/m^2) a-wave, b-wave and oscillatory potentials are small but clearly evident in Cacna1f^{nob2} mice at both intensities of stimulus

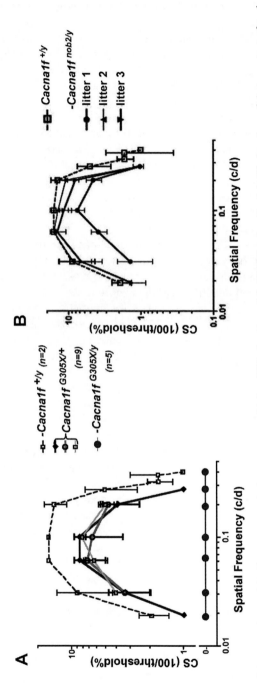

Fig. 63.3 Photopic spatial (sine-wave grating) contrast sensitivity (CS) function. (**a**) *G305X* mice Spatial CS function of heterozygous females (*Cacna1f* [+/G305X], 3 l, *n* = 9) showed reduced CS vs unaffected male (*Cacna1f* [WT]) littermates. *Cacna1f* [G305X/Y]: no response to any spatial frequency or contrast. (**b**) *nob2* mice Spatial CS function of affected males (*Cacna1f* [nob2/y], 3 l, *n* = 15). The CS was similar to that of WT (*Cacna1f* [WT]) in nob2 litters 2 and 3, but not to that of *Cacna1f* [+/G305X] in nob2 liter 1

but with peak CS and acuity about 50% less than those of wild-type mice (Fig. 63.3a; Bonfield 2009).

Cacna1f^nob2: A spontaneous mutant having no b-wave was isolated from colonies at the Jackson Laboratory. It was first reported to have an insertion of a transposable element (ETn) into exon 2 of *Cacna1f*, predicted to produce an in-frame premature stop codon (Chang et al. 2005). However, by northern blotting we identified not one but two mRNA species in *nob2* mice; ~90% of the transcripts contained the in-frame stop codon previously identified, but ~10% of the transcripts lacked this stop codon because it was removed by alternative splicing within the ETn element. Thus *nob2* mice were predicted to encode a complete (but altered) $Ca_V1.4$ protein with 22 novel amino acids in the N-terminal region (Doering et al. 2008). Biophysical analysis of channels in HEK cells transfected with this complete but altered cDNA revealed activation and inactivation characteristics indistinguishable from those of wild-type; but binding with filamin proteins, a property of the N-terminal portion of wild-type α_{1F} protein, was absent from the mutant protein (Doering et al. 2008). We also have observed: reductions in amplitude of both scotopic and photopic ERG b-waves and oscillatory potentials (Fig. 63.2) (Doering et al. 2008), reduction in thickness of the outer plexiform layer, and sprouting of rod bipolar and horizontal cell dendrites into the outer nuclear layer, as in the *G305X* mouse. Remarkably, the peak optokinetic CS was normal in most of the affected (*Cacna1f^nob2/nob2* and *Cacna1f^nob2/y*) *nob2* mice; however, their acuity was almost 50% lower than in WT mice, and CS was significantly below normal at most spatial frequencies in one of the three litters tested (Fig. 63.3b: litter 1).

63.4 Discussion

CSNB2 is a clinically variable retinal neurotransmission disorder, difficult to diagnose without detailed assessment of visual acuity, visual field, refractive error, nystagmus and strabismus, plus rigorous electroretinography (Tremblay et al. 1995; Boycott et al. 2000). Identification of the gene responsible for CSNB2 has made possible DNA-definitive diagnosis (nearly 80% of patients with the clinical features of iCSNB have mutations in *CACNA1F* [Bech-Hansen and Tobias, unpublished]). Signs and symptoms of CSNB2 are variable, not only in patients having different *CACNA1F* mutations (Lodha et al. Submitted), but also among members of families sharing the same *CACNA1F* founder mutation (Boycott et al. 2000). This variability may be due in part to mutations in modifier genes, thus altering interactions of their protein products with $Ca_V1.4$ protein and directly impairing $Ca_V1.4$ channel assembly, integrity, and function; this is suggested by the observation that the biophysical properties of some mutant *CACNA1F*-encoded channels are normal (McRory et al. 2004; Hoda et al. 2005; Peloquin et al. 2007). The functional phenotypes of the *G305X* and *nob2* mice are distinctive, even though both are due to mutations in the *Cacna1f* gene. The phenotype of *Cacna1f^G305X* mice is more severe than that of *Cacna1f^nob2* mice; the OKR, visual evoked potential, and ERG findings indicate virtually complete loss of cone function as well as cone-to-bipolar cell synaptic transmission in *Cacna1f* ^{G305X} (Mansergh et al. 2005; Bonfield et al. 2007; Orton et al. 2007), whereas the OKR and ERG indicate substantial (although diminished) cone viability and cone-bipolar cell transmission in *Cacna1f* ^{nob2} (Bonfield et al. 2007; Doering et al. 2008). Loss and disorganization of rod and cone ribbon synapses is accompanied by thinning of the outer plexiform layer in both mutants; however, cone ribbon synapses are completely lost in *G305X* mice, while some survive in *nob2* mice (Chang et al. 2006; Raven et al. 2008). The presumably small fraction of complete (though abnormal) $Ca_V1.4$ protein in *Cacna1f* ^{nob2} may sustain sufficient binding with critical protein partners that *nob2* cones survive and function at near-normal levels, and cone synaptic transmission in *nob2* retinas may be defective because of the loss of $Ca_V1.4$-protein interactions that are critical for the normal development and functioning of ribbon synapses. It is noteworthy that knockouts of genes for bassoon, CABP4, and calcium-channel β2-subunits cause similar defects in the development and function of photoreceptor ribbon synapses (Ball and Gregg 2002; Dick et al. 2003; Haeseleer et al. 2004), suggesting that the formation of functional ribbon synapses depends on the assembly of microdomains containing key proteins. Furthermore, accumulation of abnormal proteins (such as α_{1F}) may cause endoplasmic reticulum (ER) stress, leading to an unfolded protein response and cell death (Xia and Link 2008). Cones are likely to be more susceptible to ER stress, because each cone has ~20–40 times as many synaptic ribbon complexes as each rod (Haverkamp et al. 2000) and therefore is likely to be stressed by a much larger synthetic load of any abnormal ribbon synapse-related proteins. Cones may be spared in *Cacna1f* ^{nob2} mice, because even though the complete $Ca_V1.4/\alpha_{1F}$ protein is somewhat abnormal in structure and amount, it is less likely to remain unfolded in the ER than the truncated protein.

How do the differences in mutations account for the differences in optokinetic behavior of the two mouse strains? Because of random inactivation of most genes on the X-chromosome, ~50% of cones in *Cacna1f* $^{G305X/+}$ females should express the normal, and ~50% the truncation-encoding, *Cacna1f* gene; the loss of 50% of cones is the most economical explanation for the 50% reduction in photopic contrast sensitivity and acuity of females heterozygous for the G305X mutation. *Nob2* mice, on the other hand, may have enough 'complete' $Ca_V1.4$ channel protein to support normal assembly of ribbon synapse proteins, in all cones thus maintaining quasi-normal synaptic transmission to cone bipolar cells. Despite their superior performance under photopic conditions, however, *nob2* mice should perform as poorly as *G305X* mice under scotopic conditions, because of the massive loss of rod ribbon synapses in both. However, the optokinetic contrast sensitivity functions of both mutants are velocity-tuned for photopic vision (when present), indicating that velocity-tuning is dependent on the unaffected circuitry of the inner plexiform layer rather than the mutation-altered circuitry of the outer plexiform layer.

Our findings in these two mutant mice highlight the importance of $Ca_V1.4$ protein in the structure and function of photoreceptor ribbon synapses and synaptic transmission. Even minor expression of a *Cacna1f* transcript, and presumably a reduced amount of $Ca_V1.4$ protein, are sufficient to support some visual function (OKR).

Table 63.1 Summary of characteristics of *Cacna1f* ^{G305X} and *Cacna1f* ^{nob2} CSNB2 models

Trait	Cacna1f ^{G305X}	Cacna1f ^{nob2}
Mutation	Truncation of protein at codon G305 – true knockout	Early truncation (25) + small amount abnormal but functional Ca$_V$1.4
Histology	Diminished OPL	Diminished POL
Immunology	No α$_{1F}$ protein	Little α$_{1F}$ protein
OPL synapses	Absent/markedly diminished	Diminished
2nd order neuron	ONL sprouting, ectopic synapses	ONL sprouting, ectopic synapses
Rods	Rods survive, synapses lost	Rods survive, synapses lost
ERG, scotopic	Intact a-wave, b-wave abolished	Intact a-wave, b-wave present at higher intensities
Cones	Severe loss (apoptosis)	Moderate cone loss
ERG, photopic	Absent	a-wave intact, b-wave reduced ∼50%
RGCs	Not tested	Loss ON-resp; other abnormal
OKR, homozyg	Blind	Almost normal CS, acuity∼60%
OKR, hetero	Peak CS & acuity down ∼50%	Not tested
Ca^{++} Channel	No detectable Ca^{++} Current	Channels normal in HEK cells

OPL = outer plexiform layer, neur = neuron, ERG = electroretinogram, RGCs = retinal ganglion cells, resp = response, OKR = optokinetic response, homozyg = homozygous, hetero = heterozygous, CS = contrast sensitivity (Manserg et al. 2005; Doering et al. 2009).

On the other hand, we also recognize that patients with the same founder mutation show extensive clinical variability, raising the suspicion that modifier genes also contribute to the phenotypic variability seen in CSNB2 patients.

63.5 Conclusion

Ca$_V$1.4 plays key roles in photoreceptor synaptogenesis and synaptic function in the mouse retina. *Cacna1f* ^{G305X} is a true knockout model for human CSNB2, with prominent defects in cone function, whereas *Cacna1f* ^{nob2} is not a true knockout model for CSNB2, because the synthesis of some functional Ca$_V$1.4 protein such as to maintain cone survival and photopic visual function. Differences in Ca$_V$1.4 synthesis and cone survival might explain some of the phenotypic variability seen in human CSNB2, as well as in these two murine models.

Acknowledgments Supported by: FFB-Canada, CIHR, NSERC, and AHFMR.

References

Ball SL, Gregg RG (2002) Using mutant mice to study the role of voltage-gated calcium channels in the retina. Adv Exp Med Biol 514:439–450

Baumann L, Gerstner A et al (2004) Functional characterization of the L-type Ca^{2+} channel Cav1.4alpha1 from mouse retina. Invest Ophthalmol Vis Sci 45(2):708–713

Bayley PR, Morgans CW (2007) Rod bipolar cells and horizontal cells form displaced synaptic contacts with rods in the outer nuclear layer of the nob2 retina. J Comp Neurol 500(2):286–298

Bech-Hansen NT, Naylor MJ et al (1998) Loss-of-function mutations in a calcium-channel alpha1-subunit gene in Xp11.23 cause incomplete X-linked congenital stationary night blindness. Nat Genet 19(3):264–267

Bonfield S, Tejedor J et al (2007) Spatiotemporal contrast sensitivity characteristics of optokinetic responses in chicks and in normal and Cacna1f-mutant mice, Invest Ophthalmol Vis Sci: (ARVO Abstracts), Program #2988

Bonfield S, Tejedor J et al (2009) Spatiotemporal contrast sensitivity characteristics of optokinetic responses in chicks and in normal and Cacna1f-mutant mice in neuroscience. University of Calgary.

Boycott KM, Pearce WG et al (2000) Clinical variability among patients with incomplete X-linked congenital stationary night blindness and a founder mutation in Cacna1f. Can J Ophthalmol 35(4):204–213

Chang B, Hawes NL et al (2005) Mouse models of ocular diseases. Vis Neurosci 22(5):587–593

Chang B, Heckenlively JR et al (2006) The nob2 mouse, a null mutation in Cacna1f: anatomical and functional abnormalities in the outer retina and their consequences on ganglion cell visual responses. Vis Neurosci 23(1):11–24

Dick O, tom Dieck C et al (2003) The presynaptic active zone protein bassoon is essential for photoreceptor ribbon synapse formation in the retina. Neuron 37(5):775–786

Doering CJ, Rehak R et al (2008) Modified Ca(v)1.4 expression in the Cacna1f(nob2) mouse due to alternative splicing of an ETn inserted in exon 2. PLoS ONE 3(7):e2538

Haeseleer F, Imanishi Y et al (2004) Essential role of Ca^{2+}-binding protein 4, a Cav1.4 channel regulator, in photoreceptor synaptic function. Nat Neurosci 7(10):1079–1087

Haverkamp S, Grünert U et al (2000) The cone pedicle, a complex synapse in the retina. Neuron 27(1):85–95

Hoda JC, Zaghetto F et al (2005) Congenital stationary night blindness type 2 mutations S229P, G369D, L1068P, and W1440X alter channel gating or functional expression of Ca(v)1.4 L-type Ca^{2+} channels. J Neurosci 25(1):252–259

Lodha N et al (2009) Phenotypic variability in genetically defined X-linked congenital stationary night blindness. Investigative Ophthalmology and Vis Sci Invest Ophthalmol, p. (ARVO Abstracts), Program # 3721

Mansergh F, Orton NC et al (2005) Mutation of the calcium channel gene Cacna1f disrupts calcium signaling, synaptic transmission and cellular organization in mouse retina. Hum Mol Genet 14(20):3035–3046

McRory JE, Hamid J et al (2004) The Cacna1f gene encodes an L-type calcium channel with unique biophysical properties and tissue distribution. J Neurosci 24(7):1707–1718

Miyake Y (2002) Establishment of the concept of new clinical entities-complete and incomplete form of congenital stationary night blindness. Nippon Ganka Gakkai Zasshi 106(12):737–755; discussion 756

Miyake Y, Yagasaki K et al (1986) Congenital stationary night blindness with negative electroretinogram. A new classification. Arch Ophthalmol 104(7):1013–1020

Morgans CW, Bayley PR et al (2005) Photoreceptor calcium channels: insight from night blindness. Vis Neurosci 22(5):561–568

Orton NC, Stell WK, Bech-Hansen NT (2007) The Cacna1f-Mutant Retina Shows Evidence of Failed Synaptogenesis, Abnormal Synaptic Ribbon Structure and Increased Photoreceptor Cell Death. Investigative Ophthalmology and Visual Science Invest Ophthalmol, p. (ARVO Abstract), Program # 4466

Peloquin JB, Rehak R et al (2007) Functional analysis of congenital stationary night blindness type-2 CACNA1F mutations F742C, G1007R, and R1049W. Neuroscience 150(2): 335–345

Prusky GT, Douglas RM (2004) Characterization of mouse cortical spatial vision. Vis Res 44(28):3411–3418

Raven ME, Orton NC et al (2008) Early afferent signaling in the outer plexiform layer regulates development of horizontal cell morphology. J Comp Neurol 506(5):745–758

Strom TM, Nyakatura G et al (1998) An L-type calcium-channel gene mutated in incomplete
    X-linked congenital stationary night blindness. Nat Genet 19(3):260–263
Tremblay F, Laroche RG et al (1995) The electroretinographic diagnosis of the incomplete form
    of congenital stationary night blindness. Vis Res 35(16):2383–2393
Umino Y, Solessio E et al (2008) Speed, spatial, and temporal tuning of rod and cone vision in
    mouse. J Neurosci 28(1):189–198
Xia J, Link DC (2008) Severe congenital neutropenia and the unfolded protein response. Curr Opin
    Hematol 15(1):1–7

Chapter 64
Protection of Photoreceptors in a Mouse Model of RP10

Lawrence C. S. Tam, Anna-Sophia Kiang, Naomi Chadderton, Paul F. Kenna, Matthew Campbell, Marian M. Humphries, G. Jane Farrar, and Pete Humphries

Abstract Recombinant adeno-associated viral (rAAV) vectors have recently been widely used for the delivery of therapeutic transgenes in preclinical and clinical studies for inherited retinal degenerative diseases. Interchanging capsid genes between different AAV serotypes has enabled selective delivery of transgene into specific cell type(s) of the retina. The RP10 form of autosomal dominant retinitis pigmentosa (adRP) is caused by missense mutations within the gene encoding inosine $5'$-monophosphate dehydrogenase type 1. Here, we report that the use of rAAV2/5 vectors expressing shRNA targeting mutant IMPDH1 prevents photoreceptor degeneration, and preserves synaptic connectivity in a mouse model of RP10.

64.1 Introduction

Over the past decade, tremendous progress has been made in the field of therapeutic gene-based strategies for acquired and inherited ocular diseases. In particular, the commencement of three clinical trials in the United Kingdom and the United States for the autosomal recessive retinal dystrophy, Leber congenital amaurosis (LCA), has transcended the field of gene-mediated therapy for retinal diseases (Bainbridge et al. 2008; Maguire et al. 2008; Hauswirth et al. 2008). The advance from proof-of principle study into human clinical trials has been made possible by extensive efforts placed in tackling one of the major obstacles in retinal gene therapy, namely to achieve specific, high level and long-term expression of therapeutic transgenes in the affected cell type(s). However, this has been made exceptionally difficult by the fact that the retina is composed of a complex arrangement of different cell types that are intricately networked together. In addition, the target tissues to which the therapy must be delivered depends on the disease. For example, recessively inherited retinal diseases such as LCA would require a gene replacement strategy focusing

L.C.S. Tam (✉)
The Ocular Genetics Unit, Department of Genetics, Trinity College Dublin, Dublin 2, Ireland
e-mail: lawrenct@tcd.ie

R.E. Anderson et al. (eds.), *Retinal Degenerative Diseases*, Advances in Experimental Medicine and Biology 664, DOI 10.1007/978-1-4419-1399-9_64,
© Springer Science+Business Media, LLC 2010

on the delivery of functional transgenes to the retinal pigment epithelium (RPE). Similarly in retinitis pigmentosa (RP), which is mainly caused by mutations in genes expressed exclusively in rod photoreceptor cells, specific delivery into the outer segment (OS) and outer nuclear layer (ONL) of the retina would be required. Furthermore, acquired retinopathies such as diabetic retinopathy or age-related macular degeneration (AMD), which are caused by complex pathological mechanisms, would require delivery into multiple cell types. Recently, adeno-associated viral (AAV) vectors have become one of the most successful delivery systems because of the wide variety of retinal cell types that can be selectively transduced using these vectors without causing significant toxicity over a long period of time in small and large animal models. Furthermore, the capsid genes can be interchanged between different AAV serotypes to create hybrid AAV vectors that benefit from enhanced in vivo efficacy and unique cellular tropism of the various serotypes (Auricchio et al. 2001; Rabinowitz et al. 2002). Therefore, one can package the best studied genome of AAV2 into the capsid of any AAV serotype (Rabinowitz et al. 2002). Currently there are many examples in the literature illustrating the use of AAV pseudotyping strategy to achieve specific cellular transduction within the retina. For example, recombinant AAV2/1 and 2/4 vectors (rAAVs) have been shown to transduce the pigment epithelium efficiently in rodents, canines and nonhuman primates (Auricchio et al. 2001; Weber et al. 2003; Acland et al. 2005; Le Meur et al. 2007), while rAAV2/5 was reported to be ideal for photoreceptor transduction (Auricchio et al. 2001; Lotery et al. 2003; O'Reilly et al. 2007)

Here in this report, we describe the development of a therapeutic strategy that combines the use of recombinant AAV vectors and RNA interference (RNAi) for treating the RP10 form of RP. The molecular elucidation of RP10 began in 1993, when an autosomal dominant RP gene (RP10 locus) that segregated in a large Spanish family was mapped to chromosome 7 through genetic linkage mapping (Jordan et al. 1993). Twelve years later, comparative transcriptional profiling between wild-type (WT) and degenerating mouse retinas (Rho$^{-/-}$ and Crx$^{-/-}$) (Kennan et al. 2002; Bowne et al. 2002) identified mutations in the gene encoding inosine 5'-monophosphate dehydrogenase type 1 (IMPDH1) to be associated with the disease. Further studies on the molecular pathology of the disease indicated that combined suppression of both normal and mutant IMPDH1 transcripts in the human form of the disease may hold great therapeutic potential (Aherne et al. 2004). We therefore explored the feasibility of using rAAV2/5 vectors for the delivery of IMPDH1-targeting shRNAs in vivo to alleviate the pathological effect of mutant IMPDH1.

64.2 Results

64.2.1 Evaluation of Optimal IMPDH1 Suppressors

Initially a series of short hairpin RNAs (shRNAs) targeting distinct regions of human and mouse IMPDH1 transcripts were evaluated in mammalian cell cultures.

Quantitative Real-Time RT-PCR and western blot analysis showed that one particular shRNA, shImp1, was capable of eliciting up to 84% suppression of IMPDH1 at both the mRNA and protein levels in HeLa cells, as compared to non-targeting controls. Furthermore, the use of a dual expression vector system directing the synthesis of shImp1 and enhanced green fluorescent protein (EGFP) demonstrated efficient knockdown of endogenous IMPDH1 transcripts following in vitro electroporation in murine retinal explants. Following this, rAAV2/5 vectors carrying shImp1 and EGFP were generated to evaluate suppression efficiency in vivo. Similar to previous observations, subretinal inoculation of rAAV2/5 vectors expressing shImp1 ($3 \mu l$ of 6.85×10^{12} vp/ml per eye) into WT mice resulted in greater than 70% suppression of IMPDH1 at both the mRNA (Fig. 64.1a) and protein (Fig. 64.1b) levels in vivo. Moreover, rAAV2/5 vectors specifically transduced the outer segment and outer nuclear layer of WT mouse retinas as shown in Fig. 64.1c.

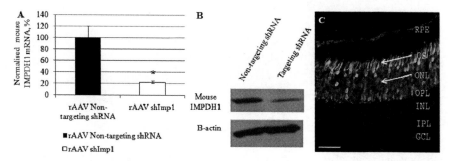

Fig. 64.1 rAAV-mediated suppression of IMPDH1 in vivo. (**a**) Quantitative Real-time RT-PCR analysis showing shRNA significant reduced IMPDH1 mRNA expression to $22 \pm 3\%$ following subretinal injection of rAAV targeting shRNA. *$P<0.05$. Error bar: standard error of the mean. (**b**) Western blot analysis illustrating potent suppression of mouse IMPDH1 (55 kDa) in vivo. (**c**) Specific transduction of the OS and ONL (*pointed arrows*) in mouse retinal sections (12 μm) following subretinal inoculation of rAAV2/5 expressing shRNA and EGFP. Scale bar, 40 μm. RPE: retinal pigment epithelium; OS: outer segment; ONL: outer nuclear layer; OPL; outer plexiform layer; INL: inner nuclear layer; IPL: inner plexiform layer; GCL: ganglion cell layer

64.2.2 RP10 Mouse Model

Animal models are valuable tools to study disease pathogenesis and to evaluate experimental therapies. A mouse model displaying the pathological effect of mutant IMPDH1 was generated by subretinal inoculation of rAAV2/5 expressing human mutant IMPDH1 bearing the missense mutation (Arg224Pro) in adult WT mice ($3 \mu l$ of 1.4×10^{12} vp/ml per eye). Four weeks post-injection, mice receiving rAAV2/5 expressing WT IMPDH1 showed normal retinal structure (Fig. 64.2a). In stark contrast, delivery of mutant IMPDH1 completely ablated the outer nuclear layer (Fig. 64.2b). rAAV-mediated delivery of human mutant IMPDH1 via

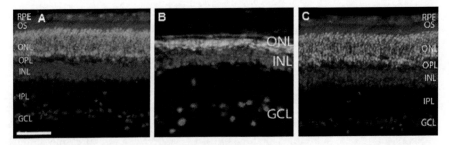

Fig. 64.2 Protection of ONL structure by rAAV-mediated suppression of mutant IMPDH1. (**a**) Representative images of eyes treated with rAAV WT IMPDH1 displayed normal ONL structure, (**b**) whereas eyes treated with rAAV mutant IMPDH1 alone, or with non-targeting shRNA showed dramatic ONL degeneration. (**c**) In contrast, eyes treated with rAAV mutant IMPDH1 and targeting shRNA protected the ONL from degeneration. Scale bar, 40 μm. RPE: retinal pigment epithelium; OS: outer segment; ONL: outer nuclear layer; OPL; outer plexiform layer; INL: inner nuclear layer; IPL: inner plexiform layer; GCL: ganglion cell layer

subretinal inoculation induced a rapid and aggressive retinopathy in WT mice, and thus provided a rapid method for generating a disease animal model for RP10.

64.2.3 Rescue of Photoreceptor Cells by rAAV-Mediated Downregulation of Mutant IMPDH1

In the final stage of this study, we tested our hypothesis namely that the photoreceptor cells could be rescued through RNAi-mediated downregulation of mutant IMPDH1 protein. rAAV2/5 vectors carrying human mutant IMPDH1 cDNA or shImp were co-injected subretinally at an experimentally derived viral particle

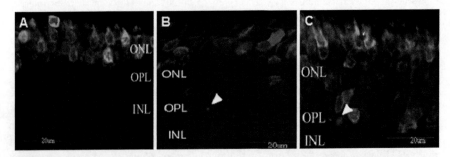

Fig. 64.3 Synaptic connectivity in RP10 mice following rAAV inoculation. (**a**) Eyes treated with rAAV mutant IMPDH1 and non-targeting shRNA showed an absence of synaptic marker staining. (**b**) In contrast, eyes treated with rAAV mutant IMPDH1 and shImp1 stained positively for synaptophysin (*pointed arrow*) and (**c**) bassoon (pointed arrow) across the outer plexiform layer (OPL). Scale bar, 20 μm. ONL: outer nuclear layer; OPL: outer plexiform layer; INL: inner nuclear layer

ratio of 1:5 (i.e. 1 μl of rAAV mutant IMPDH1 at 1.4×10^{12} vp/ml: 2 μl of rAAV shImp1 at 3.3×10^{12} vp/ml) in eight WT mice, and control eyes were injected with non-targeting shRNAs. Four weeks post-injection, all eyes receiving a simultaneous delivery of mutant IMPDH1 and shImp1, as compared to control eyes (Fig. 64.2b), showed significant protection of photoreceptor structure (Fig. 64.2c). Furthermore, immunostaining with pre- and post- synaptic markers such as synaptophysin (Fig. 64.3b) and bassoon (Fig. 64.3c) suggested intact synaptic integrity along the outer plexiform layer in rescued retinas as compared to controls (Fig. 64.3a).

64.3 Discussion

For autosomal dominant retinitis pigmentosa, the ability to attain long-term and stable suppression of mutant protein is essential to achieve therapeutic benefits. In this study, we used rAAV2/5 vectors as the delivery vehicle for shRNA in vivo. The choice for this AAV serotype combination was established by the fact that IMPDH1 expression was shown to be predominantly localised in murine outer segments (Aherne et al. 2004; Bowne et al. 2006), and other studies have demonstrated the effectiveness of this rAAV combination in transducing photoreceptor cells in mouse retinas (Auricchio et al. 2001; O'Reilly et al. 2007). Histological analysis carried out in this study clearly demonstrated the persistence of rAAV expression in the targeted retinal layers four weeks post-injection, and also showed effective knockdown of IMPDH1 at both the mRNA and protein levels. Previous preclinical studies in the canine and primate retina have even reported rAAV-mediated expression of transgenes for up to two years and beyond (Narfstrom et al. 2003; Stieger et al. 2008). Another important observation made in this study was that rAAV-mediated expression of human mutant IMPDH1, but not WT IMPDH1 in WT mouse retinas, induced rapid photoreceptor degeneration within four weeks of injection. Although the underlying pathological mechanism of this effect has not yet been fully deciphered, Aherne et al. (2004) have shown that mutant IMPDH1 has a high tendency to form protein aggregates that may have a negative pathological effect in photoreceptor cells. This hypothesis is supported by observations in other retinal diseases caused by protein aggregation, such as the Pro23His mutation in rhodopsin that causes adRP (Illing et al. 2002), and the R14W mutation in carbonic anhydrase IV that causes the RP17 form of RP (Rebello et al. 2004). Regardless of the disease-causing mechanism, simultaneous delivery of rAAV human mutant IMPDH1 with rAAV shRNA targeting IMPDH1 by subretinal injection in WT mice provided significant protection of photoreceptor structure, as compared to controls. Furthermore, immunostaining with pre-synaptic markers such as bassoon, which labels photoreceptor ribbons in both cone pedicles and rod spherules, and synaptophysin which labels pre-synaptic elements of cone pedicles and rod spherules, illustrated the protection of synaptic connectivity between neuronal sensory cell layers in treated eyes, as compared to control eyes. These observations provided proof-of-principle of the potential for rAAV-mediated downregulation of mutant IMPDH1 in vivo as a therapeutic strategy to combat RP10. Nonetheless, a number of issues regarding the safety of this approach, such as toxic effects, if any, as regards long-term rAAV delivery of shRNA in vivo, will need to be addressed. Furthermore it remains a considerable challenge to translate the results from murine models to large animals, and ultimately to human patients.

Acknowledgments This work was supported by grants from Science Foundation Ireland (G20026); The Health Research Board of Ireland (PRO262001); European Union-RETNET (MRTN-CT-2003-504003); European Union-EviGenoRET (LSHG-CT-2005-512036); The British RP Society and Fighting Blindness Ireland. The authors thank Dr. Sara Bowne (University of Texas, Houston) for providing the IMPDH1 antibody, and Dr. Arpad Palfi (Trinity College Dublin, Ireland) for providing the EGFP Dual-Expression plasmid vector.

References

Acland GM, Aguirre GD, Bennett J et al (2005) Long-term restoration of rod and cone vision by single dose rAAV-mediated gene transfer to the retina in a canine model of childhood blindness. Mol Ther 12:1072–1082

Aherne A, Kennan A, Kenna PF et al (2004) On the molecular pathology of neurodegeneration in IMPDH1-based retinitis pigmentosa. Hum Mol Gen 13:641–650

Auricchio A, Kobinger G, Anand V et al (2001) Exchange of surface proteins impacts on viral vector cellular specificity and transduction characteristics: the retina as a model. Hum Mol Gen 10:3075–3081

Bainbridge JW, Smith AJ, Barker SS et al (2008) Effect of gene therapy on visual function in Leber's congenital amaurosis. N Engl J Med 358:2231–2239

Bowne SJ, Liu Q, Sullivan LS et al (2006) Why do mutations in the ubiquitously expressed housekeeping gene IMPDH1 cause retina-specific photoreceptor degeneration? Invest Ophthalmol Vis Sci 47:3754–3765

Bowne SJ, Sullivan LS, Blanton SH et al (2002) Mutations in the inosine monophosphate dehydrogenase 1 gene (IMPDH1) cause the RP10 form of autosomal dominant retinitis pigmentosa. Hum Mol Gen 11:559–568

Hauswirth W, Aleman TS, Kaushal S et al (2008) Phase I trial of Leber congenital amaurosis due to RPE65 mutations by ocular subretinal injection of adeno-associated virus gene vector: short-term results. Hum Gene Ther 7:7

Illing ME, Rajan RS, Bence NF et al (2002) A rhodopsin mutant linked to autosomal dominant retinitis pigmentosa is prone to aggregate and interacts with the ubiquitin proteasome system. J Biol Chem 277:34150–34160

Jordan SA, Farrar GJ, Kenna PF et al (1993) Localization of an autosomal dominant retinitis pigmentosa gene to chromosome 7q. Nat Genet 4:54–58

Kennan A, Aherne A, Palfi A et al (2002) Identification of an IMPDH1 mutation in autosomal dominant retinitis pigmentosa (RP10) revealed following comparative microarray analysis of transcripts derived from retinas of wild-type and Rho–/– mice. Hum Mol Gen 11:547–557

Le Meur G, Stieger K, Smith AJ et al (2007) Restoration of vision in RPE65-deficient Briard dogs using an AAV serotype 4 vector that specifically targets the retinal pigmented epithelium. Gene Ther 14:292–303

Lotery AJ, Yang GS, Mullins RF et al (2003) Adeno-associated virus type 5: transduction efficiency and cell type specificity in the primate retina. Hum Gen Ther 14:1663–1671

Maguire AM, Simonelli F, Pierce EA et al (2008) Safety and efficacy of gene transfer for Leber's congenital amaurosis. N Engl J Med 358:2240–2248

Narfström K, Katz ML, Ford M et al (2003) In vivo gene therapy in young and adult RPE65–/– dogs produces long-term visual improvement. J Hered 94:31–37

O'Reilly M, Palfi A, Chadderton N et al (2007) RNA interference-mediated suppression and replacement of human rhodopsin in vivo. Am J Hum Genet 81:127–135

Rabinowitz JE, Rolling F, Li C et al (2002) Cross-packaging of a single adeno-associated virus (AAV) type 2 vector genome into multiple AAV serotypes enables transduction with broad specificity. J Virol 76:791–801

Rebello G, Ramesar R, Vorster A et al (2004) Apoptosis inducing signal sequence mutation in carbonic anhydrase IV indentified in patients with the RP17 form of retinitis pigmentosa. PNAS 101:6617–6622

Stieger K, Schroeder J, Provost N et al (2008) Detection of intact rAAV particles up to 6 years after successful gene transfer in the retina of dogs and primates. Mol Ther doi:10.1038/mt.2008.283

Weber M, Rabinowitz J, Provost N et al (2003) Recombinant adeno-associated virus serotype 4 mediates unique and exclusive long-term transduction of retinal pigmented epithelium in rat, dog, and nonhuman primate after subretinal delivery. Mol Ther 7:774–781

Chapter 65
Correlation Between Tissue Docosahexaenoic Acid Levels and Susceptibility to Light-Induced Retinal Degeneration

Masaki Tanito, Richard S. Brush, Michael H. Elliott, Lea D. Wicker, Kimberly R. Henry, and Robert E. Anderson

Abstract In a mouse model of acute light-induced retinal degeneration, positive correlations between the levels of DHA, the levels of n3 PUFA lipid peroxidation, and the vulnerability to photooxidative stress were observed. On the other hand, higher sensitivity of the electroretinogram a-wave response, a measure of the amplification of the phototransduction cascade, was correlated with higher retinal DHA levels. These results highlight the dual roles of DHA in cellular physiology and pathology.

65.1 Introduction

Docosahexaenoic acid (DHA; 22:6n3) is more abundant in rod photoreceptor outer segments (ROS) than in any other mammalian membrane (Fliesler and Anderson 1983). Studies in rodents and monkeys have demonstrated that DHA plays an important role in retinal function (Benolken et al. 1973; Wheeler et al. 1975; Birch et al. 1992; Bush et al. 1994; Jeffrey et al. 2002; Mitchell et al. 2003; Anderson and Penn 2004; Niu et al. 2004). Animals cannot synthesize n3 or n6 fatty acids de novo and must rely on a dietary source of these essential fatty acids. The fat-1 gene, cloned from C. elegans (Spychalla et al. 1997), encodes an n6 desaturase that converts n6 to n3 polyunsaturated fatty acids (PUFA). This transgene has been expressed in mice (Kang et al. 2004), which were found to produce n3 PUFA when fed a diet containing only n6 PUFA.

Acute light exposure to rats and mice causes photoreceptor and retinal pigment epithelial (RPE) cell damage (Tytell et al. 1989). Exposure of the retina to intense light causes lipid peroxidation of retinal tissues (Wiegand et al. 1983; Organisciak

M. Tanito (✉)
Department of Ophthalmology, Shimane University Faculty of Medicine, Enya 89-1, Izumo, Shimane, 693-8501, Japan
e-mail: tanito-oph@umin.ac.jp

R.E. Anderson et al. (eds.), *Retinal Degenerative Diseases*, Advances in Experimental Medicine and Biology 664, DOI 10.1007/978-1-4419-1399-9_65, © Springer Science+Business Media, LLC 2010

et al. 1992; Tanito et al. 2006a) and lipid peroxidation is propagated by free radicals, especially lipid radicals (De La Paz and Anderson 1992; Winkler et al. 1999). Thus, double bonds in PUFA are target substrates to propagate oxidative stress in photoreceptors.

65.2 Methods

All procedures were carried out according to the ARVO Statement for the Use of Animals in Ophthalmic and Vision Research and the University of Oklahoma Health Sciences Center (OUHSC) Guidelines for Animals in Research. The breeding pairs of fat-1 transgenic mice carrying a fat-1 gene of Caenorhabditis elegans and wildtype C57BL/6 J were kindly provided from Dr. Jing Kang (Department of Medicine, Massachusetts General Hospital and Harvard Medical School, Boston, MA) (Kang et al. 2004). Fat-1 C57BL/6 J mice were bred onto a Balb/c background and both C57BL/6 J and Balb/c fat-1 animals were independently utilized alongside their fat-1 negative wildtype siblings (wt animals). Fat-1 and wt males expressing the fat-1 gene were bred to wild type females that, prior to breeding, had been placed on a semi-synthetic, modified AIN-76A diet (#180465; Dyets, Bethlehem, PA) containing 10% (wt/wt) safflower oil (n6/n3 ratio of 274). Mice were born and raised under a cyclic light environment (< 30 lux, 12 h on/off, 7AM-7PM) in the Dean A. McGee Eye Institute vivarium and weaned onto the SFO diet (SFO animals).

Fatty acid profiles were analyzed in ROS, cerebellum, plasma, and liver from fat-1-SFO and wt-SFO of both C57BL/6 J and Balb/c strains. Purified lipid extracts from plasma, liver, and cerebellum were resolved into neutral lipid classes using one-dimensional thin-layer chromatography (TLC). Fatty acids from scraped TLC spots and from purified lipid extracts from ROS were derivatized to form fatty acid methyl esters (FAMES) and analyzed using gas-liquid chromatography (GLC) (Morrison and Smith 1964).

For the damaging light exposure experiments, 6-week-old Balb/c fat-1 and wt mice fed with a safflower oil diet (fat-1-SFO and wt-SFO, respectively) were exposed to 3,000 lux diffuse, cool, white fluorescent light for 24 h as described previously (Tanito and Anderson 2006) with slight modifications. After light exposure [light (+) animals], the mice were kept under the cyclic light environment (< 30 lux, 12 h on/off, 7AM-7PM) for up to 1 wk, after which electroretinograms (ERGs) were recorded and eyes were enucleated for morphometric and biochemical analyses. The outer nuclear layer (ONL) thickness was measured in retinal sections as described previously (Tanito et al. 2007). TUNEL was performed on paraffin-embedded sections using an Apoptag Peroxidase In Situ Apoptosis Detection Kit (Chemicon, Temecula, CA) according to the manufacturer's instructions. Western dot blot analyses for 4-hydroxynonenal (4-HNE)- and 4-hydroxyhexenal (4-HHE)-modified retinal proteins were performed as previously described (Tanito et al., 2005) with slight modification.

65.3 Results

Figure 65.1 shows the n6/n3 PUFA ratios of lipids from the ROS, cerebellum, plasma and liver of C57BL/6 J and Balb/c fat-1 transgenic mice and control siblings all maintained on a diet consisting of 10% safflower oil. Figure 65.2 shows the polyunsaturated fatty acid levels in ROS from both Balb/c and C57BL/6 J strains. When animals were maintained on a 10% safflower oil (SFO) diet deficient in n3 and enriched in n6 PUFA, fat-1 transgenic animals (fat-1-SFO) showed significantly elevated levels of total n3 PUFA and lower levels of total n6 PUFA compared to wild type siblings (wt-SFO) for each tissue analyzed from both mouse strains. The fat-1-SFO in both strains had significantly higher percentages of 20:5n3, 22:5n3, and 22:6n3, and significantly lower percentages of 20:4n6, 22:4n6, and 22:5n6, compared to the wt-SFO siblings, in ROS.

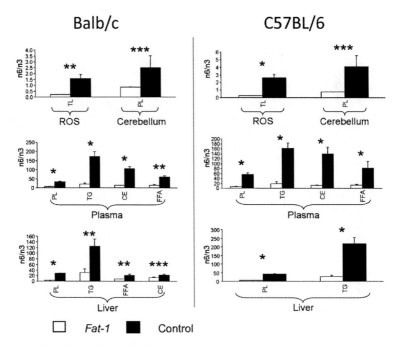

Fig. 65.1 The n6/n3 PUFA ratios of lipids from the rod outer segments, cerebellum, plasma and liver of C57BL/6 J and Balb/c fat-1 transgenic mice and control siblings all maintained on a diet consisting of 10% safflower oil. (ROS, rod outer segments; TL, total lipid; PL, phospholipid; TG, triglyceride; CE, cholesterol ester; FFA, free fatty acid). *$p<0.001$, **$p<0.01$, ***$p<0.05$; Multivariant ANOVA with post-hoc Neuman-Keuls test (Balb/c $n=3$; C57BL/6 J $n=3–5$). This figure is reproduced from Tanito et al., Journal of Lipid Research 2008 Nov 20 with permission from the American Society for Biochemistry and Molecular Biology

Retinal function and morphology were examined in Balb/c wt-SFO and fat-1-SFO, following exposure to damaging light [light (+)]. In light (+) animals 7 days after light exposure, ERG a- and b-waves were significantly lower in the fat-1-SFO

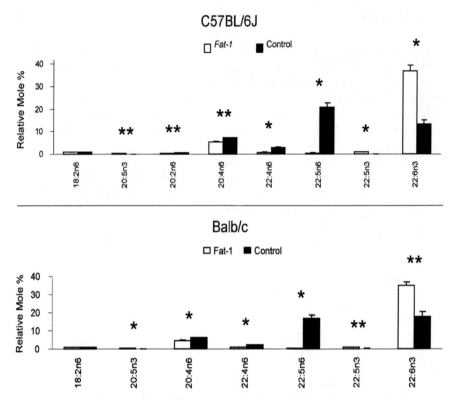

Fig. 65.2 Relative mole percentage of n-3 and n-6 PUFA from total lipid extracts of rod outer segments from C57BL/6 J and Balb/c fat-1 transgenic mice and control siblings all maintained on a diet consisting of 10% safflower oil. *$p<0.001$, **$p<0.01$, ***$p<0.05$; Multivariant ANOVA with post-hoc Neuman-Keuls test ($n=3$). This figure is reproduced from Tanito et al., Journal of Lipid Research 2008 Nov 20 with permission from the American Society for Biochemistry and Molecular Biology

group compared to those in the wt-SFO group (Tanito et al. 2009). The ONL thickness was significantly reduced in fat-1-SFO compared to wt-SFO light (+) animals (Tanito et al. 2009). In light (+) animals, larger numbers of TUNEL positive ONL cell nuclei were observed in retinal sections from the fat-1-SFO group compared to those from the wt-SFO (Tanito et al. 2009).

The levels of proteins modified by 4-HNE and 4-HHE, reactive aldehydes derived from non-enzymatic oxidation of n6 and n3 PUFAs, respectively, were tested in Balb/c wt-SFO and fat-1-SFO retinas from light (−) and light (+) animals by Western dot blot. In light (+) animals, the levels of 4-HNE protein modifications increased significantly in both groups compared to the corresponding light (−) animals, but no differences were detected between the 2 light-exposed groups (Tanito et al. 2009). However, in light (+) animals, the levels of 4-HHE protein modification increased significantly in the fat-1-SFO group compared to corresponding light (−)

animals, whereas no significant increase was observed between light (–) and light (+) animals in the wt-SFO group (Tanito et al. 2009).

65.4 Discussion

The fat-1 transgene encodes an n3 fatty acid desaturase that converts n6 to n3 PUFA (Spychalla et al. 1997; Kang et al. 2004). In this study, we demonstrated that expression of the fat-1 transgene enables mice fed an n3-deficient diet to endogenously synthesize and incorporate n3 fatty acids into ROS membranes (as well as other tissues), resulting in significantly lower n6/n3 ratios (Figs. 65.1 and 65.2).

The functional and morphological analyses in the light-damage experiments revealed that retinas from animals with low n6/n3 ratios (i.e., fat-1-SFO) were severely damaged. Several previous studies using dietary deprivation of n3 PUFA in albino rats have reported a positive relationship between n3-PUFA levels and susceptibility to light damage (Bush et al. 1991; Koutz et al. 1995; Organisciak et al. 1996). Our results strongly suggest that the levels of n3 PUFA are related to the vulnerability of the retina to photooxidative stress.

Due to facile reactivity with histidine, cysteine, or lysine residues of proteins (Uchida and Stadtman 1992), the reactive aldehydes exhibit a variety of cytopathological effects such as inhibition of enzyme activity; inhibition of protein, RNA, and DNA synthesis; cell cycle arrest; and apoptosis (Toyokuni 1999; Awasthi et al. 2004). Our earlier work suggests that modifications by lipid aldehydes of a specific set of retinal proteins are molecular events that precede light-induced photoreceptor cell apoptosis (Tanito et al. 2005, 2006b). Collectively, with the morphological and functional analyses, current results strongly suggest causal relationships between n3 PUFA levels, n3 PUFA oxidation, and the vulnerability of the retina to photooxidative stress.

The long chain PUFA DHA is more abundant in ROS than in any other mammalian membrane (Fliesler and Anderson 1983) and photoreceptors have a robust mechanism to conserve it (Wiegand et al. 1991). We showed a number of years ago that the fatty acid composition of ROS membranes is an important determinant for optimal retinal function in rodents (Benolken et al. 1973; Wheeler et al. 1975) and DHA deficiency results in the reduction of ERG response, with a-wave amplitudes affected more profoundly.

The roles of DHA in the retina are potentially conflicting in the literature. In the present study, we provide clear evidence that fat-1-SFO mice are more susceptible to light damage than wt-SFO mice and that the levels of DHA, the major n3 PUFA in the retina, and protein modifications by its oxidation products 4-HHE, are positively related to the vulnerability. These results highlight the ying and yang roles of n3 PUFA and DHA in retinal physiology and pathology.

Acknowledgments Financial support from the Foundation Fighting Blindness, Research to Prevent Blindness, Inc., the National Eye Institute (EY12190, EY04149, and EY00871), and National Center for Research Resources (RR17703) is gratefully acknowledged.

References

Anderson RE, Penn JS (2004) Environmental light and heredity are associated with adaptive changes in retinal DHA levels that affect retinal function. Lipids 39:1121–1124

Awasthi YC, Yang Y, Tiwari NK et al (2004) Regulation of 4-hydroxynonenal-mediated signaling by glutathione S-transferases. Free Radic Biol Med 37:607–619

Benolken RM, Anderson RE, Wheeler TG (1973) Membrane fatty acids associated with the electrical response in visual excitation. Science 182:1253–1254

Birch DG, Birch EE, Hoffman DR et al (1992) Retinal development in very-low-birth-weight infants fed diets differing in omega-3 fatty acids. Invest Ophthalmol Vis Sci 33: 2365–2376

Bush RA, Reme CE, Malnoe A (1991) Light damage in the rat retina: the effect of dietary deprivation of N-3 fatty acids on acute structural alterations. Exp Eye Res 53:741–752

Bush RA, Malnoe A, Reme CE et al (1994) Dietary deficiency of N-3 fatty acids alters rhodopsin content and function in the rat retina. Invest Ophthalmol Vis Sci 35:91–100

De La Paz MA, Anderson RE (1992) Lipid peroxidation in rod outer segments. Role of hydroxyl radical and lipid hydroperoxides. Invest Ophthalmol Vis Sci 33:2091–2096

Fliesler SJ, Anderson RE (1983) Chemistry and metabolism of lipids in the vertebrate retina. Prog Lipid Res 22:79–131

Jeffrey BG, Mitchell DC, Gibson RA et al (2002) n-3 fatty acid deficiency alters recovery of the rod photoresponse in rhesus monkeys. Invest Ophthalmol Vis Sci 43:2806–2814

Kang JX, Wang J, Wu L et al (2004) Transgenic mice: fat-1 mice convert n-6 to n-3 fatty acids. Nature 427:504

Koutz CA, Wiegand RD, Rapp LM et al (1995) Effect of dietary fat on the response of the rat retina to chronic and acute light stress. Exp Eye Res 60:307–316

Mitchell DC, Niu SL, Litman BJ (2003) Enhancement of G protein-coupled signaling by DHA phospholipids. Lipids 38:437–443

Morrison WR, Smith LM (1964) Preparation of fatty acid methyl esters and dimethylacetals from lipids with boron fluoride–methanol. J Lipid Res 5:600–608

Niu SL, Mitchell DC, Lim SY et al (2004) Reduced G protein-coupled signaling efficiency in retinal rod outer segments in response to n-3 fatty acid deficiency. J Biol Chem 279: 31098–31104

Organisciak DT, Darrow RM, Jiang YL et al (1996) Retinal light damage in rats with altered levels of rod outer segment docosahexaenoate. Invest Ophthalmol Vis Sci 37:2243–2257

Organisciak DT, Darrow RM, Jiang YI et al (1992) Protection by dimethylthiourea against retinal light damage in rats. Invest Ophthalmol Vis Sci 33:1599–1609

Spychalla JP, Kinney AJ, Browse J (1997) Identification of an animal omega-3 fatty acid desaturase by heterologous expression in Arabidopsis. Proc Natl Acad Sci U S A 94:1142–1147

Tanito M, Anderson RE (2006) Bright cyclic light rearing-mediated retinal protection against damaging light exposure in adrenalectomized mice. Exp Eye Res 83:697–701

Tanito M, Kaidzu S, Anderson RE (2007) Delayed loss of cone and remaining rod photoreceptor cells due to impairment of choroidal circulation after acute light exposure in rats. Invest Ophthalmol Vis Sci 48:1864–1872

Tanito M, Elliott MH, Kotake Y et al (2005) Protein modifications by 4-hydroxynonenal and 4-hydroxyhexenal in light-exposed rat retina. Invest Ophthalmol Vis Sci 46:3859–3868

Tanito M, Yoshida Y, Kaidzu S et al (2006a) Detection of lipid peroxidation in light-exposed mouse retina assessed by oxidative stress markers, total hydroxyoctadecadienoic acid and 8-iso-prostaglandin F(2alpha). Neurosci Lett 398:63–68

Tanito M, Brush RS, Elliott MH et al (2009) High levels of retinal membrane docosahexaenoic acid increase susceptibility to stress-induced degeneration. J Lipid Res 50(5):807–819

Tanito M, Haniu H, Elliott MH et al (2006b) Identification of 4-hydroxynonenal-modified retinal proteins induced by photooxidative stress prior to retinal degeneration. Free Radic Biol Med 41:1847–1859

Toyokuni S (1999) Reactive oxygen species-induced molecular damage and its application in pathology. Pathol Int 49:91–102

Tytell M, Barbe MF, Gower DJ (1989) Photoreceptor protection from light damage by hyperthermia. Prog Clin Biol Res 314:523–538

Uchida K, Stadtman ER (1992) Modification of histidine residues in proteins by reaction with 4-hydroxynonenal. Proc Natl Acad Sci U S A 89:4544–4548

Wheeler TG, Benolken RM, Anderson RE (1975) Visual membranes: specificity of fatty acid precursors for the electrical response to illumination. Science 188:1312–1314

Wiegand RD, Giusto NM, Rapp LM et al (1983) Evidence for rod outer segment lipid peroxidation following constant illumination of the rat retina. Invest Ophthalmol Vis Sci 24:1433–1435

Wiegand RD, Koutz CA, Stinson AM et al (1991) Conservation of docosahexaenoic acid in rod outer segments of rat retina during n-3 and n-6 fatty acid deficiency. J Neurochem 57: 1690–1699

Winkler BS, Boulton ME, Gottsch JD et al (1999) Oxidative damage and age-related macular degeneration. Mol Vis 5:32

Chapter 66
Activation of Müller Cells Occurs During Retinal Degeneration in RCS Rats

Tong Tao Zhao, Chun Yu Tian, and Zheng Qin Yin

Abstract Müller cells can be activated and included in different functions under many kinds of pathological conditions, however, the status of Müller cells in retinitis pigmentosa are still unknown. Using immunohistochemisty, Western blots and co-culture, we found that Müller cells RCS rats, a classic model of RP, could be activated during the progression of retinal degeneration. After being activated at early stage, Müller cells began to proliferate and hypertrophy, while at later stages, they formed a local 'glial seal' in the subretinal space. As markers of Müller cells activation, the expression of GFAP and ERK increased significantly with progression of retinal degeneration. Co-cultures of normal rat Müller cells and mixed RCS rat retinal cells show that Müller cells significantly increase GFAP and ERK in response to diffusable factors from the degenerting retina, which implies that Müller cells activation is a secondary response to retinal degeneration.

66.1 Introduction

Retinal degeneration is a group of severe diseases leading to blindness, which lack effective therapeutic measures. Among the retinal degenerative diseases, retinitis pigmentosa is the most common inherited retinal disease, and features a progressive apoptosis of photoreceptors and dysfunction of the retinal pigmented epithelium (RPE) (Lund et al., 2001).

Z.Q. Yin (✉)
Southwest Hospital, Southwest Eye Hospital, Third Military Medical University, Chongqing, 400038, China
e-mail: qinzyin@yahoo.com.cn

The authors Tong Tao Zhao and Zheng Qin Yin contributed equally to this work.

R.E. Anderson et al. (eds.), *Retinal Degenerative Diseases*, Advances in Experimental Medicine and Biology 664, DOI 10.1007/978-1-4419-1399-9_66,
© Springer Science+Business Media, LLC 2010

Müller cells are the principal glial cells of the retina playing important roles in normal retinal physiological activities. Under pathological conditions such as retinal detachment, PVR (proliferative vitreous retinopathy) and PDR (peripheral diabetic retinopathy), Müller cells can be activated to perform a series of changes in morphology, as well as protein expression and production (Bringmann and Reichenbach 2001; Ortrud et al. 2003; Steven and Geoffrey 2003; Clyde 2005). However, it is still unclear whether Müller cells were also activated during retinitis pigmentosa. Royal College of Surgeons (RCS) rats, an animal model of retinitis pigmentosa, possess a naturally occurring deletion mutation in the receptor tyrosine kinase gene, which impairs the ability of the retinal pigmented epithelium (RPE) to phagocytose the photoreceptor outer segments, resulting in a buildup of debris in the subretinal space ultimately leading to photoreceptors death (Steven and Geoffrey 2003). Our aim was to determine if RCS rat Müller cells are activated during retinal degeneration and any changes in Müller cell morphology and protein expression.

66.2 Materials and Methods

66.2.1 Animal

All experiments were carried out in accordance with applicable Chinese laws and with the ARVO Statement for the Use of Animals in Ophthalmic and Vision Research. RCS rats at different developmental stages (postnatal days, PND15, PND30, PND60, PND90 and PND120, 3 rats at each age) were deeply anesthetized with urethane (2.0 g/kg) before decapitation and enucleation. Take the RCS-rdy rats of same age and quantity as control.

66.2.2 Immunohistochemical Staining

After fixation in 4% paraformaldehyde for 24 h and cryosectioning (thickness of 10um), immunostaining on sections or cover slips was performed as following: several washes in phosphate-buffered saline (PBS), followed by incubation in 10% normal goat serum plus 0.3% Triton X-100 in saline for 1 h, then incubation with a primary antibody overnight at 4°C. Sections were washed several times and incubated with a secondary antibody for 1 h at 37°C, washed in PBS, counterstained with DAPI, and then mounted with fluorescent mounting medium (Dako corporation) and examined under a confocal microscope (Zeiss, Germany). The following antibodies were used: mouse anti-vimentin (1:100; Sigma-Aldrich), mouse anti-extracellular signal-regulated kinase (ERK) (1:100; Santa Cruz), rabbit anti-GFAP (1:100; Sigma-Aldrich). Appropriate fluorescence conjugated secondary antibodies were used. Müller cells count: count those vimentin positive processes with the length over 1/2 of the retina thickness as number of Müller cells.

66.2.3 Western Blot Test

The retinal tissues (4 eyes for each age) were treated with test substances for 10 minutes before harvesting. The tissues were washed twice with cold PBS (pH 7.4; Biochrom), and moved into 200 μl of lysis buffer (Mammalian Cell Lysis-1 Kit; Sigma). The total lysates were centrifuged at 10,000 rpm for 10 min, and the supernatant then analyzed by immunoblotting. Equal amounts of protein (30 μg) were separated by 12% SDS-polyacrylamide gel electrophoresis. Immunoblots were probed with primary and secondary antibodies, and immunoreactive bands visualized with diaminobenzidine (peroxidase substrate kit; Vector Laboratories) or 5-bromo-4-chloro-3-indolyl phosphate/nitro blue tetrazolium (Sigma-Aldrich). Chemiluminescence development and software Labworks 4.6 were used to analyze the gray scale of protein electrophoresis.

66.2.4 Müller Cell Cultures

Müller cells were isolated according to an established protocol (Hicks and Courtois 1990). Ten PND15 control rats were killed by decapitation and their eyes were removed and stored overnight at room temperature in the dark in Dubelcco's Modified Eagles medium (DMEM) containing 2 mM glutamine and 1/1000 penicillin/streptomycine. The intact globes were incubated in DMEM containing 0.1% trypsin at 37°C for 45 min. The retinas were isolated, chopped into $\sim$1 mm^2 pieces and cultured in DMEM with 10% fetal bovine serum (FBS) and 1% penicilline/streptomycine. The use of pigmented eyes in all experiments permitted easy monitoring of any possible contaminating tissue such as the RPE or ora serrata. The cultures were maintained at 37°C in a 5% CO_2/95% air in a humidified incubator. To obtain a purified cell population, retinal aggregates and non-adherent cells were removed by vigorous rinsing and fresh medium added when cell outgrowth had acquired semiconfluence. Medium was changed every 3–4 days. When the cells became fully confluent the cultures were washed twice with DMEM, twice with Ca^{2+}-free PBS and incubated in D-Hank's with 1% trypsin for 1 min at 37°C. The action of trypsin was stopped by adding 10% FBS in DMEM. The suspension was centrifuged at 1,000g for 10 min at room temperature, the pellet re-suspended and the Müller cells cultured on poly-L-lysine-coated coverslips until they became adherent. Coverslips containing normal Müller cells were co-cultured in a transwell system with mixed cell cultures from PND30 RCS rat retinas.

66.2.5 Data Analysis

Quantitative analysis of the data was preformed using SPSS13.0 software. Mean values with standard deviations are given in the text. Unless stated otherwise, statistical analysis was performed using a Student's t-test. Differences with a P-value $\leq$0.05 were considered significant.

66.3 Results

66.3.1 Morphology and Quantity Changes of Müller Cells

At PND15, RCS rats Müller cells had formed long processes spanning the entire thickness of the retina. This Müller cell arrangement became disorganized by PND60 and by PND90 the Müller processes had became hypertrophic and extended processes into the subretinal space; note this was not found in control retinas. Müller cell counts at PND- 60, 90, 120, showed that the number of cells in RCS rats retinas were significantly higher than control ($P < 0.05$) (Fig. 66.1).

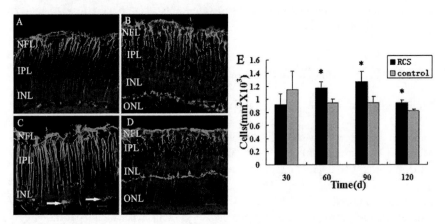

Fig. 66.1 Müller cell morphology and numbers in RCS and control rat retinas. (**a–d**) Vimentin(green) stained the processes of Müller cells in RCS retina at different postnatal days (**a**: RCS PND60; **b**: control PND60; **c**: RCS PND120; **d**: control PND120, respectively). Müller processes became hypertrophic and extended processes into the subretinal space (*white arrow*) (**e**) Müller cell numbers were quantified at different postnatal days. The numbers of Müller cells in RCS rats were significantly higher (*$P < 0.05$) at all ages after PND30 compared with control rats ($n = 27$) Scale bar = 20 μm

66.3.2 Expression of GFAP and ERK in RCS Rat Müller Cells

GFAP (glial fibrillary acidic protein) and ERK (extracellular signal – regulated kinase) are the activation-related proteins of Müller cell. At early age, the stain of GFAP and ERK in Müller cells was rare, with the progression of retinal degeneration, the stain of GFAP and ERK increased dramatically (Figs. 66.2 and 66.3). Western blots showed that at PND-30, 60, 120, the expression of GFAP and ERK in RCS rat retinas(GFAP:0.24±0.06, 0.32±0.07, 0.33±0.06; ERK: 0.11±0.03, 0.17±0.04, 0.18±0.04) was significantly higher compared with control(GFAP: 0.19±0.05, 0.24±0.04, 0.23±0.06; ERK: 0.08±0.03, 0.11±0.04, 0.11±0.03) ($P < 0.05$; Figs. 66.2–66.4).

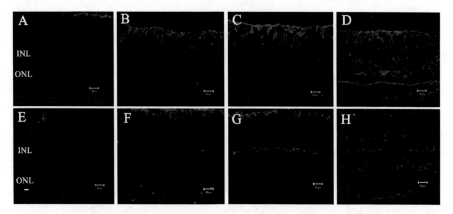

Fig. 66.2 Expression of GFAP in Müller cells. (**a–d**) The GFAP staining intensity of RCS rat Müller cells increased with the progression of retinal degeneration (PND- 15, 30, 60, 120, respectively). Note the staining in the vitreal endfeet compared to control rat retinas at similar ages (**e–h**). Scale bars 20 μm

66.3.3 Effect of Mixed Retinal Cells of RCS Rats on Normal Müller Cells

After one day of co-culturing, few Müller cells expressed GFAP, and no ERK positive cells were found. At 3 d and 7 d after co-culture, the number of GFAP and ERK positive cells increased dramatically, in contrast GFAP and ERK expression was not found in control cultures. Western-blot test confirmed that after 3 days the quantity of GFAP and ERK protein expressed by Müller cells (GFAP: 0.59 ± 0.16; ERK: 0.59 ± 0.14) was significantly higher ($P<0.05$) than in control cultures (GFAP: 0.39 ± 0.11; ERK: 0.25 ± 0.06) (Fig. 66.5).

66.4 Discussion

As a chronic retinal degenerative disease, retinitis pigmentosa, which features a progressive loss of photoreceptors, also shows remarkable changes of other retinal neurons, such as bipolar and retinal ganglion cells. However, Müller cell changes have not been characterised morphologically. Müller cells are connected to almost all the retinal neurons by their specialized morphology, which is the foundation of normal retinal function (Reichenbach et al., 1995; Newman 1996). Müller cells are involved in many retinal physiological activities including glycometabolism, blood regulation, neurotransmitter cycling, homeostasis and control of neuronal excitability (Newman and Zahs 1998; Stevens et al., 2003; Bringmann et al., 2004). Therefore, when Müller cells are activated, the changed function may dramatically affect the retinal pathophysiologic processes.

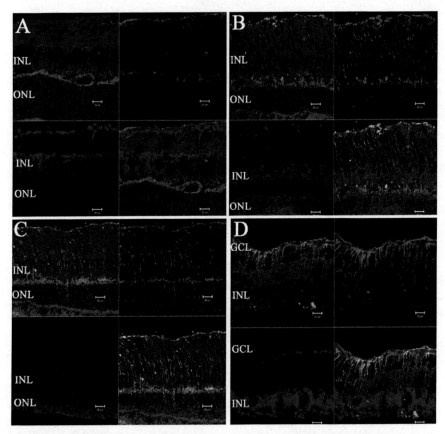

Fig. 66.3 Expression of Vimentin and ERK in RCS rat Müller cells. (**a–d**) Each set of four micrographs shows the labeling for ERK (*upper left*) vimentin (*upper right*), DAPI (*lower left*) and the merged images (*lower right*) at PND15d (**a**), PND30 (**b**), PND60 (**c**), and PND120 (**d**). Note the increased intensity of ERK staining with the progression of retinal degeneration (Scale bar 20 μm)

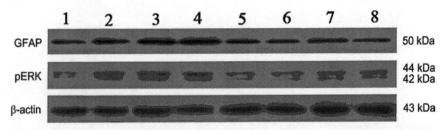

Fig. 66.4 Western blots of GFAP and ERK expression in RCS and normal rats. Western blots showed that the expression of GFAP and ERK in RCS rats retinas was significantly higher than that seen in control animals ($P < 0.05$, $n=3$ samples). Lanes 1–4 show RCS rat data at PND- 15, 30, 60, and 120, respectively; lanes 5–8 show data of control rats at the same ages

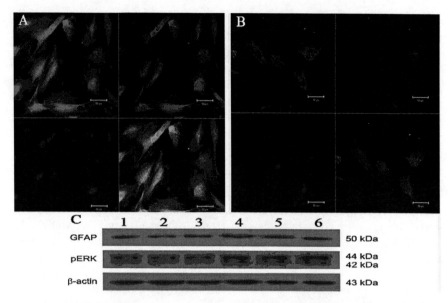

Fig. 66.5 Expression GFAP (green) and ERK (red) in response to co-cultures of RCS retinal tissue. (**a–b**) Each set of four micrographs shows the labeling for GFAP (*upper left*) ERK (*upper right*), DAPI (*lower left*) and the merged images (*lower right*) after 7 days RCS co-culture (**a**) and control co-culture (**b**). Scale bar 20 μm. (**c**) Western-blot confirmed the increase expression of GFAP and ERK in Müller cells at different co-cultured days. Lanes 1, 3 and 5 represent Müller cells co-cultured with controls after 1, 3, and 7 days respectively; lanes 2, 4, and 6 show expression of Müller cells co-cultured with mixed RCS rat retinal cells after 1, 3, and 7 days respectively. After 3 days coculture the quantity of GFAP and ERK protein expressed by Müller cells was significantly higher ($P < 0.05$) than in control cultures ($n = 3$ samples)

At an early stage of embryonic development, the immature Müller cells play an important role in the formation of retinal neural circuitry by supplying framework for neuronal migration. When mature Müller cells are activated, they may resume this kind of function (Willbold et al., 1997; Stier and Schlosshauer 1998). We found that Müller cells showed remarkable change in the progress of RCS rat retinal degeneration. In response to the simulation induced by retinal degeneration, Müller cells develop morphologically more rapidly than cells in normal animals, which may be considered as the beginning of compensation. With the progress of retinal degeneration, RCS rat Müller cells become hypertrophic and disorganized and as degeneration proceeds part of their processes extend into the subretinal space. This invasion of the subretinal space might be a major component of the 'glial seal' and an attempt at retinal reconstruction. Studies on AMD (age-related macular degeneration) and retinal detachment showed that when activated, Müller cells began to proliferate, and may extend their processes into other layers of the retina including the subretinal space (Steven and Geoffrey 2003; Sullivan et al., 2003; Robert et al., 2003). The formation of the glial seal blocks the connection between RPE and photoreceptors thus exacerbating the disease process. In this study, we have seen both the initial proliferation of Müller cells and the formation of a similar glial seal composed of Müller cell processes (immunostaining) in RCS rats with advanced retinal degeneration.

Our Western blot analysis confirmed that the expression of proteins related to Müller cell activation are indeed upregulated. GFAP and ERK are activation-related proteins of Müller cell. Under many pathological conditions, the expression of GFAP in Müller cells increases, thus establishing GFAP as a marker of Müller cell activation (Malhotra et al., 1990; Vijay 2007). In other animal models such as glaucoma, retinal detachment and diabetes retinopathy, Müller cells were activated at early stage of injury by showing an increased expression of GFAP (Francke et al., 2001; Fletcher et al., 2005; Xue et al., 2006). ERK is also a marker of glial cell proliferation and differentiation (Yang et al., 2008). In the retina, ERK is prominently expressed in Müller cells, and in many retinal disease models its increased expression is coincident with an increase in GFAP, thus suggesting that Müller cells initiate proliferation and differentiation (Scott et al., 2001; Masumi et al., 2002; Gulgun et al., 2003). The significant increase of GFAP and ERK protein seen in this study supports the data showing proliferation of Müller cells and their activated in response to the progression of retinal degeneration in the of RCS rats.

To determine whether the Müller cell activation is a primary reaction or a secondary response to the retinal degeneration, we co-cultured mixed retinal cells of RCS rats with Müller cells from control animals. The results showed a significant increase of GFAP and ERK expression in response to the degenerative PND30 RCS rat retina. From that under the effect of mixed retinal cells of RCS rats, this suggests that normal Müller cells are activated by a diffusible factor(s) in the RCS rat retina.

We have shown by both in vivo and in vitro techniques that Müller cells were activated in the progress of RCS rats retinal degeneration and underwent dramatic changes in morphology and protein expression. Determining the factors that initiate this process and ways to control this process may significantly improve the rehabilitation of the degenerating retina.

Acknowledgments The authors thank Dr. T. Fitz Gibon for comments on earlier drafts of the paper; Yu Xiao Zeng, Dong Ning Liu, Li Feng Chen, Yan Hua Wang for excellent technical support. This work was supported by the National Basic Research Program of China (Grant No. 2007CB512203), and the funds from a Nature Science Foundation of China (Grant No. 30772371).

References

Bringmann A, Reichenbach A (2001) Role of Müller cells in retinal degenerations. Front Biosci 6:E72–E92

Bringmann A, Reichenbach A, Wiedemann P (2004) Pathomechanisms of cystoid macular edema. Ophthalm Res 36:241–249

Clyde G (2005) The role of Müller cells in fibrocontractive retinal disorders. Prog Retin Eye Res 24:75–86

Fletcher EL, Phipps JA, Wilkinson-Berka JL (2005) Dysfunction of retinal neurons and glia during diabetes. Clin Exp Optom 88:132–145

Francke M, Faude F, Pannicke T et al (2001) Electrophysiology of rabbit Müller (glial) cells in experimental retinal detachment and PVR. Invest Ophthalmol Vis Sci 42:1072–1079

Gulgun T, Balwantray CC, Raymond PL et al (2003) Immunohistochemical assessment of the glial mitogen-activated protein kinase activation in glaucoma. Invest Ophthalmol Vis Sci 44: 3025–3033

Hicks D, Courtois Y (1990) The growth and behaviour of rat retinal Müller cells in vitro. 1. An improved method for isolation and culture. Exp Eye Res 51:119–129

Lund RD, Kwan ASL, Keegan DJ (2001) Cell transplantation as a treatment for retinal disease. Prog Retin Eye Res 20(4):415–449

Malhotra S, Shnitka T, Elabrink J (1990) Reactive astrocytes. A review. Cytobios 61(1):133

Masumi T, Akira T, Akitoshi Y et al (2002) Extracellular signal-regulated kinase activation predominantly in Müller cells of retina with endotoxin-induced uveitis. Invest Ophthalmol Vis Sci 43:907–911

Newman EA (1996) Acid efflux from retinal glial cells generated by sodium bicarbonate cotransport. J Neurosci 16:159–168

Newman EA, Zahs KR (1998) Modulation of neuronal activity by glial cells in the retina. J Neurosci 18:4022–4028

Ortrud U, Susann U, Michael W et al (2003) Upregulation of purinergic P2Y receptor-mediated calcium responses in glial cells during experimental detachment of the rabbit retina. Neurosci Lett 338:131–134

Reichenbach A, Stolzenburg J-U, Wolburg H et al (1995) Effects of enhanced extracellular ammonia concentration on cultured mammalian retinal glial (Müller) cells. Glia 13:195–208

Robert EM, Bryan WJ, Carl BW et al (2003) Neural remodeling in retinal degeneration. Prog Retin Eye Res 22:607–655

Scott FG, Geoffrey PL, Steven KF (2001) FGFR1, signaling and AP-1 expression after retinal detachment: reactive Müller and RPE cells. Invest Ophthalmol Vis Sci 42:1363–1369

Steven KF, Geoffrey PL (2003) Müller cell and neuronal remodeling in retinal detachment and reattachment and their potential consequences for visual recovery: a review and reconsideration of recent data. Vis Res 43:887–897

Stevens ER, Esguerra M, Kim PM et al (2003) D-serine and serine racemase are present in the vertebrate retina and contribute to the physiological activation of NMDA receptors. Proc Natl Acad Sci USA 100:6789–6794

Stier H, Schlosshauer B (1998) Different cell surface areas of polarized radial glia having opposite effects on axonal outgrowth. Eur J Neurosci 10:1000–1010

Sullivan R, Penfold P, Pow DV (2003) Neuronal migration and glial remodeling in degenerating retinas of aged rats and in nonneovascular AMD. Invest Ophthalmol Vis Sci 44:856–865

Vijay S (2007) Focus on molecules: glial fibrillary acidic protein (GFAP). Exp Eye Res 84:381–382

Willbold E, Berger J, Reinicke M et al (1997) On the role of Müller glia cells in histogenesis: only retinal spheroids, but not tectal, telencephalic and cerebellar spheroids develop histotypical patterns. J Hirnforsch 38:383–396

Xue LP, Lu J, Cao Q et al (2006) Müller glial cells express nestin coupled with gilal fibrillary acidic protein in experimentally induced glaucoma in the rat retina. Neuroscience 139:723–732

Yang JY, Zong CS, Xia W et al (2008) ERK promotes tumorigenesis by inhibiting FOXO3a via MDM2-mediated degradation. Nat Cell Biol 10(2):138–148

Chapter 67
Effect of 3′-Daidzein Sulfonic Sodium on the Anti-oxidation of Retinal Ischemia/Reperfusion Injury in Rats

Huang Zhihua, Li Liangdong, Li Xiao, Cheng Fang, and Zeng Jing

Abstract

Objective: To research the 3′-daidzein sulfonic sodium's (DSS) effect on anti-oxidation of retinal ischemia/reperfusion (RI/R) injury in rats.

Methods: RI/R in rats was made by reperfusion for 1 h after occlusion of common carotid artery (CCA) for 1 h and the rats were divided into four groups randomly, including sham control group, model group of RI/R injury, low-dosage DSS group and high-dosage DSS group. 1 ml/kg NS was injected through sublingual vein after CCA was dissociated in sham group. Other groups were treated with normal saline, low-dosage DSS (1 mg/kg) and high-dosage DSS (2 mg/kg) through sublingual vein respectively before occlusion of CCA. After occlusion of CCA for 1 h and reperfusion for 1 h, blood was put out and separated into the serum. Then detect the contents of MDA and NO, the activity of SOD and GSH-PX.

Result: (1) The content of MDA was increased in model group ($P<0.05$), and low-dosage DSS can reverse it ($P<0.05$). (2) The content of serum NO in model group was lower than in sham group ($P<0.001$). The content of serum NO in model group is lower than in low-dosage DSS group ($P<0.05$) and high-dosage DSS group ($P<0.01$) respectively. (3) The activity of GSH-PX in high-dosage group was higher than in model group ($P<0.05$). (4) The activity of SOD in low-dosage group was higher than in model group ($P<0.05$).

Conclusion: DSS can decrease the cellular damage and protect the optical function in RI/R injury through elevating the content of NO, the activity of SOD and GSH-PX, and increasing anti-oxidation.

Z. Jing (✉)
Preclinical Medical College, Gannan Medical University, Ganzhou, Jiangxi Province 341000, China
e-mail: zengjing61@hotmail.com

R.E. Anderson et al. (eds.), *Retinal Degenerative Diseases*, Advances in Experimental Medicine and Biology 664, DOI 10.1007/978-1-4419-1399-9_67,
© Springer Science+Business Media, LLC 2010

67.1 Introduction

Retinal ischemia/reperfusion (RI/R) injury is one of the common ocular diseases in clinical medicine, mainly seen in the ocular ischemic diseases caused by retinal vascular occlusion in such cases as central retinal vein or artery occlusion, acute angel-closure glaucoma and diabetic retinopathy. Its symptom is that many patients, after the reperfusion, find their retina seriously damaged and their visual function worsened even further. RI/R is the result of multiple factors, such as lack of energy, intracellular calcium overload, the exploding growth of free radicals, the excessive release of excitatory amino acid and the lack of neurotrophic factors, which turns on the gene monitoring apoptosis, leading to the apoptosis of retinal neural cells (Neal et al. 1994; Romano et al. 1993).

3′-daidzein sulfonate sodium (DSS) is a newly compounded and strongly water-soluble substance, produced by modifying the structure of daidzein, the main active ingredient of the Chinese herbal medicine Radix Puerariae. Earlier researches of our team have shown that DSS can help an organism anti-hypoxia, expand blood vessels and anti-oxidation (Zeng et al. 2005; Li, Zeng and Qiu 2005). Can DSS alleviate RI/R injury by enhancing an organism's anti-oxidative ability? To find the answer, we produce RI/R models through the method of common carotid artery occlusion, so as to examine the protective effect of DSS on RI/R injuries, and explore the relationship between its protective effect and the anti-oxidative ability.

67.2 Materials and Methods

67.2.1 Animals and Reagents

Sprague Dawley (SD) rats (male, 250~280 g, age: 8~10 weeks) were obtained from Jiangxi traditional Chinese medical college and maintained in the Center of Laboratory Animal Resources at Gannan Medical College.

DSS was a white crystal powder produced by Shenyang Pharmaceutical University, with 99% purity. It is diluted to the needed concentration with NS before animal experiment. LDH, SOD and GSH-PX reagent kits were bought from Nanjing Jiancheng Biological Engineering Company.

67.2.2 Induction of RI/R

Twenty-four male SD rats, weighing 250–280 g, were randomly divided into four groups ($n = 6$/group), including sham control group, model group of RI/R injury, low dosage DSS (1 mg/kg) group and high-dosage DSS (2 mg/kg) group. The animals were anaesthetized with 10% Chloral hydrate solution (350 mg/kg, ip). Then, RI/R injury was induced by occluding common carotid artery on the left side. First, the skin on the neck was sterilized with 75% alcohol. Cut open the skin, the subcutaneous tissue and the muscularis along the middle of the neck, find the lamina praetrachealis and cut it open. Find the common carotid artery; then occlude the artery with an artery clip. Dilate the eye pupil adequately, and use fluorescence fundus angiography (FFA) to ensure retinal ischemia has occurred. After 60 min of occlusion, remove the artery clip and again use the FFA to ensure reperfusion has occurred. Repeat all the steps for the sham group, except for occluding the common carotid artery. 1 ml/kg NS was injected through sublingual vein after CCA was dissociated in sham group. Other groups were treated with normal saline, low-dosage DSS and high-dosage DSS through sublingual vein respectively before occlusion of CCA.

67.2.3 Detection of MDA and NO Concentration, SOD and GSH-PX Activity

After 60 min of reperfusion, blood was taken from the rats' abdominal vein, then put on the centrifuge for 10 min at 3,000 rpm and 4°C. The serum was separated and kept at –80°C. Strictly following the instruction of the reagent kits, use Xanthine oxidase (the hydroxylamine method) to detect the activity of SOD, use the colorimetric method to detect the activity of GSH-PX, use the Thibabituric acid to detect the concentration of MDA, and use the method of Nitrate Reductase to detect the concentration of NO.

67.2.4 Statistical Analysis

All experimental data are expressed as means ± SEM. Statistical comparisons between the control and treatment groups were carried out using one-way analysis of variance (ANOVA) followed by Newman-Keuls *post-hoc* test. Probability levels of 0.05 or smaller were used for reporting statistical significance.

67.3 Results

67.3.1 The Effect of DSS on the Concentration of MDA in Serum After RI/R Injury

As shown in Fig. 67.1, the MDA concentration of the model group was higher than that of the sham operation group ($P<0.05$), while after the treatment of low-dosage DSS, the concentration of MDA decreased ($P<0.05$).

Fig. 67.1 Concentration of
MDA in serum

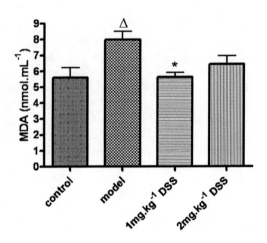

67.3.2 The Effect of DSS on the Activity of SOD in Serum After RI/R Injury

As shown in Fig. 67.2, the activity of serum SOD enhance after low-dosage DSS treatment ($P<0.05$).

Fig. 67.2 Activity of SOD in
serum

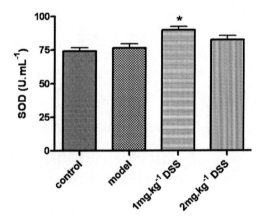

67.3.3 The Effect of DSS on the Activity of Serum GSH-PX After RI/R Injury

As shown in Fig. 67.3, the activity of serum GSH-PX was increased significantly after high-dosage DSS treatment ($P<0.05$).

Fig. 67.3 Activity of
GSH-PX in serum

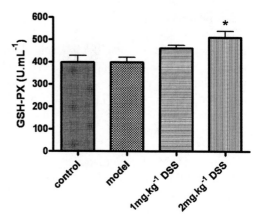

67.3.4 The Effect of DSS on the Concentration of Serum NO After RI/R Injury

As shown in Fig. 67.4, the concentration of serum NO of the model group is lower than that of the sham operation group ($P<0.001$), while in both the low-dosage ($P<0.05$) and high-dosage treatment group ($P<0.001$), the concentration of serum NO increased, with the extent of increase dependent on the dosage.

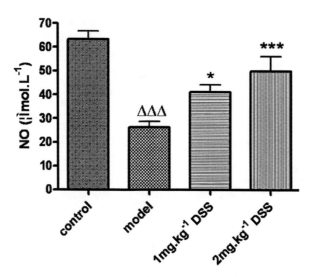

Fig. 67.4 Concentration of NO in serum

67.4 Discussion

Ischemia and reperfusion (I/R) injury is a serious problem in many diseases that result in blindness. Ischemic injury results when the blood supply to a tissue is interrupted, but, paradoxically, a more severe tissue injury occurs when blood flow is restored on reperfusion (Tsujikawa et al. 1999).

Oxygen-derived free radicals (OFR) can cause cell damage in biological systems. OFR generation has been implicated as a major mediator in RI/R injury (Veriac et al. 1993; Ophir et al. 1993; Szabo et al. 1991). During the process of RI/R, OFR and other free radical increase (Szabo et al. 1997; Song et al. 2008). The appearance of these harmful products is related to the activation of the Xanthine oxidase and the increased activity of the neutrophil leucocyte. After the ischemia and reperfusion, the newly arrived oxygen reacts with the xanthine oxidase, producing OFR and other free radical (Peachey et al. 1993). Ischemia also can inhibit the activities of the anti-oxidant enzymes, and weaken the body's ability to eliminate oxygen free radicals, leading to the accumulation of free radicals in the body. OFR can not only cause the apoptosis of cells through a series of chain reactions, but also impair the cells with lipid peroxides (such as MDA) (Aydemir et al. 2004; Pannicke et al. 2005). Our experiments have found that DSS can help prevent the increase of MDA, pointing to its ability to inhibit the lipid peroxidation process induced by RI/R.

SOD and GSH-PX are naturally developed anti-oxidant enzymes in an organism. They are able to eliminate oxygen free radicals in the body, and prevent the lipid peroxidation chain reaction (Rios et al. 1999). Our experiments have shown that, after the DSS treatment, the activities of both SOD and GSH-PX in the serum were enhanced. This is a sign that DSS can strengthen the activities of the anti-oxidant enzymes, abate the lipid peroxidation induced by oxygen free radicals, and thus mitigate the damage of I/R on retinal cells.

Acknowledgments This work was supported by National Nature Science Fund (NO.30760284); Department of Education of Jiangxi Province (NO.GJJ08394); Department of Health Care of Jiangxi Province (NO.20072034).

References

Aydemir O, Naziroglu M, Celebi S et al (2004) Antioxidant effects of alpha-, gamma- and succinate – tocopherols in guinea pig retina during ischemia-reperfusion injury. Pathophysiology 11: 167–171

Li L, Zeng J, Qiu F (2005) Effect of 3′-Daidzein sulfonate sodium on contractle of rabbit thoracic aortic strips. Drug Dev Res 66:243

Neal MJ, Cunningham JR, Hutson PH et al (1994) Effects of ischaemia on neurotransmitter release from the isolated retina. J Neurochem 62:1025–1033

Ophir A, Berenshtein E, Kitrossky N et al (1993) Hydroxyl radical generation in the cat retina during reperfusion following ischemia. Exp Eye Res 57:351–357

Pannicke T, Uckermann O, Iandiev I et al (2005) Altered membrane physiology in Muller glial cells after transient ischemia of the rat retina. Glia 50:1–11

Peachey NS, Green DJ, Ripps H (1993) Ocular ischemia and the effects of allopurinol on functional recovery in the retina of the arterially perfused cat eye. Invest Ophthalmol Vis Sci 34:58–65

Rios L, Cluzel J, Vennat JC et al (1999) Comparison of intraocular treatment of DMTU and SOD following retinal ischemia in rats. Ocul Pharmacol Ther 15:547–556

Romano C, Price M, Bai HY et al (1993) Neuroprotectants in Honghua: glucose attenuates retinal ischemic damage. Invest Ophthalmol Vis Sci 34:72–80

Song Y, Gong YY, Xie ZG et al (2008) Edaravone (MCI-186), a free radical scavenger, attenuates retinal ischemia/reperfusion injury in rats. Acta Pharmacol Sin 29:823–828

Szabo ME, Droy-Lefaix MT, Doly M et al (1991) Free radical-mediated effects in reperfusion injury: a histologic study with superoxyde dismutase and Egb 761 in rat retina. Ophthalmic Res 23:225–234

Szabo ME, Droy-Lefaix MT, Doly M (1997) Direct measurement of free radicals in ischemic/reperfused diabetic rat retina. Clin Neurosci 4:240–245

Tsujikawa A, Ogura Y, Hiroshiba N et al (1999) Retinal ischemia-reperfusion injury attenuated by blocking of adhesion molecules of vascular endothelium. Invest Ophthalmol Vis Sci 40: 1183–1190

Veriac S, Tissie G, Bonne C (1993) Oxygen free radicals adversely affect the regulation of vascular tone by nitric oxide in the rabbit retina under high intraocular pressure. Exp Eye Res 56:85–88

Zeng J, Zeng Z, Huang Z et al (2005) Anti-hypoxia effect of 3'-daidzein. J Clin Rehabil 10: 130–132

Chapter 68
Structural and Functional Phenotyping in the Cone-Specific Photoreceptor Function Loss 1 (*cpfl1*) Mouse Mutant – A Model of Cone Dystrophies

M. Dominik Fischer, Naoyuki Tanimoto, Susanne C. Beck, Gesine Huber, Karin Schaeferhoff, Stylianos Michalakis, Olaf Riess, Bernd Wissinger, Martin Biel, Michael Bonin, and Mathias W. Seeliger

Abstract

Purpose: We performed a comprehensive in vivo assessment of retinal morphology and function in *cpfl1* (*cone photoreceptor function loss 1*) mice to better define the disease process in this model of cone dystrophies.

Methods: Mice were examined using electroretinography (ERG), confocal scanning laser ophthalmoscopy (cSLO), and spectral domain optical coherence tomography (SD-OCT). Cross-breeding *cpfl1* mutants with mice expressing green fluorescent protein (GFP) under control of red-green cone opsin promoter allowed for an in vivo timeline analysis of number and distribution of cone photoreceptors using the autofluorescence (AF) mode of the cSLO.

Results: Light-evoked responses of cone origin were practically absent in *cpfl1* mice, whereas rod system function appeared normal. In vivo imaging revealed a progressive loss of cone photoreceptors with a major decline between PW4 and PW8, while retinal architecture and layering remained essentially intact.

Discussion: While the absence of substantial light-evoked cone responses in the *cpfl1* mice is evident from early on, the course of physical cone degeneration is protracted and has a major drop between PW4 and PW8. However, these changes do not lead to significant alterations in retinal architecture, probably due to the relatively low number and wide dissemination of cone photoreceptor cells within the afoveate mouse retina.

M.D. Fischer (✉)
Division of Ocular Neurodegeneration, Institute for Ophthalmic Research, Centre
for Ophthalmology, University of Tuebingen Schleichstr. 12-16, 72070 Tuebingen, Germany
e-mail: dominik.fischer@med.uni-tuebingen.de

R.E. Anderson et al. (eds.), *Retinal Degenerative Diseases*, Advances in Experimental
Medicine and Biology 664, DOI 10.1007/978-1-4419-1399-9_68,
© Springer Science+Business Media, LLC 2010

68.1 Introduction

Cone dystrophies are an important group of inherited retinal degenerations as they affect visual acuity and color vision due to a functional impairment and subsequent physical loss of cone photoreceptors. In contrast to many other inherited degenerations, rod function and morphology is not affected. The *cpfl1* (*cone photoreceptor function loss 1*) mutant is a naturally arising mouse model featuring a mutation (116-bp insertion) in the cGMP-phosphodiesterase subunit (*PDE6C*) gene of the cone photoreceptors (Chang et al. 2002). The phenotype was first described as lacking cone-mediated light responses combined with a progressive loss of cone photoreceptors, and thus the *cpfl1* mouse was proposed to comprise a model for congenital achromatopsia (Chang et al. 2001). In this study, we provide evidence that the *cpfl1* mouse is a valid model for cone dystrophies, based on in vivo functional and morphological data.

68.2 Materials and Methods

68.2.1 Animals

Animals were housed under fluorescent lights in a 12-h light - dark cycle, had free access to food and water, and were used irrespective of gender. All procedures were performed in accordance with the local ethics committee, German laws governing the use of experimental animals, and the ARVO statement for the use of animals in ophthalmic and visual research.

68.2.2 Functional Testing

Electroretinography (ERG) was performed according to previously described procedures (Seeliger et al. 2001). The ERG equipment consisted of a Ganzfeld bowl, a direct current amplifier, and a PC-based control and recording unit (Multiliner Vision; VIASYS Healthcare GmbH, Hoechberg, Germany). Mice were dark-adapted overnight and anaesthetised with ketamine (66.7 mg/kg) and xylazine (11.7 mg/kg). The pupils were dilated and single flash ERG recordings were obtained under dark-adapted (scotopic) and light-adapted (photopic) conditions. Light adaptation was accomplished with a background illumination of 30 cd/m^2 starting 10 min before recording. Single white-flash stimulation ranged from –4 to 1.5 log cd^*s/m^2, divided into 10 steps of 0.5 and 1 log cd^*s/m^2. Ten responses were averaged with an inter-stimulus interval (ISI) of either 5 s or 17 s (for 0, 0.5, 1, and 1.5 log cd^*s/m^2). For additional photopic bright flash experiments, we used a Mecablitz 60CT4 flash gun (Metz, Germany) added to the Ganzfeld bowl. The intensity used in this photopic bright flash protocol was 4.1 log cd^*s/m^2.

68.2.3 In Vivo Imaging

Confocal scanning laser ophthalmoscopy (cSLO) was performed as previously described (Seeliger et al. 2005). Briefly, cSLO imaging was performed using the HRA I (Heidelberg Engineering, Heidelberg, Germany) featuring two argon wavelengths (488 and 514 nm) in the short wavelength range and two infrared diode lasers (795 and 830 nm) in the long wavelength range. The laser wavelength of 795 nm was used for indocyanine-green (ICG) angiography with a barrier filter at 800 nm. The 488 nm wavelength was used for fundus autofluorescence analysis and detection of GFP expression using a barrier filter at 500 nm. Mouse eyes were subjected to spectral domain OCT (SD-OCT) using the Spectralis^{TM} device (Heidelberg Engineering) featuring a broadband superluminescent diode at $\lambda =$ 880 nm as low coherent light source. Each high resolution two-dimensional B-Scan recorded at 30° field of view consists of 1536 A-Scans, which are acquired at a speed of 40,000 scans per second. Optical depth resolution is ca. 7 μm with digital resolution reaching 3.5 μm (Wolf-Schnurrbusch et al. 2008). Resulting data were exported as 8 bit color image files and processed in Adobe Photoshop CS2 (Adobe Systems, San Jose, CA).

68.3 Results

68.3.1 Function

To investigate functional properties in *cpfl1* mice, flash ERGs were recorded from 4-week-old wild type and *cpfl1* mice under dark-adapted (Fig. 68.1a) and light-adapted (Fig. 68.1b and e) conditions. The ERG results were generally matching those in *Cnga3*$^{-/-}$ mice (deficient of the cone cyclic nucleotide-gated channel α subunit, Biel et al. 1999), suggesting a strongly reduced cone system but regular rod system function. While dark-adapted ERG responses up to approximately -2 log cd*s/m^2 intensity are evoked exclusively by the rod system (Tanimoto et al. 2009), the cone system begins to respond to stimuli brighter than -2 log cd*s/m^2 (Jaissle et al. 2001), and contributes to the trailing part of the scotopic b-wave (Biel et al. 1999). Consequently, the scotopic a-wave and the leading part of the scotopic b-wave do not change significantly in mice with selective loss of cone function (Biel et al. 1999). Indeed, we found a normal b-wave up to -2 log cd*s/m^2 intensity and a normal a-wave at all light intensities (Fig. 68.1a), but a reduction of the trailing edge of the b-wave especially at high intensities (arrow in Fig. 68.1c).

As the *cpfl1* mouse line was named after its deficient cone system function (Chang et al. 2002), the photopic ERGs were strongly reduced as anticipated. However, unlike in *Cnga3*$^{-/-}$ mice (Biel et al. 1999), photopic responses were not completely absent in *cpfl1* mice (arrows in Fig. 68.1b). To confirm that these changes

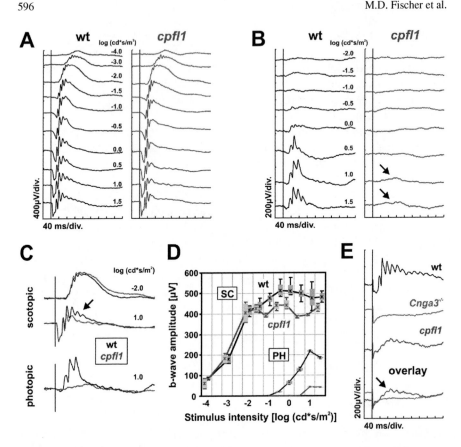

Fig. 68.1 Electroretinographic data from wild type and *cpfl1* mice at 4 weeks of age. (**a**) Scotopic (dark-adapted) single flash ERG intensity series of a wild type (*left*) and a cpfl1 mouse (*right*). *Vertical line* crossing each trace shows the timing of the light flash. (**b**) Photopic (light-adapted) single flash ERG intensity series of a wild type (*left*) and a cpfl1 mouse (*right*). The photopic responses are strongly reduced but not completely absent (*arrows* in **b**). (**c**) Overlay of selected scotopic (*top*) and photopic (*bottom*) waveforms from the intensity series. The alteration of the trailing edge of the scotopic b-wave at high stimulus intensities is illustrated (*arrow* in **c**). (**d**) Scotopic (SC) and photopic (PH) b-wave amplitudes from wild-type and *cpfl1* mice as a function of the logarithm of the flash intensity. *Boxes* indicate the 25–75% quantile range, whiskers indicate the 5 and 95% quantiles, and the *asterisk* indicates the median of the data. (**e**) Photopic bright flash ERG responses obtained from a wild-type and a *cpfl1* mouse, and also from a functionally all-rod mouse (*Cnga3$^{-/-}$*, cone cyclic nucleotide-gated channel deficient). Small response was detected in *cpfl1* mice (*arrow* in **e**), indicating some remaining cone system function at 4 weeks of age

truly reflect residual cone system function, we performed a photopic bright flash ERG using a light stimulus of 4.1 log cd*s/m^2 intensity (Fig. 68.1e). Although response amplitudes are initially masked by a flash artefact, a small but distinct light-evoked response could be demonstrated in 4-week-old *cpfl1* mice (arrow in Fig. 68.1e).

68.3.2 Morphology

Cpfl1 mice undergo a progressive selective degeneration of cone photoreceptor cells with age. To analyse morphological changes in the retina, in vivo cSLO and SD-OCT analyses were performed. Since only about 3% of the murine photoreceptors are cones and these are widely spaced, no differences between *wt* and *cpfl1* mice could be detected in native en face (cSLO) and cross sectional imaging (SD-OCT). In particular, no enhanced fundus autofluorescence as indicator of cumulative photoreceptor degeneration (Seeliger et al. 2005) was detected. To specifically analyse the fate of the cone photoreceptor cells in vivo, we cross-bred *cpfl1* mice with the RG-GFP mouse line selectively expressing green fluorescent protein under control of a red-green opsin promotor (Fei and Hughes 2001). This allowed non-invasive imaging of individual cone photoreceptors in the autofluorescence mode of the cSLO. Timeline analysis of numbers and distribution of GFP positive cone photoreceptors in wild type and double mutant RG-GFP/*cpfl1* mice revealed no change in the control animals (Fig. 68.2, top row), but a marked decrease in GFP expression over time in the RG-GFP/*cpfl1* animals, leading to an almost complete loss of GFP expressing cells in the ventral region and a strong reduction in the dorsal region (Fig. 68.2, bottom row).

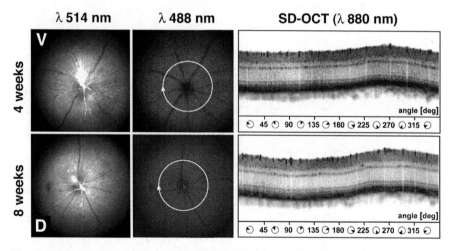

Fig. 68.2 Time course of GFP expression in RG-GFP mice and RG-GFP/*cpfl1* mice analyzed by cSLO. In RG-GFP mice, the GFP expression remains constant between 3 and 8 weeks of age. Conversely, the expression decreases considerably over time in RG-GFP/*cpfl1* mice with some reduction visible at 4 weeks and drastic changes at 6 weeks of age. At 8 weeks only few cones can be detected by GFP expression. V = ventral; D = dorsal

68.4 Discussion

The *cpfl1* mouse model is known for a lack of cone mediated ERG responses (Chang et al. 2001; Chang et al. 2002). However, stringent ERG testing revealed a minimally intense photopic response indicating a low degree of residual cone photoreceptor

function. Latter contrasts this line from an established functional rod-only model
such as the $Cnga3^{-/-}$ mice (Biel et al. 1999).

In vivo imaging of *cpfl1* mice demonstrated progressive cone photoreceptor
degeneration with a marked reduction between 4 and 8 weeks of age, i.e. the functional deficit and the physical loss are independent in time. Already at 4 weeks of
age, the cone system functions were strongly reduced in *cpfl1* mice, although only
a slight decrease in GFP expression could be observed in cSLO imaging of double
mutant RG-GFP/*cpfl1* mice at 4 weeks of age. This also explains why the respective
human disease due to mutations in the *PDE6C* gene is usually classified as achromatopsia, clinically manifesting as a lack of cone function from birth (Wissinger
et al. 2007), and not as a cone dystrophy, where cone function more closely follows
the actual physical loss. Nevertheless, the processes involved may well be studied
in the *cpfl1* mouse model.

Structurally, the impact of cone degeneration on general retinal morphology
remains limited. In cSLO and in the SD-OCT derived virtual cross sections, retinal architecture was seemingly unchanged (Fig. 68.3). This can at least partly be
explained by the relatively slow degenerative process and the low number and sparse
distribution of cones in the afoveate murine retina, whose remains may be removed
without persistent degradation products often seen in rod degenerations as areas of
enhanced fundus autofluorescence.

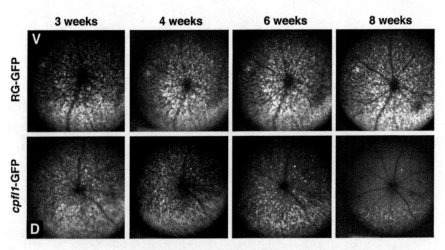

Fig. 68.3 In vivo imaging of *cpfl1* mouse retinae shows essentially normal retinal configuration
in the course of progressive cone photoreceptor degeneration. *Left panels* show normal fundus
appearance of *cpfl1* mice aged 4 (*top*) and 8 (*bottom*) weeks similar to WT mice (not shown)
in native cSLO imaging modes. V = ventral; D = dorsal; λ 514 nm = argon laser (reflectance
mode); λ 488 nm = argon laser (autofluorescence mode); *white circles* indicate orientation of
respective SD-OCT scans shown in the *right panels*. SD-OCT derived virtual cross sections display
essentially intact retinal architecture in *cpfl1* mice at both time points similar to WT mice (not
shown)

In this work, we present in vivo functional and structural characteristics of the retina in the *cpfl1* mouse model for cone dystrophy. In addition, we present a non-invasive method to follow the fate of single photoreceptors over time in individual mice and provide new aspects of residual cone function in the *cpfl1* mouse model.

References

Chang B, Hawes NL, Hurd RE et al (2002) Retinal degeneration mutants in the mouse. Vis Res 42:517–525

Chang B, Hawes NL, Hurd RE et al (2001) A new mouse model of cone photoreceptor function loss (cpfl1) Invest Ophthalmol Vis Sci 42:ARVO E-Abstract S527

Seeliger MW, Grimm C, Stahlberg F et al (2001) New views on RPE65 deficiency: the rod system is the source of vision in a mouse model of Leber congenital amaurosis. Nat Genet 29:70–74

Seeliger MW, Beck SC, Pereyra-Munoz N et al (2005) In vivo confocal imaging of the retina in animal models using scanning laser ophthalmoscopy. Vis Res 45:3512–3519

Wolf-Schnurrbusch UE, Enzmann V, Brinkmann CK et al (2008) Morphological changes in patients with geographic atrophy assessed with a novel spectral OCT-SLO combination. Invest Ophthalmol Vis Sci 49:3095–3099

Biel M, Seeliger M, Pfeifer A et al (1999) Selective loss of cone function in mice lacking the cyclic nucleotide-gated channel CNG3. Proc Natl Acad Sci U S A 96:7553–7557

Jaissle GB, May CA, Reinhard J et al (2001) Evaluation of the rhodopsin knockout mouse as a model of pure cone function. Invest Ophthalmol Vis Sci 42:506–513

Fei Y, Hughes TE (2001) Transgenic expression of the jellyfish green fluorescent protein in the cone photoreceptors of the mouse. Vis Neurosci 18:615–623

Tanimoto N, Muehlfriedel RL, Fischer MD et al (2009) Vision tests in the mouse: functional phenotyping with electroretinography. Front Biosci 14:2730–2737

Wissinger B, Chang B, Dangel S et al. (2007) Cone phosphodiesterase defects in the murine cpfl1 mutant and human achromatopsia patients Invest Ophthalmol Vis Sci 48:ARVO E-Abstract B122

Chapter 69
The Differential Role of Jak/Stat Signaling in Retinal Degeneration

C. Lange, M. Thiersch, M. Samardzija, and C. Grimm

Abstract Retinal degenerative diseases are a major cause of severe visual impairment or blindness in humans. To develop therapeutic strategies it is of particular importance to understand the molecular mechanisms taking place during the progression of the disease. Genes and proteins of the Janus kinase/Signal Transducer and Activator of Transcription (Jak/STAT) signaling pathway have been shown to play an important role in models of retinal degeneration (RD). Here we investigated the expression of additional genes involved in the Jak/STAT pathway in an induced (light exposure) and an inherited (rd1 mouse) model of RD. We show that STAT mRNAs as well as the Jak2/shp-1 pathway are differentially regulated in the two models. In contrast, we show that Jak3 mRNA is upregulated in both, the light damaged and the degenerative retina of the rd1 mouse. This common answer to probably different apoptotic stimuli suggests a prominent role for Jak3 in the damaged retina and could therefore be interesting for further investigations.

69.1 Introduction

Retinal degenerative diseases like retinitis pigmentosa (RP) are a frequent cause of severe visual impairment or blindness in human patients. They are characterized by the progressive loss of visual cells by apoptosis. Understanding the molecular mechanisms underlying the processes of photoreceptor degeneration and identifying endogenous rescue pathways is of fundamental importance to develop successful therapeutic strategies for this group of diseases.

There are various animal models, induced as well as inherited, to study retinal degenerations. In one model for induced retinal degeneration mice are exposed to bright light which causes photoreceptors to die by apoptosis (Reme et al. 1998; Grimm et al. 2000; Wenzel et al. 2005). Depending on the light intensity used and

C. Lange (✉)
Lab for Retinal Cell Biology, Department of Ophthalmology, University of Zurich, Zurich, Switzerland
e-mail: christina.lange@usz.ch

R.E. Anderson et al. (eds.), *Retinal Degenerative Diseases*, Advances in Experimental Medicine and Biology 664, DOI 10.1007/978-1-4419-1399-9_69, © Springer Science+Business Media, LLC 2010

the duration of exposure, more or less photoreceptors die and are cleared from the subretinal space until 10 days post exposure. The rd1 (retinal degeneration 1) mouse is a model for autosomal recessive RP. It carries a null mutation in the β-subunit of the cGMP-phosphodiesterase. Lack of cGMP-phosphodiesterase activity leads to accumulation of cGMP and Ca^{2+} in the outer segment of rod-photoreceptors (Bowes et al. 1990). In this model, photoreceptors start to die around postnatal day (PND) 10 with nearly no photoreceptors left at PND 21. Although photoreceptors die by an apoptotic process in both models, it is not yet clear how induced models compare to inherited models for retinal degeneration. Understanding the cell death mechanisms that these models share or in which they are different is important in order to develop treatment strategies, which aim at the inhibition of cell death mechanisms or at the activation of cell survival strategies.

Gene expression analysis in mouse retinas has shown that the expression of different genes of the Janus kinase/Signal Transducer and Activator of Transcription (Jak/STAT) signaling pathway changes during retinal degeneration after light exposure and in the rd1 mouse (Samardzija et al. 2006). This points to an important role of individual members of this pathway for cell death or cell survival in injured retinas.

Here we investigated additional genes from the Jak/STAT pathway and analyzed their potential involvement in the induced (light) and the inherited (rd1) model for retinal degeneration.

69.2 Materials and Methods

69.2.1 Mice and Light Exposure

Animals were treated in accordance with the regulations of the Veterinary Authority of Zurich and with the statement of 'The Association for Research in Vision and Ophthalmology' for the use of animals in research. About 6- to 8-week old Balb/c mice (from Harlan) were dark adapted over night (16h) and exposed to white fluorescent light (5,000 lux) for 1 h. After light exposure mice were kept in darkness for different periods of time before sacrifice and removal of the retina. After 24 h in darkness they were returned to cyclic (12 h: 12 h) light. Mice that were dark-adapted but not exposed to light served as controls. Rd1 mice (Harlan) were sacrificed at different ages (PND10 to PND37) for removal of the retina. Here, wild-type Bl/6 mice (from a breeding colony in the animal facility of the University Hospital Zurich) served as controls for normalization.

69.2.2 Semi-Quantitative Real Time Polymerase Chain Reaction (PCR)

Retinas were removed through a slit in the cornea and immediately frozen in liquid nitrogen. Total RNA was prepared using the RNeasy RNA isolation kit (Qiagen) according to the manufacture's directions including a DNase treatment to digest residual genomic DNA. Equal amounts of RNA were used for reverse transcription using oligo(dT) and M-MLV reverse transcriptase (Promega). Relative quantification of cDNA was carried out by real-time PCR using the LightCycler 480 Sybr Green I Master kit, a LightCycler 480 instrument (Roche) and specific primer pairs (Table 69.1). Three animals per time point were analyzed in duplicates and compared to the expression of the bipolar cell marker visual system homeobox 2 (CHX10) by relative quantification using the Light Cycler 480 software (Roche). CHX10 was chosen because it is expressed in the inner nuclear layer and should not be affected by photoreceptor apoptosis during retinal degeneration. Light exposure samples were normalized to the dark control (DC). Rd1 samples were normalized to the wild-type and to 10 day old rd1 (PND10).

Table 69.1 PCR primers used for real time PCR

Gene	Upstream	Downstream	Product (bp)
Jak1	tgagctttgatcggatcctt	gcagggtcccagaatagatatg	90
Jak2	gaacctacagatacggagtgtcc	caaaatcatgccgccact	96
Jak3	cacagtgcatggcctatgat	aggtgtggggtctgagagg	110
Shp-1	tgactaccagagaggtggagaaagg	agagaccatagacacgctgagtgc	84
STAT1	ttgtgttgaatcccgaacct	tcgaaccactgtgacatcct	95
STAT2	attggaagttgcagcgagag	tgcgccatttggactctt	67
STAT3	caaaaccctcaagaagccaagg	tcactcacaatgcttctccgc	139
STAT4	ttcagagcagctcaacatgc	ggtgaggtgaccatcattgtag	70
STAT5a	aagatcaagctggggcacta	catgggacagcggtcatac	60
STAT5b	cgagctggtctttcaagtca	ctggctgccgtgaacaat	64
Tyk2	cctgtgtcaccttgctctca	ggaatgagggatgcagttct	85

69.3 Results

69.3.1 STATs Are Induced Differently in Retinas of Light-Exposed and rd1 Mice

After light exposure STAT1 and STAT2 were induced with peaks at 12–24 h (4- to 5-fold). STAT3 expression was activated earlier with an induction peak at 6–12 h (5- to 7-fold). STAT4 showed only a minor induction at 6–12 h (2-fold) and STAT5a and b did not change in expression (STAT5a) or were slightly downregulated (STAT5b). In the rd1 mouse none of the STATs showed a major differential expression during the degeneration. Only STAT3 was mildly induced at postnatal day 16 (2- to 3-fold). Of note and in contrast to the light-induced model, STAT5b was rather upregulated than downregulated (Table 69.2).

Table 69.2 Real time semi-quantitative PCR. Given are means ± standard deviation (SD) of 3 retinas per time-point amplified in duplicates. After light exposure STAT1, 2 and 3 were induced. In the rd1 mouse in contrast there was no induction of STATs. DC: dark control. Im: immediately after light exposure. 6h-30d (light exposure): time-point after light exposure. 10d-37d (rd1): day after birth

	STAT1	STAT2	STAT3	STAT4	STAT5a	STAT5b
DC	1.00±0.49	1.00±0.20	1.00±0.16	1.00±0.90	1.00±0.23	1.00±0.12
Im	0.74±0.27	0.93±0.03	0.91±0.07	0.64±0.44	1.03±0.19	0.83±0.15
6h	1.96±0.05	1.58±0.18	6.53±0.81	2.13±2.64	1.18±0.16	0.80±0.13
12 h	4.73±0.28	4.51±0.62	5.95±1.05	2.05±2.49	1.09±0.33	0.63±0.04
24 h	4.69±0.30	4.73±0.66	4.28±0.82	0.75±0.26	1.18±0.12	0.63±0.12
2d	1.78±0.31	1.16±0.04	1.68±0.54	0.63±0.36	0.92±0.23	0.49±0.10
3d	2.27±1.52	1.80±0.97	1.69±0.61	1.05±0.32	1.12±0.12	0.71±0.21
5d	0.82±0.38	0.64±0.21	0.76±0.07	0.59±0.42	0.70±0.06	0.59±0.14
10d	0.88±0.16	1.02±0.07	0.88±0.08	0.45±0.11	1.10±0.23	0.91±0.15
20d	0.61±0.06	0.81±0.11	0.84±0.03	0.77±0.23	1.32±0.14	0.88±0.08
30d	0.64±0.04	0.84±0.11	0.75±0.12	0.87±0.43	1.25±0.26	0.87±0.08
Rd1						
10d	1.00±0.00	1.00±0.00	1.00±0.00	1.00±0.00	1.00±0.00	1.00±0.00
14d	0.78±0.34	1.04±0.29	1.79±0.44	0.85±0.24	1.38±0.24	2.01±0.35
16d	0.81±0.17	0.91±0.22	2.42±0.11	0.57±0.07	1.85±0.10	1.77±0.11
21d	0.73±0.16	0.90±0.16	1.45±0.34	1.43±0.67	1.95±0.29	1.97±0.68
28d	0.82±0.23	0.80±0.08	1.38±0.46	0.66±0.13	1.51±0.14	1.59±0.35
37d	0.56±0.22	0.71±0.35	1.24±0.54	2.37±1.10	1.44±0.68	1.49±0.70

69.3.2 Shp-1 Is Induced After Light Exposure But Not in the rd1 Mouse

After light exposure scr-homology containing phosphatase 1 (shp-1) was induced with a peak (7-fold) at 3 days post exposure. In contrast, shp-1 was not induced and showed rather a tendency for downregulation in the rd1 mouse (Table 69.3).

69.3.3 Jak3 mRNA Is Induced Similarly in the Model of Light Induced Photoreceptor Cell Death and the rd1 Mouse Model

Jak3 showed an induction with a peak (11-fold) at 24 h after light exposure (Table 69.4). The expression of other Janus kinases remained nearly unchanged. Also in the rd1 mouse induction of Jak3 was prominent at the time of the peak of photoreceptor death (14 days after birth) (5-fold). It stayed induced (2- to 3-fold) at least until all photoreceptors have disappeared (37 days after birth) (Table 69.4). Here the expression of the other Janus kinases tended to be downregulated.

Table 69.3 Real time semi-quantitative PCR for shp-1. Given are means ± standard deviation (SD) of 3 retinas per time-point amplified in duplicates. After light exposure shp-1 was induced. In the rd1 mouse there was no induction of shp-1. DC: dark control. Im: immediately after light exposure. 6h-30d (light exposure): time-point after light exposure. 10d-37d (rd1): day after birth

	Shp-1
DC	1.00±0.41
Im	1.18±0.16
6h	1.63±1.14
12 h	2.14±1.09
24 h	3.17±0.63
2d	4.17±0.84
3d	7.42±1.52
5d	2.17±0.14
10d	2.72±0.72
20d	1.73±0.09
30d	2.12±0.54
10d	1.00±0.03
14d	0.87±0.13
16d	0.52±0.05
21d	0.36±0.01
28d	0.49±0.10
37d	0.14±0.02

Table 69.4 Real time semi-quantitative PCR. Given are means ± standard deviation (SD) of 3 retinas per time-point amplified in duplicates. Jak3 was induced in both models. It peaked at 24 h after light exposure and was induced from PND 14 on in the rd1 mouse. DC: dark control. Im: immediately after light exposure. 6h-30d (light exposure): time-point after light exposure. 10d-37d (rd1): day after birth

	Jak1	Jak2	Jak3	Tyk2
DC	1.00±0.22	1.00±0.09	1.00±0.00	1.00±0.31
Im	1.05±0.18	1.44±0.15	0.80±0.06	1.42±0.07
6h	1.31±0.09	1.79±0.24	5.53±0.58	1.35±0.14
12 h	1.10±0.32	1.45±0.18	9.75±1.75	1.47±0.11
24 h	0.63±0.07	1.18±0.09	11.50±2.58	1.71±0.30
2d	0.45±0.03	0.80±0.04	4.07±1.00	1.64±0.42
3d	0.59±0.04	0.75±0.05	4.75±1.17	1.61±0.47
5d	0.47±0.09	0.83±0.17	0.98±0.11	0.99±0.35
10d	1.04±0.10	0.90±0.23	1.34±0.10	1.66±0.27
20d	0.67±0.40	0.69±0.11	1.08±0.10	1.32±0.29
30d	0.81±0.13	0.74±0.17	1.00±0.05	1.19±0.21
Rd1				
10d	1.00±0.00	1.00±0.09	1.00±0.00	1.00±0.09
14d	0.65±0.12	0.93±0.18	5.33±2.74	0.69±0.07
16d	0.43±0.04	0.76±0.07	5.04±0.53	0.67±0.10
21d	0.54±0.02	0.72±0.05	2.84±0.61	0.51±0.01
28d	0.30±0.00	0.60±0.06	2.35±0.38	0.48±0.10
37d	0.21±0.00	0.48±0.17	3.14±1.54	0.31±0.05

69.4 Discussion

Jak2 and STAT3, proteins from the Jak/STAT signaling pathway, have been shown to be involved in photoreceptor apoptosis during retinal degeneration (Samardzija et al. 2006). To further increase our understanding of the role of Jak/STAT signaling in this process, we analyzed the expression profiles of additional Jak/STAT related genes in the light-induced and the inherited rd1 model for retinal degeneration.

Although there were similarities between the two models of retinal degeneration, significant differences support the existence of model-specific signaling systems.

Expression of STAT1, 2 and 3 was upregulated after light exposure but only STAT3 was induced in the rd1 mouse (Table 69.2).

Similarly, the phosphatase shp-1, was induced after light exposure but not in the rd1 mouse (Table 69.3). Shp-1 is known to bind to activated Jak2 to dephosphorylate and therefore inhibit it (Akagi et al. 2004; Minoo et al. 2004; Lyons et al. 2006; Chong and Maiese 2007). We have shown that Jak2 is transiently phosphorylated in response to light peaking at 12 h after light exposure (Samardzija et al. 2006). Thereafter, levels of p-Jak2 are gradually reduced reaching basal levels at 2 days post exposure. During this decline of p-Jak2 levels, expression of shp-1 started to rise. It is therefore likely that shp-1 is upregulated to inhibit Jak2 in the light damaged retina. In the rd1 mouse Jak2 does not appear to be phosphorylated during photoreceptor degeneration (Samardzija et al. 2006). Therefore, a molecular control of Jak2 activity may not be needed which may explain the lack of shp-1 upregulation in the rd1 retina. A different signaling between the rd1 and the light damaged retina has been observed earlier. Whereas erythropoietin (EPO) protects photoreceptors against light damage it does not inhibit the inherited degeneration caused by the rd1 mutation (Grimm et al. 2004). Since EPO is reported to trigger the Jak2/shp-1 pathway (Akagi et al. 2004), lack of protection in the rd1 mouse may indicate that the Jak2 signaling system may be severely disturbed early in the degenerating rd1 retina.

Although both the light damaged and the degenerative rd1 retina upregulate STAT3 expression and phosphorylation (Samardzija et al. 2006), the up- and downstream signaling cascades are not yet clear. A likely candidate up- or downstream is Jak3, which was induced at least from PND 14 on in the rd1 mouse and with a peak at 24 h after light exposure (Table 69.4). Since Jak3 activity is mainly regulated on the gene expression level (Mangan et al. 2006), the strong induction of mRNA levels suggest a prominent role of this kinase in the injured retina. It is possible that Jak3 is part of an immune-related response induced by retinal damage. This response may be responsible for the attraction of immune-cells entering the retina in both models of retinal degeneration (Zeng et al. 2005; Zhang et al. 2005). Jak3 was described to be important for lymphoid development and to be primarily expressed in immune-cells (Leonard and O'Shea 1998). Lack of Jak3 leads to a severe combined immunodeficiency. Preliminary results from laser-capture experiments (data not shown), however, suggest that Jak3 is also expressed in the outer nuclear layer and the ganglion cell layer of the healthy retina. Whether its expression is indeed relevant for immune-related signaling or whether Jak3 may have other roles for example in the survival of retinal cells is not known and will be studied in detail using Jak3 knockout animals.

Acknowledgments   The authors thank Coni Imsand, Hedwig Wariwoda and Philipp Huber for excellent technical assistance. This work was supported by the Swiss National Science Foundation (SNF).

References

Akagi S, Ichikawa H et al (2004) The critical role of SRC homology domain 2-containing tyrosine phosphatase-1 in recombinant human erythropoietin hyporesponsive anemia in chronic hemodialysis patients. J Am Soc Nephrol 15(12):3215–3224

Bowes C, Li T et al (1990) Retinal degeneration in the rd mouse is caused by a defect in the beta subunit of rod cGMP-phosphodiesterase. Nature 347(6294):677–680

Chong ZZ, Maiese K (2007) The Src homology 2 domain tyrosine phosphatases SHP-1 and SHP-2: diversified control of cell growth, inflammation, and injury. Histol Histopathol 22(11): 1251–1267

Grimm C, Wenzel A et al (2000) Gene expression in the mouse retina: the effect of damaging light. Mol Vis 6:252–260

Grimm C, Wenzel A et al (2004) Constitutive overexpression of human erythropoietin protects the mouse retina against induced but not inherited retinal degeneration. J Neurosci 24(25): 5651–5658

Leonard WJ, O'Shea JJ (1998) Jaks and STATs: biological implications. Annu Rev Immunol 16:293–322

Lyons BL, Smith RS et al (2006) Deficiency of SHP-1 protein-tyrosine phosphatase in "viable motheaten" mice results in retinal degeneration. Invest Ophthalmol Vis Sci 47(3):1201–1209

Mangan JK, Tantravahi RV et al (2006) Granulocyte colony-stimulating factor-induced upregulation of Jak3 transcription during granulocytic differentiation is mediated by the cooperative action of Sp1 and Stat3. Oncogene 25(17):2489–2499

Minoo P, Zadeh MM et al (2004) A novel SHP-1/Grb2-dependent mechanism of negative regulation of cytokine-receptor signaling: contribution of SHP-1 C-terminal tyrosines in cytokine signaling. Blood 103(4):1398–1407

Reme CE, Grimm C et al (1998) Apoptotic cell death in retinal degenerations. Prog Retin Eye Res 17(4):443–464

Samardzija M, Wenzel A et al (2006) Differential role of Jak-STAT signaling in retinal degenerations. FASEB J 20(13):2411–2413

Wenzel A, Grimm C et al (2005) Molecular mechanisms of light-induced photoreceptor apoptosis and neuroprotection for retinal degeneration. Prog Retin Eye Res 24(2):275–306

Zeng HY, Zhu XA et al (2005) Identification of sequential events and factors associated with microglial activation, migration, and cytotoxicity in retinal degeneration in rd mice. Invest Ophthalmol Vis Sci 46(8):2992–2999

Zhang C, Shen JK et al (2005) Activation of microglia and chemokines in light-induced retinal degeneration. Mol Vis 11:887–895

Part VI
Neuroprotection and Gene Therapy

Chapter 70
Gene Therapy in the *Retinal Degeneration Slow* Model of Retinitis Pigmentosa

Xue Cai, Shannon M. Conley, and Muna I. Naash

Abstract Human blinding disorders are often initiated by hereditary mutations that insult rod and/or cone photoreceptors and cause subsequent cellular death. Generally, the disease phenotype can be predicted from the specific mutation as many photoreceptor genes are specific to rods or cones; however certain genes, such as *Retinal Degeneration Slow* (*RDS*), are expressed in both cell types and cause different forms of retinal disease affecting rods, cones, or both photoreceptors. RDS is a transmembrane glycoprotein critical for photoreceptor outer segment disc morphogenesis, structural maintenance, and renewal. Studies using animal models with *Rds* mutations provide valuable insight into *Rds* gene function and regulation; and a better understanding of the physiology, pathology, and underlying degenerative mechanisms of inherited retinal disease. Furthermore, these models are an excellent tool in the process of developing therapeutic interventions for the treatment of inherited retinal degenerations. In this paper, we review these topics with particular focus on the use of *rds* models in gene therapy.

70.1 Introduction

Inherited retinal degenerations can be caused by mutations in over 100 different genes, and in many cases, the structure, function, and regulation of these genes are well documented. Among them, the *RDS* (retinal degeneration slow, also known as peripherin/rds or prph2) gene is an important target of study because: (1) over 80 different disease causing mutations have been identified in *RDS* (http://www.retina-international.com/sci-news/rdsmut.htm), (2) these mutations account for a substantial fraction of inherited retinal diseases, and (3) the variety in *RDS*-associated

M.I. Naash (✉)
Department of Cell Biology, University of Oklahoma Health Sciences Center, Oklahoma City, OK 73104, USA
e-mail: muna-naash@ouhsc.edu

R.E. Anderson et al. (eds.), *Retinal Degenerative Diseases*, Advances in Experimental Medicine and Biology 664, DOI 10.1007/978-1-4419-1399-9_70, © Springer Science+Business Media, LLC 2010

disease phenotypes provides critical insight into the biological function of rod and cone photoreceptors (Boon et al. 2008).

RDS is located in the rim region of rod and cone outer segment (OS) discs and is critical for OS disc formation, orientation, renewal and structural stability (Connell et al. 1991; Molday et al. 1987). Interestingly though, the protein has been shown to play different roles in rod vs. cone OS morphogenesis (Farjo et al. 2006b; Nour et al. 2004).

70.2 Diseases Associated with *RDS* Mutations

Disease causing mutations in the human *RDS* gene were first reported in 1991 and were associated with an autosomal dominant retinitis pigmentosa (adRP) phenotype (Farrar et al. 1991; Kajiwara et al. 1991). Further investigation found that different mutations in the *RDS* gene cause not just adRP, but a wide spectrum of both cone- and rod-dominant retinal diseases including a variety of macular dystrophies, cone and cone-rod dystrophy, central areolar chroidal dystrophy, retinitis punctata albescens, and autosomal recessive Stargardt disease (Boon et al. 2008). While the phenotypes of *RDS*-associated diseases vary in severity, age of onset, and clinical presentation, most lead to debilitating blindness, and all are currently uncurable.

70.3 Current Animal Models

Animal models carrying *Rds* mutations are of great value in the investigation of the physiology and pathology of *RDS*-associated disease and for the establishment of potential therapies. The initial *Rds* animal model to be characterized was the *rds* mouse which has been studied for over 30 years (Farjo and Naash 2006; van Nie et al. 1978). This mouse contains a spontaneous 9 kb insertion into exon II of the mouse *Rds* gene and produces two large and stable *Rds* messages that cannot be translated to protein. The heterozygous mouse ($rds^{+/-}$) has a striking adRP-like haploinsufficiency phenotype characterized by malformed OSs, a deficit in ERG function, and a progressive, slow loss of rods and cones (Cheng et al. 1997; Nour et al. 2004; Stricker et al. 2005). The homozygous mouse ($rds^{-/-}$) does not form OSs and has little or no detectable ERG function accompanied by retinal degeneration (Farjo and Naash 2006). So far, several other animal models carrying deletion or missense mutations in *Rds* on either a wild-type (WT) or $rds^{-/-}$ background have been studied including nmf193 (Nystuen et al. 2008), P216L (Kedzierski et al. 1997), C214S (Nour et al. 2008; Stricker et al. 2005) and R172W (Conley et al. 2007; Ding et al. 2004). All these mice exhibit photoreceptor degeneration, abnormalities in OS structure, and reduction in ERG amplitudes. The mutant mice frequently share similar phenotypes to their human counterparts; e.g. C214S-RDS mice show an adRP like phenotype (Stricker et al. 2005) while R172W-RDS mice display a macular dystrophy phenotype (Conley et al. 2007; Ding et al. 2004).

70.4 Gene Therapy in *rds* Models

Gene therapy for the treatment of the diseased eye has become a common strategy; however, there are many factors which can influence its efficacy. Depending on the disease, a therapeutically beneficial effect can be achieved by directly targeting the primary genetic defect using gene replacement therapy (for loss-of-function phenotypes) or by suppressing mutant transcripts by RNA-based ribozymes or RNAi (shRNA). Alternatively, the desired effect may be achieved indirectly by modulating a secondary effect associated with the disease. Examples of this type of gene therapy in the eye include delivery of neurotrophic factors and anti-apoptotic genes to protect and improve photoreceptor survival in the presence of a degenerative insult (Danos 2008; Farrar et al. 2002; Hauswirth and Lewin 2000). Based on the characteristics of the delivery vehicles, gene therapies are commonly classified into two broad categories: viral and non-viral.

70.5 Viral Gene Therapy Approaches

Viral methods have been utilized quite successfully in the eye. Retrovirus, lentivirus, adenovirus, and adeno-associated virus (AAV) have all been used to transfer therapeutic genes to the retina (Hauswirth and Lewin 2000), but AAV vectors have been the most effective thus far. They are small in size, can efficiently and stably transduce a variety of dividing and non-dividing cell types, and site-specifically integrate without pathogenicity or immune response. AAV vectors are associated with high transduction efficiency, long term gene expression, and after therapeutic delivery to the eye, improvement in retinal function and vision (Acland et al. 2005; Acland et al. 2001). The only limitation of AAV vectors is capacity; traditional AAV vectors usually hold no more than 4.5–4.7 kb. Recently, however, one study reported that rAAV2/5 can incorporate up to 8.9 kb DNA (Allocca et al. 2008). So far, ocular AAV-mediated gene therapy in animals and humans has a good safety record (Mueller and Flotte 2008). For example, in several recent clinical trials, one in which rAAV-PEDF was delivered to treat age-related macular degeneration (AMD) (Campochiaro et al. 2006), and three in which rAAV-RPE65 was used to treat Leber's Congenital Amaurosis (LCA) (Bainbridge et al. 2008; Cideciyan et al. 2008; Maguire et al. 2008), patients reported no severe side effects and some improvement in visual function.

Several viral approaches have been adopted for the treatment of *Rds*-associated disease. Ali's group used the gene replacement approach, delivering *Rds* cDNA to the retinas of neonatal and adult $rds^{-/-}$ mice. They reported restoration of retinal ultrastructure and function; however, transduction efficiency was about 10%, gene expression decreased over time, and the treatment did not significantly ameliorate cell death (Ali et al. 2000; Sarra et al. 2001; Schlichtenbrede et al. 2003).

The neuroprotection approach has also been applied to *rds* models (Buch et al. 2006; LaVail et al. 1998). Combination therapy with glial cell line-derived neurotrophic factor (AAV.CBA.GDNF) and *Rds* (AAV.Rho.Prph2) delivered to the *rds*[−/−] retina was significantly more effective than gene replacement therapy alone (AAV.Rho.Prph2), but the positive effects did not persist beyond 3 months (Buch et al. 2006). Neonatal or adult delivery of ciliary neurotrophic factor (rAAV-CNTF) to the subretinal or the intravitreal space of P216L-RDS mice in either the *rds*[+/−] or *rds*[−/−] background significantly reduced photoreceptor death, increased rhodopsin expression in surviving rods, improved expression of key phototransduction genes, and improved rod ERG responses (Bok et al. 2002; Cayouette et al. 1998; Liang et al. 2001; Rhee et al. 2007). However, there is some controversy regarding the benefits of treatment with CNTF. Subsequent studies reported a dose-dependent reduction in retinal function and an abnormal nuclear phenotype in P216L-RDS mice after CNTF delivery (Bok et al. 2002; Buch et al. 2006; Rhee et al. 2007; Schlichtenbrede et al. 2003, 2003). The mechanisms underlying this deleterious effect are not understood and may be species specific. However the ability to attenuate photoreceptor cell death is clearly beneficial and further study of the effects of neurotrophic factors on *Rds*-associated retinal disease should be undertaken.

A final viral gene therapy approach which may be quite useful in the future, but has not yet been applied to the treatment of *Rds*-associated diseases is gene knockdown therapy. This approach will likely be a critical one to the successful treatment of *Rds*-associated macular diseases in particular since they tend to be associated with toxic, gain-of-function mutations. Ribozymes can reduce the production of mutated proteins by selectively cleaving the mutant mRNA molecules with a high degree of specificity (Hauswirth and Lewin 2000). Ribozymes have been successfully used to treat rhodopsin-associated adRP: AAV-ribozyme delivered to rhodopsin rats carrying the P23H mutation significantly decreased P23H transgene mRNA level, significantly reduced photoreceptor loss, increased outer nuclear layer (ONL) thickness, and improved scotopic b-wave amplitudes (Gorbatyuk et al. 2007a; Hauswirth et al. 2000; LaVail et al. 2000). An alternative knockdown strategy is delivery of shRNAs. This technology can be used to selectively knock down mutant alleles or more broadly to knock down both mutant and WT alleles, and has been applied to several different rhodopsin adRP models (Allen et al. 2007; Gorbatyuk et al. 2007b). While selective knockdown of a mutant allele may appear to be the ideal option for this type of therapy, this approach would require development of separate therapies for each individual mutation. In the case of *RDS*, the sheer number of different dominant mutations would likely make this cost-prohibitive. As an alternative, RNAi knockdown of both mutant and WT message (knockdown based on a recognition sequence not associated with the mutation) with concurrent administration of supplementary RNAi-resistant WT protein has been successfully tested in P23H rhodopsin mutant rats and would likely be a good strategy for dominant *RDS* mutations (O'Reilly et al. 2007).

70.6 Non-viral Approaches

As an alternative to traditional viral-based gene delivery, non-viral vectors have recently become popular. The most common limitations encountered when using non-viral vectors is low transfection efficiency and transient gene expression. Many non-viral methods have been used in the eye including nanoparticles; liposomes; dendrimers; and plasmid DNA, with or without electroperation or ionotophoresis (Andrieu-Soler et al. 2006). In spite of the varying degrees of success associated with these strategies, so far, no non-viral vectors have been used clinically to treat ocular diseases. Recently, compacted-DNA nanoparticles (CK30PEG) were shown to be safe and effective in delivering the cystic fibrosis transmembrane receptor to the airways of cystic fibrosis patients in a type I/IIa clinical trial (Konstan et al. 2004). Given these positive results, we decided to investigate the utility of these nanoparticles in the eye. We subretinally injected CK30PEG nanoparticles containing a CMV-GFP vector into adult mice and demonstrated transfection of almost 100% of retinal cells beginning as early as two days post injection (PI) without any adverse effect on retinal structure or function. Since our ultimate goal is to use nanoparticles to treat *Rds*-associated adRP, we next generated nanoparticles containing the *Rds* cDNA with the P341Q modification at the C-terminus to enable specific recognition of the transferred protein with mAb 3B6. *Rds* cDNA expression was directed to rods and cones by the photoreceptor specific promoter IRBP (interphotoreceptor retinoid binding protein). We chose to deliver the treatment at postnatal day (P) 5, before the normal onset of RDS expression (P7) and OS formation (P8-10) (Cepko et al. 1996). As shown in Fig. 70.1a (qRT-PCR) and Fig. 70.1b (immunohistochemistry), after P5 injection into WT mice, the nanoparticles induced high levels of transgene expression as early as PI-2. In contrast to our results with the CMV-GFP nanoparticles (Farjo et al. 2006), IRBP nanoparticles drove sustained expression to PI-30 (the latest time point examined). At all timepoints, expression of the transferred protein (labeled with 3B6) was limited to the OS or developing OS layer, similar to the localization of the WT (RDS-CT) protein (Fig. 70.1b). To determine whether the nanoparticles could drive gene expression earlier than endogenous gene expression begins, a subset of animals was injected at

Fig. 70.1 (continued) IRBP nanoparticles can drive persistent and elevated transgene expression in the WT Retina. WT mice were injected at P5 (**a**, **b**) or P2 (**c**) with IRBP nanoparticles. At various timepoints whole eyes were harvested and processed for qRT-PCR using *Rds* primers (**a**) or immunohistochemistry using mAB 3B6-green (specific for transferred/transgenic RDS) or RDS-CT polyclonal antibody-red (for endogenous RDS) with DAPI counterstain-blue (**b–d**). (**a**) Nanoparticle injection results in *Rds* message levels several fold higher than in uninjected contralateral control eyes. Levels remain elevated to PI-30. (**b**) Transferred RDS is detected at PI-2 in the nascent OS layer and co-localizes with the endogenous RDS at all timepoints examined. When nanoparticles are injected at P2, transferred protein is detected prior to the onset of endogenous RDS (**c**) although in stable transgenic mice generated using the same construct as the nanoparticle, transgenic RDS is not detectable until P12 (equivalent to PI-7) (**d**). Scale bar, 20 μm

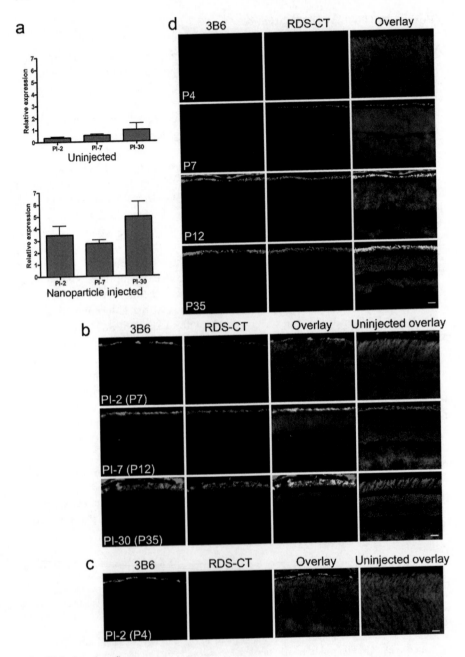

Fig. 70.1 (continued)

P2. As shown in Fig. 70.1c, immunohistochemistry revealed that nanoparticle transferred protein (3B6) is detected at PI-2 after P2 injection, while endogenous protein is not apparent this early. Interestingly, when we used this same IRBP construct to generate stable transgenic mice, the transgenic RDS protein was not detected before the endogenous protein (Fig. 70.1d). Our data shown here and previously (Farjo et al. 2006) demonstrate that CK30PEG nanoparticles can efficiently transfect both mitotic and post-mitotic cells and induce rapid-onset and sustain gene expression. When the *Rds* gene is delivered, nanoparticles are capable of driving gene expression earlier than the native RDS without ectopic expression outside the photoreceptor OS layer. Our current studies are focused on determining whether these nanoparticles can rescue the *rds*[+/-] adRP disease phenotype, thus making them potential candidates for clinical use in the eye.

References

Acland GM, Aguirre GD, Bennett J et al (2005) Long-term restoration of rod and cone vision by single dose rAAV-mediated gene transfer to the retina in a canine model of childhood blindness. Mol Ther 12:1072–1082

Acland GM, Aguirre GD, Ray J et al (2001) Gene therapy restores vision in a canine model of childhood blindness. Nat Genet 28:92–95

Ali RR, Sarra GM, Stephens C et al (2000) Restoration of photoreceptor ultrastructure and function in retinal degeneration slow mice by gene therapy. Nat Genet 25:306–310

Allen D, Kenna PF, Palfi A et al (2007) Development of strategies for conditional RNA interference. J Gene Med 9:287–298

Allocca M, Doria M, Petrillo M et al (2008) Serotype-dependent packaging of large genes in adeno-associated viral vectors results in effective gene delivery in mice. J Clin Invest 118:1955–1964

Andrieu-Soler C, Bejjani RA, de Bizemont T et al (2006) Ocular gene therapy: a review of nonviral strategies. Mol Vis 12:1334–1347

Bainbridge JW, Smith AJ, Barker SS et al (2008) Effect of gene therapy on visual function in Leber's congenital amaurosis. N Engl J Med 358:2231–2239

Bok D, Yasumura D, Matthes MT et al (2002) Effects of adeno-associated virus-vectored ciliary neurotrophic factor on retinal structure and function in mice with a P216L rds/peripherin mutation. Exp Eye Res 74:719–735

Boon CJ, den Hollander AI, Hoyng CB et al (2008) The spectrum of retinal dystrophies caused by mutations in the peripherin/RDS gene. Prog Retin Eye Res 27:213–235

Buch PK, MacLaren RE, Duran Y et al (2006) In contrast to AAV-mediated Cntf expression, AAV-mediated Gdnf expression enhances gene replacement therapy in rodent models of retinal degeneration. Mol Ther 14:700–709

Campochiaro PA, Nguyen QD, Shah SM et al (2006) Adenoviral vector-delivered pigment epithelium-derived factor for neovascular age-related macular degeneration: results of a phase I clinical trial. Hum Gene Ther 17:167–176

Cayouette M, Behn D, Sendtner M et al (1998) Intraocular gene transfer of ciliary neurotrophic factor prevents death and increases responsiveness of rod photoreceptors in the retinal degeneration slow mouse. J Neurosci 18:9282–9293

Cepko CL, Austin CP, Yang X et al (1996) Cell fate determination in the vertebrate retina. Proc Natl Acad Sci U S A 93:589–595

Cheng T, Peachey NS, Li S et al (1997) The effect of peripherin/rds haploinsufficiency on rod and cone photoreceptors. J Neurosci 17:8118–8128

Cideciyan AV, Aleman TS, Boye SL et al (2008) Human gene therapy for RPE65 isomerase deficiency activates the retinoid cycle of vision but with slow rod kinetics. Proc Natl Acad Sci U S A 105:15112–15117

Conley S, Nour M, Fliesler SJ et al (2007) Late-onset cone photoreceptor degeneration induced by R172W mutation in Rds and partial rescue by gene supplementation. Invest Ophthalmol Vis Sci 48:5397–5407

Connell G, Bascom R, Molday L et al (1991) Photoreceptor peripherin is the normal product of the gene responsible for retinal degeneration in the rds mouse. Proc Natl Acad Sci U S A 88:723–726

Danos O (2008) AAV vectors for RNA-based modulation of gene expression. Gene Ther 15:864–869

Ding XQ, Nour M, Ritter LM et al (2004) The R172W mutation in peripherin/rds causes a cone-rod dystrophy in transgenic mice. Hum Mol Genet 13:2075–2087

Farjo R, Naash MI (2006) The role of Rds in outer segment morphogenesis and human retinal disease. Ophthalmic Genet 27:117–122

Farjo R, Skaggs JS, Nagel BA et al (2006b) Retention of function without normal disc morphogenesis occurs in cone but not rod photoreceptors. J Cell Biol 173:59–68

Farjo R, Skaggs J, Quiambao AB et al (2006a) Efficient non-viral ocular gene transfer with compacted DNA nanoparticles. PLoS ONE 1:e38

Farrar GJ, Kenna PF, Humphries P (2002) On the genetics of retinitis pigmentosa and on mutation-independent approaches to therapeutic intervention. EMBO J 21:857–864

Farrar GJ, Kenna P, Jordan SA et al (1991) A three-base-pair deletion in the peripherin-RDS gene in one form of retinitis pigmentosa. Nature 354:478–480

Gorbatyuk M, Justilien V, Liu J et al (2007a) Preservation of photoreceptor morphology and function in P23H rats using an allele independent ribozyme. Exp Eye Res 84:44–52

Gorbatyuk M, Justilien V, Liu J et al (2007b) Suppression of mouse rhodopsin expression in vivo by AAV mediated siRNA delivery. Vis Res 47:1202–1208

Hauswirth WW, LaVail MM, Flannery JG et al (2000) Ribozyme gene therapy for autosomal dominant retinal disease. Clin Chem Lab Med 38:147–153

Hauswirth WW, Lewin AS (2000) Ribozyme uses in retinal gene therapy. Prog Retin Eye Res 19:689–710

Kajiwara K, Hahn LB, Mukai S et al (1991) Mutations in the human retinal degeneration slow gene in autosomal dominant retinitis pigmentosa. Nature 354:480–483

Kedzierski W, Lloyd M, Birch DG et al (1997) Generation and analysis of transgenic mice expressing P216L-substituted rds/peripherin in rod photoreceptors. Invest Ophthalmol Vis Sci 38:498–509

Konstan MW, Davis PB, Wagener JS et al (2004) Compacted DNA nanoparticles administered to the nasal mucosa of cystic fibrosis subjects are safe and demonstrate partial to complete cystic fibrosis transmembrane regulator reconstitution. Hum Gene Ther 15:1255–1269

LaVail MM, Yasumura D, Matthes MT et al (1998) Protection of mouse photoreceptors by survival factors in retinal degenerations. Invest Ophthalmol Vis Sci 39:592–602

LaVail MM, Yasumura D, Matthes MT et al (2000) Ribozyme rescue of photoreceptor cells in P23H transgenic rats: long-term survival and late-stage therapy. Proc Natl Acad Sci U S A 97:11488–11493

Liang FQ, Aleman TS, Dejneka NS et al (2001) Long-term protection of retinal structure but not function using RAAV.CNTF in animal models of retinitis pigmentosa. Mol Ther 4:461–472

Maguire AM, Simonelli F, Pierce EA et al (2008) Safety and efficacy of gene transfer for Leber's congenital amaurosis. N Engl J Med 358:2240–2248

Molday RS, Hicks D, Molday L (1987) Peripherin. A rim-specific membrane protein of rod outer segment discs. Invest Ophthalmol Vis Sci 28:50–61

Mueller C, Flotte TR (2008) Clinical gene therapy using recombinant adeno-associated virus vectors. Gene Ther 15:858–863

Nour M, Ding XQ, Stricker H et al (2004) Modulating expression of peripherin/rds in transgenic mice: critical levels and the effect of overexpression. Invest Ophthalmol Vis Sci 45:2514–2521

Nour M, Fliesler SJ, Naash MI (2008) Genetic supplementation of RDS alleviates a loss-of-function phenotype in C214S model of retinitis pigmentosa. Adv Exp Med Biol 613:129–138

Nystuen AM, Sachs AJ, Yuan Y et al (2008) A novel mutation in Prph2, a gene regulated by Nr2e3, causes retinal degeneration and outer-segment defects similar to Nr2e3 (rd7/rd7) retinas. Mamm Genome 9:623–633

O'Reilly M, Palfi A, Chadderton N et al (2007) RNA interference-mediated suppression and replacement of human rhodopsin in vivo. Am J Hum Genet 81:127–135

Rhee KD, Ruiz A, Duncan JL et al (2007) Molecular and cellular alterations induced by sustained expression of ciliary neurotrophic factor in a mouse model of retinitis pigmentosa. Invest Ophthalmol Vis Sci 48:1389–1400

Sarra GM, Stephens C, de Alwis M et al (2001) Gene replacement therapy in the retinal degeneration slow (rds) mouse: the effect on retinal degeneration following partial transduction of the retina. Hum Mol Genet 10:2353–2361

Schlichtenbrede FC, MacNeil A, Bainbridge JW et al (2003) Intraocular gene delivery of ciliary neurotrophic factor results in significant loss of retinal function in normal mice and in the Prph2Rd2/Rd2 model of retinal degeneration. Gene Ther 10:523–527

Schlichtenbrede FC, da Cruz L, Stephens C et al (2003) Long-term evaluation of retinal function in Prph2Rd2/Rd2 mice following AAV-mediated gene replacement therapy. J Gene Med 5: 757–764

Stricker HM, Ding XQ, Quiambao A et al (2005) The Cys214–>Ser mutation in peripherin/rds causes a loss-of-function phenotype in transgenic mice. Biochem J 388:605–613

van Nie R, Ivanyi D, Demant P (1978) A new H-2-linked mutation, rds, causing retinal degeneration in the mouse. Tissue Antigens 12:106–108

Chapter 71
PEDF Promotes Retinal Neurosphere Formation and Expansion In Vitro

Anna De Marzo, Claudia Aruta, and Valeria Marigo

Abstract The retina is subject to degenerative conditions leading to blindness. Although retinal regeneration is possible in lower vertebrates, it does not occur in the adult mammalian retina. Retinal stem cell (RSC) research offers unique opportunities for developing clinical application for therapy. The ciliary body of adult mammals represents a source of quiescent RSC. These neural progenitors have a limited self-renewal potential in vitro but this can be improved by mitogens. Pigment Epithelium Derived Factor (PEDF), a member of the serpin gene family, is synthesized and secreted by retinal pigment epithelium (RPE) cells. We tested combinations of PEDF with fibroblast growth factor (FGF) during RSC growth to evaluate self-renewal and subsequent differentiation into retinal-like neuronal cell types. Medium supplemented with FGF + PEDF enhanced the RSC yield and more interestingly allowed expansion of the culture by increasing secondary retinal neurospheres after the 1st passage. This effect was accompanied by cell proliferation as revealed by BrdU incorporation. PEDF usage did not affect rod-like differentiation potential. This was demonstrated by immunofluorescence analysis of Rhodopsin and Pde6b that were found similarly expressed in cells derived from FGF or FGF + PEDF cultured RSC. Our studies suggest a possible application of PEDF in Retinal Stem Cell culture and transplantation.

71.1 Introduction

Many forms of blindness arise from photoreceptor degeneration and to date have no satisfactory solutions to rescue retinal tissues.

Mammalian eyes do not have a regenerative capability characteristic of lower vertebrates but recent evidences have demonstrated that ciliary body (CB), a

A. De Marzo (✉)
Department of Biomedical Sciences, University of Modena and Reggio Emilia, Modena, Italy
e-mail: anna.demarzo@unimore.it

R.E. Anderson et al. (eds.), *Retinal Degenerative Diseases*, Advances in Experimental Medicine and Biology 664, DOI 10.1007/978-1-4419-1399-9_71,
© Springer Science+Business Media, LLC 2010

structure analogous to the CMZ of lower vertebrates, contains retinal stem cells (RSC) (Moshiri et al. 2004; Nishiguchi et al. 2008; Tropepe et al. 2000; Ahmad et al. 2000; Coles et al. 2004; Inoue et al. 2005).

Multipotent retinal stem or progenitor cells can be isolated from the ciliary body of an adult mammalian retina using a neurosphere culture. Tropepe et al. have demonstrated that one out of 500 CB cells gives rise to a clonal aggregate called neurosphere consisting of ~12,000 pigmented cells and that each neurosphere can generate six to eight daughter neurosphere colonies.

Although the presence and the function of retinal stem cells (RSCs) in vivo remains unknown RSCs proliferate in vitro; they differentiate into cell subtypes expressing markers of certain mature retinal neurons such as bipolar cells, photoreceptor cells or Mueller glia suggesting the possibility that these cells may represent a potential cell source in transplantation therapy for retinal diseases (Tropepe et al. 2000; Giordano et al. 2007). Differentiation is induced by plating the cells on an extracellular matrix substrate and exposing the cells to 1% Fetal Bovine Serum (FBS). In these conditions the percentage of cells that undertake a rod-like fate is about 30–40% as assessed by rhodopsin and the Pde6b co-expression. Growth of neurospheres with FGF without EGF before differentiation favors rod-like differentiation (Giordano et al. 2007).

Primary cultures of cells collected from the CB are in FBS free medium and the formation of neurospheres takes about 5–7 days. The number of neurospheres is dependent upon the growth factors to which cells are exposed, such as FGF or EGF. A limitation in the culture of RSC comes from low ability of these cells to be expanded in vitro. In fact, a single retinal neurosphere composed of about 12,000 cells upon passaging does not give rise to 12,000 new spheres but only an average of 3. Furthermore, no expansion of the culture has been obtained from the third passage (Giordano et al. 2007). Amelioration of the culture condition is therefore a fundamental aspect that needs to be addressed if we want to bring RSC to therapeutic applications.

Previous works have shown that pigment epithelium-derived factor (PEDF) secreted by the murine subventricular zone (SVZ) promotes self-renewal and activation of slowly dividing adult neural stem cells (NSC) in vitro (Ramirez-Castillejo et al. 2006). PEDF is a neurotrophic antiangiogenic factor initially purified from conditioned media of retinal pigment epithelial cells (Tombran-Tink et al. 1991; Becerra et al. 1995). PEDF is secreted from many different cells and can modulate cell cycle progression (Pignolo et al. 2003). Thus PEDF may have positive effects on RSC culture.

Here we show that the treatment of RSC with PEDF together with FGF increases the neurosphere yield and, ameliorates self-renewal in neurosphere passaging. We then tested whether PEDF could affect differentiation to rod-like fate. This improvement does not decrease the number of cells expressing rhodopsin and Pde6b. Moreover, cells differentiated from a FGF+PEDF culture did not express bipolar cell markers.

71.2 Materials and Methods

71.2.1 Retinal Stem Cell Isolation and Culture

All procedures on mice (including their euthanasia) were performed in accordance with the ARVO Statement for the Use of Animals in Ophthalmic and Vision Research and with institutional guidelines for animal research. In this study we used C57BL/6 mice purchased from Charles River Italy (Calco, Italy) and housed them under standard conditions with a 12-hour light/dark cycle. We dissected eyes from 12-week-old C57BL6 mice in artificial cerebral spinal fluid (ACSF) containing 124 mM NaCl, 5 mM KCl, 100 nM CaCl2, 1.3 mM MgCl2, 26 mM NaHCO3 and 10 mM D-glucose. Eyes were cut in two hemispheres and the lens and the neural retina were carefully removed. The ciliary body was separated from the retinal pigment epithelium (RPE), treated with trypsin and hyaluronidase and the ciliary margin cells were scraped from the sclera according to the procedures described in the paper (Giordano et al. 2007). The isolated cells were grown in a serum free medium (0.6% glucose and N2 hormone mix in DMEM-F12) containing either 20 ng/ml basic FGF (FGF) supplemented with 2 μg/ml heparin (Sigma, Milan, Italy) or both FGF + 20 ng/ml PEDF (Chemicon). Cells were seeded at a concentration of 40,000 cells/ml and incubated for 6 days until floating spheres formed.

71.2.2 Single Sphere Passaging

A single sphere was placed in a microcentrifuge tube and incubated in enzyme solution (ACSF containing 1.33 mg/ml trypsin, 0.67 mg/ml hyaluronidase, 0.5 mg/ml collagenase type I-A, 0.5 mg/ml collagenase XI, 0.13 mg/ml kynurenic acid) for 1 h at 37°C. After centrifugation at 400g for 5 min the supernatant was replaced with 1 mg/ml of trypsin inhibitor in medium and the sphere was mechanically dissociated. Collected cells from each sphere were seeded into a 96-well plate in serum-free medium containing FGF or FGF+PEDF and incubated for 6 days.

71.2.3 Bromodeoxyuridine Labeling

Retinal floating spheres at 5 days of culture were treated with 10 mM bromodeoxyuridine (BrdU) for 3 h, washed with PBS, allowed to attach to a slide and fixed in 4% paraformaldehyde (PFA). Spheres were treated with 2 N HCl at 30°C for 30 min, placed in a 0.1 M borate buffer pH 8.5 for 15 min and then washed with PBS. Blocking was performed in a 3% bovine serum albumin (BSA), 1% glycine and 0.3% Triton-X 100 for 30 min at room temperature followed by incubation with 1:8000 anti-BrdU monoclonal antibody (Developmental Hybridoma,

Iowa City, IA) overnight at 4°C. Slides were washed with PBS, incubated with 1:1000 Alexa Fluor® 568 goat anti-mouse secondary antibody (Molecular Probes) for 1 h, washed and nuclei were labeled with 1 µg/ml Dapi (Roche) and treated with 2.5 mg/ml RNAse A at 37°C for 1 h. Slides were mounted with Moviol mounting solution (Sigma) and BrdU positive cells were counted in a stack of 20 images (5 µm) at a Leica laser confocal microscope system (Leica SP2, Wetzlar Gmbh Germany) of the CIGS University of Modena, Italy.

71.2.4 Retinal Stem Cell Differentiation

In differentiation experiments retinal floating spheres were plated on glass coverslips coated with extracellular matrix (ECM, Sigma). Cells were cultured in DMEM-F12 supplemented with either 20 ng/ml FGF and 2 µg/ml heparin or FGF + 20 ng/ml PEDF. The cells were allowed to proliferate and migrate out of the sphere over the course of 4 days. The medium was then replaced with 1% FBS (Gibco, San Giuliano Milanese, Italy) containing medium and cultured for 15 days.

71.2.5 Immunofluorescence

Cells grown on glass coverslips were fixed in 4% paraformaldehyde for 15 min at room temperature. Permeabilization and blocking was performed with 0.2% TritonX-100 and 3% bovine serum albumin (BSA) (Sigma, St Louis, MO) in PBS for 1 h followed by incubation with primary antibodies overnight at 4°C. Cells underwent five washes with PBS and then were incubated with fluorescent-conjugated secondary antibodies for 1 h at room temperature. Primary antibodies used were as follows: 1:1500 anti-Pkc-α rabbit polyclonal (Sigma), 1:100 anti-Pde6b rabbit polyclonal (ABCAM, Cambridge, UK), 1:100 anti-rhodopsin mouse monoclonal 1D4 (Sigma), 1:400 anti-G0α mouse monoclonal (Chemicon), 1:750 anti-syntaxin mouse monoclonal (Sigma), 1:1000 anti-calbindin D 28 K mouse monoclonal (Sigma). Secondary antibodies were as follows: 1:1000 Oregon Green® 488 goat anti-mouse (Molecular Probes, San Giuliano Milanese, and Italy) and 1:1000 Alexa Fluor® 568 goat anti-rabbit (Molecular Probes). Finally slides were mounted in moviol and analyzed using immunofluorescence microscopy Axiocam (Zeiss).

71.3 Results

71.3.1 PEDF Promotes Retinal Neurospheres Growth and Self-Renewal

Previous studies showed that retinal neurospheres had a limited ability to proliferate and to be expanded in vitro (Giordano et al. 2007; Gu et al. 2007). In all the

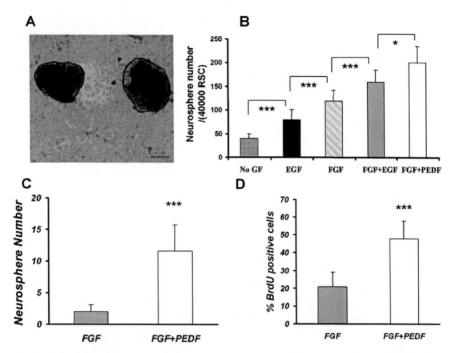

Fig. 71.1 Retinal neurospheres growth and proliferation. (**a**) RSCs grow clonally at low density to form neurospheres. Progenitor cells within the sphere proliferate for 7 days giving rise to a progeny of pigmented and non-pigmented cells. Scale bar, 50 μm. (**b**) Differences in neurosphere yield by culturing 40,000 cells with different growth factor combinations. (**c**) Secondary neurosphere number after single sphere passage grown with FGF or FGF + PEDF. The student t-Test was used. ***$p < 0.001$; ** $p < 0.01$; * $p < 0.05$. (**d**) Proliferation was evaluated in neurosphere by labeling with BrdU for 3 hrs at the 5th day of neurosphere formation. When cells were grown in FGF + PEDF medium a higher number of cells in proliferation (BrdU+) was counted

different conditions retinal neurospheres appeared with a similar morphology and pigmented (Fig. 71.1a). Cells were seeded at low density (40,000 cells/ml) in the growth medium and neurospheres were counted for each growth factor (GF) treatment. As shown in Fig. 71.1b, exposure to EGF doubled the floating sphere number compared to the cells plated in the absence of GF, while addictions of FGF increased this number of 3-fold. Moreover, the combination of FGF + EGF enhanced the neurosphere formation of 4 folds compared to the culture without GF. Because PEDF is a neurotrophic factor for some neural population, we set out to test whether the combination of PEDF + FGF enriches the neurosphere population and/or self renewal. The addiction of PEDF (20 ng/ml) to the FGF culture media resulted in a 60% increase of neurospheres when compared to FGF alone and 20% more neurospheres than FGF+EGF ($n=3$, $p < 0.01$).

Our previous studies have shown that EGF alone has a reduced ability to generate secondary neurospheres after passaging while cultures with FGF and EGF+FGF doubled the number of neurospheres at the first cell passage. In order to evaluate

whether the positive effect of PEDF was not limited to the primary culture in RSC
but could be extended also to RSC self renewal we dissociated single primary generation neurospheres to single cells and re-plated them in the same culture media
containing FGF+PEDF. The number of cells capable of generating a secondary
neurosphere population increased in the presence of PEDF (Fig. 71.1c). We could
measure a 5 time increase of passaged neurospheres when exposed to PEDF+FGF
compared to FGF alone ($n=4$, $p < 0.001$). Altogether these data suggest that PEDF
favors growth of retinal stem cells in primary cultures and enhances the chances of
self-renewal in culture expansions.

71.3.2 Retinal Neurosphere Proliferation

A previous study carried on in our lab demonstrated that EGF in the culture medium
of RSC favors proliferation during the first days of culture and then proliferation
stops. On the other hand, FGF allows high proliferation to be maintained with time
in culture. This observation may explain also the positive effect that FGF has on cell
passaging. In order to evaluate if the increase in self-renewal properties we observed
with PEDF was correlated with enhanced cell proliferation during the neurosphere
growth, we labeled retinal spheres with BrdU at the sixth day of the retinal stem
cell culture. BrdU positive (BrdU$^+$) and BrdU negative (BrdU$^-$) cells were counted
and compared in FGF and FGF+PEDF culture conditions (Fig. 71.2). The presence of PEDF during neurosphere growth promoted cell proliferation more than

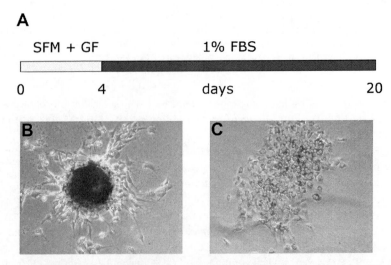

Fig. 71.2 RSC differentiation. (**a**) Schematic representation of the protocol for RSC differentiation: retinal neurospheres were plated onto an ECM substrate to let progenitor cells to exit for 4
days. The GF minimal medium was then replaced with 1% FBS and cells were differentiated up to
20 days. (**b**) Light microscope image of RSC at 4 days of differentiation where cells growing out
of the dark sphere (centre) can be seen. (**c**) RSC at 7 days of differentiation

FGF alone. In particular, FGF gave an average of 20% of BrdU⁺ cells within each retinal sphere while supplementation with PEDF increased this value up to 45% (Fig. 71.1d). This result indicates that the observed enhanced retinal neurosphere generation is accompanied by increased cell proliferation when RSCs are grown in presence of FGF+PEDF.

71.3.3   Differentiation of Retinal Cells Precursors from RSCs

The interest in the evaluation of RSC culture treatment correlates with the need of setting the favorable culture conditions to obtain rod photoreceptor differentiation. Several studies have indicated the possibility of using RSCs as a donor source.

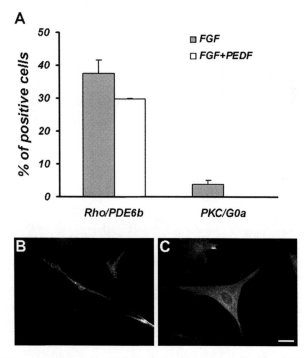

Fig. 71.3 Rod-like cell differentiation from PEDF treated retinal neurospheres. All the RSCs were differentiated in a 1% FBS culture medium. Differentiation was evaluated by immunofluorescence identifying rod-like cells and bipolar-like cells by co-expression of Rho/Pde6b and Pkcα/G₀α respectively. (**a**) *Grey bar* represents the amount of cells positive for markers derived from neurospheres grown in FGF medium; the *white bar* represents the amount of cells positive for markers derived from neurospheres grown in FGF + PEDF medium. Rod-like cells amount was similar when cells derived from spheres grown in either culture media while bipolar-like cells decreased when neurospheres were cultured in FGF + PEDF. The student t-Test was used for statistical analysis. *** $p< 0.001$; ** $p< 0.01$; * $p< 0.05$. (**b**) Co-immunolocalization of Rho and Pde6b markers in rod-like cells. (**c**) Co-immunolocalization of Pkc α and G₀α , markers of bipolar cells. Scale bar in C represents 10 μm

We investigated the ability of differentiated RSCs to express typical markers of adult retinal cells. In our previous work we have evaluated the effect of different GF combinations on retinal cell differentiation. After 6 days of growth, retinal spheres were plated onto an extracellular matrix substrate for 4 days to allow progenitor cells to exit, attach and start differentiation (Fig. 71.2a–c). After 4 days the culture medium was replaced with media containing 1% FBS. Retinal progenitor cells (RPCs) were cultured up to 20 days and then underwent expression analysis by immunofluorescence labeling. Rod photoreceptor-like cells were elongated and defined by the co-expression of specific rod markers: Rhodopsin and Pde6b (an example of Rhodopsin distribution is shown in Fig. 71.3b). Rod-like cells were also characterized by smaller cell size accompanied by smaller nuclei compared to the Rho/Pde6b negative cells. Bipolar-like cells were identified by co-expression of $G_0\alpha$ and Pkcα (an example of Pkcα distribution is shown in Fig. 71.3c). Our culture condition was also favorable for expression of horizontal and amacrine markers like calbindin and syntaxin respectively (data not shown). Generation of neurospheres in the presence of FGF+PEDF did not significantly alter the number of rod-like cells that reached 30–40% of the total cultured cells (Fig. 71.3a). In turn, we were not able to detect bipolar-like cells in the FGF+PEDF culture while 5% of cells treated with FGF only were positive to $G_0\alpha$/Pkcα.

Altogether, results on retinal cell differentiation indicate that PEDF does not significantly affect rod-like differentiation.

71.4 Discussion

Few cells in the mammalian adult ciliary body have the ability to proliferate when subjected to the appropriate stimuli (Tropepe et al. 2000; Ahmad et al. 2000; Zhao et al. 2002). This capability, which resides in less than 1% of the ciliary body cells, can be ameliorated with exposure to growth factors in the culture media. In our previous work we have demonstrated that addiction of FGF + EGF gave the highest neurosphere yield and that this property is maintained also over daughter neurosphere generation after sphere passage (Giordano et al. 2007). Despite the enhanced neurosphere yield, the presence of EGF decreased the rod-like cell number during RSC differentiation and increased the bipolar-like marker expression. This latter result prompted us to investigate alternative GF combinations in order to maximize the RSC self-renewal without affecting the photoreceptor-like cell amount during the following differentiation. Here we report that PEDF in combination with FGF ameliorates the neurosphere formation, likewise acting on the self-renewal capability of the RSCs. This property already described by PEDF on NSC derived from the adult SVZ (Ramirez-Castillejo et al. 2006), was also confirmed during retinal neurosphere passaging. Self-renewal involves both proliferation and maintenance of undifferentiated state, although this process is still poorly understood at molecular levels. We propose here that PEDF might be a modulator during cell division likely promoting generation of two identical stem cells or one stem cell and one committed progenitor instead of two committed progenitor cells. Unlike NSC,

(Ramirez-Castillejo et al. 2006) we find that PEDF has a mitogen effect on RSC as indicated from BrdU incorporation during neurosphere growth. This might be due to cell-intrinsic mechanisms (Arsenijevic 2003) or due to the lack of some external cues such as growth promoting NSC culture conditions.

Upon differentiation, PEDF does not interfere with rod-like cell marker expression giving a similar amount of ~35% to those cells differentiated in the FGF only medium. However, the true identity of photoreceptor-like cells with further molecular and functional analysis remains to be investigated.

Although PEDF has no influence on the rod-like cells number, it causes a lack in bipolar-like cell amount. This effect suggests a possible role of PEDF on Chx10 gene regulation since it has been reported in the involvement of this transcription factor in bipolar cell differentiation (Livne-Bar et al. 2006; Kokkinopoulos et al. 2008). The fact that loss of bipolar-like cells is not accompanied by an increase in other interneuron or rod-like cells may lead to enrichment in progenitor cells still capable of being addressed toward a diverse retinal cell fate, however, this needs to be documented by further studies.

Taken together, these findings indicate that PEDF may contribute to ameliorate RSC expansion, offering a source of alternative therapy in regenerative medicine.

Acknowledgments We are grateful to Fondazione Cassa di Risparmio di Modena for Dr De Marzo fellowship support and XIII International Symposium on Retinal Degeneration for her travel award grant. We acknowledge the CIGS of University of Modena for providing confocal microscopy assistance. This work was supported by research grants EVI-GENORET: LSHG-CT-2005-512036 from the European Community, by research grant GGP06096 from Fondazione Telethon and PRIN 2006053302_003.

References

Ahmad I, Tang L, Pham H (2000) Identification of neural progenitors in the adult mammalian eye. Biochem Biophys Res Commun 270:517–521

Arsenijevic Y (2003) Mammalian neural stem-cell renewal: nature versus nurture. Mol Neurobiol 27(1):73–98

Becerra SP, Sagasti A, Spinella P et al (1995) Pigment epithelium-derived factor behaves like a noninhibitory serpin. Neurotrophic activity does not require the serpin reactive loop. J Biol Chem 270:25992–25999

Coles BL, Angénieux B, Inoue T, Del Rio-Tsonis K, Spence JR, McInnes RR, Arsenijevic Y, van der Kooy D (2004) Facile isolation and the characterization of human retinal stem cells. Proc Natl Acad Sci U S A 101(44):15772–15777

Giordano F, De Marzo A, Vetrini F et al (2007) Facile isolation and the characterization of human retinal stem cells. Mol Vis 13:1842–1850

Gu P, Harwood LG, Zhang X et al (2007) Isolation of retinal progenitor and stem cells from the porcine eye. Mol Vis 13:1045–1057

Inoue Y, Yanagi Y, Tamaki Y et al (2005) Clonogenic analysis of ciliary epithelial derived retinal progenitor cells in rabbits. Exp Eye Res 81(4):437–445

Kokkinopoulos I, Pearson RA, Macneil A, Dhomen NS, Maclaren RE, Ali RR, Sowden JC (2008) Isolation and characterisation of neural progenitor cells from the adult Chx10(orJ/orJ) central neural retina. Mol Cell Neurosci 38(3):359–373

Livne-Bar I, Pacal M, Cheung MC et al (2006) Chx10 is required to block photoreceptor differentiation but is dispensable for progenitor proliferation in the postnatal retina. Proc Natl Acad Sci U S A 103(13):4988–4993

Moshiri A, Close J, Reh TA (2004) Retinal stem cells and regeneration. J Dev Biol 48(8–9): 1003–1014

Nishiguchi KM, Kaneko H, Nakamura M et al (2008) Identification of photoreceptor precursors in the pars plana during ocular development and after retinal injury. Invest Ophthalmol Vis Sci 49(1):422–428

Pignolo RY, Francis MK, Rotemberg MO et al (2003) Putative role for EPC-1/PEDF in the G0 growth arrest of human diploid fibroblasts. J Cell Physiol 195(1):12–20

Ramirez-Castillejo C, Sanchez-Sanchez F, Andreu-Agullo C et al (2006) Pigment epithelium-derived factor is a niche signal for neural stem cell renewal. Nat Neurosci 9(3):331–338

Tombran-Tink J, Chader GG, Johnson LV (1991) PEDF: a pigment epithelium-derived factor with potent neuronal differentiative activity. Exp Eye Res 53:411–414

Tropepe V, Coles BL, Chiasson BJ et al (2000) Retinal stem cells in the adult mammalian eye. Science 287:2032–2036

Zhao X, Liu J, Ahmad I (2002) Differentiation of embryonic stem cells into retinal neurons. Biochem Biophys Res Commun 297(2):177–84

Chapter 72
A Multi-Stage Color Model Revisited: Implications for a Gene Therapy Cure for Red-Green Colorblindness

Katherine Mancuso, Matthew C. Mauck, James A. Kuchenbecker, Maureen Neitz, and Jay Neitz

Abstract In 1993, DeValois and DeValois proposed a 'multi-stage color model' to explain how the cortex is ultimately able to deconfound the responses of neurons receiving input from three cone types in order to produce separate red-green and blue-yellow systems, as well as segregate luminance percepts (black-white) from color. This model extended the biological implementation of Hurvich and Jameson's Opponent-Process Theory of color vision, a two-stage model encompassing the three cone types combined in a later opponent organization, which has been the accepted dogma in color vision. DeValois' model attempts to satisfy the long-remaining question of how the visual system separates luminance information from color, but what are the cellular mechanisms that establish the complicated neural wiring and higher-order operations required by the Multi-stage Model? During the last decade and a half, results from molecular biology have shed new light on the evolution of primate color vision, thus constraining the possibilities for the visual circuits. The evolutionary constraints allow for an extension of DeValois' model that is more explicit about the biology of color vision circuitry, and it predicts that human red-green colorblindness can be cured using a retinal gene therapy approach to add the missing photopigment, without any additional changes to the post-synaptic circuitry.

72.1 Introduction

In 1993, DeValois and DeValois proposed a 'multi-stage color model' to explain how the cortex is ultimately able to deconfound the responses of neurons receiving input from three cone types – short- (S-), middle- (M-), and long- (L-) wavelength

K. Mancuso (✉)
Department of Ophthalmology, University of Washington, Seattle, WA, USA
e-mail: kmancuso@u.washington.edu

R.E. Anderson et al. (eds.), *Retinal Degenerative Diseases*, Advances in Experimental Medicine and Biology 664, DOI 10.1007/978-1-4419-1399-9_72,
© Springer Science+Business Media, LLC 2010

sensitive – to produce separate red-green and blue-yellow systems, as well as segregate luminance percepts (black-white) from color (DeValois and DeValois 1993). This model extended the biological implementation of Hurvich and Jameson's Opponent-Process Theory of color vision (Hurvich and Jameson 1957), a two-stage model encompassing the three cone types combined in a later opponent organization, which has been the accepted dogma in color vision. The DeValois' model attempts to satisfy the long-remaining question of how the visual system separates luminance information from color, but what are the cellular mechanisms that establish the complicated neural wiring and higher-order operations required by the Multi-Stage Model? Throughout the last decade and a half, results from molecular biology have shed new light on the evolution of primate color vision, thus constraining the possibilities for the circuitry underlying each of the six main hue percepts – red, green, blue, yellow, black, and white. The evolutionary constraints allow for an extension of DeValois' model that is more explicit about the biology of the circuitry, and it predicts that human red-green colorblindness can be cured using a retinal gene therapy approach to add the missing cone photopigment (M or L), without further modifications that would be required to transform neural circuits for luminance into ones for color.

72.2 A Brief History of Color Vision Theory

Prior to the emergence of modern biological techniques, breakthroughs in color vision research stemmed from careful consideration of perceptual experiences. The three-component theories of Young and Helmholtz, as well as Hering's conflicting hypothesis of three paired, opponent color processes were developed in the 1800s, long before the three types of cone photopigment were isolated and characterized within the retina. In the 1950s Hurvich and Jameson proposed a resolution to the apparent conflict between earlier models by combining them in a two-stage theory of color vision (Hurvich and Jameson 1957). The first stage was comprised of three cone types, the outputs of which were combined in an opponent organization at the second stage. Their model accounted for observations that there are four main hue percepts arranged in opponent pairs, red-green and blue-yellow, in addition to achromatic black-white opponency. Shortly thereafter, L/M 'ON-' and 'OFF-type' opponent cells were, indeed, discovered in the lateral geniculate nucleus (LGN) (DeValois et al. 1966; Wiesel and Hubel 1966), providing a physiological substrate for the red-green circuitry proposed by Hurvich and Jameson. However, in later experiments, identifying a corresponding number of opponent cells with appropriate response characteristics for blue-yellow color vision, as would be expected based on the similar acuities of red-green and blue-yellow vision, has proved troublesome. To date, only a small percentage of cells responding with S-ON characteristics have been described (Dacey and Lee 1994), and a corresponding number of S-OFF-type cells has remained elusive.

An additional problem with the two-stage model is that most cells in the LGN respond to both color and luminance variations, and confound them, because of the spatial arrangement of their inputs from different cone types. That is, L/M ON- and OFF-opponent cells respond similarly to black-white luminance signals and to red-green chromatic signals, but logic tells us that the visual system is able to separate these confounded responses; otherwise, any time we are presented with a black-white pattern we would have spurious color percepts and vice versa. Furthermore, the idea that red-green color vision is based on comparisons between only L and M cones does not account for data from human psychophysics, which indicates that there is an S-cone contribution to red-green, as well as blue-yellow color perception. These considerations lead DeValois and DeValois to use a bottom-up approach, based on anatomically-suggested connections known at the time, in proposing a third stage of cortical processing in which signals from S-opponent cells were added to, or subtracted from, the L- and M-opponent units to split and rotate the geniculate L/M response axis into separate red-green and yellow-blue color channels, and separate luminance from color (DeValois and DeValois 1993). While an additional stage of higher-level cortical processing is one possibility, understanding how such complicated neural circuitry could have arisen during evolution has been difficult.

72.3 Color Vision from an Evolutionary Perspective

Our dichromatic, or red-green colorblind, primate ancestors had only two types of cone, S and L cones and, presumably, they also had similar circuits underlying their vision as modern-day dichromats. Results from molecular genetics indicate that trichromatic color vision arose relatively recently from a gene duplication event that added M cones. In order for this low-probability genetic event to get passed-on and eventually confer routine trichromacy to Old World primates, including humans, it must have produced an immediate advantage for the primate ancestor by adapting some pre-existing visual circuit for a new purpose. One candidate circuit would have been the high-acuity spatial vision circuit; the primate midget system or its precursor, which compared L vs. L cones to provide achromatic luminance signals. A second candidate would have been the pre-existing color vision circuit which compared S vs. L cones to provide blue-yellow color vision. If the first possibility is correct, then additional changes in the post-synaptic circuitry would have been required over time to separate red-green color signals from achromatic luminance signals. However, the ancient, pre-existing blue-yellow circuitry had already evolved mechanisms for filtering-out luminance signals and only responding to color. Thus, a more plausible explanation is that rather than 'hijacking' pre-existing luminance circuitry, the new class of M cone changed the input to the pre-existing blue-yellow circuit such that it automatically gave rise to a new dimension of red-green color vision. That is, in a dichromat with only S and L cones, any circuits across the retina that compared spectrally different cones would have the same S vs. L opponency, but the addition of M cones would introduce a variety of possible comparisons, providing two different L/M receptive field organizations. When combined with S cones in the existing chromatic pathway, they produced two different chromatic signatures, one corresponding to red-green and another to blue-yellow color vision. This idea implies that luminance and color information become segregated as early as the initial inputs into primary visual cortex, and that the specialized functions of the higher-order cortical circuits are imposed by the character of the peripheral receptor mosaic.

72.4 Evolutionary Constraints Lead to an Extension of Devalois' Model

Short wavelength cones are an evolutionarily ancient photoreceptor type and blue-yellow color vision, based on comparisons between S cones and longer-wavelength cones, appears to be the ancestor from which all other color vision evolved. DeValois and DeValois explained their multi-stage model in terms of S-cone input being either added to or subtracted from the red-green system. However, from an evolutionary perspective, it was actually a new M cone input that was either added to the 'center' or the 'surround' of pre-existing blue-yellow opponent receptive fields, in order to give rise to separate red-green and blue-yellow systems. In primates, the S cones have only two significant outputs: (1) a straight-through output to the receptive field center of S-cone-specific bipolars which, in turn, output to the small bistratified ganglion cells (Fig. 72.1, upper panels) providing a 'blue-on' signal (Dacey and Lee 1994), and (2) input via H2 horizontal cells to adjacent cones (Dacey et al. 1996), which then output to ganglion cells via L/M cone specific bipolar cells (Fig. 72.1, lower panels). The blue-ON bistratified ganglion cell is considered to be a candidate for providing the basis for blue-yellow color vision. However, this cell type would have been little affected in its spectral response characteristics by the addition of M cones to the retina; the center would remain unaltered due to the S-cone specific connections made by small bistratified cells, and the surround would be transformed from 'L' to 'M+L.' Thus, the simple addition of a third cone type would not 'split' this ganglion cell class into two spectral types, as required by the evolutionary constraint that the addition of a third cone type produced an immediate advantage for primate ancestors by adding a new dimension of color vision.

From an anatomical perspective, there is only one other plausible circuit that could be the basis for blue-yellow perception: L/M midget ON and OFF ganglion cells that receive S-cone input in their receptive field surrounds via H2 horizontal cells. Most retinal electrophysiologists would argue from recordings in both the retina and LGN that this type of S-cone input is not observed. Given the paucity of S cones in the retina, it is conceivable that the S-inputs that are transmitted by a correspondingly small percentage of midget cells may have been overlooked in earlier electrophysiological recordings; however, midget cells with these response characteristics have recently been reported by Tailby and colleagues (Tailby et al.

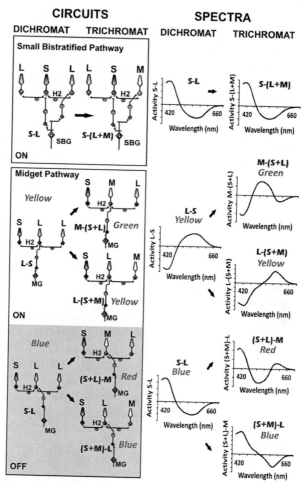

Fig. 72.1 The addition of M cones to a dichromat only changes the 'surrounds' of small bistratified ganglion (SBG) cell receptive fields, and all SBGs continue to have similar spectral response properties, making them an unlikely substrate for hue sensations of red, green, blue, and yellow. In contrast, both the 'center' and 'surround' of midget ganglion (MG) cell receptive fields become altered by the addition of M cones, splitting the pre-existing blue and yellow circuits each into two organizations with distinct spectral response properties and providing a biological basis for separate blue-yellow and red-green systems, with only a single change in the cone mosaic. H2 horizontal cells are labeled

2008). If midget ganglion cells with S-cone-surround input are the basis for the primordial blue-yellow system, the evolutionary steps leading to a new dimension of red-green color vision were as follows. In the dichromatic primate fovea, each L cone has a private connection with two different bipolar cells and two midget ganglion cells, providing an ON- and OFF-pathway for each L cone. The cones are also interconnected by an inhibitory network in which lateral connections are provided by horizontal cells. This is the functional unit of the retina; it acts to compare the light absorption of a single cone to the average light absorption of its neighbors. It is set in such a way that if the activity of a cone is equal to its neighbors, then the antagonistic interaction between center and surround results in no signal. If the center cone is more active than the surrounding cells, then a signal is sent through the ON pathway, and if the center is less active than the surround, the OFF pathway becomes activated. This initial round of lateral inhibition between adjacent cones gives rise to two classes of midget ganglion cells. One class receiving input from an L-center, L-surround receptive field would be spatially-opponent and responsible for signaling high resolution spatial luminance contrast; presumably, 'whiteness' through the ON-pathway and 'blackness' through the OFF-pathway. These signals are then propagated to the lateral geniculate nucleus and then on to primary visual cortex. In order for this luminance system to function properly, there must also be a second round of lateral antagonism at the level of the visual cortex. The reason for this is that intrinsic noise is very high in cone photoreceptors and ganglion cells produce random action potentials at a high rate in the dark. If cortical-level antagonism did not filter-out these random signals, they would produce a constant pattern of white noise that would be interpreted as a constantly changing blotchy luminance pattern.

In the same dichromatic primate, the second, smaller population of midget ganglion cells that receives input from an L-center, S + L surround receptive field would be spectrally-opponent. Diffuse blue light would cause the L-OFF midget ganglion cell to become activated via S-cone input from the surround, which is inverted at the H2 horizontal cell synapse; thus paradoxically, this OFF-cell would also be carrying an S-ON signal. Likewise, diffuse yellow light would cause the L-ON midget ganglion cell to fire, and it would have an S-OFF response characteristic due to the sign-reversal via H2 horizontal cells. In the circuitry proposed here, there is a total of four midget cell types – luminance 'ON' and 'OFF,' and S 'ON' and 'OFF' cells – exactly as is required as the substrate for the sensations of white, black, blue, and yellow, respectively. In contrast to the 'blue-ON' small bistratified ganglion cells discussed above, the opponent midget ganglion cells satisfy the evolutionary constraint that the addition of a third class of cone produced the immediate advantage of a new dimension of red-green color vision. That is, when M cones were randomly added to the pre-existing midget system, the spectrally-opponent ganglion cells would have automatically become segregated into two different classes. The center of the receptive field would become either 'L' or 'M;' accordingly, the receptive field surrounds were transformed to either 'M + S' or 'L + S,' automatically producing midget cells with two different spectral response characteristics–one corresponding to red-green and the other to blue-yellow color vision (Fig. 72.1, lower panels).

Following the DeValois and DeValois multi-stage color model, all four hue percepts are the result of circuits with input from S cones, and the relationship between cone inputs and hue is as follows: the perception of red comes from a neural comparison between (S+L)-M; green from M-(S+L); blue from (S+M)-L; and yellow from L-(S+M). As explained above, it is possible to extend DeValois' model in proposing a straightforward mechanism to form these circuits. Simply, midget ganglion cells that have inhibitory S-cone input in their surround become the basis for hue circuits in the cortex. The cone forming the receptive field center can be either L or M, and the ganglion cells can be either ON or OFF center. The resulting four possible combinations correspond to the four main hue perceptions. An ON-center ganglion cell receiving input from an M cone center with S and L cones in the surround makes M-(S+L) – green; the same receptive field through an OFF-center ganglion cell makes (S+L)-M – red. An L cone center with an M and S surround makes L-(S+M) – yellow; that same receptive field through an OFF-center ganglion cell produces (S+M)-L – blue. Accordingly, cortical neurons receiving input from receptive fields containing only M and L cones are the basis for luminance circuitry and give rise to achromatic white percepts through the ON pathway and black percepts via the OFF pathway. Thus, even though L/M opponent receptive fields result in midget ganglion cells and LGN cells that respond both to color and luminance, the second round of lateral antagonism at the level of visual cortex nulls the spurious color signals, leaving this circuit dedicated to the original purpose for which it evolved – responding to luminance signals only.

72.5 The Possibility of Gene Therapy to Cure Red-Green Colorblindness

An important implication of the color vision model described here is that it should be possible to cure human red-green colorblindness, even in adults. A rapidly progressing field in molecular biology has been viral vector-mediated gene therapy, with great strides being made in the area of vision disorders, in particular. We have recently demonstrated that it is possible to target therapeutic transgenes specifically to cone photoreceptors in primates (Mancuso et al. 2007). Because all of the circuitry required for taking advantage of a third cone type is already present in dichromatic individuals, it should be possible to transform an adult dichromat to a trichromat with full red-green color vision through the simple addition of the missing photopigment to the retina. The model described here implies that gene therapy would recapitulate what occurred during the evolution of trichromatic color vision in our primate ancestors, and the addition of a third cone type would split the dichromat's existing blue-yellow circuits into two classes, one for red-green and the other for blue-yellow color vision.

As discussed above, an unresolved problem in color vision has stemmed from the fact that most cells in the lateral geniculate nucleus respond to both color and luminance variations and confound them. When considering this problem, DeValois and DeValois commented, 'The Standard Model [i.e., the two-stage opponent-process theory] has one color system (the RG system) based on the outputs of the L and M cones, some 90–95% of the cone population, whereas the whole YB system is centered on just the remaining 5–10% of the cones, the S cones. Such an imbalance seems inherently implausible, and one of the considerations that led us to our current model was that of attempting to arrive at a more balanced arrangement between the inputs to the red-green and the yellow-blue color systems. One can reasonably argue that the preponderance of L and M cones reflects the fact that these cone types alone are used for luminance detection. However, with current color models, this still leaves one with either an imbalance between the two chromatic systems or the equally distasteful suggestion that only a fraction of the spectrally-opponent information from L and M cones contributes to color vision.' A key difference between our model and DeValois' model is that evolutionary constraints force us to the notion (albeit 'distasteful') that most of the spectrally-opponent information from L and M cones is disregarded by the visual system and that all LGN cells that receive input from L and M, but not S cones, ultimately give rise to achromatic luminance percepts. Consideration of known retinal anatomy and observations from human color perception has guided us to the conclusion that both the red-green and blue-yellow systems are based on the S cones; all four hue percepts require S-cone input early in the visual pathway, rectifying the apparent imbalance between each color system. In summary, trichromats have six different circuits that extract six distinct percepts from an original mosaic containing three cone types. All six circuits arise as the natural consequence of generic cortical circuitry that indiscriminately compares the activity of a cell in the center of its cortical receptive field with the receptive fields of its immediate neighbors. Therefore, the specialized functions of the cortical circuits are imposed by the character of the peripheral receptor mosaic and by post-receptoral elements early in the neural pathway.

Acknowledgments Supported by the National Institutes of Health grants R01EY016861, R01EY09303, and Research to Prevent Blindness.

References

Dacey DM, Lee BB (1994) The blue-ON opponent pathway in primate retina originates from a distinct bistratified ganglion cell type. Nature 367:731–735

Dacey DM, Lee BB, Stafford DK et al (1996) Horizontal cells of the primate retina: cone specificity without spectral opponency. Science 271:656–659

DeValois RL, Abramov I, Jacobs GH (1966) Analysis of response patterns of LGN cells. J Opt Soc Am 56:966–977

DeValois RL, DeValois KK (1993) A multi-stage color model. Vis Res 33(8):1053–1065

Hurvich LM, Jameson D (1957) An opponent process theory of color vision. Psychol Rev 64: 384–404

Mancuso K, Hendrickson AE, Connor TB Jr et al (2007) Recombinant adeno-associated virus targets passenger gene expression to cones in primate retina. J Opt Soc Am A Opt Image Sci Vis 24:1411–1416

Tailby C, Solomon SG, Lennie P (2008) Functional asymmetries in visual pathways carrying S-cone signals in macaque. J Neurosci 28(15):4078–4087

Wiesel TN, Hubel DH (1966) Spatial and chromatic interactions in the lateral geniculate body of the rhesus monkey. J Neurophysiol 29(6):1115–1156

Chapter 73
Achromatopsia as a Potential Candidate for Gene Therapy

Ji-Jing Pang, John Alexander, Bo Lei, Wentao Deng, Keqing Zhang, Qiuhong Li, Bo Chang, and William W. Hauswirth

Abstract Achromatopsia is an autosomal recessive retinal disease involving loss of cone function that afflicts approximately 1 in 30,000 individuals. Patients with achromatopsia usually have visual acuities lower than 20/200 because of the central vision loss, photophobia, complete color blindness and reduced cone-mediated electroretinographic (ERG) amplitudes. Mutations in three genes have been found to be the primary causes of achromatopsia, including *CNGB3* (beta subunit of the cone cyclic nucleotide-gated cation channel), *CNGA3* (alpha subunit of the cone cyclic nucleotide-gated cation channel), and *GNAT2* (cone specific alpha subunit of transducin). Naturally occurring mouse models with mutations in *Cnga3* (*cpfl5* mice) and *Gnat2* (*cpfl3* mice) were discovered at The Jackson Laboratory. A natural occurring canine model with *CNGB3* mutations has also been found. These animal models have many of the central phenotypic features of the corresponding human diseases. Using adeno-associated virus (AAV)-mediated gene therapy, we and others show that cone function can be restored in all three models. These data suggest that human achromatopsia may be a good candidate for corrective gene therapy.

73.1 Human Achromatopsia

The human retina has approximately 6 million cone photoreceptors and 100 million rod photoreceptors. Cones are primarily responsible for central, fine resolution and color vision while operating in low to very bright light; they are primarily concentrated in the central macula comprising nearly 100% of the fovea. In contrast, rods are responsible for peripheral, low light and night vision, and are primarily found in the peripheral retina and perimacular region. Achromatopsia, or rod monochromatism, is a recessive genetic condition characterized by cone dysfunction, thus leaving the patient with only rod mediated vision. There are two clinical forms of

J.-J. Pang (✉)
Department of Ophthalmology, College of Medicine, University of Florida, 1600 SW Archer Road, Gainesville, FL 32610, USA
e-mail: jpang@ufl.edu

R.E. Anderson et al. (eds.), *Retinal Degenerative Diseases*, Advances in Experimental Medicine and Biology 664, DOI 10.1007/978-1-4419-1399-9_73,

achromatopsia: complete and incomplete. The complete form results in serious visual deficits and affects approximately 1:30,000 Americans (Kohl et al. 2002). Those achromats exhibit total color vision loss, relatively stable central vision loss, and visual acuity of 20/200 or worse (Kohl et al. 2005), usually making them legally blind. Since these individuals see the world only with their rods, they experience photophobia or 'daytime blindness' because their rods become light-saturated in normal bright light conditions.

73.1.1 Clinical Manifestations

Clinically, the first signs of achromatopsia in infants are the presence of nystagmus, a pendular quivering of the eyes, and photophobia as evidenced by squinting in bright light (Kohl et al. 2005). Infants can be tested by the cone ERG, and, as they mature they can be given specific tests such as the Sloan Achromatopsia Test.

73.1.2 Current Achromatopsia Treatments

There are no treatments available that correct cone function in achromats to any degree. Current standard of care consists of managing symptoms by limiting retinal light exposure with tinted contact lenses (Park and Sunness 2004), and (or) very darkly tinted sunglasses (Young et al. 1982, 1983). Tinted central contact lenses typically transmitting light at wavelengths between 400 and 480 nm (Park and Sunness 2004) are an improvement over simple cutoff filters in alleviating photophobia (Schornack et al. 2007). Additionally, these contacts have reduced the stigma of wearing dark wraparound sunglasses indoors. However, such red central contacts only reduce the amount of light entering the retina and do nothing to improve high-resolution vision or color sensitive tasks. A partial solution is to use tinted contact lenses with magnification to boost what central vision is still present from functional photoreceptors (Fonda and Thomas 1974). With respect to visual acuity, improvement can be obtained by employing microscopic eyewear, enlarged print and closed circuit TV. Even with the best external aid techniques in place, daily tasks such as driving and going to school present significant obstacles. This is especially problematic for school age children because of the usual color-based curriculum; in this context tinted lenses have been tested (Schiefer et al. 1995). A common result of these symptoms is that achromats often gravitate towards activities normally performed in the evening or in low light.

73.2 Genetics of Human Achromatopsia

Autosomal recessive mutations in predominantly three genes, *CNGB3*, *CNGA3*, and *GNAT2*, cause achromatopsia (Kohl et al. 1998, 2000, 2002, 2005; Sundin et al.

2000; Aligianis et al. 2002). *CNGB3* encodes the beta subunit of the cone cyclic nucleotide-gated cation channel and *CNGA3* encodes the alpha subunit. *GNAT2* encodes the cone specific alpha subunit of transducin. Of all mutations that cause complete achromatopsia, those in *CNGB3* account for about 50% of cases whereas *CNGA3* mutations account for about 23% and *GNAT2* mutations for about 2% (Wissinger et al. 2001; Kohl et al. 2002, 2005; Aligianis et al. 2002). The majority of *CNGB3* mutations result no protein or protein truncations that are functionally null (Kohl et al. 2005). In contrast, *CNGA3* mutations are predominantly missense (Wissinger et al. 2001; Kohl et al. 2005). Recently, a Japanese patient with congenital achromatopsia was identified with compound heterozygous mutations in *CNGA3* (Goto-Omoto et al. 2006).

73.2.1 *GNAT2 Achromatopsia*

Genetic analysis points to several classes of mutations in the *GNAT2* gene that give rise to the similar phenotypes. Kohl et al. (2002) analyzed 77 achromatopsia patients with *GNAT2* mutations and identified six distinct disease-related sequence alterations that segregated in five apparently independent families of European descent. There was one nonsense mutation, four small deletion and/or insertion mutations and a sixth mutation containing a large intragenic deletion of 2,019 bp including exon 4 and flanking intron sequences. All mutations resulted in premature translation termination or in mutant polypeptides that lack considerable portions of the carboxyl terminus. In rods the conserved carboxyl terminus of the corresponding rod α-transducin contains major sites of interaction with photo-excited rhodopsin (Cai et al. 2001). Considering the high conservation between the rod and cone transducin α-subunits, a similar structural function is likely to exist in the cone system, and thus explain the carboxy-terminal mutations. Accordingly, Kohl et al. (2002) suggest that all mutations in these achromatopsia families represent effectively null alleles of *GNAT2*, which prevent either the formation of a functional heterotrimeric G-protein complex or its interaction with excited photopigments. Additionally, Aligianis et al. (2002) identified a consanguineous Pakistani family with six members having autosomal recessive achromatopsia. The deduced frameshift mutation in exon 7 of *GNAT2* is different from the one described by Kohl et al. (2002), suggesting that the complete spectrum of *GNAT2* mutations causing achromatopsia is not yet known. Additionally, it is important to note that not all mutations in what would appear to be 'important' *GNAT2* domains cause disease. Although lysine 270 of GNAT2 has been suggested by modeling to play a key role in fixing the purine ring of GTP in the nucleotide binding cleft of GNAT2, when Pina et al. (2004) examined the phenotype of a K270 deletion in homozygous carriers, segregation analysis showed that the deletion is not co-inherited with the disease phenotype and, therefore, is not the disease causing mutation. Presumably, GNAT2 function is not altered by K270 deletion possibly because of a compensatory effect of K271. Thus, GNAT2 is able to structurally and functionally tolerate a K270 deletion as shown by its ability to support normal cone function.

73.2.2 CNG Achromatopsia

Cones like rods rely on cyclic nucleotide gated (CNG) channels for membrane hyperpolarization and signal transduction upon light absorption. Heterotetrameric cation channels in rods and cones form a central pore, with the occupancy of cGMP binding sites on each subunit regulating pore formation. Six genes control CNG expression in mammals, four alpha subunits (CNGA1-4) and two beta subunits (CNGB1 and CNGB3) (Bradley et al. 2001). CNGA subunits can form functional homomeric proteins, while CNGB subunits must be associated with CNGA subunits to form functional channels (Kaupp and Seifert 2002). Two classes of CNGA subunits are found in vertebrate retinas: CNGA1 is expressed in rod outer segments and CNGA3 is expressed in cones. The latter is also expressed in sperm, kidney, cardiac and brain cells. Cone CNG channels consist of two A3 subunits and two B3 subunits (Bradley et al. 2005; Peng et al. 2004).

In humans, cone photoreceptor function loss due to *CNGB3* gene mutations is known as achromatopsia 1 (Khan et al. 2007). Achromatopsia 2 is caused by *CNGA3* gene mutation. In European populations about 25% of patients with complete achromatopsia have *CNGA3* mutations (Kaupp and Seifert 2002; Kohl et al. 2005), and another 50% have *CNGB3* mutations (Wissinger et al. 2001).

73.2.3 Achromatopsia Gene Therapy

Thus far mutations causing achromatopsia disrupt either G-protein signaling (*GNAT2*) or cGMP gated cation channel function (*CNGB3* and *CNGA3*). Since these mutations appear to result in a relatively stationary cone phenotype and therefore human achromats do not generally experience severe retinal degeneration as is seen with other diseases such as Leber's Congenital Amaurosis. However, recent adaptive optics analysis of achromats with *CNGB3* mutation suggests foveal structural abnormalities (Carroll et al. 2008). Taken together, achromatopsia is a potentially viable candidate for gene therapy where animal models exist for all three major genetic forms of disease in which to test this hypothesis.

73.3 The Mutant Gnat2 Mouse and Gene Therapy

The *Gnat2^{cpfl3}* mouse carries a recessive mutation in its cone α-transducin gene that results in cone mediated vision loss, little or no cone-mediated ERG and poor visual acuity, all of which are similar to the corresponding human form of achromatopsia (Chang et al. 2006; Alexander et al. 2007). Homozygous *Gnat2^{cpfl3}* mice were treated with a single subretinal injection of an AAV serotype 5 vector (4×10^{10} vector genome containing particles) carrying a wild type mouse *Gnat2* cDNA under control of a human red cone opsin promoter that targets vector transgene expression to cones in mice (Alexander et al. 2007). In treated eyes, light-adapted (cone specific) ERG responses were stably restored to within the normal amplitude range for at least 7 months (Alexander et al. 2007). Cone ERG amplitudes in untreated eyes remained undetectable. Furthermore, visual acuity was restored to normal levels as deduced through optomotor behavioral testing. These encouraging results suggest that long term, effective cone-targeted therapy is possible, providing a basis for treating a variety of related diseases. Additional testing has revealed that treated eyes also respond to cone isolating flicker ERG stimuli more robustly than untreated contralateral eyes (Fig. 73.1) further confirming the efficacy to cone-target gene therapy in this model of achromatopsia.

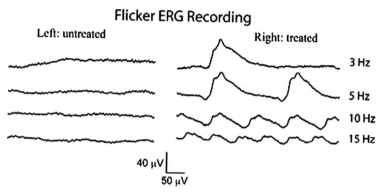

Fig. 73.1 Light-adapted flicker ERGs recorded from a *cpfl3* mouse (homozygous recessive Gnat2 mutation) at 7 months after subretinal injection of AAV vector. The *right eye* was vector treated and the *left eye* was untreated as a control. For the flicker ERG series, mice were exposed to flashes of 2.5 cd·s/m^2 at 3, 5, 10, and 15 Hz in the presence of a 30 cd s/m^2 background light

73.3.1 The Cnga3 Mutant Mouse and Gene Therapy

Recently a new mouse with a cone function loss, *cpfl5* (Cone Photoreceptor Function Loss 5) mice, that has an ocular phenotype similar to human achromatopsia was discovered in The Jackson Laboratory. *Cpfl5* is a naturally occurring mouse model of autosomal recessive achromatopsia as defined by a missense mutation in exon 5 of the *Cnga3* gene (Hawes et al. 2006). Functional studies found no cone ERG response. Histological and immunohistochemical analysis revealed a migration of cone cell bodies into the outer plexiform layer of the retina from as early as postnatal week 3 suggesting early pathogenesis.

To test whether AAV-mediated *Cnga3* gene therapy could restore cone function to *cpfl5* mice, we delivered an AAV vector encoding the wild type mouse *Cnga3* gene driven by a human blue cone promoter (HB570) that preferentially targeted transgene expression to cones to *cpfl5* mice. About 1 μl of AAV5-HB570-*Cnga3* vector (1 × 10¹⁰ genome containing viral particles) was injected subretinally into one eye of 10 *cpfl5* mice and the untreated contralateral eyes were used as controls. Treatment was at postnatal day 14 (P14) before the cone degeneration initiated. Dark- and light-adapted ERGs were recorded periodically from 3 to 10 weeks after injections. In the treated eyes, measurable light-adapted ERG signals were observed at 3 weeks after vector administration. This restored light-adapted ERGs remained stable for at least 2 months after treatment (Fig. 73.2) with b-wave amplitudes about half of that recorded in normal *C57BL/6 J* mice. In the contralateral untreated eyes, cone-driven ERGs remained unrecordable. Dark-adapted ERG analysis confirmed that the rod function is normal and unaffected by vector treatment in *cpfl5* mice at this age (Fig. 73.2).

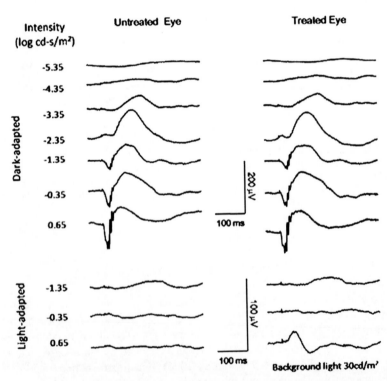

Fig. 73.2 Subretinal administration of AAV5-HB570-cnga3 vector restores the cone-driven function in *cpfl5* mouse. Representative ERGs recorded at 2 months after treatment at P14. The *left column* shows ERGs of an untreated control eye and the *right column* shows ERGs of the contralateral vector treated eye. Comparison between eyes demonstrates that gene transfer restored cone-driven function. Dark-adapted ERGs of the two eyes are comparable, suggesting the treatment had minimal effects on normal rod-driven ERGs in these mice

73.3.2 *The Cngb3 Mutant Dog and Gene Therapy*

One autosomal recessive canine disease that occurs naturally in the Alaskan Malamute has been found to be related to *CNGB3* mutations. Its phenotype is similar to human achromatopsia, and is characterized by day-blindness and absence of retinal cone function (Sidjanin et al. 2002). Since *CNGB3* mutations account for 50% of human achromatopsia, this dog provides a valuable large animal model for exploring disease mechanisms and evaluating potential genetic therapeutic intervention (Sidjanin et al. 2002).

AAV-mediated gene therapy in this canine model of achromatopsia has achieved major therapeutic effect (Komaromy et al. 2008). ERG restoration has been observed and maintained for over 14 months in the *CNGB3* Malamute following a subretinal injection of an AAV5 vector containing human *CNGB3* cDNA controlled by a truncated human red cone opsin promoter (Komaromy et al. 2008).

73.4 Prospects for Achromatopsia Gene Therapy

AAV mediated gene transfer of the corresponding wild type gene corrects cone functional deficiencies in two mouse models and one dog model representing all three (*Gnat3, Cnga3* and *CNGB3*) genetic forms of human achromatopsia. Such intervention effectively restores cone system function as demonstrated by ERGs and/ or by visually elicited behavior. These data suggests achromatopsia may be a viable candidate for gene-based therapy.

Acknowledgment This research is supported by NIH grants, EY018331, EY13729, EY11123, NS36302, EY08571, EY007758 and FFB, MVRF, RPB, Lions of Central NY.

References

Alexander JJ, Yumiko Umino Y, Everhart D et al (2007) Restoration of cone vision in a mouse model of achromatopsia. Nat Med 13:685–687

Aligianis IA, Forshew T, Johnson S et al (2002) Mapping of a novel locus for achromatopsia (ACHM4) to 1p and identification of a germline mutation in the alpha subunit of cone transducin (GNAT2). J Med Genet 39:656–660

Bradley J, Frings S, Yau KW et al (2001) Nomenclature for ion channel subunits. Science 294:209–2096

Bradley J, Reisert J, Frings S (2005) Regulation of cyclic nucleotide gated channels. Curr Opin Neurobiol 15:343–349

Cai K, Itoh Y, Khorana HG (2001) Mapping of contact sites in complex formation between transducin and light-activated rhodopsin by covalent crosslinking: use of a photoactivatable reagent. PNAS 98:4877–4882

Carroll J, Choi SS, Williams DR (2008) In vivo imaging of the photoreceptor mosaic of a rod monochromat. Vis Res 48(26):2564–2568

Chang B, Dacey MS, Hawes NL et al (2006) Cone photoreceptor function loss-3, a novel mouse model of achromatopsia due to a mutation in Gnat2. Invest Ophthalmol Vis Sci 47:5017–5021

Fonda G, Thomas H (1974) Correction of low visual acuity in achromatopsia. Use of corrective lenses as an aid to educational and vocational placement. Arch Ophthalmol 91:20–23

Goto-Omoto S, Hayashi T, Gekka T et al (2006) Compound heterozygous CNGA3 mutations (R436W, L633P) in a Japanese patient with congenital achromatopsia. Vis Neurosci 23:395–402

Hawes NL, Wang X, Hurd RE et al (2006) A point mutation in the *Cnga3* gene causes cone photoreceptor function loss (cpfl5) in mice. Paper presented at ARVO, E Abstract–4579, Fort Lauderdale, April 30 to May 4, 2006

Kaupp UB, Seifert R (2002) Cyclic nucleotide gated ion channels. Physiol Rev 82:769–824

Khan NW, Wissinger B, Kohl S et al (2007) *CNGB3* achromatopsia with progressive loss of residual cone function and impaired rod-mediated function. Invest Ophthalmol Vis Sci 48:3864–3871

Kohl S, Baumann B, Broghammer M et al (2000) Mutations in the CNGB3 gene encoding the beta-subunit of the cone photoreceptor cGMP-gated channel are responsible for achromatopsia (ACHM3) linked to chromosome 8q21. Hum Mol Genet 9:2107–2116

Kohl S, Baumann B, Rosenberg T et al (2002) Mutations in the cone photoreceptor G-protein alpha-subunit gene GNAT2 in patients with achromatopsia. Am J Hum Genet 71:422–425

Kohl S, Marx T, Giddings I et al (1998) Total color blindness is caused by mutations in the gene encoding the alpha-subunit of the cone photoreceptor cGMP-gated cation channel. Nat Genet 19:257–259

Kohl S, Varsanyi B, Antunes GA et al (2005) CNGB3 mutations account for 50% of all cases with autosomal recessive achromatopsia. Eur J Hum Genet 13:302–308

Komaromy AM, Alexander JJ, Chiodo AV et al (2008) Long-term rescue of cone function in a canine model of achromatopsia by rAAV-mediated gene therapy. Paper presented at ARVO, E Abstract–1131, Fort Lauderdale, April 27 to May 1, 2008

Park WL, Sunness JS (2004) Red contact lenses for alleviation of photophobia in patients with cone disorders. Am J Ophthalmol 137:774–775

Peng C, Rich ED, Varnum MD (2004) Subunit configuration of heteromeric cone cyclic nucleotide gated channels. Neuron 42:401–410

Pina AL, Baumert U, Loyer M et al (2004) A three base pair deletion encoding the amino acid (lysine-270) in the alpha-cone transducin gene. Mol Vis 10:265–271

Schiefer U, Kurtenbach A, Braun E et al (1995) Centrally tinted contact lenses. A useful visual aid for patients with achromatopsia. Ger J Ophthalmol 4:52–56

Schornack MM, Brown WL, Siemsen DW (2007) The use of tinted contact lenses in the management of achromatopsia. Optometry 78:17–22

Sidjanin DJ, Lowe JK, McElwee JL et al (2002) Canine *CNGB3* mutations establish cone degeneration as orthologous to the human achromatopsia locus ACHM3. Hum Mol Genet 11:1823–1833

Sundin OH, Yang JM, Li Y et al (2000) Genetic basis of total colorblindness among the Pingelapese islanders. Nat Genet 25:289–293

Wissinger B, Gamer D, Jagle H et al (2001) CNGA3 mutations in hereditary cone photoreceptor disorders. Am J Hum Genet 69:722–737

Young RS, Krefman RA, Anderson RJ et al (1983) Two additional benefits of dark glasses on rod vision in patients with congenital achromatopsia. Am J Optom Physiol Opt 60:56–60

Young RS, Krefmanm RA, Fishman GA (1982) Visual improvements with red-tinted glasses in a patient with cone dystrophy. Arch Ophthalmol 100:268–271

Chapter 74
Function and Mechanism of CNTF/LIF Signaling in Retinogenesis

Kun Do Rhee and Xian-Jie Yang

Abstract Ciliary neurotrophic factor (CNTF) and leukemia inhibitory factor (LIF) exhibit multiple biological effects in the developing vertebrate retina. CNTF/LIF inhibits rod photoreceptor, and promotes bipolar cells and Muller glia differentiation. In addition, CNTF/LIF has been shown to have proliferative and apoptotic effects. Moreover, LIF also inhibits retinal vascular development. CNTF/LIF signaling components CNTFRα, LIFRβ, gp130, and a number of STAT proteins are expressed in the retina. CNTF/LIF activates Jak-STAT, ERK, and Notch pathways during retinal development. Perturbation of CNTF induced signal transduction reveals that different combinations of CNTF/LIF signaling pathways regulate differentiation of retinal neurons and glia. Gene expression studies show that CNTF/LIF affects retinogenesis by regulating various genes involved in transcription, signal transduction, protein modification, apoptosis, protein localization, and cell ion homeostasis. Most past studies have deployed ectopic expression or addition of exogenous CNTF/LIF, thus further analysis of mice with conditional mutations in CNTF/LIF signaling components will allow better understanding of in-vivo functions of CNTF/LIF associated signaling events in retinogenesis.

74.1 Introduction

The mature vertebrate retina consists of seven major neuronal cell types generated from a common progenitor pool. Lineage tracing analyses using retrovirus infection and fluorescent dye single cell injection have shown that retinal progenitor cells are multipotent and cell fates are specified during or after their terminal mitosis (Wetts and Fraser 1988; Turner et al. 1990). Molecular genetic studies have further

K.D. Rhee (✉)
Jules Stein Eye Institute, Molecular Biology Institute, University of California, Los Angeles, CA, USA
e-mail: kdrhee@ucla.edu

R.E. Anderson et al. (eds.), *Retinal Degenerative Diseases*, Advances in Experimental Medicine and Biology 664, DOI 10.1007/978-1-4419-1399-9_74,
© Springer Science+Business Media, LLC 2010

647

demonstrated that retinal cell fates are regulated by both cell intrinsic and extrinsic mechanisms. A proposed model suggests that progenitors pass through a series of intrinsically determined competence states, and under each state, progenitors are capable of giving rise to a limited subset of cell types under the influence of extrinsic signals (Livesey and Cepko 2001). Various signal molecules have been shown to influence retinal cell differentiation either positively or negatively (Levine et al. 2000; Yang 2004). Among them, ciliary neurotrophic factor (CNTF) and leukemia inhibitory factor (LIF), members of the interleukin (IL)-6 family of cytokines, exhibit multiple biological effects in the developing vertebrate retina.

CNTF/LIF family of cytokines bind to a tripartite receptor complex consisting of two single membrane spanning beta-receptor subunits and an additional alpha receptor specific for certain members of the cytokine family (Ip, 1998). CNTF/LIF triggers multiple intracellular signaling events, including activation of the Janus kinases (Jak)-Signal Transducer and Activator of Transcription (STAT), the extracellular signal-regulated kinases (ERK) (Boulton et al. 1994) and the phosphatidylinositol 3 kinase (PI3K)-Akt pathways (Oh et al. 1998).

74.2 Effects of CNTF/LIF on Photoreceptor and Bipolar Neuron Differentiation

CNTF/LIF has been shown to strongly inhibit differentiation of rod photoreceptors in both mouse and rat retinas (Ezzeddine et al. 1997; Neophytou et al. 1997; Kirsch et al. 1998; Schulz-Key et al. 2002; Sherry et al. 2005; Elliott et al. 2006). Both CNTFRα and LIFRβ knockout retinas display increased proportions of rod photoreceptors when cultured as explants for 10 days in-vitro starting from postnatal day 0 (Ezzeddine et al. 1997). In contrast, in a chicken retinal culture, CNTF appears to promote the differentiation of a subclass of cone photoreceptors (Fuhrmann et al. 1995; Xie and Adler 2000). Consistent with the observed influence of CNTF/LIF on photoreceptor development in-vitro, retinas of transgenic mice that misexpress LIF from the alpha crystallin promoter during embryonic development show dose-dependent disruption of photoreceptor differentiation (Graham et al. 2005).

In addition to their effects on photoreceptor development, CNTF/LIF also regulates other late born retinal cell types. Concomitant to suppression of rod differentiation, CNTF/LIF promotes the expression of several bipolar cell markers in the postnatal retina (Ezzeddine et al. 1997; Schulz-Key et al. 2002; Bhattacharya et al. 2004; Zahir et al. 2005). By tracking cell birthdates and analyzing proportions of different cell markers, Ezzeddine et al. (1997) concluded that the bipolar marker-positive cells are derived from cells that would normally give rise to rod photoreceptors. This result indicates that CNTF/LIF affects the differentiation process of immature postmitotic neuronal precursors. They also observed that once rod cells begin to express rhodopsin protein, they become increasingly resistant to the inhibitory effects of CNTF. Consistent with this observation, Schulz-Key et al. (2002) showed that retinal explants treated with CNTF contain bipolar marker-positive cells in the outer nuclear layer and greatly reduced opsin-positive cells. Yet, the suppression of rhodopsin and upregulation of bipolar markers are reversible (Schulz-Key et al. 2002). This effect is interesting as rod and bipolar cells are derived from common postnatal progenitor cells that share key transcription factors including Otx2 and Crx (Furukawa et al. 1997; Koike et al. 2007). Nonetheless, transgenic mice that overexpress LIF during embryogenesis do not overproduce bipolar cells in-vivo (Sherry et al. 2005), suggesting that timing and/or duration of signaling may play a role in the cellular effects.

In contrast to in-vitro studies where rod photoreceptor differentiation is blocked, Elliott et al. (2006) reports that misexpressing CNTF during development in-vivo causes reduction of photoreceptors resulting from the cell death of postmitotic rod precursors. In this study, mouse retinas were infected at P2 with an adenovirus encoding a secretable CNTF. When analyzed at P32, the outer nuclear layer (ONL) was considerable thinner than the control and TUNEL positive apoptotic cells were observed in ONL. The authors argue that the enhanced cell death was due to activation of cytokine signaling, which positively regulates nitric oxide production to influence developmental programmed cell death. Unlike the previous studies, there was no change in the number of bipolar cells. Interestingly, embryonic misexpression of LIF results in broad defects of multiple retinal cell types and abnormal synaptogenesis, including disruption of bipolar cells and ganglion cells (Sherry et al. 2005).

74.3 Effects of CNTF/LIF on Muller Glia Genesis and Late Progenitor Proliferation

CNTF promotes astrocyte development in the central nervous system (Bonni et al. 1993; Rajan and McKay 1998). In the mouse retina, CNTF enhances the production of Muller glia in-vitro up to 3-folds (Goureau et al. 2004). As Muller glial cells are the last born cells in the vertebrate retina, this Muller glia promotion effect maybe linked to the proliferative effects of CNTF detected during the late neurogenic phase. Goureau et al. (2004) observe a 2- to 3-fold increase in BrdU-positive cells only when retinal explants were labeled with BrdU from P5-P6, but not from P0 to P3, despite a continuous exposure to CNTF from P0. Furthermore, BrdU-positive cells were found to co-label with Muller glial markers GFAP and CRALBP. Therefore, CTF/LIF may promote cell proliferation of the residual progenitors before the completion of retinogenesis, leading to an increased number of progenitor cells adopting Muller glial fate.

74.4 Effects of LIF Misexpression on Retinal Vasculature Development

The development of retinal vasculature involves multiple cell types including endothelial cells, astrocytes, pericytes, and Muller glia. Developing retinal ganglion cells are known to express vascular endothelial growth factor (VEGF) (Yang and Cepko 1996; Hashimoto et al. 2003) among other growth factors. In transgenic mice overexpressing LIF from the embryonic lens, the retinal vascular development is severely retarded and the expression of VEGF is aberrantly elevated (Ash et al. 2005). The potential normal functions of LIF-like cytokines in retinal vessel development remain to be explored.

74.5 Expression of CNTF/LIF Signaling Components in the Developing Retina

Multiple CNTF/LIF signaling components are detected in the developing vertebrate retina (Kirsch and Hofmann 1994; Kirsch et al. 1997; Rhee and Yang 2003; Zhang et al. 2003; Hertle et al. 2008). In the postnatal mouse retina, immunolabeling has detected the expression of gp130, CNTFRα, Jak kinases, STAT1, and STAT3 proteins at low levels in the proliferative zone and at higher levels in the plexiform layers as well as in the ganglion cell layer and horizontal cells (Rhee and Yang 2003). In addition to STAT1 and STAT3, STAT2, 4, 5, 6 are also expressed in the developing retina (Zhang et al. 2003). Thus, the necessary components required for cytokine signaling are present in the retina.

CNTFRα has been defined as the specific receptor required for CNTF binding and signaling. However, its location in the retina remains controversial. In the mouse retina, CNTFRα protein was detected at low levels in the proliferative zone and localized to the inner and outer segments of mature photoreceptor cells (Rhee and Yang 2003). Hertle et al. (2008) analyzed presumptive and differentiating ONL using laser-caption and RT-PCR, and showed that both LIFRβ and CNTFRα are expressed in the immature rat photoreceptors. Using immunocytochemistry and several anti-CNTFRα antibodies, Beltran et al. (2005) detected CNTFRα localization to the photoreceptors of adult non-rodent mammalian retinas but not to the rodent retinas. Using laser caption and single cell RT-PCR, Wahlin et al. (2004) detected CNTFRα expression in the mouse Muller cells but not in photoreceptors.

74.6 Signaling Events Triggered by CNTF/LIF During Retinogenesis

Analysis of CNTF/LIF signal transduction involved in retinogenesis has revealed activation of different signaling pathways, including Jak-STAT, ERK, and Notch pathways. Both in-vitro and in-vivo results demonstrate that only the Jak-STAT pathway is involved in the inhibition of rod photoreceptor differentiation by CNTF/LIF (Ozawa et al. 2004; Rhee et al. 2004; Zhang et al. 2004). Using antibodies that recognizing phosphorylated STAT proteins (pSTAT) and serine/threonine phosphorylated ERK1/2 (pERK1/2), we provide evidence that both STAT and ERK are rapidly activated by CNTF in the neonatal mouse retina (Rhee et al. 2004).

Interestingly, the pSTAT3 and pERK1/2 are distributed differently in the retina, with pERK1/2 predominantly activated in progenitor cells and pSTAT3 primarily activated in postmitotic ganglion cells and amacrine cells. In addition, STAT3 is activated by CNTF in newly postmitotic Crx-positive rod precursors located near the ventricular surface. Disruption of the two signaling pathways in-vitro using pharmacological inhibitors and dominant negative STAT mutant showed that CNTF/LIF inhibition of rod differentiation requires activation of the Jak-STAT, but not the ERK pathway (Rhee et al. 2004; Zhang et al. 2004). Consistent with the in-vitro findings, in mice that carry conditional deletion of STAT3 in the peripheral retina, CNTF inhibition of photoreceptor differentiation is blocked (Ozawa et al. 2004). In contrast, in the gp130 ^{F759} knockin mouse, which encodes a SHP2 binding site mutant (gp130^{F759}) that blocks the PI3K and ERK pathways without interfering with the Jak-STAT pathway, CNTF inhibition of rod differentiation is not affected (Ozawa et al. 2004).

In contrast to the inhibitory effect on rod differentiation, promotion of Muller glial development by CNTF/LIF appears to involve several signaling pathways. Blocking signaling by pathway specific inhibitors or STAT mutant indicates that activation of both Jak-STAT and ERK are involved in gliogenesis (Goureau et al. 2004). Recently, Bhattacharya et al. (2008) reports that CNTF/LIF regulates neuronal versus glial differentiation of progenitors in the neural sphere culture via ERK, Jak-STAT, and Notch signaling pathways. Their results show that low concentrations of CNTF activates ERK pathway to promote bipolar cell differentiation, whereas high concentrations activates Jak-STAT pathway to promote Muller glia differentiation. In addition, dominant negative MAPK (dnMAPK) abolished bipolar cell differentiation and dominant negative STAT3 (dnSTAT3) abolished Muller glia differentiation. Furthermore, Notch pathway activation plus CNTF treatment inhibited bipolar differentiation, but promoted Muller glia differentiation. Moreover, disruption of Notch and Jak-STAT pathways promoted differentiation of rod photoreceptors. These results are consistent with previously reported functions of CNTF and Notch effectors in Muller glia genesis (Furukawa et al. 2000; Hojo et al. 2000; Satow et al. 2001). In addition, Zhang et al. (2005) showed that Hes1 was upregulated with STAT3 overexpresseion, and perturbation of Jak-STAT pathway using dnSTAT3 eliminated co-labeling of pSTAT3 with progenitor marker Hes1. These results are further supported by the recent finding that STAT3 co-oscillates with Hes1 (Yoshiura et al. 2007).

74.7 CNTF/LIF Regulate Numerous Genes Involved in Retinogenesis

CNTF/LIF regulates broad categories of genes during retinal development. Real-time RT-PCR shows that CNTF/LIF inhibits phototransduction genes, Crx, Nrl and Nr2e3 (Ozawa et al. 2004; Graham et al. 2005). Low levels of CNTF promote bipolar differentiation, and upregulate transcription factors Ath3, Chx10 and mGluR6, while down regulate both Hes1 and Hes5 (Bhattacharya et al. 2004, 2008). As expected, high levels of CNTF promote Muller glia genesis and upregulate vimentin, Notch1, GFAP, GS, and Hes5. When perturbation of both Jak-STAT and Notch pathways increased rod photoreceptor differentiation, both Nrl and Otx transcription factors were elevated.

Subtractive hybridization has identified pleiotrophin (Ptn), which is upregulated when P0 retinal explants are exposed to CNTF/LIF (Roger et al. 2006). Overexpression of Ptn inhibits rod differentiation and promotes bipolar cell differentiation mimicking CNTF/LIF effects in retinogenesis. Further analysis revealed 7 genes upregulated and 17 genes downregulated after 6 days of CNTF treatment and these were classified into six categories involving in transcription regulation, signal transduction, protein modification, apoptosis, protein localization and cell ion homeostasis (Roger et al. 2007). These studies show that CNTF/LIF potently influences retinogenesis via regulation of numerous genes.

74.8 Perspective

Despite studies showing effects of CNTF/LIF in retinogenesis, the majority of the studies involves misexpression of genes or addition of exogenous CNTF/LIF in-vitro or in-vivo. Thus, endogenous functions of CNTF/LIF signaling events in retinogenesis remain to be examined by using advanced molecular genetic approaches. Nonetheless, current evidence establishes CNTF/LIF as potent growth factor agents that can affect retinal neuronal differentiation and survival.

References

Ash J, McLeod DS, Lutty GA (2005) Transgenic expression of leukemia inhibitory factor (LIF) blocks normal vascular development but not pathological neovascularization in the eye. Mol Vis 11:298–308

Beltran WA, Rohrer H, Aguirre GD (2005) Immunolocalization of ciliary neurotrophic factor receptor alpha (CNTFRalpha) in mammalian photoreceptor cells. Mol Vis 11:232–244

Bhattacharya S, Das AV, Mallya KB et al (2008) Ciliary neurotrophic factor-mediated signaling regulates neuronal versus glial differentiation of retinal stem cells/progenitors by concentration-dependent recruitment of mitogen-activated protein kinase and Janus kinase-signal transducer and activator of transcription pathways in conjunction with Notch signaling. Stem Cells 26:2611–2624

Bhattacharya S, Dooley C, Soto F et al (2004) Involvement of Ath3 in CNTF-mediated differentiation of the late retinal progenitors. Mol Cell Neurosci 27:32–43

Bonni A, Frank DA, Schindler C et al (1993) Characterization of a pathway for ciliary neurotrophic factor signaling to the nucleus. Science 262:1575–1579

Boulton TG, Stahl N, Yancopoulos GD (1994) Ciliary neurotrophic factor/leukemia inhibitory factor/interleukin 6/oncostatin M family of cytokines induces tyrosine phosphorylation of a common set of proteins overlapping those induced by other cytokines and growth factors. J Biol Chem 269:11648–11655

Elliott J, Cayouette M, Gravel C (2006) The CNTF/LIF signaling pathway regulates developmental programmed cell death and differentiation of rod precursor cells in the mouse retina in vivo. Dev Biol 300:583–598

Ezzeddine ZD, Yang X, DeChiara T et al (1997) Postmitotic cells fated to become rod photoreceptors can be respecified by CNTF treatment of the retina. Development 124:1055–1067

Fuhrmann S, Kirsch M, Hofmann HD (1995) Ciliary neurotrophic factor promotes chick photoreceptor development in vitro. Development 121:2695–2706

Furukawa T, Morrow EM, Cepko CL (1997) Crx, a novel otx-like homeobox gene, shows
photoreceptor-specific expression and regulates photoreceptor differentiation. Cell 91:
531–541

Furukawa T, Mukherjee S, Bao ZZ et al (2000) rax, Hes1, and notch1 promote the formation of
Muller glia by postnatal retinal progenitor cells. Neuron 26:383–394

Goureau O, Rhee KD, Yang XJ (2004) Ciliary neurotrophic factor promotes muller glia differentiation from the postnatal retinal progenitor pool. Dev Neurosci 26:359–370

Graham DR, Overbeek PA, Ash JD (2005) Leukemia inhibitory factor blocks expression of Crx
and Nrl transcription factors to inhibit photoreceptor differentiation. Invest Ophthalmol Vis Sci
46:2601–2610

Hashimoto T, Zhang XM, Yang XJ (2003) Expression of the Flk1 receptor and its ligand VEGF in
the developing chick central nervous system. Gene Expr Patterns 3:109–113

Hertle D, Schleichert M, Steup A et al (2008) Regulation of cytokine signaling components in
developing rat retina correlates with transient inhibition of rod differentiation by CNTF. Cell
Tissue Res 334:7–16

Hojo M, Ohtsuka T, Hashimoto N et al (2000) Glial cell fate specification modulated by the bHLH
gene Hes5 in mouse retina. Development 127:2515–2522

Ip NY (1998) The neurotrophins and neuropoietic cytokines: two families of growth factors acting
on neural and hematopoietic cells. Ann N Y Acad Sci 840:97–106

Kirsch M, Hofmann HD (1994) Expression of ciliary neurotrophic factor receptor mRNA and
protein in the early postnatal and adult rat nervous system. Neurosci Lett 180:163–166

Kirsch M, Lee MY, Meyer V et al (1997) Evidence for multiple, local functions of ciliary neurotrophic factor (CNTF) in retinal development: expression of CNTF and its receptors and in
vitro effects on target cells. J Neurochem 68:979–990

Kirsch M, Schulz-Key S, Wiese A et al (1998) Ciliary neurotrophic factor blocks rod photoreceptor
differentiation from postmitotic precursor cells in vitro. Cell Tissue Res 291:207–216

Koike C, Nishida A, Ueno S et al (2007) Functional roles of Otx2 transcription factor in postnatal
mouse retinal development. Mol Cell Biol 27:8318–8329

Levine EM, Fuhrmann S, Reh TA (2000) Soluble factors and the development of rod photoreceptors. Cell Mol Life Sci 57:224–234

Livesey FJ, Cepko CL (2001) Vertebrate neural cell-fate determination: lessons from the retina.
Nat Rev Neurosci 2:109–118

Neophytou C, Vernallis AB, Smith A et al (1997) Muller-cell-derived leukaemia inhibitory factor arrests rod photoreceptor differentiation at a postmitotic pre-rod stage of development.
Development 124:2345–2354

Oh H, Fujio Y, Kunisada K et al (1998) Activation of phosphatidylinositol 3-kinase through glycoprotein 130 induces protein kinase B and p70 S6 kinase phosphorylation in cardiac myocytes.
J Biol Chem 273:9703–9710

Ozawa Y, Nakao K, Shimazaki T et al (2004) Downregulation of STAT3 activation is required for
presumptive rod photoreceptor cells to differentiate in the postnatal retina. Mol Cell Neurosci
26:258–270

Rajan P, McKay RD (1998) Multiple routes to astrocytic differentiation in the CNS. J Neurosci
18:3620–3629

Rhee KD, Goureau O, Chen S et al (2004) Cytokine-induced activation of signal transducer
and activator of transcription in photoreceptor precursors regulates rod differentiation in the
developing mouse retina. J Neurosci 24:9779–9788

Rhee KD, Yang XJ (2003) Expression of cytokine signal transduction components in the postnatal
mouse retina. Mol Vis 9:715–722

Roger J, Brajeul V, Thomasseau S et al (2006) Involvement of pleiotrophin in CNTF-mediated
differentiation of the late retinal progenitor cells. Dev Biol 298:527–539

Roger J, Goureau O, Sahel JA et al (2007) Use of suppression subtractive hybridization to identify genes regulated by ciliary neurotrophic factor in postnatal retinal explants. Mol Vis 13:206–219

Satow T, Bae SK, Inoue T et al (2001) The basic helix-loop-helix gene hesr2 promotes gliogenesis in mouse retina. J Neurosci 21:1265–1273

Schulz-Key S, Hofmann HD, Beisenherz-Huss C et al (2002) Ciliary neurotrophic factor as a transient negative regulator of rod development in rat retina. Invest Ophthalmol Vis Sci 43:3099–3108

Sherry DM, Mitchell R, Li H et al (2005) Leukemia inhibitory factor inhibits neuronal development and disrupts synaptic organization in the mouse retina. J Neurosci Res 82:316–332

Turner DL, Snyder EY, Cepko CL (1990) Lineage-independent determination of cell type in the embryonic mouse retina. Neuron 4:833–845

Wahlin KJ, Lim L, Grice EA et al (2004) A method for analysis of gene expression in isolated mouse photoreceptor and Muller cells. Mol Vis 10:366–375

Wetts R, Fraser SE (1988) Multipotent precursors can give rise to all major cell types of the frog retina. Science 239:1142–1145

Xie HQ, Adler R (2000) Green cone opsin and rhodopsin regulation by CNTF and staurosporine in cultured chick photoreceptors. Invest Ophthalmol Vis Sci 41:4317–4323

Yang XJ (2004) Roles of cell-extrinsic growth factors in vertebrate eye pattern formation and retinogenesis. Semin Cell Dev Biol 15:91–103

Yang X, Cepko CL (1996) Flk-1, a receptor for vascular endothelial growth factor (VEGF), is expressed by retinal progenitor cells. J Neurosci 16:6089–6099

Yoshiura S, Ohtsuka T, Takenaka Y et al (2007) Ultradian oscillations of Stat, Smad, and Hes1 expression in response to serum. Proc Natl Acad Sci U S A 104:11292–11297

Zahir T, Klassen H, Young MJ (2005) Effects of ciliary neurotrophic factor on differentiation of late retinal progenitor cells. Stem Cells 23:424–432

Zhang SS, Liu MG, Kano A et al (2005) STAT3 activation in response to growth factors or cytokines participates in retina precursor proliferation. Exp Eye Res 81:103–115

Zhang SS, Wei JY, Li C et al (2003) Expression and activation of STAT proteins during mouse retina development. Exp Eye Res 76:421–431

Zhang SS, Wei J, Qin H et al (2004) STAT3-mediated signaling in the determination of rod photoreceptor cell fate in mouse retina. Invest Ophthalmol Vis Sci 45:2407–2412

Chapter 75
gp130 Activation in Müller Cells is Not Essential for Photoreceptor Protection from Light Damage

Yumi Ueki, Srinivas Chollangi, Yun-Zheng Le, and John D. Ash

Abstract Members of IL-6 family cytokines, such as leukemia inhibitory factor (LIF) and ciliary neurotrophic factor (CNTF), activate the common signal-transducing receptor gp130. We and others have previously shown that application of exogenous gp130 ligands promotes photoreceptor survival in light-induced and inherited retinal degeneration in animal models. While there is strong evidence that gp130 plays an essential role in photoreceptor protection, it is not clear whether protection is cell-autonomous in photoreceptors or an effect of Müller cell activation. To investigate the role of Müller cells in gp130-mediated photoreceptor protection, we have generated conditional *gp130* knockout (KO) mice in retinal Müller cells using the Cre/*lox* system. Western blot and immunohistochemical analyses show that in our conditional *gp130* KO mice, approximately 50% Müller cells no longer respond to LIF with activation of known downstream signaling proteins, STAT3 and ERK1/2. Despite the loss of gp130 activity in many Müller cells, intravitreal injection of LIF still induced significant degree of photoreceptor protection that was comparable to normal littermates. These data suggest that Müller cell activation of gp130 is not essential for photoreceptor protection, and support the hypothesis that the protection is mediated by cell-autonomous mechanisms in photoreceptors.

75.1 Introduction

Signal-transducing receptor gp130 is a common receptor for interleukin (IL)-6 family of cytokines, such as ciliary neurotrophic factor (CNTF), leukemia inhibitory factor (LIF), and cardiotropin-like cytokine (CLC). Application of exogenous gp130 ligands has been shown to promote photoreceptor survival in both light-induced and

Y. Ueki (✉)
Oklahoma Center for Neuroscience, University of Oklahoma Health Sciences Center, Oklahoma City, OK, USA

R.E. Anderson et al. (eds.), *Retinal Degenerative Diseases*, Advances in Experimental Medicine and Biology 664, DOI 10.1007/978-1-4419-1399-9_75,
© Springer Science+Business Media, LLC 2010

inherited models of retinal degeneration (LaVail et al. 1992; Cayouette et al. 1998; LaVail et al. 1998; Chong et al. 1999; Liang et al. 2001; Bok et al. 2002; Song et al. 2003).

We have shown that activation of gp130 by intravitreal injection of LIF preserves photoreceptor function and prevents photoreceptor cell death against light-induced oxidative stress (light damage) in dose-dependent manner (Ueki et al. 2008). While there is strong evidence that gp130 plays an essential role in survival of photoreceptors, the mechanism by which this is accomplished is not well established.

Activated gp130 signals through the Jak/STAT3, ERK1/2, and PI3K/Akt pathways (Boulton et al. 1994; Heinrich et al. 2003; Oh et al. 1998). In the rodent retina, activation of STAT3 and/or ERK1/2 is detected in Müller cells shortly after the injection of gp130 ligands (Wahlin et al. 2000; Peterson et al. 2000; Wen et al. 2006), suggesting that Müller cell activation of gp130 is essential for photoreceptor protection. On the other hand, our previous study has demonstrated that all retinal cells, including photoreceptors activate STAT3 at the time of light damage (Ueki et al. 2008), suggesting photoreceptor protection requires direct gp130 activation in photoreceptors. Thus, it is not known whether protection is cell autonomous in photoreceptors or an effect of Müller cell activation. The purpose of this study was to investigate whether photoreceptor protection by gp130 ligands requires activation of gp130 in Müller cells. To accomplish this, we generated conditional $gp130$ knockout mice in Müller cells using the Cre/lox system.

75.2 Conditional $gp130$ Knockout in the Retinal Müller Cells

In order to study Müller cell-specific roles of gp130 in photoreceptor protection, we have generated conditional $gp130$ knockout (KO) mice using the Cre/lox system. We have mated mice homozygous for floxed $gp130$ allele ($gp130^{f/f}$) (Betz et al. 1998) with $VMD2$-cre transgenic line (Ueki et al. 2009). $gp130^{f/f}$/$VMD2$-cre^+ mice were viable and had no apparent phenotypic abnormalities. All mice used for experiments were albino and 6- to 7-week old.

To assess the extent of cell-specific $gp130$ deletion in the retina, intravitreal injection of a gp130 ligand, leukemia inhibitory factor (LIF) was performed, and activation of known downstream signaling proteins was detected by immunohistochemistry (IHC) (Fig. 75.1). Our previous study has shown that injection of LIF can induce robust STAT3 and ERK1/2 activation in Müller cell 30 min after the injection (Ueki et al. 2008). As a result of Cre-mediated recombination of $gp130$, STAT3 and ERK1/2 activation was significantly reduced in $gp130^{f/f}$/$VMD2$-cre^+ mice 30 min after the injection and the loss was localized to Müller cells by IHC (Fig. 75.1; ERK1/2 data not shown). Our data show that approximately 50% Müller cells in $gp130^{f/f}$/$VMD2$-cre^+ retinas do not respond to gp130 ligands as a result of Cre-mediated knockout of $gp130$ (Fig. 75.1).

Fig. 75.1 Localization of activated STAT3 (pSTAT3) 30 min after intravitreal injection of LIF. PBS injection did not induce detectable activation of STAT3 (**b**). While pSTAT3 was detected in all Müller cell nuclei in the *gp130$^{f/f}$/VMD2-cre$^-$* retinas (**c**), apparent loss of STAT3 activation was observed in the *gp130$^{f/f}$/VMD2-cre$^+$* retinas (*arrowheads* in **d**). Approximately 50% of Müller cell nuclei were no longer positive for pSTAT3. onl, outer nuclear layer; inl, inner nuclear layer; gcl, ganglion cell layer. Representative images were shown (*n* = 4)

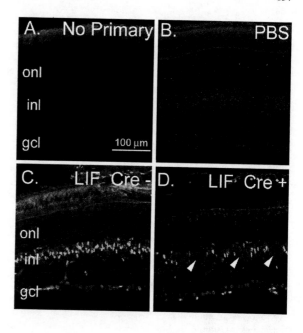

75.3 Effect of Impaired gp130 Activation in Müller Cells on LIF-Induced Photoreceptor Protection

Our previous study has demonstrated that activation of gp130 by LIF preserves photoreceptor function and prevents photoreceptor cell death from acute light damage (Ueki et al. 2008). The same acute light damage paradigm was used here to determine the role of Müller cell activation of gp130 in photoreceptor protection. Briefly, 6-week old *gp130$^{f/f}$/VMD2-cre$^+$* mice were injected intravitreally with 0.5 μg/μl of LIF (1 μl volume) into the right eyes. Phosphate-buffered saline (PBS) was injected into the left eyes, serving as an internal control. *gp130$^{f/f}$/VMD2-cre$^-$* littermates were used as controls. Mice were then exposed to 3,000 lux of white fluorescent light for 4 hours (light damage) to determine the degree of gp130-induced photoreceptor protection. ERG and histological analyses were performed after 4 days of recovery under dim cyclic light.

The scotopic ERG a-waves from 8 animals per group were averaged at each flash intensity and were plotted in Fig. 75.2. In this light damage model, *gp130$^{f/f}$/VMD2-cre$^-$* mice injected with PBS retained approximately 30% of the photoreceptor function of untreated mice (compare closed triangles and squares in Fig. 75.2). Eyes injected with LIF had significantly higher a-wave amplitudes than PBS-injected eyes (compare closed diamonds and triangles in Fig. 75.2), demonstrating LIF-induced protection of photoreceptor function. Interestingly, loss of gp130 activation in approximately 50% of Müller cells did not have any effect in protective ability of LIF (compare closed and open diamonds in Fig. 75.2).

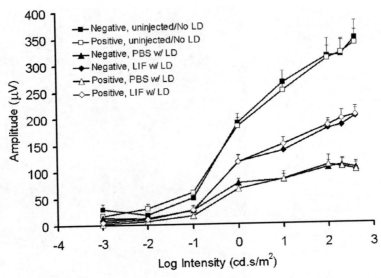

Fig. 75.2 Scotopic a-wave amplitudes. ERGs were recorded from at least 8 mice per group and the average a-wave amplitudes were plotted versus the intensity of each light flash. Compared to the normal retina (uninjected/no LD; *rectangles*), PBS-injected control group with light exposure had approximately 70% decrease in the a-wave amplitude (*triangles*). LIF-injected group (*diamonds*) preserved the a-wave amplitude significantly after the light damage compared to PBS-injected group (*triangles*). Loss of gp130 activity in Müller cells did not affect the LIF-induced preservation of photoreceptor function from light damage (compare *closed and open diamonds*). Negative, $gp130^{f/f}/VMD2\text{-}cre^-$ mice (*closed symbols*); positive, $gp130^{f/f}/VMD2\text{-}cre^+$ mice (*open symbols*); LD, light damage. Values are the means ± SEM

In order to determine the degree of light-induced cell death, eyes were collected and cross sections were obtained for histological evaluation (Fig. 75.3). Consistent with the a-wave amplitudes of scotopic ERG, loss of gp130 activation in Müller cells did not have any effect on ability of LIF to prevent photoreceptor cell death. The number of photoreceptors in $gp130^{f/f}/VMD2\text{-}cre^+$ retinas subjected to LIF injection followed by light damage was not different from that in $gp130^{f/f}/VMD2\text{-}cre^-$ controls (compare open and closed diamonds in Fig. 75.3b). Together, these results suggest that Müller cell activation of gp130 is not essential for photoreceptor protection.

75.4 Discussion

We have successfully demonstrated that approximately 50% of Müller cells in $gp130^{f/f}/VMD2\text{-}cre^+$ mice lost gp130-dependant activation of STAT3. Our data clearly demonstrate that this loss of gp130 activation in Müller cells does not impair LIF-induced photoreceptor protection from light damage. Many studies have

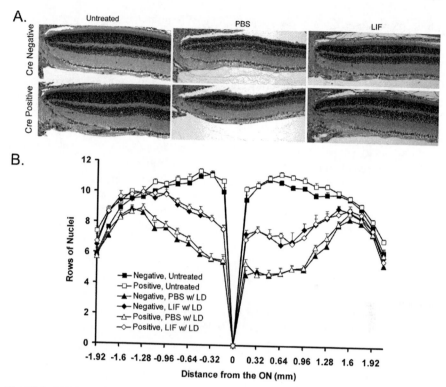

Fig. 75.3 LIF protects photoreceptors from light-induced cell death even after the loss of gp130 activity in Müller cells. (**a**) Representative histological sections through the superior retina near the optic nerve head are shown. (**b**) The number of photoreceptors lying in a single column (rows of photoreceptors) in the outer nuclear layer was counted along the vertical meridian of the eye at the optic nerve head. Untreated retinas are neither injected nor exposed to bright light. The number of photoreceptors present after light exposure was significantly higher in the LIF-injected groups (*diamonds*) compared to PBS-injected controls (*triangles*). Loss of gp130 activity in Müller cells did not affect the LIF-induced protection of photoreceptors from light-induced cell death (compare *closed and open diamonds*). Values are the means ± SEM (*n* = 8 per group)

focused on robust activation of signaling pathways in Müller cells immediately following the injection of gp130 ligands. Robust activation of ERK1/2 and STAT3 was detected in Müller cells in response to CNTF (Wahlin et al. 2000; Peterson et al. 2000; Wen et al. 2006) or LIF (Ueki et al. 2008), suggesting a possibility of indirect mechanisms of photoreceptor protection through Müller cell activation of gp130. On the other hand, our recent study demonstrated a possibility for direct mechanism of gp130-mediated photoreceptor protection through STAT3 activation in photoreceptors. While Müller cells are the first to respond to gp130 ligands, sustained activation of STAT3 was also detected progressively over time in all the retinal cells, including photoreceptors (Ueki et al. 2008). This delay in STAT3 activation in photoreceptors could be simply due to the rate of LIF diffusion through the retina. In addition, STAT3, but not ERK1/2 or Akt pathway, was active in the retina at the time of the photoreceptor protection, further suggesting a cell-autonomous mechanism of photoreceptor protection through STAT3 activation (Ueki et al. 2008). In this current study, we observed loss of both STAT3 and ERK1/2 signaling in at least 50% of Müller cells in the $gp130^{f/f}/VMD2\text{-}cre^+$ retina (Fig. 75.2; ERK1/2 data not shown). However, this loss of signaling did not affect the gp130-mediated photoreceptor protection against light-induced cell death (Figs. 75.2 and 75.3). These data support the hypothesis that the protection is mediated by cell autonomous mechanism in photoreceptors.

In summary, impaired activation of gp130 in Müller cells does not diminish gp130-mediated photoreceptor protection from light damage. A caveat to this study is that our conditional $gp130$ KO is not complete and some Müller cells still express gp130. Data from these $VMD2\text{-}cre$ mice cannot be used to conclusively rule out the possibility that remaining activated Müller cells compensate for the loss of gp130 in gp130-negative Müller cells. However, in another study to be published separately, knockout of gp130 in photoreceptors does impair gp130-mediated protection. In total, these studies provide clear evidence that gp130 activation in photoreceptors is the direct mechanism of LIF-mediated protection.

Acknowledgments This work was supported by funding from National Institute of Health (R01 EY016459, P20 RR017703, P30 EY012190), The Foundation Fighting Blindness, and an Unrestricted grant from Research to Prevent Blindness.

References

Betz UA, Bloch W, van den BM et al (1998) Postnatally induced inactivation of gp130 in mice results in neurological, cardiac, hematopoietic, immunological, hepatic, and pulmonary defects. J Exp Med 188:1955–1965

Bok D, Yasumura D, Matthes MT et al (2002) Effects of adeno-associated virus-vectored ciliary neurotrophic factor on retinal structure and function in mice with a P216L rds/peripherin mutation. Exp Eye Res 74:719–735

Boulton TG, Stahl N and Yancopoulos GD (1994) Ciliary neurotrophic factor/leukemia inhibitory factor/interleukin 6/oncostatin M family of cytokines induces tyrosine phosphorylation of a common set of proteins overlapping those induced by other cytokines and growth factors. J Biol Chem 269:11648–11655

Cayouette M, Behn D, Sendtner M et al (1998) Intraocular gene transfer of ciliary neurotrophic factor prevents death and increases responsiveness of rod photoreceptors in the retinal degeneration slow mouse. J Neurosci 18:9282–9293

Chong NH, Alexander RA, Waters L et al (1999) Repeated injections of a ciliary neurotrophic factor analogue leading to long-term photoreceptor survival in hereditary retinal degeneration. Invest Ophthalmol Vis Sci 40:1298–1305

Heinrich PC, Behrmann I, Haan S et al (2003) Principles of interleukin (IL)-6-type cytokine signalling and its regulation. Biochem J 374:1–20

LaVail MM, Unoki K, Yasumura D et al (1992) Multiple growth factors, cytokines, and neurotrophins rescue photoreceptors from the damaging effects of constant light. Proc Natl Acad Sci U S A 89:11249–11253

LaVail MM, Yasumura D, Matthes MT et al (1998) Protection of mouse photoreceptors by survival factors in retinal degenerations. Invest Ophthalmol Vis Sci 39:592–602

Liang FQ, Dejneka NS, Cohen DR et al (2001) AAV-mediated delivery of ciliary neurotrophic factor prolongs photoreceptor survival in the rhodopsin knockout mouse. Mol Ther 3:241–248

Oh H, Fujio Y, Kunisada K et al (1998) Activation of phosphatidylinositol 3-kinase through glyco-protein 130 induces protein kinase B and p70 S6 kinase phosphorylation in cardiac myocytes. J Biol Chem 273:9703–9710

Peterson WM, Wang Q, Tzekova R et al (2000) Ciliary neurotrophic factor and stress stimuli activate the Jak-STAT pathway in retinal neurons and glia. J Neurosci 20:4081–4090

Song Y, Zhao L, Tao W et al (2003) Photoreceptor protection by cardiotrophin-1 in transgenic rats with the rhodopsin mutation s334ter. Invest Ophthalmol Vis Sci 44:4069–4075

Ueki Y, Ash JD, Zhu M et al (2009) Expression of Cre recombinase in retinal Muller cells. Vis Res 49:621–651

Ueki Y, Wang J, Chollangi S et al (2008) STAT3 activation in photoreceptors by leukemia inhibitory factor is associated with protection from light damage. J Neurochem 105:784–796

Wahlin KJ, Campochiaro PA, Zack DJ et al (2000) Neurotrophic factors cause activation of intracellular signaling pathways in Muller cells and other cells of the inner retina, but not photoreceptors. Invest Ophthalmol Vis Sci 41:927–936

Wen R, Song Y, Kjellstrom S et al (2006) Regulation of rod phototransduction machinery by ciliary neurotrophic factor. J Neurosci 26:13523–13530

Chapter 76
Neuroprotectin D1 Modulates the Induction of Pro-Inflammatory Signaling and Promotes Retinal Pigment Epithelial Cell Survival During Oxidative Stress

Jorgelina M. Calandria and Nicolas G. Bazan

Abstract Retinal pigment epithelial (RPE) cells are the most restrictive layer of the three components of the outer Blood-Retina Barrier, preventing the passage of biomolecules in relation to size and charge and thus preserving a controlled environment for the photoreceptors. The retinal pigment epithelium is a tight structure that, when disrupted as a cause or consequence of pathological conditions, deeply affects the neural retina. Since adult human RPE cells are not replicative cells, their preservation is of major interest for the biomedical field due to their loss in many retino-degenerative pathologies. There are several triggers that elicit reactive oxygen species (ROS) formation in normal and pathological circumstances. When the production of these species overwhelms the scavenging and detoxifying systems, their activity results in programmed cell death. Docosahexaenoic acid (DHA) is an essential lipid that is conspicuously accumulated in photoreceptors and RPE cells in the retina. DHA and its oxygenation product, neuroprotectin D1 (NPD1), are major players in the protection of these cells and the retina. NPD1 promotes the synthesis of anti-apoptotic proteins of certain members of the Bcl-2 family and blocks the expression of pro-inflammatory proteins like cyclooxygenase-2.

76.1 The Importance of RPE Cell Function and Integrity for Photoreceptor Survival

The outer Blood-Retinal Barrier (oBRB) mediates the exchange of small molecules and solutes and other metabolites from the blood stream to the neural-retina (Strauss 2005). Specifically, the retinal pigment epithelium is the most restrictive layer of the three components of the oBRB, preventing the passage of biomolecules regarding size and charge and thus preserving a controlled environment for the

N.G. Bazan (✉)
Neuroscience Center of Excellence and Department of Ophthalmology, Louisiana State University Health Sciences Center, 2020 Gravier Street, Suite D, New Orleans, LA 70112, USA
e-mail: nbazan@lsuhsc.edu

R.E. Anderson et al. (eds.), *Retinal Degenerative Diseases*, Advances in Experimental Medicine and Biology 664, DOI 10.1007/978-1-4419-1399-9_76,
© Springer Science+Business Media, LLC 2010

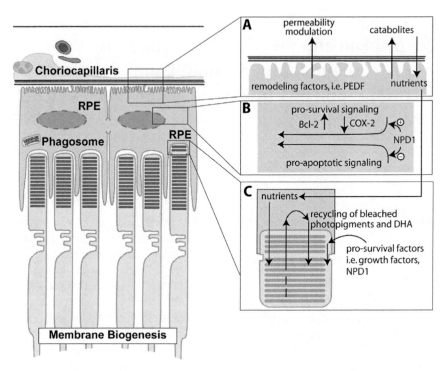

Fig. 76.1 RPE role in the preservation of the retinal structure and NPD1 signaling. Retinal pigment epithelial (RPE) cells interact with photoreceptors in the neural retina. (**a**) They are actively involved in the remodeling and permeability of blood vessels in the choriocapillaries, which in turn provides them with nutrients such as docosahexaenoic acid (DHA). (**b**) Within the retinal pigment epithelium, neuroprotectin D1 (NPD1) signaling is transmitted and pro- and anti-apoptotic cues are integrated to decide the cell fate. (**c**) RPE cells also contribute to daily maintenance by recycling oxidized and bleached pigments and membranes, and then returning DHA, other lipids, and pro-survival factors, such as NPD1

photoreceptors (see Fig. 76.1). The retinal pigment epithelium is a tight structure in which cells are communicated laterally through tight junctions (see Fig. 76.1B). These cells present an elaborate trans-cellular transport system and a high polarization that allows the two different surfaces to have different functions (Pournaras et al. 2008). The selective permeability of the oBRB depends on its integrity, and retinal pigment epithelial (RPE) cells are also involved in the preservation of this structure by interacting reciprocally in cell formation and maintenance. TRP2-FGF9 transgenic mice, in which embryonic RPE cells are forced to become neural retinal cells through the ectopic expression of FGF9, fail to form blood vessels in the choroid layers adjacent to those regions where RPE cells are absent. Instead, blood vessels are found in the vicinity of patch where RPE cells are present (Zhao and Overbeek 2001). The dependency between RPE cells and endothelial vascular cells continues during the adult life through the regulation of neovascularization.

Compelling evidence links RPE cells with the secretion of several angiogenic-related factors. In particular, RPE cells from transgenic ApoE2 mice, which express human ApoE2 protein and whose eyes present several common features with those of age-related macular degeneration (AMD) patients, show reciprocal unbalanced expression of pigment epithelium-derived factor (PEDF) and vascular endothelial growth factor (VEGF), indicating that neovascularization may be increased (Lee et al. 2007). Furthermore, autocrine VEGF signaling in RPE cells stimulate VEGF-related gene expression as well as PEDF modulation, which is a potent angiogenic inhibitor.

Apart from these, RPE cells are capable of producing a wide variety of growth factors (Tanihara et al. 1997), including ciliary neurotrophic factor (CNTF), platelet-derived growth factor (PDGF), insulin-like growth factor-1 (IGF-1) and transforming growth factor-beta (TGF-β) and other molecules such as different types of tissue inhibitor of matrix metalloproteases (TIMPs) (Strauss 2005).

In addition, the structural apico-basal polarization evidenced by deep basal folds and apical microvilli, which have functionally pronounced differences, are found on both sides of the epithelium (see Fig. 76.1). The long apical processes are specialized phagocytic surfaces that engulf shed photoreceptor outer segments in a daily rhythmic cycle to scavenge bleached photopigments, proteins and lipids. During this cycle, a large amount of docosahexaenoic acid (DHA) is incorporated into the RPE cells and is either transformed into neuroprotectin D1 (NPD1), which acts in a paracrine and autocrine manner, or is returned to the photoreceptor to serve as a substrate in the biogenesis of disc membranes (Bazan 2007). Concomitantly with the photoreceptor survival effect of outer segment phagocytosis, the retinal pigment epithelium benefits from this process, which provides resistance to oxidative stress (Mukherjee et al. 2007b). Furthermore, the dependence between RPE cells and photoreceptors is significant in Usher type 1B syndrome. The lack of myosin VIIa in this progressive disease affects the ability of RPE cells to phagocytize the photoreceptor outer segment, which resulted in retinal degeneration in a mouse model (Gibbs et al. 2003). Similar to what was proposed to happen in the Blood Brain Barrier in the neurovascular hypothesis of Alzheimer's disease (AD) (Zlokovic 2005), defective clearance of certain molecules across the barrier may initiate a series of faulty maintenance functions that could lead to a retino-vascular inflammatory response, contributing to the development of AMD.

It was recently proposed that some reactive oxygen species (ROS) may have specific targets that affect certain signaling pathways, a property that makes these reactive species signaling molecules, as is the case of Nitric Oxide (NO) (D'Autreaux and Toledano 2007). Accordingly, redox systems are a part of the normal cell milieu, and thus are tightly regulated. If this were not the case, the disturbed equilibrium may lead to fatal consequences for the cell.

The context in which RPE cells are immersed is highly destructive due to the presence of disposal sub-products of retinal activity. Photochemical reactions take place in the retina under normal conditions to produce ROS by the absorption of photons in the presence of oxygen (Boulton et al. 2001). Moreover, unlike in other cell types in the retina, oxygen consumption and oxidative enzymatic activity is highest in RPE cells. Consequently, the regulation of those processes is of major importance in the prevention of oxidative stress. In particular, anomalous functions of mitochondria produce abnormalities in the mitochondrial electron transport system, which are implicated as a cause of oxidative stress (Lenaz et al. 2002). Likewise, within the membranes of some epithelial cells the activity of 12-lipoxygenase (LOX) is linked with Nox-1 ROS production, a part of the NADPH oxidase complex (de Carvalho et al. 2008).

The production ROS is a double-edged sword because of their high reactivity. On one hand they are necessary to maintain several pathways, but on the other hand their synthesis needs to be strictly controlled; that is to say, after their formation there should be mechanisms that remove them or their products. In normal conditions, excess ROS are scavenged either by enzymatic methods (Superoxide dismutase, catalase, etc.) or by non-enzymatic antioxidants (Vitamin E, etc.) (Margrain et al. 2004). Therefore, RPE cells are exposed to noxious stimuli either due to their environment or to their own function, making these cells especially susceptible to oxidative stress-induced cell death.

In summary, RPE cells are involved in nutrition, intercellular and intra/intertissue communication and remodeling, scavenging of sub-products produced by retinal function, and promotion of neurotrophic signaling, all of which depends to a large extent on the preservation of their epithelium structure (see Fig. 76.1).

76.2 The Loss of RPE Cells in Retinal Degeneration

As key scavenger and filter cells in the oBRB, RPE cells maintain vital life cycles in photoreceptors and the neural retina milieu. In this sense, the slowdown of RPE cell detoxification and filtering functions not only represent a problem for the recycling of the photoreceptors, but also for the retinal pigment epithelium itself. In this sense, disappearance of RPE cells may cause subsequent photoreceptor degeneration. As it occurs with oxidative stress caused by hyperglycemia in diabetes patients, the aberrant formation of advanced glycation end-products (AGE) may be involved in the evolving deregulation of the neural retina milieu through the ablation of the oBRB, which in turn fails to clear internal toxic sub-products, such as lipofuscins capable of inducing the production of ROS in the retinal pigment epithelium (Sparrow and Boulton, 2005). AGE promotes pro-inflammatory signaling that results in nuclear factor-kinase beta (NF-kβ)-dependent gene activation (Bierhaus et al. 2001).

Recent evidence, however, suggests the starvation-dependent disappearance of photoreceptors as the initial cause of retinal pigment epithelium breakdown in retinitis pigmentosa, an inherited retinal degeneration. These findings propose that metabolic defects induce the death of photoreceptors that disrupt the structure of the RPE layer, making the neural-retina permeable to external toxic factors that act as a positive loop to enhance the death of more photoreceptors, just as if it were a house of cards (Punzo et al. 2009).

In any case, the structural or toxic disruption of the retinal pigment epithelium is of great importance for the preservation of retinal functionality, and RPE cells in particular are key elements that contribute to neural-retina homeostasis. The adult retinal pigment epithelium is a non-dividing layer of cells, and thus its protection becomes essential in the prevention of retinal degenerative diseases. This idea is supported by the impracticability of retinal pigment epithelium monolayer replacement, which makes the idea of prevention very attractive (Sheridan et al. 2009).

76.3 DHA and NPD1 Properties and Neuroprotection

DHA is a major component of the structural lipids of photoreceptor outer segment membranes and discs and is incorporated and retained with high efficiency (Bazan et al. 1993; Niemoller et al. 2009). DHA was proposed to be important in influencing the photoreceptor outer segment membranes, biophysically altering permeability fluidity and thickness that, for instance, modulates membrane-bound protein interactions (Clandinin et al. 1994; Jumpsen and Clandinin 1997). In the past, however, DHA was also attributed to biochemical actions involving the direct modulation of gene expression by inducing changes in mRNA processing, transport and stabilization (Uauy et al. 2001).

Even though DHA was proposed to be responsible for neuroprotection, it was recently demonstrated that a stereospecific oxidation derivative, neuroprotectin D1 (NPD1, 10R,17S-dihydroxy-docosa-4Z,7Z,11E,13E,15Z,19Z-hexaenoic acid), possesses the ability to promote cell survival upon stress-induced apoptotic cellular damage. RPE cells, when confronted with oxidative stress in vitro, enhance production of NPD1 as a homeostatic survival mechanism (Mukherjee et al. 2004). Although the exact biosynthetic pathway is unclear, recent evidence points to 15-lipoxygenase-1 (15-LOX-1) as being responsible for the conversion of DHA into NPD1. 15-lipoxygenase-1 catalyzes the formation of NPD1 in T-helper lymphocytes, where the silencing of 15-LOX-1 leads to reduced production of NPD1 (Ariel et al. 2005). Moreover, 15-LOX-1 knock-down cells show, in addition to decreased production of NPD1, an increased susceptibility to apoptosis, which is only rescued by the addition of exogenous NPD1 (unpublished observations).

15-LOX-1, a nonheme iron-containing dioxygenase, stereospecifically inserts oxygen in arachidonic acid, dually forming 15(S)-hydroxyeicosatetraenoic acid (HETE), 12(S)-HETE, and lipoxin A4, a product of its joint activity with 5-lipoxygenase. 15-LOX-1 also has the capability to oxygenate linoleic acid into 13-hydroxyoctadecadienoic acid (13-HODE) (Kühn et al. 1993). Human 15-LOX-1 and 12-LOX are highly homologous proteins (65% identity) encoded by different genes, and their messenger RNAs are similar (little more than 70% identity). On the other hand, 15-LOX-2 is a different lipoxygenase that shares only 39% identity with human 15-LOX-1 (Brash et al. 1997). 15-LOX-2 and human 12-LOX differ from 15-LOX-1 in the ratio of 15-HETE and 12-HETE produced from arachidonic acid. This means that they possess different selective product formation, and thus their activities contribute to different pools of lipid mediators. These compensatory functions of lipoxygenases do not affect the production of NPD1. In fact, when 15-LOX-1 is knocked down, this reveals only NPD1 and lipoxin A$_4$ depletion, whereas other oxygenation products are modified, but to a lesser extent. 15-LOX is inducible by Ca^{++} signaling (Brinkmann et al. 1998; Walther et al. 2004); thus, it is highly possible that its activity may also be induced by the initiation of oxidative stress-mediated pro-inflammatory signaling as a way for the cell to counteract the pro-apoptotic process in the integration of antagonist pathways.

76.4 NPD1 Modulates the Expression of Survival and Apoptotic-Related Proteins

NPD1 is a potent neuroprotective lipid mediator that inhibits the expression of pro-inflammatory genes and enhances the expression of anti-apoptotic proteins of the Bcl-2 family (Mukherjee et al. 2004; Lukiw et al. 2005). Moreover, NPD1 signaling is involved in neurotrophin-mediated RPE cell survival (Mukherjee et al. 2007a). Although the exact molecular mechanisms responsible for this decision are not yet clear, some evidence links the consequent pro-survival response of ARPE-19 cells after NPD1-pathway induction with the decrease in the activation of caspase-3. A DNA array-based human mRNA expression profiling in the central nervous system (CNS) shows that NPD1 'turns off' pro-inflammatory and anti-apoptotic genes, whereas these genes elicit the opposite effect of that produced by the amyloid β peptide, Aβ42 (Lukiw et al. 2005).

In summary, NPD1 is involved in the preservation of the retinal pigment epithelium through the promotion of pro-survival signaling, at which point these cells decide whether to continue along the pro-apoptotic pathway or counteract this process by activating the pro-survival mode.

Acknowledgments Supported by NIH/NEI grant R01 EY005121, NIH/NCRR grant P20 RR016816, the Edward G. Schlieder Educational Foundation, the Eye, Ear, Nose and Throat Foundation, and the Ernest C. and Yvette C. Villere Chair for Research in Retinal Degeneration (NGB).

References

Ariel A, Li PL, Wang W et al (2005) The docosatriene protectin D1 is produced by TH2 skewing and promotes human T cell apoptosis via lipid raft clustering. J Biol Chem 280:43079–43086

Bazan NG (2007) Homeostatic regulation of photoreceptor cell integrity: significance of the potent mediator neuroprotectin D1 biosynthesized from docosahexaenoic acid. Invest Ophthalmol Vis Sci 48:4866–4881

Bazan NG, Rodriguez de Turco EB, Gordon WC (1993) Pathways for the uptake and conservation of docosahexaenoic acid in photoreceptors and synapses: biochemical and autoradiographic studies. Can J Physiol Pharmacol 71:690–698

Bierhaus A, Schiekofer S, Schwaninger M et al (2001) Diabetes-associated sustained activation of the transcription factor nuclear factor-kappaB. Diabetes 50:2792–2808

Boulton M, Rozanowska M, Rozanowski B (2001) Retinal Photodamage. J Photochem Photobiol B 64:144–161

Brash AR, Boeglin WE, Chang MS (1997) Discovery of a second 15S-lipoxygenase in humans. Proc Natl Acad Sci U S A 94:6148–6152

Brinckmann R, Schnurr K, Heydeck D et al (1998) Membrane translocation of 15-lipoxygenase in hematopoietic cells is calcium-dependent and activates the oxygenase activity of the enzyme. Blood 91:64–74

Clandinin MT, Jumpsen J, Suh M (1994) Relationship between fatty acid accretion, membrane composition, and biologic functions. J Pediatr 125:S25–S32

D'Autreaux B, Toledano MB (2007) ROS as signaling molecules: mechanisms that generate specificity in ROS homeostasis in a physiologically controlled environment. Nature Review Mol Cell Biol 8:813–824

de Carvalho DD, Sadock A, Bourgarel-Rey V et al (2008) Nox1 downstream of 12-Lipoxygenase controls cell proliferation but not cell spreading of colon cancer cells. Int J Cancer 122:1757–1764

Gibbs D, Kitamoto J, Williams DS (2003) Abnormal phagocytosis by retinal pigmented epithelium that lacks myosin VIIa, the Usher syndrome 1B protein. Proc Natl Acad Sci U S A 100:6481–6486

Jumpsen JA, Lien EL, Goh YK et al (1997) During neuronal and glial cell development diet n – 6 to n – 3 fatty acid ratio alters the fatty acid composition of phosphatidylinositol and phosphatidylserine. Biochim Biophys Acta 1347:40–50

Kühn H, Thiele BJ, Ostareck-Lederer A et al (1993) Bacterial expression, purification and partial characterization of recombinant rabbit reticulocyte 15-lipoxygenase. Biochim Biophys Acta 1168:73–78

Lee SJ, Kim JH, Kim JH et al (2007) Human apolipoprotein E2 transgenic mice show lipid accumulation in retinal pigment epithelium and altered expression of VEGF and bFGF in the eyes. J Microbiol Biotechnol 17:1024–1030

Lenaz G, Bovina C, D'Aurelio M et al (2002) Role of mithocondria in oxidative stress and aging. Ann NY Acad Sci 959:199–213

Lukiw WJ, Cui JG, Marcheselli VL et al (2005) A role for docosahexaenoic acid-derived neuroprotectin D1 in neural cell survival and Alzheimer disease. J Clin Invest 115:2774–2783

Margrain TH, Boulton M, Marshall J et al (2004) Do blue light filters confer protection against age-related macular degeneration? Prog Retin Eye Res 23:523–531

Mukherjee PK, Marcheselli VL, Barreiro S et al (2007a) Neurotrophins enhance retinal pigment epithelial cell survival through neuroprotectin D1 signaling. Proc Natl Acad Sci U S A 104:13152–13157

Mukherjee PK, Marcheselli VL, de Rivero Vaccari JC et al (2007b) Photoreceptor outer segment phagocytosis attenuates oxidative stress-induced apoptosis with concomitant neuroprotectin D1 synthesis. Proc Natl Acad Sci U S A 104:13158–13163

Mukherjee PK, Marcheselli VL, Serhan CN et al (2004) Neuroprotectin D1: a docosahexaenoic acid-derived docosatriene protects human retinal pigment epithelial cells from oxidative stress. Proc Natl Acad Sci U S A 101:8491–8496

Niemoller TD, Stark DT, Bazan NG (2009) Omega-3 fatty acid docosahexaenoic acid is the precursor of neuroprotectin D1 in the nervous system. World Rev Nutr Diet 99:46–54

Pournaras CJ, Rungger-Brändle E, Riva CE et al (2008) Regulation of retinal blood flow in health and disease. Prog Retin Eye Res 27:284–330

Punzo C, Kornacker K, Cepko CL (2009) Stimulation of the insulin/mTOR pathway delays cone death in a mouse model of retinitis pigmentosa. Nat Neurosci 12:44–52

Sheridan CM, Mason S, Pattwell DM et al (2009) Replacement of the RPE monolayer. Eye 23:1910–1915

Sparrow JR, Boulton M (2005) RPE lipofuscins and its role in retina pathobiology. Exp Eye Res 80:595–606

Strauss O (2005) The retinal pigment epithelium in visual function. Phisiol Rev 85:845–881

Tanihara H, Inatani M, Honda Y (1997) Growth factors and their receptors in the retina and pigment epithelium. Prog Retin Eye Res 16:271–301

Uauy R, Hoffman DR, Peirano P et al (2001) Essential fatty acids in visual and brain development. Lipids 36:885–895

Walther M, Wiesner R, Kuhn H (2004) Investigations into calcium-dependent membrane association of 15-lipoxygenase-1. Mechanistic roles of surface-exposed hydrophobic amino acids and calcium. J Biol Chem 279:3717–3725

Zhao S, Overbeek PA (2001) Regulation of choroid development by the retinal pigment epithelium. Mol Vis 2:277–282

Zlokovic BV (2005) Neurovascular mechanisms of Alzheimer's neurodegeneration. Trends Neurosci 28:202–208

Chapter 77
Adeno-Associated Virus Serotype-9 Mediated Retinal Outer Plexiform Layer Transduction is Mainly Through the Photoreceptors

Bo Lei, Keqing Zhang, Yongping Yue, Arkasubhra Ghosh, and Dongsheng Duan

Abstract Due to its high ocular transduction, low immune clearance and capability to bypass the brain blood barrier, adeno-associated virus-9 (AAV9) has been regarded as a promising vector for retinal disease gene therapy. We recently demonstrated that AAV9 efficiently transduces the retinal outer plexiform layer (OPL). The OPL consists of synapses formed between axons of the rod and cone photoreceptors (cell bodies in the outer nuclear layer, ONL) and dendrites of bipolar and horizontal cells (cell bodies in the inner nuclear layer, INL). It is not clear whether AAV9 transduces the OPL through the photoreceptors in the ONL or through bipolar and horizontal cells in the INL. To map the subcelluar pathway(s) involved in AAV9-mediated OPL transduction, we delivered subretinally AAV9.CMV.eGFP, an AAV vector carrying the enhanced green fluorescent protein gene (eGFP, 1×10^{10} viral genome particles in microliter), to young (21-day-old) and adult (2- to 3-month-old) *C57BL/6* mice. Four weeks after subretinal injection, eGFP expression was examined on retinal cryosections. PSD95 (postsynaptic density protein, a marker for photoreceptor terminals), CtBP2 (C-terminal binding protein 2, a marker for the photoreceptor synaptic ribbon), PKCalpha (protein kinase Cα, a marker for rod bipolar cells), and calbindin (a marker for horizontal cells) were localized by immunofluorescence staining. In AAV9 infected retina, eGFP expression was seen in the retinal pigment epithelia, photoreceptor inner segments, ONL, OPL, Müller cells in the INL, inner plexiform layer and ganglion cell layer. Interestingly, eGFP expression co-localized with PSD95 and CtBP2, but not with PKCalpha and calbindin. Our results suggest that AAV9 transduces the photoreceptor side of the synapses in the OPL rather than the dendrites of bipolar and horizontal cells.

B. Lei (✉)
Department of Ophthalmology, The First Affiliated Hospital of Chongqing Medical University, 1 You Yi Road, Yu Zhong District, Chongqing 400016, China
e-mail: bolei99@126.com

R.E. Anderson et al. (eds.), *Retinal Degenerative Diseases*, Advances in Experimental Medicine and Biology 664, DOI 10.1007/978-1-4419-1399-9_77,
© Springer Science+Business Media, LLC 2010

77.1 Introduction

In the past decade, the world has witnessed tremendous progress in the treatment of inherited retinal degenerations. While no long ago such conditions were regarded untreatable and incurable by any means, gene therapy has preserved retinal morphology and restored retinal functions in several animal models of retinal degenerations (Ali et al. 2000; Acland et al. 2001; Allocca et al. 2006; Alexander et al. 2007). Promising results have also been reported recently in Leber's Congenital Amaurosis (LCA) patients (Bainbridge et al. 2008; Cideciyan et al. 2008; Hauswirth et al. 2008; Maguire et al. 2008).

To develop more efficient and safe vectors for retinal gene therapy, many groups have begun to evaluate new gene vectors. Among the newly described AAV serotypes, AAV serotype-9 (AAV9) stands out as a particularly attractive vehicle because of its superior performance (Gao et al. 2004, 2005). It was recently reported that AAV9 transduction efficiency can be 200-fold higher than that of other AAV serotypes (Inagaki et al. 2006; Limberis and Wilson 2006; Pacak et al. 2006; Bostick et al. 2007; Vandendriessche et al. 2007). In addition, AAV9 is capable to bypass the brain blood barrier (Foust et al. 2009), an important feature that may be utilized to treat a wide range of neural degenerations in the central never system. Therefore, it is imperative to understand details of this novel AAV vector.

In the eye, two previous studies suggest that subretinal administration of AAV9 lead to robust transduction in the retinal pigment epithelium (RPE), the photoreceptors (including the outer and inner segments, the cell bodies in the outer nuclear layer, ONL), the Müller cells in the inner nuclear layer (INL), and the retinal ganglion cell (RGC) layer (Allocca et al. 2007; Lebherz et al. 2008). Using three different genes and two different promoters, we found that AAV9 also transduces the two retinal synaptic layers (the outer plexiform layer OPL, and the inner plexiform layer IPL), a special characteristic that was rarely documented with all AAV serotypes (Lei et al. 2009). Here, we further showed that AAV9-mediate expression co-localized with two photoreceptor terminal markers PSD95 and CtBP2, but not with rod ON bipolar cell and horizontal cell markers. Our results suggest that AAV9 mediated OPL transduction is through the photoreceptors but not the neurons in the INL.

77.2 AAV9-Mediated Gene Transfer in the Retina

Two recent studies evaluated AAV9 transduction in the retina following subretinal administration (Allocca et al. 2007; Lebherz et al. 2008). Both studies demonstrated efficient transduction of the RPE and Müller cells (Allocca et al. 2007; Lebherz et al. 2008). However, one group found photoreceptor transduction (Allocca et al. 2007), whereas the other group did not detect photoreceptor transduction (Lebherz et al. 2008). The reasons for these differences are unknown but may relate to experimental designs such as animal age, the promoter, the reporter gene and the time frame of observation.

To further characterize AAV9 mediated transduction in the retina, we performed a comprehensive study in mice. First, we injected subretinally an RSV promoter driving alkaline phosphatase (AP) reporter gene vector (AAV9.RSV.AP, 1 μl, 1 × 10^9 viral genome particles). We found widespread (peripheral-central-peripheral) and throughout (from RPE to RGC) transduction in mice ranging from 3- to 12-week-old. AP expression was observed in the RPE, ONL, INL, OPL, IPL, RGC layer and Müller cells but not the outer and inner segments of the photoreceptor. Remarkably, two retinal synaptic layers (OPL and IPL) were highly transduced (Lei et al. 2009).

To exclude the potential bias from the transgene and/or the promoter, we performed another study with the AAV9.CMV.eGFP vector (1 μl, 1 × 10^{10} viral genome particles). Four weeks after subretinal injection, we observed intense eGFP expression in the RPE, ONL and to less extent in the OPL, Müller cells in the INL, IPL, and RGC layer in all experimental mice (3- to 12-week-old) (Fig. 77.1). Similar

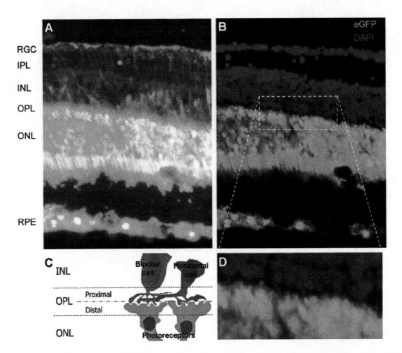

Fig. 77.1 Mouse retinal eGFP expression 4 weeks after subretinal delivery of 1 μl AAV9.CMV.eGFP vector (1 × 10^{10} viral genome particles). **Panels A and B** were from the same field except that **panel B** was taken with a shorter exposure time. **Panel C** shows schematic outline of the OPL synapse structure. **Panel D** shows an enlarge view of the *boxed* area in **panel B**. The highest eGFP expression was seen in the ONL and RPE layers. Substantial eGFP expression was also found in the OPL, INL, IPL, and RGC layers and the Müller cells. In **panels B and D**, eGFP expression is mainly localized to the distal portion of the OPL. (RGC, retinal ganglion cell; IPL, inner plexiform layer; INL, inner nuclear layer; OPL, outer plexiform layer; ONL, outer nuclear layer)

Table 77.1 Retinal tropism of AAV9 in mouse

	RPE	Photoreceptors	OPL	Müller cells	IPL	RGC layer
AP expression	+++++	+++	+++	+++	+++	++
eGFP expression	+++++	+++++	+++	++	+	+

to those observed in AAV9.RSV.AP injected eyes (Lei et al. 2009), eGFP expression was widespread and throughout the retina. Our results are consistent with those of Allocca et al and confirm that AAV9 indeed transduces the photoreceptors (Allocca et al. 2007). Similar to our findings with the AV.RSV.AP vector, we observed eGFP expression in the OPL and IPL, the two retinal synaptic layers. Table 77.1 summarizes the retinal tropism of AAV9 mediated gene transduction after subretinal injection.

77.3 The Sub-Cellular Location of AAV9 Transduction in the OPL

The finding that AAV9 mediated efficient expression in the OPL is intriguing. Pathology in the OPL is associated with a wide range of retinal diseases (Miyake et al. 1986; Alexander et al. 1992; Fitzgerald et al. 1994; Dryja et al. 2005; Chang et al. 2006). Therefore, AAV9 may be a candidate gene therapy vector for these disorders. Unfortunately, few studies have thoroughly evaluated AAV transduction in the OPL.

To investigate the pattern of AAV9-mediated OPL transduction, we stained AAV9.CMV.eGFP infected eyes with CtBP2 (C-terminal binding protein 2, a marker for the photoreceptor synaptic ribbon), PSD95 (postsynaptic density protein, a marker for the photoreceptor terminals), PKCα (protein kinase C alpha, a marker for the rod bipolar cells), and calbindin (a marker for the horizontal cells). Nuclei were revealed with 4′, 6 diamidino-2-phenylindole dihydrocholoride (DAPI). With shorter exposure time eGFP expression was only seen in the RPE and photoreceptors. Interestingly eGFP co-localized with CtBP2 (Lei et al. 2009) and PSD95 but not with PKCα and calbindin (Fig. 77.2). These results strongly suggest that the observed eGFP expression in the OPL is from the photoreceptor terminals, while the rod bipolar cell and horizontal cell dendrites play minimal role.

77.4 AAV9-Mediated Retinal Gene Transfer in mdx^{3cv} Mice

Mdx^{3cv} mice are models for Duchene muscular dystrophy (DMD), a lethal childhood genetic disease caused by mutations in the dystrophin gene (Pillers et al. 1995; Pillers et al. 1999). Besides muscle disease, DMD patients also suffer from pathology in other tissues including the retina. A 260 kD dystrophin isoform (Dp260) is

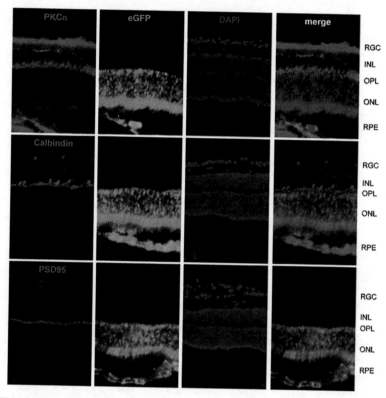

Fig. 77.2 Subcellular localization of AAV9 transduction in the OPL. Immunofluorescence staining of PKCα, calbindin and PSD95 in AAV9.CMV.eGFP infected retina (1×10^{10} viral genome particles). PKCα and calbindin are the markers for the rod bipolar cells and horizontal cells (and their dendrites in the proximal portion of the OPL) respectively. PSD95 is a marker for the photoreceptor terminals (distal portion of the OPL). In the overlay images eGFP only co-localize with PSD95

normally expressed in the photoreceptor terminals in the OPL. Dp260 expression is lost in the eyes of DMD patients and mdx^{3cv} mice (Pillers et al. 1993; Schmitz and Drenckhahn 1997; Jastrow et al. 2006). Absence of Dp260 has been associated with the abnormal electroretinogram seen in DMD patients, such as reduced b-wave amplitude and prolonged implicit time.

To determine whether AAV9 can be used to deliver a therapeutic gene to the OPL, we performed subretinal injection of AAV9.CMV.△R4/△C vector in mdx^{3cv} mice. The 3.8 kb △R4/△C microgene encodes a truncated dystrophin. This microgene has been extensively studied as a candidate gene for DMD gene therapy (Harper et al. 2002). At 5 weeks after subretinal injection, we examined dystrophin expression by immunofluorescence staining. Two epitope-specific antibodies were used in the study. The Dys-2 antibody recognizes endogenous Dp260 in the wild type retina, the Dys-3 antibody only reacts with micro-dystrophin. Consistent with our findings with the reporter AAV vectors, we observed robust microgene expression in the OPL of the injected mdx^{3cv} mice (Lei et al. 2009). These results raise the hope of using AAV9 to treat retinal diseases that are associated with defects in the photoreceptor terminals.

77.5 Subretinal Injection of AAV9 Vector Did Not Cause Acute Retinal Damage

We also examined whether subretinal injection of AAV9 vector causes acute damages to the retina. At 5 weeks after delivery of AAV9.RSV.AP or a saline control, we examined retinal histology and recorded dark- and light-adapted electroretinogram in the mouse eyes. Compared with untreated eyes, neither saline nor AAV9 RSV.AP resulted in appreciable morphology alterations. We obtained similar measurements in the thresholds and amplitudes of the dark-adapted ERG a-wave, b-wave and light-adapted b-wave in AAV injected and saline injected eyes (Lei et al. 2009). Our results suggest that rod and cone photoreceptor and bipolar cell functions are not affected by subretinal delivery of AAV9 vectors.

77.6 Conclusions

Using three different genes and two different promoters, we confirmed that subretinal delivery of AAV9 mediates robust photoreceptor gene transduction. AAV9 vectors also efficiently ferry transgene products to the photoreceptor terminals in the OPL. Our data indicated that AAV9 may be a promising vector for retinal disease gene therapy, especially for disorders that primarily affect the RPE, photoreceptors and the OPL.

Acknowledgments This work was supported in part by Research Board of the University of Missouri; National Institutes of Health grant NIH AR49419, and a grant from the Muscular Dystrophy Association. We thank Mrs. Chun Long for technical assistant, Drs. Guangping Gao and James Wilson for providing the AAV9 packaging plasmid pRep2/Cap9.

References

Acland GM, Aguirre GD, Ray J et al (2001) Gene therapy restores vision in a canine model of childhood blindness. Nat Genet 28:92–95

Alexander JJ, Umino Y, Everhart D et al (2007) Restoration of cone vision in a mouse model of achromatopsia. Nat Med 13:685–687

Alexander KR, Fishman GA, Peachey NS et al (1992) 'On' response defect in paraneoplastic night blindness with cutaneous malignant melanoma. Invest Ophthalmol Vis Sci 33:477–483

Ali RR, Sarra GM, Stephens C et al (2000) Restoration of photoreceptor ultrastructure and function in retinal degeneration slow mice by gene therapy. Nat Genet 25:306–310

Allocca M, Mussolino C, Garcia-Hoyos M et al (2007) Novel adeno-associated virus serotypes efficiently transduce murine photoreceptors. J Virol 81:11372–11380

Allocca M, Tessitore A, Cotugno G et al (2006) AAV-mediated gene transfer for retinal diseases. Expert Opin Biol Ther 6:1279–1294

Bainbridge JW, Smith AJ, Barker SS et al (2008) Effect of gene therapy on visual function in Leber's congenital amaurosis. N Engl J Med 358:2231–2239

Bostick B, Ghosh A, Yue Y et al (2007) Systemic AAV9 transduction in mice is influenced by animal age but not by the route of administration. Gene Ther 14:1605–1609

Chang B, Heckenlively JR, Bayley PR et al (2006) The nob2 mouse, a null mutation in Cacna1f: anatomical and functional abnormalities in the outer retina and their consequences on ganglion cell visual responses. Vis Neurosci 23:11–24

Cideciyan AV, Aleman TS, Boye SL et al (2008) Human gene therapy for RPE65 isomerase deficiency activates the retinoid cycle of vision but with slow rod kinetics. Proc Natl Acad Sci U S A 105:15112–15117

Dryja TP, McGee TL, Berson EL et al (2005) Night blindness and abnormal cone electroretinogram ON responses in patients with mutations in the GRM6 gene encoding mGluR6. Proc Natl Acad Sci U S A 102:4884–4889

Duan D, Yue Y, Yan Z et al (2000) Endosomal processing limits gene transfer to polarized airway epithelia by adeno-associated virus. J Clin Invest 105:1573–1587

Fitzgerald KM, Cibis GW, Giambrone SA et al (1994) Retinal signal transmission in Duchenne muscular dystrophy: evidence for dysfunction in the photoreceptor/depolarizing bipolar cell pathway. J Clin Invest 93:2425–2430

Foust KD, Nurre E, Montgomery CL et al (2009) Intravascular AAV9 preferentially targets neonatal neurons and adult astrocytes. Nat Biotechnol 27:59–65

Gao G, Vandenberghe LH, Alvira MR et al (2004) Clades of Adeno-associated viruses are widely disseminated in human tissues. J Virol 78:6381–6388

Gao G, Vandenberghe LH, Wilson JM (2005) New recombinant serotypes of AAV vectors. Curr Gene Ther 5:285–297

Harper SQ, Hauser MA, DelloRusso C et al (2002) Modular flexibility of dystrophin: implications for gene therapy of Duchenne muscular dystrophy. Nat Med 8:253–261

Hauswirth WW, Aleman TS, Kaushal S, et al. (2009) Treatment of leber congenital amaurosis due to RPE65 mutations by ocular subretinal injection of adeno-associated virus gene vector: short-term results of a phase I trial. 19(10):979–990

Inagaki K, Fuess S, Storm TA et al (2006) Robust systemic transduction with AAV9 vectors in mice: efficient global cardiac gene transfer superior to that of AAV8. Mol Ther 14:45–53

Jastrow H, Koulen P, Altrock WD et al (2006) Identification of a beta-dystroglycan immunoreactive subcompartment in photoreceptor terminals. Invest Ophthalmol Vis Sci 47: 17–24

Lebherz C, Maguire A, Tang W et al (2008) Novel AAV serotypes for improved ocular gene transfer. J Gene Med 10:375–382

Lei B, Zhang K, Yue Y et al (2009) Adeno-associated virus serotype-9 efficiently transduces the retinal outer plexiform layer. Mol Vis 15:1374–1382.

Limberis MP, Wilson JM (2006) Adeno-associated virus serotype 9 vectors transduce murine alveolar and nasal epithelia and can be readministered. Proc Natl Acad Sci U S A 103:12993–12998

Maguire AM, Simonelli F, Pierce EA et al (2008) Safety and efficacy of gene transfer for Leber's congenital amaurosis. N Engl J Med 358:2240–2248

Miyake Y, Yagasaki K, Horiguchi M et al (1986) Congenital stationary night blindness with negative electroretinogram. A new classification. Arch Ophthalmol 104:1013–1020

Pacak CA, Mah CS, Thattaliyath BD et al (2006) Recombinant adeno-associated virus serotype 9 leads to preferential cardiac transduction in vivo. Circ Res 99:e3–e9

Pillers DA, Bulman DE, Weleber RG et al (1993) Dystrophin expression in the human retina is required for normal function as defined by electroretinography. Nat Genet 4:82–86

Pillers DA, Weleber RG, Green DG et al (1999) Effects of dystrophin isoforms on signal transduction through neural retina: genotype-phenotype analysis of duchenne muscular dystrophy mouse mutants. Mol Genet Metab 66:100–110

Pillers DM, Weleber RG, Woodward WR et al (1995) mdxCv3 mouse is a model for electroretinography of Duchenne/Becker muscular dystrophy. Invest Ophthalmol Vis Sci 36:462–466

Schmitz F, Drenckhahn D (1997) Localization of dystrophin and beta-dystroglycan in bovine reti-
    nal photoreceptor processes extending into the postsynaptic dendritic complex. Histochem Cell
    Biol 108:249–255
Vandendriessche T, Thorrez L, Acosta-Sanchez A et al (2007) Efficacy and safety of adeno-
    associated viral vectors based on serotype 8 and 9 vs. lentiviral vectors for hemophilia B gene
    therapy. J Thromb Haemost 5:16–24
Zhang SH, Wu JH, Wu XB et al (2008) Distinctive gene transduction efficiencies of commonly
    used viral vectors in the retina. Curr Eye Res 33:81–90

Index